Pharmacotherapy Casebook

A Patient-Focused Approach

Tenth Edition

Editors

Terry L. Schwinghammer, PharmD, FCCP, FASHP, FAPhA, BCPS

Professor and Chair
Department of Clinical Pharmacy
School of Pharmacy
West Virginia University
Morgantown, West Virginia

Julia M. Koehler, PharmD, FCCP

Professor and Associate Dean for Clinical Education and
External Affiliations
College of Pharmacy and Health Sciences
Butler University
Ambulatory Care Clinical Pharmacist
Methodist Hospital of Indiana University Health
Indianapolis, Indiana

Jill S. Borchert, PharmD, BCACP, BCPS, FCCP

Professor and Vice Chair
Department of Pharmacy Practice
Director, PGY2 Ambulatory Care Residency Program
Midwestern University Chicago College of Pharmacy
Downers Grove, Illinois

Douglas Slain, PharmD, BCPS, FCCP, FASHP

Professor
Department of Clinical Pharmacy
School of Pharmacy
West Virginia University
Infectious Diseases Clinical Specialist
WVU Medicine and Ruby Memorial Hospital
Morgantown, West Virginia

Sharon K. Park, PharmD, BCPS

Assistant Professor
Department of Clinical and Administrative Sciences
School of Pharmacy
Notre Dame of Maryland University
Clinical Pharmacy Specialist
Drug Information and Medication Use Policy
The Johns Hopkins Hospital
Baltimore, Maryland

A companion workbook for: Pharmacotherapy: *A Pathophysiologic Approach*, 10th ed.
DiPiro JT, Talbert RL, Yee GC, Matzke GR, Wells BG, Posey ML, eds. New York, NY: McGraw-Hill Education, 2017.

New York   Chicago   San Francisco   Athens   London   Madrid   Mexico City
Milan   New Delhi   Singapore   Sydney   Toronto

Pharmacotherapy Casebook: A Patient-Focused Approach, Tenth Edition

1 2 3 4 5 6 7 8 9 LOV 21 20 19 18 17 16

ISBN 978-1-259-64091-9
MHID 1-259-64091-4

This book was set in Minion by Cenveo® Publisher Services.
The editors were Michael Weitz and Peter J. Boyle.
The production supervisor was Richard Ruzycka.
Project management was provided by Anju Joshi, Cenveo Publisher Services.
The designer was Alan Barnett.
LSC Communications was the printer and binder.

This book was printed on acid-free paper.

NOTICE

Medicine is an ever-changing science. As new research and clinical experience broaden our knowledge, changes in treatment and drug therapy are required. The authors and the publisher of this work have checked with sources believed to be reliable in their efforts to provide information that is complete and generally in accord with the standards accepted at the time of publication. However, in view of the possibility of human error or changes in medical sciences, neither the authors nor the publisher nor any other party who has been involved in the preparation or publication of this work warrants that the information contained herein is in every respect accurate or complete, and they disclaim all responsibility for any errors or omissions, or for the results obtained from use of the information contained in this work. Readers are encouraged to confirm the information contained herein with other sources. For example and in particular, readers are advised to check the product information sheet included in the package of each drug they plan to administer to be certain that the information contained in this work is accurate and that changes have not been made in the recommended dose or in the contraindications for administration. This recommendation is of particular importance in connection with new or infrequently used drugs.

Library of Congress Cataloging-in-Publication Data

Names: Schwinghammer, Terry L., editor. | Koehler, Julia M., editor. |
    Borchert, Jill S., editor. | Slain, Douglas, 1967- editor. | Park, Sharon K.,
    editor.
Title: Pharmacotherapy casebook : a patient-focused approach / editors,
    Terry L. Schwinghammer, Julia M. Koehler, Jill S. Borchert, Douglas Slain,
    Sharon K. Park.
Other titles: Complemented by (work): Pharmacotherapy. Tenth edition.
Description: Tenth edition. | New York : McGraw-Hill Education, [2017] |
    Complemented by Pharmacotherapy / [editors], Joseph T. DiPiro, Robert L.
    Talbert, Gary C. Yee, Gary R. Matzke, Barbara G. Wells, L. Michael Posey ;
    associate editors, Vicki Ellingrod, Stuart Haines, Thomas Nolin. Tenth
    edition. 2017. | Includes bibliographical references and index.
Identifiers: LCCN 2016047743| ISBN 9781259640919 (pbk.) | ISBN 1259640914
    (pbk.)
Subjects: | MESH: Drug Therapy | Patient-Centered Care | Examination
    Questions | Case Reports
Classification: LCC RM263 | NLM WB 18.2 | DDC 615.5/8—dc23 LC record available at
    https://lccn.loc.gov/2016047743

International Edition ISBN 978-1-260-08413-9; MHID 1-260-08413-2.
Copyright © 2017. Exclusive rights by McGraw-Hill Education for manufacture and export. This book cannot be re-exported from the country to which it is consigned by McGraw-Hill Education. The International Edition is not available in North America.

McGraw-Hill Education books are available at special quantity discounts to use as premiums and sales promotions or for use in corporate training programs. To contact a representative, please visit the Contact Us pages at www.mhprofessional.com.

CONTENTS

SECTION 1

Principles of Patient-Focused Therapy
Section Editor: *Terry L. Schwinghammer*

SECTION 2

Cardiovascular Disorders
Section Editor: *Julia M. Koehler*

SECTION 3

Respiratory Disorders
Section Editor: *Julia M. Koehler*

SECTION 4

Gastrointestinal Disorders
Section Editor: *Jill S. Borchert*

SECTION 5

Renal Disorders
Section Editor: *Jill S. Borchert*

SECTION 6

Neurologic Disorders
Section Editor: *Sharon K. Park*

SECTION 7

Psychiatric Disorders
Section Editor: *Sharon K. Park*

SECTION 8

Endocrinologic Disorders
Section Editor: *Julia M. Koehler*

SECTION 17

Oncologic Disorders
Section Editor: Terry L. Schwinghammer

CONTRIBUTORS

Marie A. Abate, BS, PharmD

Professor of Clinical Pharmacy; Director, West Virginia Center for Drug and Health Information; Director of Programmatic Assessment, West Virginia University School of Pharmacy, Morgantown, West Virginia

Nicole P. Albanese, PharmD, CDE, BCACP

Clinical Assistant Professor, Department of Pharmacy Practice, University at Buffalo, School of Pharmacy and Pharmaceutical Sciences; Clinical Pharmacist in Ambulatory Care, Buffalo Medical Group, Buffalo, New York

Kwadwo Amankwa, PharmD, BCPS

Assistant Professor, Notre Dame of Maryland University, Baltimore, Maryland

Jarrett R. Amsden, PharmD, BCPS

Associate Professor, Department of Pharmacy Practice, Butler University College of Pharmacy and Health Sciences; Infectious Diseases Clinical Pharmacist, Department of Clinical Pharmacy, Community Health Network, Indianapolis, Indiana

Alexander J. Ansara, PharmD, BCPS (AQ Cardiology)

Associate Professor, Department of Clinical Pharmacy Practice, Butler University College of Pharmacy and Health Sciences; Clinical Pharmacist in Advanced Heart Care, Indiana University Health Methodist Hospital, Indianapolis, Indiana

Sally A. Arif, PharmD, BCPS (AQ Cardiology)

Associate Professor, Department of Pharmacy Practice, Midwestern University, Chicago College of Pharmacy, Downers Grove; Clinical Pharmacist, Rush University Medical Center, Chicago, Illinois

Lori T. Armistead, PharmD

Clinical Instructor, UNC Eshelman School of Pharmacy, The University of North Carolina at Chapel Hill, Chapel Hill, North Carolina

Jessica J. Auten, PharmD, BCPS, BCOP

Clinical Pharmacy Specialist (Inpatient Malignant Hematology), Department of Pharmacy, North Carolina Cancer Hospital, Chapel Hill, North Carolina

Melissa Badowski, PharmD, BCPS, AAHIVP

Clinical Assistant Professor, Section of Infectious Diseases, University of Illinois at Chicago, College of Pharmacy; Illinois Department of Corrections HIV Telemedicine Program, Chicago, Illinois

Jacquelyn L. Bainbridge, PharmD, FCCP

Professor, Department of Clinical Pharmacy, Skaggs School of Pharmacy and Pharmaceutical Sciences, University of Colorado, Aurora, Colorado

Gina M. C. Baugh, PharmD

Clinical Associate Professor, Department of Clinical Pharmacy, School of Pharmacy, West Virginia University, Robert C. Byrd Health Sciences Center, Morgantown, West Virginia

Scott J. Bergman, PharmD, BCPS (AQ-ID)

Southern Illinois University Edwardsville School of Pharmacy, Edwardsville, Illinois

Christopher M. Bland, PharmD, BCPS, FIDSA

Clinical Assistant Professor, Department of Clinical and Administrative Pharmacy, University of Georgia College of Pharmacy; Critical Care/Infectious Diseases Clinical Pharmacist, St. Joseph's/Candler Health System, Savannah, Georgia

Meghan M. Bodenberg, PharmD, BCPS

Associate Professor and Director of Site-Based Experiential Education, Butler University College of Pharmacy & Health Sciences, Indianapolis, Indiana

Scott Bolesta, PharmD, BCPS, FCCM

Associate Professor, Department of Pharmacy Practice, Nesbitt School of Pharmacy, Wilkes University, Wilkes-Barre; Investigator, Center for Pharmacy Innovation and Outcomes, Geisinger Health System, Danville; Clinical Pharmacist in Internal Medicine/Critical Care, Pharmacy Department, Regional Hospital of Scranton, Scranton, Pennsylvania

Larissa N. H. Bossaer, PharmD, BCPS

Associate Professor, Department of Pharmacy Practice, Bill Gatton College of Pharmacy, East Tennessee State University; Adjunct Professor, Department of Family Medicine, Quillen College of Medicine, East Tennessee State University, Johnson City, Tennessee

Bonnie L. Boster, PharmD, BCOP

Clinical Pharmacy Specialist—Breast Medical Oncology, Division of Pharmacy, The University of Texas MD Anderson Cancer Center, Houston, Texas

Jessica H. Brady, PharmD, BCPS

Clinical Associate Professor, Department of Clinical Sciences, School of Pharmacy, University of Louisiana at Monroe; Adult Medicine Clinical Pharmacist, University Health Conway, Monroe, Louisiana

Trisha N. Branan, PharmD, BCCCP

Clinical Assistant Professor, Department of Clinical & Administrative Pharmacy, University of Georgia College of Pharmacy; Critical Care Clinical Pharmacist, Athens Regional Medical Center, Athens, Georgia

Amie D. Brooks, PharmD, FCCP, BCPS, BCACP

Professor, Department of Pharmacy Practice, St. Louis College of Pharmacy, St. Louis, Missouri

Gretchen M. Brophy, PharmD, BCPS, FCCP, FCCM, FNCS

Professor of Pharmacotherapy & Outcomes Science and Neurosurgery, School of Pharmacy, Virginia Commonwealth University, Richmond, Virginia

Kristen L. Bunnell, PharmD, BCPS

Infectious Diseases Pharmacotherapy Fellow, University of Illinois at Chicago, School of Pharmacy, Chicago, Illinois

Rodrigo M. Burgos, PharmD, AAHIVP

Clinical Assistant Professor, Section of Infectious Diseases, Department of Pharmacy Practice, College of Pharmacy, University of Illinois at Chicago, Chicago, Illinois

Karim A. Calis, PharmD, MPH, FASHP, FCCP

Adjunct Senior Clinical Investigator, Eunice Kennedy Shriver National Institute of Child Health and Human Development; Clinical Professor, University of Maryland School of Pharmacy, Baltimore, MD; Clinical Professor, Virginia Commonwealth University School of Pharmacy, Richmond, Virginia

Lauren Camaione, BS, PharmD

Pediatric Pharmacotherapy Specialist, The Brooklyn Hospital Center; Clinical Assistant Professor of Pharmacy Practice, Long Island University, Arnold and Marie Schwartz College, Brooklyn, New York

Krista D. Capehart, PharmD, MSPharm, AE-C

Clinical Associate Professor, Department of Clinical Pharmacy, School of Pharmacy, West Virginia University, Morgantown; Director of the Wigner Institute for Advanced Pharmacy Practice, Education, and Research, Charleston, West Virginia

Katie E. Cardone, PharmD, BCACP, FNKF, FASN

Associate Professor, Department of Pharmacy Practice; Albany College of Pharmacy and Health Sciences, Albany, New York

Diana H. Cauley, PharmD, BCOP

Clinical Pharmacy Specialist, Genitourinary Medical Oncology, Division of Pharmacy, The University of Texas MD Anderson Cancer Center, Houston, Texas

Juliana Chan, PharmD, FCCP, BCACP

Clinical Associate Professor, Colleges of Pharmacy and Medicine, University of Illinois at Chicago; Clinical Pharmacist—Gastroenterology/Hepatology, Illinois Department of Corrections Hepatology Telemedicine, Sections of Hepatology, Digestive Diseases and Nutrition, Chicago, Illinois

Sheh-Li Chen, PharmD, BCOP

Clinical Pharmacy Specialist in Benign Hematology, University of North Carolina Medical Center; Assistant Professor of Clinical Education, UNC Eshelman School of Pharmacy, Chapel Hill, North Carolina

Amber N. Chiplinski, PharmD, BCPS

Clinical Pharmacy Coordinator, Meritus Medical Center, Hagerstown, Maryland

Kevin W. Cleveland, PharmD, ANP

Director of Student Services and Assistant Dean for Experiential Education; Associate Professor, Idaho State University College of Pharmacy, Meridian, Idaho

Jennifer Confer, PharmD, BCPS, BCCCP

Clinical Associate Professor, Department of Clinical Pharmacy, School of Pharmacy, West Virginia University, Morgantown; Clinical Pharmacist in Critical Care, Cabell Huntington Hospital, Huntington, West Virginia

Tracy J. Costello, PharmD, BCPS

Assistant Professor of Pharmacy Practice, Butler University College of Pharmacy and Health Sciences; Clinical Pharmacy Specialist, Family Medicine, Community Health Network, Indianapolis, Indiana

Elizabeth A. Coyle, PharmD, FCCM, BCPS

Assistant Dean of Assessment, Clinical Professor, University of Houston College of Pharmacy, Houston, Texas

Brian L. Crabtree, PharmD, BCPP

Professor and Chair, Department of Pharmacy Practice, Eugene Applebaum College of Pharmacy and Health Sciences, Wayne State University, Detroit, Michigan

Daniel J. Crona, PharmD, PhD

Assistant Professor, Division of Pharmacotherapy and Experimental Therapeutics, Eshelman School of Pharmacy; Clinical Pharmacy Specialist (Genitourinary Malignancies), Department of Pharmacy, North Carolina Cancer Hospital, Chapel Hill, North Carolina

Nicole S. Culhane, PharmD, FCCP, BCPS

Director of Experiential Education; Professor, Clinical and Administrative Sciences, School of Pharmacy, Notre Dame of Maryland University, Baltimore, Maryland

Aaron Cumpston, PharmD, BCOP

Clinical Specialist, Department of Pharmacy, West Virginia University Medicine, Morgantown, West Virginia

Kendra M. Damer, PharmD

Associate Professor, Department of Pharmacy Practice, College of Pharmacy and Health Sciences, Butler University, Indianapolis, Indiana

Lisa E. Davis, PharmD, FCCP, BCPS, BCOP

Professor, Department of Pharmacy Practice & Science, College of Pharmacy, University of Arizona, Tucson, Arizona

Christopher M. Degenkolb, PharmD, BCPS

Clinical Pharmacy Specialist in Internal Medicine, Richard L. Roudebush VA Medical Center, Indianapolis, Indiana

Paulina Deming, PharmD, PhC

Associate Professor of Pharmacy, University of New Mexico College of Pharmacy, Albuquerque, New Mexico

Margarita V. DiVall, PharmD, MEd, BCPS

Clinical Professor & Director of Assessment, Northeastern University School of Pharmacy, Boston, Massachusetts

Holly S. Divine, PharmD, BCACP, CGP, CDE, FAPhA

Clinical Associate Professor, Department of Pharmacy Practice and Science, University of Kentucky College of Pharmacy, Lexington, Kentucky

Ernest J. Dole, PharmD, PhC, FASHP, BCPS

Clinical Pharmacist; University of New Mexico Hospitals Pain Consultation & Treatment Center; Clinical Associate Professor, University of New Mexico College of Pharmacy, Albuquerque, New Mexico

Jennifer A. Donaldson, PharmD

Clinical Pharmacist Specialist, Riley Hospital for Children at Indiana University Health, Indianapolis, Indiana

Gabriella A. Douglass, PharmD, BCACP

Assistant Professor, Department of Pharmacy Practice, Harding University College of Pharmacy, Searcy; Clinical Pharmacist in Ambulatory Care, ARcare, Augusta, Arkansas

Scott R. Drab, PharmD, CDE, BC-ADM

Associate Professor of Pharmacy & Therapeutics, University of Pittsburgh, School of Pharmacy; Director, University Diabetes Care Associates, Pittsburgh, Pennsylvania

Sharon M. Erdman, PharmD

Clinical Professor, Department of Pharmacy Practice, College of Pharmacy, Purdue University, West Lafayette; Infectious Diseases Clinical Pharmacist, Eskenazi Health, Indianapolis, Indiana

Kathryn Eroschenko, PharmD

Clinical Assistant Professor, Department of Pharmacy Practice, Idaho State University, Meridian; Clinical Pharmacist in Ambulatory Care, Saint Alphonsus Medical Group Clinic, Boise, Idaho

Brian E. Erstad, PharmD, FCCP, FCCM, FASHP

Professor and Head, Department of Pharmacy Practice and Science, The University of Arizona College of Pharmacy, Tucson, Arizona

John S. Esterly, PharmD, BCPS AQ-ID

Scientific Director, Hepatitis C/HIV, Merck Research Laboratories, Chicago, Illinois

Jeffery D. Evans, PharmD

Clinical Associate Professor, Department of Clinical Pharmacy, School of Pharmacy, University of Louisiana at Monroe, Monroe, Louisiana

Virginia Fleming, PharmD, BCPS

Clinical Assistant Professor, Clinical and Administrative Pharmacy, University of Georgia College of Pharmacy, Athens, Georgia

Rachel W. Flurie, PharmD, BCPS

Assistant Professor, Internal Medicine, Department of Pharmacotherapy and Outcomes Science, School of Pharmacy, Virginia Commonwealth University, Richmond, Virginia

Michelle Fravel, PharmD, BCPS

Clinical Assistant Professor, Department of Pharmacy Practice and Science, University of Iowa College of Pharmacy, Iowa City, Iowa

Mary E. Fredrickson, PharmD, BCPS

Clinical Pharmacy Specialist, St. Joseph Warren Hospital, Warren, Ohio

Michelle D. Furler, BSc Pharm, PhD, CDE

Pharmacist, Kingston, Ontario, Canada

Lisa R. Garavaglia, PharmD, BCPS, BCPPS

Clinical Specialist in Pediatric Hematology/Oncology, Department of Pharmacy, West Virginia University Medicine; Adjunct Assistant Professor, West Virginia University School of Pharmacy, Morgantown, West Virginia

Sharon B. S. Gatewood, PharmD, FAPhA

Associate Professor, Department of Pharmacotherapy and Outcomes Sciences, School of Pharmacy, Virginia Commonwealth University, Richmond, Virginia

Amanda Geist, PharmD

Neonatal Intensive Care Unit Clinical Pharmacist, The Western Pennsylvania Hospital, Pittsburgh, Pennsylvania

Jane M. Gervasio, PharmD, BCNSP, FCCP

Professor, Department of Pharmacy Practice
Butler University, College of Pharmacy and Health Sciences, Indianapolis, Indiana

Ashley Glode, PharmD, BCOP

Assistant Professor, Department of Clinical Pharmacy, University of Colorado Skaggs School of Pharmacy and Pharmaceutical Sciences, Denver; Clinical Pharmacy Specialist, University of Colorado Cancer Center, Aurora, Colorado

Michael J. Gonyeau, BS Pharm, PharmD, MEd, FNAP, FCCP, BCPS, RPh

Clinical Professor; Acting Chair, Department of Pharmacy and Health Systems Sciences, Director of Undergraduate and Professional Programs, Northeastern University School of Pharmacy; Clinical Pharmacist, Integrated Teaching Unit, Brigham and Women's Hospital, Boston, Massachusetts

Jean-Venable "Kelly" R. Goode, PharmD, BCPS, FAPhA, FCCP

Professor and Director, Community Pharmacy Residency Program, School of Pharmacy, Virginia Commonwealth University, Richmond, Virginia

Anthony J. Guarascio, PharmD, BCPS

Assistant Professor, Department of Pharmacy, Practice, Mylan School of Pharmacy, Duquesne University, Pittsburgh, Pennsylvania

Wayne P. Gulliver, MD, FRCPC

Professor of Medicine and Dermatology; Faculty of Medicine, Memorial University of Newfoundland, Newfoundland, Canada

John G. Gums, PharmD, FCCP

Professor of Pharmacy and Medicine, Departments of Pharmacotherapy & Translational Research and Community Health & Family Medicine, Colleges of Pharmacy and Medicine, University of Florida; Associate Dean of Clinical Affairs, College of Pharmacy, University of Florida; Director of Clinical Research, Department of Community Health and Family Medicine, University of Florida, Gainesville, Florida

Jennifer R. Guthrie, MPAS, PA-C

Assistant Professor; Director of Experiential Education, Physician Assistant Program; College of Pharmacy and Health Sciences, Butler University, Indianapolis, Indiana

Deanne L. Hall, PharmD, CDE, BCACP

Associate Professor of Pharmacy and Therapeutics, University of Pittsburgh School of Pharmacy; Clinical Pharmacy Specialist—Ambulatory Care, UPMC Presbyterian/Shadyside, Pittsburgh, Pennsylvania

Felecia Hart, PharmD, MSCS

Clinical Neurology Research Fellow, Skaggs School of Pharmacy and Pharmaceutical Sciences, University of Colorado, Aurora, Colorado

Deborah A. Hass, PharmD, BCOP, BCPS

Oncology Pharmacist, Mt. Auburn Hospital, Cambridge, Massachusetts

Keith A. Hecht, PharmD, BCOP

Associate Professor, Department of Pharmacy Practice, School of Pharmacy, Southern Illinois University Edwardsville; Clinical Pharmacy Specialist, Hematology/Oncology, Mercy Hospital St. Louis, St. Louis, Missouri

Brian A. Hemstreet, PharmD, FCCP, BCPS

Assistant Dean for Student Affairs; Associate Professor of Pharmacy Practice, Regis University School of Pharmacy, Denver, Colorado

Sarah D. Hittle, PharmD, BCPS, BCCCP

Critical Care Clinical Pharmacy Specialist, St. Vincent Hospital, Indianapolis, Indiana

Brian M. Hodges, PharmD, BCPS, BCNSP

Market Clinical Director, Comprehensive Pharmacy Services, Charleston Area Medical Center; Clinical Assistant Professor, West Virginia University School of Pharmacy, Charleston, West Virginia

Brittany Hoffmann-Eubanks, PharmD, MBA

Clinical Pharmacist, Jewel-Osco Pharmacy, South Holland, Illinois

Lisa M Holle, PharmD, BCOP, FHOPA

Associate Clinical Professor, Department of Pharmacy Practice, University of Connecticut School of Pharmacy; Assistant Professor, Department of Medicine, School of Medicine, Farmington, Connecticut

Yvonne C. Huckleberry, PharmD, BCPS

Clinical Pharmacy Specialist, Critical Care, Department of Pharmacy Services, Banner University Medical Center; Clinical Assistant Professor, College of Pharmacy, The University of Arizona, Tucson, Arizona

Andrew Y. Hwang, PharmD

Postdoctoral Fellow, Departments of Pharmacotherapy & Translational Research and Community Health & Family Medicine, Colleges of Pharmacy and Medicine, University of Florida, Gainesville, Florida

Carrie L. Isaacs, PharmD, CDE

Clinical Pharmacy Specialist in Primary Care, Lexington VA Medical Center, Lexington, Kentucky

Timothy J. Ives, PharmD, MPH, FCCP, CPP

Professor of Pharmacy, UNC Eshelman School of Pharmacy; Adjunct Professor of Medicine, School of Medicine, The University of North Carolina at Chapel Hill, Chapel Hill, North Carolina

Catherine Johnson, PhD, FNP-BC, PNP-BC

Chair of Advanced Practice, School of Nursing, Duquesne University, Pittsburgh, Pennsylvania

Laura L Jung, BS Pharm, PharmD

Independent Medical Writer, Hematology/Oncology, Mount Holly, North Carolina

Teresa C. Kam, PharmD, BCOP

Clinical Pharmacist in Hematology/Stem Cell Transplantation, Indiana University Health, Indianapolis, Indiana

Michael D. Katz, PharmD

Professor, Department of Pharmacy Practice and Science, The University of Arizona College of Pharmacy, Tucson, Arizona

S. Travis King, PharmD, BCPS

Assistant Professor of Pharmacy Practice, University of Mississippi School of Pharmacy; Clinical Pharmacist in Infectious Diseases, University of Mississippi Medical Center, Jackson, Mississippi

Michael B. Kays, PharmD, FCCP

Associate Professor, Department of Pharmacy Practice, Purdue University College of Pharmacy, West Lafayette and Indianapolis; Adjunct Associate Professor, Department of Medicine, Indiana University School of Medicine, Indianapolis, Indiana

Cynthia K. Kirkwood, PharmD, BCPP

Executive Associate Dean for Academic Affairs; Professor, Department of Pharmacotherapy & Outcomes Science, School of Pharmacy, Virginia Commonwealth University, Richmond, Virginia

Julie C. Kissack, PharmD, BCPS, FCCP

Professor and Chair, Department of Pharmacy Practice, Harding University College of Pharmacy, Searcy, Arkansas

Jonathan Kline, PharmD, CACP, BCPS, CDE

Director of Pharmacy, Jefferson Medical Center, Ranson, WV; Adjunct Clinical Associate Professor, Department of Clinical Pharmacy, West Virginia University School of Pharmacy, Morgantown, West Virginia

Vanessa T. Kline, PharmD, BCPS

Clinical Pharmacy Specialist, Winchester Medical Center, Winchester, Virginia

Julia M. Koehler, PharmD, FCCP

Associate Dean for Clinical Education and External Affiliations; Professor of Pharmacy Practice, College of Pharmacy and Health Sciences, Butler University; Ambulatory Care Clinical Pharmacist, Transition Clinic and Pulmonary Rehabilitation, Indiana University Health, Indianapolis, Indiana

Cynthia P. Koh-Knox, PharmD

Clinical Associate Professor, Department of Pharmacy Practice, Purdue University College of Pharmacy, West Lafayette, Indiana

Brian J. Kopp, PharmD, BCPS, FCCM

Clinical Pharmacy Specialist—Critical Care, Department of Pharmacy Services, Banner University Medical Center—Tucson; Clinical Assistant Professor, College of Pharmacy, The University of Arizona, Tucson, Arizona

Michael D. Kraft, PharmD, BCNSP

Clinical Associate Professor, Department of Clinical Pharmacy, University of Michigan College of Pharmacy; Assistant Director—Education and Research, Department of Pharmacy Services, University of Michigan Hospitals and Health Centers, Ann Arbor, Michigan

Connie K. Kraus, PharmD, BCACP

Professor (CHS), University of Wisconsin-Madison, School of Pharmacy; Clinical Instructor, University of Wisconsin-Madison, Department of Family Medicine and Community Health, Madison, Wisconsin

Po Gin Kwa, MD

Clinical Assistant Professor, Faculty of Medicine, Memorial University of Newfoundland; Pediatrician, Eastern Health, St. John's, Newfoundland and Labrador, Canada

Kena J. Lanham, PharmD, BCPS

Clinical Pharmacy Specialist—Critical Care, Rush University Medical Center, Chicago, Illinois

Rebecca M. T. Law, BS Pharm, PharmD

Associate Professor, School of Pharmacy; Faculty of Medicine, Memorial University of Newfoundland, St. John's, Newfoundland and Labrador, Canada

Mary W. L. Lee, PharmD, BCPS, FCCP

Professor of Pharmacy Practice, Chicago College of Pharmacy; Vice President and Chief Academic Officer, Pharmacy and Optometry Education, Midwestern University, Downers Grove, Illinois

Cara Liday, PharmD, CDE

Associate Professor, Department of Pharmacy Practice and Administrative Sciences, Idaho State University; Clinical Pharmacist, InterMountain Medical Clinic, Pocatello, Idaho

Kristen L. Longstreth, PharmD, BCPS

Clinical Pharmacy Specialist, St. Elizabeth Youngstown Hospital, Youngstown; Clinical Associate Professor of Pharmacy Practice, Northeast Ohio Medical University, Rootstown, Ohio

Amy M. Lugo, PharmD, BCPS, BC-ADM, FAPhA

Clinical Pharmacy Specialist; Director—Managed Care Residency, Defense Health Agency Pharmacy Operations Division Formulary Management Branch, San Antonio, Texas

Cheen Lum, PharmD

Clinical Specialist in Behavioral Care, Community Hospital North; Ambulatory Care Pharmacist—Behavioral Care, Community Health Network, Indianapolis, Indiana

Robert MacLaren, BSc Pharm, PharmD, MPH, FCCM, FCCP

Professor, Department of Clinical Pharmacy, Skaggs School of Pharmacy and Pharmaceutical Sciences, University of Colorado, Aurora, Colorado

Erik D. Maki, PharmD, BCPS

Associate Professor, College of Pharmacy and Health Sciences, Drake University, Des Moines, Iowa

Margery H. Mark, MD

Associate Professor of Neurology and Psychiatry, UMDNJ-Robert Wood Johnson Medical School, New Brunswick, New Jersey

Joel C. Marrs, PharmD, FCCP, FASHP, FNLA, BCPS (AQ Cardiology), BCACP, CLS

Associate Professor, University of Colorado Skaggs School of Pharmacy and Pharmaceutical Sciences, Aurora, Colorado

Jay L. Martello, PharmD, BCPS

Clinical Assistant Professor, Department of Clinical Pharmacy, West Virginia University School of Pharmacy, Robert C Byrd Health Sciences Center, Morgantown, West Virginia

Lena M. Maynor, PharmD, BCPS

Clinical Associate Professor and Director of Advanced Pharmacy Practice Experiences, Department of Clinical Pharmacy, School of Pharmacy, West Virginia University, Morgantown, West Virginia

James W. McAuley, RPh, PhD, FAPhA

Professor of Pharmacy Practice and Neurology, Colleges of Pharmacy and Medicine, The Ohio State University, Columbus, Ohio

Jennifer McCann, PharmD, BCPS, BCCCP

Assistant Professor of Pharmacy Practice, Butler University College of Pharmacy and Health Sciences, Indianapolis, Indiana

William McGhee, PharmD

Clinical Pharmacy Specialist, Children's Hospital of Pittsburgh of UPMC; Adjunct Clinical Assistant Professor, School of Pharmacy, University of Pittsburgh, Pittsburgh, Pennsylvania

Ashlee McMillan, PharmD, BCACP

Director of Skills Development and Clinical Assistant Professor, Department of Clinical Pharmacy, West Virginia University School of Pharmacy, Morgantown, West Virginia

Brian McMillan, MD

Assistant Clinical Professor, Department of Ophthalmology, West Virginia University School of Medicine, Morgantown, West Virginia

Cydney E. McQueen, PharmD

Clinical Associate Professor, Department of Pharmacy Practice and Administration, School of Pharmacy, University of Missouri–Kansas City, Kansas City, Missouri

Sarah T. Melton, PharmD, BCPP, BCACP, CGP, FASCP

Associate Professor of Pharmacy Practice, Gatton College of Pharmacy at East Tennessee State University, Johnson City, Tennessee

Renee-Claude Mercier, PharmD, BCPS-AQ ID, PhC, FCCP

Professor of Pharmacy and Medicine, University of New Mexico, College of Pharmacy, Albuquerque, New Mexico

Sarah M. Michienzi, PharmD

PGY-2 HIV/ID Specialty Resident, Section of Infectious Diseases, Department of Pharmacy Practice, College of Pharmacy, University of Illinois at Chicago, Chicago, Illinois

Augusto Miravalle, MD

Associate Professor and Vice Chair of Education, Department of Neurology, University of Colorado School of Medicine, Aurora, Colorado

Marta A. Miyares, PharmD, BCPS (AQ Cardiology), CACP

Clinical Pharmacy Specialist, Internal Medicine, Jackson Memorial Hospital; Director, PGY1 Residency Program, Miami, Florida

Rima A. Mohammad, PharmD, BCPS

Clinical Assistant Professor, Department of Clinical Pharmacy, College of Pharmacy, University of Michigan; Clinical Pharmacist, University of Michigan Health System, Ann Arbor, Michigan

Scott W. Mueller, PharmD, BCCCP

Assistant Professor, Department of Clinical Pharmacy, Skaggs School of Pharmacy and Pharmaceutical Sciences, University of Colorado, Aurora, Colorado

James J. Nawarskas, PharmD, BCPS

Associate Professor, Department of Pharmacy Practice and Administrative Sciences, College of Pharmacy, University of New Mexico, University of New Mexico, Albuquerque, New Mexico

Leigh A. Nelson, PharmD, BCPP

Associate Professor, University of Missouri-Kansas City School of Pharmacy, Division of Pharmacy Practice and Administration; Associate Professor, University of Missouri-Kansas City School of Medicine, Department of Psychiatry; Clinical Pharmacist, Truman Medical Center Behavioral Health, Kansas City, Missouri

Branden D. Nemecek, PharmD, BCPS

Assistant Professor, Department of Pharmacy Practice, Mylan School of Pharmacy, Duquesne University, Pittsburgh, Pennsylvania

TuTran Nguyen, PharmD, BCPS

Adjunct Faculty, Department of Clinical Pharmacy Practice, Butler University College of Pharmacy and Health Sciences; PGY-2 Internal Medicine Pharmacy Resident, Indiana University Health Methodist Hospital, Indianapolis, Indiana

Sarah A. Nisly, PharmD, BCPS

Associate Professor, Department of Pharmacy Practice, Butler University, College of Pharmacy and Health Sciences; Clinical Specialist—Internal Medicine, Indiana University Health Methodist Hospital, Indianapolis, Indiana

Jason M. Noel, PharmD, BCPP

Associate Professor, Department of Pharmacy Practice and Science, University of Maryland School of Pharmacy, Baltimore, Maryland

Sarah Norskog, PharmD

PGY2 Oncology Pharmacy Resident, University of Colorado Hospital, Aurora, Colorado

Kimberly J. Novak, PharmD, BCPS, BCPPS

Advanced Patient Care Pharmacist—Pediatric and Adult Cystic Fibrosis, Residency Program Director—PGY2 Pharmacy Residency-Pediatrics, Nationwide Children's Hospital; Clinical Assistant Professor, The Ohio State University College of Pharmacy, Columbus, Ohio

Kelly K. Nystrom, PharmD, BCOP

Associate Professor of Pharmacy Practice, Creighton University School of Pharmacy and Health Professions, Omaha, Nebraska

Cindy L. O'Bryant, PharmD, BCOP

Associate Professor, Department of Clinical Pharmacy, University of Colorado Skaggs School of Pharmacy and Pharmaceutical Sciences; Clinical Pharmacy Specialist, University of Colorado Cancer Center, Aurora, Colorado

Dannielle C. O'Donnell, BS, PharmD

Clinical Assistant Professor, College of Pharmacy, The University of Texas at Austin; Principal Medical Science Liaison, Immunology, US Medical Affairs, Genentech, Austin, Texas

Carol A. Ott, PharmD, BCPP

Clinical Professor of Pharmacy Practice, Purdue University College of Pharmacy; Clinical Pharmacy Specialist—Psychiatry, Eskenazi Health, Indianapolis, Indiana

Manjunath (Amit) P. Pai, PharmD

Associate Professor of Clinical Pharmacy and Deputy Director of the Pharmacokinetics Core, Department of Clinical Pharmacy, University of Michigan College of Pharmacy, Ann Arbor, Michigan

Neha S. Pandit, PharmD, AAHIVP, BCPS

Associate Professor, Department of Pharmacy Practice, University of Maryland School of Pharmacy, Baltimore, Maryland

Laura M. Panko, MD, FAAP

Assistant Professor of Pediatrics, Children's Hospital of Pittsburgh of UPMC, School of Medicine, University of Pittsburgh, Pittsburgh, Pennsylvania

Emily C. Papineau, PharmD, BCPS

Associate Professor of Pharmacy Practice, Butler University, College of Pharmacy and Health Sciences; Director of Ambulatory Pharmacy Services, Community Health Network, Indianapolis, Indiana

Dennis Parker, Jr, PharmD

Neurocritical Care Clinical Pharmacist, Detroit Receiving Hospital; Clinical Associate Professor, Eugene Applebaum College of Pharmacy and Health Sciences, Detroit, Michigan

Robert B. Parker, PharmD, FCCP

Professor, Department of Clinical Pharmacy, University of Tennessee College of Pharmacy, Memphis, Tennessee

Neelam K. Patel, PharmD, BCOP

Clinical Pharmacy Specialist—Breast Medical Oncology, Division of Pharmacy, The University of Texas MD Anderson Cancer Center, Houston, Texas

Rebecca S. Pettit, PharmD, MBA, BCPS, BCPPS

Pediatric Pulmonary Clinical Pharmacy Specialist, Riley Hospital for Children at Indiana University Health, Indianapolis, Indiana

Nicole C. Pezzino, PharmD

Assistant Professor of Pharmacy Practice, Wilkes University, School of Pharmacy, Wilkes-Barre; Clinical Pharmacist in Community/Ambulatory Pharmacy, Nanticoke, Pennsylvania

Beth B. Phillips, PharmD, FCCP, BCPS

Rite Aid Professor, University of Georgia College of Pharmacy; Clinical Pharmacy Specialist, Charlie Norwood VA Medical Center, Watkinsville, Georgia

Bradley G. Phillips, PharmD, BCPS, FCCP

Milliken-Reeve Professor and Department Head, Clinical and Administrative Pharmacy, University of Georgia College of Pharmacy, Athens, Georgia

Amy M. Pick, PharmD, BCOP

Associate Professor of Pharmacy Practice, Creighton University School of Pharmacy and Health Professions, Omaha, Nebraska

Melissa R. Pleva, PharmD, BCPS, BCNSP

Clinical Pharmacist Specialist, Department of Pharmacy Services, University of Michigan Hospitals and Health Centers; Adjunct Clinical Assistant Professor, University of Michigan College of Pharmacy, Ann Arbor, Michigan

Charles D. Ponte, BS, PharmD, FAADE, FAPhA, FASHP, FCCP, FNAP

Professor of Clinical Pharmacy and Family Medicine, West Virginia University Schools of Pharmacy and Medicine, Morgantown, West Virginia

Jamie Poust, PharmD, BCOP

Oncology Pharmacy Specialist, University of Colorado Hospital, Aurora, Colorado

Amber E. Proctor, PharmD

Clinical Oncology Specialist, UNC Healthcare; Clinical Assistant Professor, UNC Eshelman School of Pharmacy, Chapel Hill, North Carolina

Darin Ramsey, PharmD, BCPS, BCACP

Associate Professor of Pharmacy Practice, Butler University College of Pharmacy & Health Sciences; Clinical Specialist in Primary Care, Richard L. Roudebush VA Medical Center, Indianapolis, Indiana

Randolph E. Regal, BS, PharmD

Clinical Associate Professor, Department of Clinical Pharmacy, College of Pharmacy, University of Michigan; Clinical Pharmacist, University of Michigan Health System, Ann Arbor, Michigan

Paul Reynolds, PharmD, BCPS

Critical Care Pharmacy Specialist, University of Colorado Hospital; Clinical Assistant Professor, Department of Clinical Pharmacy, Skaggs School of Pharmacy and Pharmaceutical Sciences, University of Colorado, Aurora, Colorado

Denise H. Rhoney, PharmD, FCCP, FCCM

Ron and Nancy McFarlane Distinguished Professor and Chair, Division of Practice Advancement and Clinical Education, UNC Eshelman School of Pharmacy, Chapel Hill, North Carolina

Christopher Roberson, MS, AGNP-BC, ACRN

Nurse Practitioner, Baltimore, Maryland

Margaret A. Robinson, PharmD

Clinical Instructor, Department of Pharmacotherapy and Outcomes Sciences, School of Pharmacy, Virginia Commonwealth University, Richmond, Virginia

Michelle L. Rockey, PharmD, BCOP

Oncology Clinical Coordinator, The University of Kansas Hospital Cancer Center, Westwood, Kansas

Julianna V. F. Roddy, PharmD, BCOP

Clinical Pharmacist Specialist, Hematology/BMT/Oncology, Arthur G. James Cancer Hospital and Richard J. Solove Cancer Institute, The Ohio State University, Columbus, Ohio

Keith A. Rodvold, PharmD, FCCP, FIDSA

Professor of Pharmacy Practice and Medicine, Colleges of Pharmacy and Medicine, University of Illinois at Chicago, Chicago, Illinois

Kelly C. Rogers, PharmD, FCCP

Professor, Department of Clinical Pharmacy, University of Tennessee College of Pharmacy, Memphis, Tennessee

Carol J. Rollins, MS, RD, CNSC, PharmD, BCNSP

Clinical Professor, College of Pharmacy, University of Arizona; Clinical Pharmacist, Banner University Medical Center, Tucson, Arizona

Rochelle Rubin, PharmD, BCPS, CDE

Senior Clinical Pharmacy Coordinator—Family Medicine; Assistant Residency Program Director—PGY1 Pharmacy Residency, The Brooklyn Hospital Center; Clinical Assistant Professor of Pharmacy Practice, Arnold and Marie Schwartz College, Long Island University, Brooklyn, New York

Laura Ruekert, PharmD, BCPP, CGP

Clinical Specialist in Behavioral Care, Community Hospital North; Associate Professor of Pharmacy Practice, Butler University, Indianapolis, Indiana

Laurajo Ryan, PharmD, MSc, BCPS, CDE

Clinical Associate Professor, Division of Pharmacotherapy, The University of Texas at Austin College of Pharmacy, UT Health Science Center San Antonio, San Antonio, Texas

Laurel Sampognaro, PharmD

Clinical Associate Professor, Department of Clinical Pharmacy, School of Pharmacy, University of Louisiana at Monroe, Monroe, Louisiana

Elizabeth J. Scharman, PharmD, DABAT, BCPS, FAACT

Director, West Virginia Poison Center; Professor, Department of Clinical Pharmacy, School of Pharmacy, West Virginia University Health Sciences Center—Charleston Division, Charleston, West Virginia

Marc H. Scheetz, PharmD, MSc

Associate Professor, Department of Pharmacy Practice, Chicago College of Pharmacy, Midwestern University; Infectious Diseases Clinical Pharmacist, Northwestern Medicine, Chicago, Illinois

Kristine S. Schonder, PharmD

Assistant Professor, Department of Pharmacy and Therapeutics, University of Pittsburgh School of Pharmacy, Pittsburgh, Pennsylvania

Natalie R. Schwarber, PharmD

Infectious Diseases Clinical Pharmacist, HSHS St. John's Hospital, Springfield; Adjunct Clinical Instructor, Southern Illinois University Edwardsville School of Pharmacy, Edwardsville, Illinois

Jacqueline Schwartz, PharmD

Assistant Professor, School of Pharmacy, Pacific University, Hillsboro, Oregon

Terry L. Schwinghammer, PharmD, FCCP, FASHP, FAPhA, BCPS

Arthur I. Jacknowitz Distinguished Chair in Clinical Pharmacy and Chair, Department of Clinical Pharmacy, West Virginia University School of Pharmacy, Morgantown, West Virginia

Mollie A. Scott, PharmD, BCACP, FASHP, CPP

Regional Associate Dean; Clinical Associate Professor, UNC Eshelman School of Pharmacy, Chapel Hill, North Carolina

Brian Sedam, PharmD, BCPS, BCACP

Ambulatory Care Clinical Specialist, Community Health Network, Indianapolis, Indiana

Roohollah R. Sharifi, MD, FACS

Professor of Urology and Surgery, University of Illinois at Chicago College of Medicine; Section Chief of Urology, Jesse Brown Veterans Administration Hospital, Chicago, Illinois

Amanda E. Shearin, PharmD, BCPS

Clinical Pharmacist, University Medical Center, University of New Mexico, Albuquerque, New Mexico

Amy H. Sheehan, PharmD

Associate Professor of Pharmacy Practice, Purdue University College of Pharmacy; Drug Information Specialist, Indiana University Health, Indianapolis, Indiana

Alexandra Shillingburg, PharmD, BCOP

Clinical Specialist in Oncology, Pharmacy Department, West Virginia University Medicine, Morgantown, West Virginia

Dane L. Shiltz, PharmD, BCPS

Associate Professor, Department of Clinical Pharmacy Practice, Butler University College of Pharmacy and Health Sciences; Clinical Pharmacist in Internal Medicine, Indiana University Health Methodist Hospital, Indianapolis, Indiana

Carrie A. Sincak, PharmD, BCPS, FASHP

Assistant Dean for Clinical Affairs; Professor of Pharmacy Practice, Chicago College of Pharmacy, Midwestern University, Downers Grove, Illinois

Douglas Slain, PharmD, BCPS, FCCP, FASHP

Professor, Department of Clinical Pharmacy, West Virginia University School of Pharmacy; Infectious Diseases Clinical Specialist, West Virginia University Medicine, Morgantown, West Virginia

Carmen B. Smith, PharmD, BCPS

Assistant Professor—Pharmacy Practice, Division of Acute Care Pharmacy, St. Louis College of Pharmacy, St. Louis, Missouri

Curtis L. Smith, PharmD, BCPS

Professor of Pharmacy Practice, Ferris State University College of Pharmacy; Clinical Pharmacy Specialist, Sparrow Health System, Lansing, Michigan

Steven M. Smith, PharmD, MPH, BCPS

Assistant Professor of Pharmacy and Medicine, Departments of Pharmacotherapy & Translational Research and Community Health & Family Medicine, Colleges of Pharmacy and Medicine, University of Florida, Gainesville, Florida

Denise R. Sokos, PharmD, BCPS

Adjunct Assistant Professor, Department of Pharmacy and Therapeutics, University of Pittsburgh School of Pharmacy, Pittsburgh, Pennsylvania

Suellyn J. Sorensen, PharmD, BCPS, FASHP

Director, Clinical Pharmacy Services, St. Vincent Hospital and Health Care Center, Indianapolis, Indiana

Robin Southwood, PharmD, CDE

Clinical Associate Professor, Clinical and Administrative Pharmacy Department, College of Pharmacy, University of Georgia, Athens, Georgia

Mikayla Spangler, PharmD, BCPS

Associate Professor, Creighton University School of Pharmacy and Health Professions; Clinical Pharmacist, CHI Health Clinic—Lakeside, Omaha, Nebraska

Tracy L. Sprunger, PharmD, BCPS

Associate Professor of Pharmacy Practice, Butler University College of Pharmacy and Health Sciences, Indianapolis, Indiana

Mary K. Stamatakis, PharmD

Professor, Department of Clinical Pharmacy; Associate Dean of Academic Affairs and Educational Innovation, West Virginia University School of Pharmacy, Morgantown, West Virginia

Jennifer L. Swank, PharmD, BCOP

Medical Oncology Clinical Pharmacist, H. Lee Moffitt Cancer Center and Research Institute, Tampa, Florida

Lynne M. Sylvia, PharmD

Senior Clinical Pharmacy Specialist—Cardiology, Tufts Medical Center; Clinical Professor, School of Pharmacy, Northeastern University, Boston, Massachusetts

Heather Teufel, PharmD, BCPS

Clinical Pharmacist—Emergency Medicine, University of Pennsylvania Health System—Chester County Hospital, West Chester, Pennsylvania

Janine E. Then, PharmD, BCPS

Lead Pharmacist—Clinical Services, UPMC Presbyterian Hospital, Pittsburgh, Pennsylvania

James E. Tisdale, PharmD, BCPS, FCCP, FAPhA, FAHA

Professor, College of Pharmacy, Purdue University, West Lafayette; Adjunct Professor, School of Medicine, Indiana University, Indianapolis, Indiana

Trent G. Towne, PharmD, BCPS (AQ-ID)

Associate Professor of Pharmacy Practice, Natural and Health Sciences, Manchester University College of Pharmacy; Infectious Diseases Clinical Pharmacist, Parkview Regional Medical Center, Fort Wayne, Indiana

Tran H. Tran, PharmD, BCPS

Associate Professor, Department of Pharmacy Practice, Chicago College of Pharmacy, Midwestern University, Downers Grove; Clinical Pharmacist, Loyola University Medical Center, Maywood, Illinois

Kevin M. Tuohy, PharmD, BCPS

Associate Professor of Pharmacy Practice, Butler University College of Pharmacy and Health Sciences; Clinical Pharmacy Specialist—Internal Medicine, Indiana University Health Methodist Hospital, Indianapolis, Indiana

Rodney B. Turner, PharmD, BCPS

Assistant Professor, School of Pharmacy, Pacific University, Hillsboro; Infectious Diseases Clinical Specialist, Legacy Health, Portland, Oregon

Joseph P. Vande Griend, PharmD, FCCP, BCPS

Associate Professor and Assistant Director of Clinical Affairs, Skaggs School of Pharmacy and Pharmaceutical Sciences, University of Colorado; Associate Professor, Department of Family Medicine, University of Colorado School of Medicine, Aurora, Colorado

Ashley H. Vincent, PharmD, BCACP, BCPS

Clinical Associate Professor, Department of Pharmacy Practice, College of Pharmacy, Purdue University, West Lafayette; Clinical Pharmacy Specialist—Ambulatory Care, IU Health Physicians Adult Ambulatory Care Center, Indianapolis, Indiana

Mary L. Wagner, PharmD, MS

Associate Professor, Department of Pharmacy Practice, Ernest Mario School of Pharmacy, Rutgers, State University of New Jersey, Piscataway, New Jersey

Alison M. Walton, PharmD, BCPS

Associate Professor of Pharmacy Practice, College of Pharmacy and Health Sciences, Butler University; Clinical Pharmacy Specialist—Ambulatory Care, St. Vincent, Indianapolis, Indiana

Zachary A. Weber, PharmD, BCPS, BCACP, CDE

Clinical Associate Professor, Department of Pharmacy Practice, Purdue University College of Pharmacy, Indianapolis, Indiana

Lydia E. Weisser, DO, MBA

Medical Director, G. Werber Bryan Psychiatric Hospital, Columbia, South Carolina

Jeffrey T. Wieczorkiewicz, PharmD, BCPS

Assistant Professor, Department of Pharmacy Practice, Chicago College of Pharmacy, Midwestern University, Downers Grove; Clinical Pharmacy Specialist—Acute Care Internal Medicine, Edward Hines Jr. VA Hospital, Hines, Illinois

Jon P. Wietholter, PharmD, BCPS

Clinical Associate Professor, Department of Clinical Pharmacy, West Virginia University School of Pharmacy; Internal Medicine Clinical Pharmacist, Ruby Memorial Hospital, West Virginia Medicine, Morgantown, West Virginia

Susan R. Winkler, PharmD, BCPS, FCCP

Professor and Chair, Department of Pharmacy Practice, Chicago College of Pharmacy, Midwestern University, Downers Grove, Illinois

Nancy S. Yunker, PharmD, FCCP, BCPS

Assistant Professor of Pharmacy, Department of Pharmacotherapy and Outcomes Science, Virginia Commonwealth University School of Pharmacy; Clinical Pharmacy Specialist—Internal Medicine, VCU Health, Richmond, Virginia

William Zamboni, PharmD, PhD

Associate Professor, UNC Eshelman School of Pharmacy, UNC Lineberger Comprehensive Cancer Center, University of North Carolina at Chapel Hill, Chapel Hill, North Carolina

PREFACE

The purpose of the *Pharmacotherapy Casebook* is to help students in the health professions and practicing clinicians develop and refine the skills required to identify and resolve drug therapy problems by using patient case studies. Case studies can actively involve students in the learning process; engender self-confidence; and promote the development of skills in independent self-study, problem analysis, decision-making, oral communication, and teamwork. Patient case studies can also be used as the focal point of discussions about pathophysiology, medicinal chemistry, pharmacology, and the pharmacotherapy of individual diseases. By integrating the biomedical and pharmaceutical sciences with pharmacotherapeutics, case studies can help students appreciate the relevance and importance of a sound scientific foundation in preparation for practice.

The patient cases in this book are intended to complement the scientific information presented in the 10th edition of *Pharmacotherapy: A Pathophysiologic Approach*. This edition of the casebook contains 157 unique patient cases, with case chapters organized into organ system sections corresponding to those of the *Pharmacotherapy* textbook. Students should read the relevant textbook chapter to become thoroughly familiar with the pathophysiology and pharmacotherapy of each disease state before attempting to make "decisions" about the care of patients described in this casebook. The *Pharmacotherapy* textbook, casebook, and other useful learning resources are also available on *AccessPharmacy.com* (subscription required). By using these realistic cases to practice creating, defending, and implementing pharmacotherapeutic care plans, students can begin to develop the skills and self-confidence that will be necessary to make the real decisions required in professional practice.

The knowledge and clinical experience required to answer the questions associated with each patient presentation vary from case to case. Some cases deal with a single disease state whereas others have multiple diseases and drug therapy problems. As a guide for instructors, each case is identified as being one of three complexity levels; this classification system is described in more detail in Chapter 1.

Casebook Section 1: Principles of Patient-Focused Therapy includes 11 chapters that provide guidance on use of the casebook as well as several patient cases for managing special patient populations (eg, pediatrics) and situations (eg, toxicology).

Chapter 1 describes the format of case presentations and the means by which students and instructors can maximize the usefulness of the casebook. A systematic approach is consistently applied to each case. The steps involved in this approach include:

1. Identifying real or potential drug therapy problems
2. Determining the desired therapeutic outcome(s)
3. Evaluating therapeutic alternatives
4. Designing an optimal individualized pharmacotherapeutic plan
5. Developing methods to evaluate the therapeutic outcome
6. Providing patient education
7. Communicating and implementing the pharmacotherapeutic plan

In Chapter 2, the philosophy and implementation of active learning strategies are presented. This chapter sets the tone for the casebook by describing how these approaches can enhance student learning. The chapter offers a number of useful active learning strategies for instructors and provides advice to students on how to maximize their learning opportunities in active learning environments.

Chapter 3 discusses the importance of patient communication and offers strategies to get the most out of the time that the clinician shares with the patient during each encounter. The information can be used as the basis for simulated counseling sessions related to the patient cases.

Chapter 4 describes the patient care process and outlines the steps in creating care plans to help ensure that the drug-related needs of patients are met. Students should be encouraged to practice writing care plans when completing the case studies in this casebook.

Chapter 5 describes two methods for documenting clinical interventions and communicating recommendations to other healthcare providers. These include the traditional SOAP note and the more pharmacy-specific FARM note. Student preparation of documentation notes for the patient cases in this casebook will be excellent practice for future practice.

Sections 2 through 18 contain patient cases organized by organ systems that correspond to those of the *Pharmacotherapy* textbook. Section 19 (Complementary and Alternative Therapies) contains patient vignettes that are directly related to patient cases that were presented earlier in this casebook. Each scenario involves the potential use of one or more dietary supplements. Additional follow-up questions are then asked to help the reader gain the scientific and clinical knowledge required to provide an evidence-based recommendation about use of the supplement in that particular patient. Sixteen different dietary supplements are discussed: garlic, fish oil (omega-3 fatty acids), ginger, coenzyme Q10, butterbur, feverfew, St. John's wort, kava, cinnamon, α-lipoic acid, black cohosh, soy, *Pygeum africanum*, glucosamine, chondroitin, and elderberry.

The focus of classroom discussions about the patient cases should be on the process of solving patient problems as much as it is on finding the actual answers to the questions themselves. Isolated scientific facts learned today may be obsolete or incorrect tomorrow. Healthcare providers who can identify patient problems and solve them using a reasoned approach will be able to adapt to the continual evolution in the body of scientific knowledge and contribute in a meaningful way to improving the quality of patients' lives.

We are grateful for the broad acceptance that previous editions of the casebook have received. In particular, it has been adopted by many schools of pharmacy and nurse practitioner programs. It has also been used in institutional staff development efforts and by individual pharmacists wishing to upgrade their pharmacotherapy skills. It is our hope that this new edition will be even more valuable in assisting healthcare practitioners to meet society's need for safe and effective drug therapy.

ACKNOWLEDGMENTS

There are five editors of the *Pharmacotherapy Casebook*, 10th edition. Drs Jill S. Borchert and Douglas Slain have changed from being Section Editors to now being full Co-Editors. We also welcome Dr Sharon K. Park as a new Co-Editor for this edition. Each editor is responsible for specific sections of the casebook, as identified in the table of contents.

The editors would like to thank the 212 case and chapter authors from more than 100 schools of pharmacy, healthcare systems, and other institutions in the United States and Canada who contributed their scholarly efforts to this casebook. We especially appreciate their diligence in meeting deadlines, adhering to the unique format of the casebook, and providing up-to-date pharmacotherapy information. The next generation of healthcare practitioners will benefit from the willingness of these clinicians to share their expertise.

We also thank the individuals at McGraw-Hill Professional whose cooperation, advice, and commitment were instrumental in maintaining the high standards of this publication: Michael Weitz, Peter Boyle, Barbara Holton, and Laura Libretti. We appreciate the meticulous attention to composition and prepress detail provided by Anju Joshi of Cenveo Publisher Services. Finally, we are grateful to our spouses for their understanding, support, and encouragement during the preparation of this new edition.

Terry L. Schwinghammer, PharmD, FCCP, FASHP, FAPhA, BCPS
Julia M. Koehler, PharmD, FCCP
Jill S. Borchert, PharmD, BCACP, BCPS, FCCP
Douglas Slain, PharmD, BCPS, FCCP, FASHP
Sharon K. Park, PharmD, BCPS

PRINCIPLES OF PATIENT-FOCUSED THERAPY

CHAPTER 1

Introduction: How to Use This Casebook

TERRY L. SCHWINGHAMMER, PharmD, FCCP, FASHP, FAPhA, BCPS

USING CASE STUDIES TO ENHANCE STUDENT LEARNING

The case method is used primarily to develop the skills of self-learning, critical thinking, problem identification, and decision making. When case studies from this Casebook are used in the curricula of the healthcare professions or for independent study by practitioners, the focus of attention should be on learning the process of solving drug therapy problems rather than simply finding scientific answers to the problems themselves. Students do learn scientific facts during the resolution of case study problems, but they usually learn more facts from their own independent study and from discussions with their peers than they do from the instructor. Working on subsequent cases with similar problems reinforces information recall. Traditional programs in the healthcare professions that rely heavily on traditional lectures tend to concentrate on dissemination of scientific content with rote memorization of facts rather than the development of higher-order thinking skills.

Case studies in the health professions provide the personal history of an individual patient and information about one or more health care problems that must be resolved. The learner's job is to work through the facts of the case, analyze the available data, gather more information, develop hypotheses, consider possible solutions, arrive at the optimal solution, and consider the consequences of one's decisions.[1] The role of the teacher is to serve as coach and facilitator rather than as the source of "the answer." In fact, in many situations there is more than one acceptable answer to a given question. Because instructors do not necessarily need to possess the correct answer, they need not be experts in the field being discussed. Rather, the students also become teachers, and both instructors and students learn from each other through thoughtful discussion of the case.

FORMAT OF THE CASEBOOK

BACKGROUND READING

The patient cases in this Casebook can be used as the focal point for independent self-learning by individual students and for in-class problem-solving discussions by student groups and their instructors. If meaningful learning and discussion are to occur, students must come to discussion sessions prepared to discuss the case material rationally, to propose reasonable solutions, and to defend their pharmacotherapeutic plans. This requires a strong commitment to independent self-study prior to the session. The cases in this book were designed to correspond with the scientific information contained in the ninth edition of *Pharmacotherapy: A Pathophysiologic Approach.*[2] For this reason, thorough understanding of the corresponding textbook chapter is recommended as the principal method of student preparation. The online learning center *AccessPharmacy* (www.AccessPharmacy.com, subscription required) contains the *Pharmacotherapy* textbook and many other resources that are beneficial in answering case questions. The cases in the Casebook can also be used with the textbook *Pharmacotherapy Principles & Practice*, 3rd ed.,[3] or other therapeutics textbooks. Primary literature should also be consulted as necessary to supplement textbook readings.

Most of the cases in the Casebook represent common diseases likely to be encountered by generalist practitioners. As a result, not all of the *Pharmacotherapy* textbook chapters have an associated patient case in the Casebook. On the other hand, some of the textbook chapters that discuss multiple disease entities have several corresponding cases in the Casebook.

LEVELS OF CASE COMPLEXITY

Each case is identified at the top of the first page as being one of the three levels of complexity. Instructors may use this classification system to select cases for discussion that correspond to the experience level of the student learners. These levels are defined as follows:

Level I—An uncomplicated case; only a single textbook chapter is required to complete the case questions. Little prior knowledge of the disease state or clinical experience is needed.

Level II—An intermediate-level case; several textbook chapters or other reference sources may be required to complete the case. Prior clinical experience may be helpful in resolving all of the issues presented.

Level III—A complicated case; multiple textbook chapters, additional readings, and substantial clinical experience may be required to solve all of the patient's drug therapy problems.

USING LEARNING OBJECTIVES

Learning objectives are included at the beginning of each case for student reflection. The focus of these outcomes is on eventually achieving clinical competence rather than simply learning isolated scientific facts. These items reflect some of the knowledge, skills, and abilities that students should possess after reading the textbook chapter, studying the case, preparing a pharmacotherapeutic plan, and defending their recommendations. Of course, true clinical competence can only be gained by direct interaction with real patients in various health care environments.

The learning objectives provided are meant to serve as a starting point to stimulate student thinking, but they are not intended to be all-inclusive. In fact, students should also generate their own personal ability outcome statements and learning objectives for each case. By so doing, students take greater control of their own learning, which serves to improve personal motivation and the desire to learn.

PATIENT PRESENTATION

The format and organization of cases reflect those usually seen in actual clinical settings. The patient's medical history and physical examination findings are provided in the following standardized outline format.

CHIEF COMPLAINT

The chief complaint (CC) is a brief statement of the reason why the patient consulted the physician, stated in the patient's own words. In order to convey the patient's symptoms accurately, medical terms and diagnoses are generally not used. The appropriate medical terminology is used only after an appropriate evaluation (ie, medical history, physical examination, laboratory and other testing) leads to a medical diagnosis.

In the United Kingdom, the term "presenting complaint" (PC) may be used. Other synonymous terms include reason for encounter (RFE), presenting problem, problem on admission, or reason for presenting.

HPI

The history of present illness is a more complete description of the patient's symptom(s). Usually included in the HPI are:

- Date of onset
- Precise location
- Nature of onset, severity, and duration
- Presence of exacerbations and remissions
- Effect of any treatment given
- Relationship to other symptoms, bodily functions, or activities (eg, activity, meals)
- Degree of interference with daily activities

PMH

The past medical history includes serious illnesses, surgical procedures, and injuries the patient has experienced previously. Minor complaints (eg, influenza, colds) are usually omitted unless they might have a bearing on the current medical situation.

FH

The family history includes the age and health of parents, siblings, and children. For deceased relatives, the age and cause of death are recorded. In particular, heritable diseases and those with a hereditary tendency are noted (eg, diabetes mellitus, cardiovascular disease, malignancy, rheumatoid arthritis, obesity).

SH

The social history includes the social characteristics of the patient as well as environmental factors and behaviors that may contribute to development of disease. Items that may be listed are the patient's marital status; number of children; educational background; occupation; physical activity; hobbies; dietary habits; and use of tobacco, alcohol, or other drugs.

MEDS

The medication history should include an accurate record of the patient's current use of prescription medications, nonprescription products, dietary supplements, and home remedies. Because there are thousands of prescription and nonprescription products available, it is important to obtain a complete medication history that includes the names, doses, routes of administration, schedules, and duration of therapy for all medications, including dietary supplements and other alternative therapies.

ALL

Allergies to drugs, food, pets, and environmental factors (eg, grass, dust, pollen) are recorded. An accurate description of the reaction that occurred should also be included. Care should be taken to distinguish adverse drug effects ("upset stomach") from true allergies ("hives").

ROS

In the review of systems, the examiner questions the patient about the presence of symptoms related to each body system. In many cases, only the pertinent positive and negative findings are recorded. In a complete ROS, body systems are generally listed starting from the head and working toward the feet and may include the skin, head, eyes, ears, nose, mouth and throat, neck, cardiovascular, respiratory, gastrointestinal, genitourinary, endocrine, musculoskeletal, and neuropsychiatric systems. The purpose of the ROS is to evaluate the status of each body system and to prevent omission of pertinent information. Information that was included in the HPI is generally not repeated in the ROS.

PHYSICAL EXAMINATION

The exact procedures performed during the physical examination vary depending on the chief complaint, medical history, and type of encounter. A complete physical examination may be performed for annual screening, employment, or insurance purposes. In most clinical situations, only a limited physical examination is performed that is focused on the reason for the encounter. In psychiatric practice, greater emphasis is usually placed on the type and severity of the patient's symptoms than on physical findings. Most of the cases in this Casebook include comprehensive physical examination data so student learners become familiar with common procedures and learn which findings are relevant to the chief complaint and which are routine, normal findings. A suitable physical assessment textbook should be consulted for the specific procedures that may be conducted for each body system. The general sections for the PE are outlined as follows:

Gen (general appearance).

VS (vital signs)—blood pressure, pulse, respiratory rate, and temperature. In hospital settings, the presence and severity of pain is included as "the fifth vital sign." For ease of use and consistency in this Casebook, weight and height are included in the vital signs section, but they are not technically considered to be vital signs.

Skin (integumentary).

HEENT (head, eyes, ears, nose, and throat).

Lungs/Thorax (pulmonary).

Cor or CV (cardiovascular).

Abd (abdomen).

Genit/Rect (genitalia/rectal).

MS/Ext (musculoskeletal and extremities).

Neuro (neurologic).

LABS

The results of laboratory tests are included with most cases in this Casebook. **Appendix A** contains common conversion factors and anthropometric information that will be helpful in solving many case answers. Normal (reference) ranges for the laboratory tests used throughout the Casebook are included in **Appendix B**. Values in the appendix are provided in both traditional units and SI units (*le système International d'Unités*). The normal range for a given laboratory test is determined from a representative sample of the general population. The upper and lower limits of the range usually encompass two standard deviations from the population mean, which includes a range within which about 95% of healthy persons would fall. The term *normal range* may therefore be misleading, because a test result may be abnormal for a given individual even if it falls within the "normal" range. Furthermore, given the statistical methods used to calculate the range, about 1 in 20 normal, healthy individuals may have a value for a test that lies outside the range. For these reasons, the term *reference range* is preferred over normal range. Reference ranges differ among laboratories, so the values given in Appendix B should be considered only as a general guide. Institution-specific reference ranges should be used in actual clinical settings.

All of the cases include some physical examination and laboratory findings that are within normal limits. For example, a description of the cardiovascular examination may include a statement that the point of maximal impulse is at the fifth intercostal space; laboratory evaluation may include a serum sodium level of 140 mEq/L (140 mmol/L). The presentation of actual findings (rather than simple statements that the heart examination and the serum sodium were normal) reflects what will be seen in actual clinical practice. More importantly, listing both normal and abnormal findings requires students to carefully assess the complete database and identify the pertinent positive and negative findings for themselves. A valuable portion of the learning process is lost if students are only provided with findings that are abnormal and are known to be associated with the disease being discussed.

The patients described in this Casebook have fictitious names in order to humanize the situations and to encourage students to remember that they will one day be caring for patients, not treating disease states. However, in the actual clinical setting, patient confidentiality is of utmost importance, and real patient names should not be used during group discussions in patient care areas unless absolutely necessary. To develop student sensitivity to this issue, instructors may wish to avoid using these fictitious patient names during class discussions. In this Casebook, patient names are usually given only in the initial presentation; they are used infrequently in subsequent questions or other portions of the case.

The issues of race, ethnicity, and gender also deserve thoughtful consideration. The traditional format for case presentations usually begins with a description of the patient's age, race, and gender, as in: "The patient is a 65-year-old white male…." Single-word racial labels such as "black" or "white" are actually of limited value in many cases and may actually be misleading in some instances.[4] For this reason, racial descriptors are usually excluded from the opening line of each presentation. When ethnicity is pertinent to the case, this information is presented in the social history or physical examination. Adult patients in this Casebook are referred to as men or women, rather than males or females, to promote sensitivity to human dignity.

The patient cases in this Casebook include medical abbreviations and both generic and proprietary drug names, just as medical records do in actual practice. Although abbreviations and brand names are sometimes the source of clinical problems, the intent of their inclusion is to make the cases as realistic as possible. **Appendix C** lists the medical abbreviations used in the Casebook. This list is limited to commonly accepted abbreviations; thousands more exist, which makes it difficult for novice practitioners to efficiently assess patient databases. Most healthcare institutions have an approved list of accepted abbreviations; these lists should be consulted in practice to facilitate one's understanding and to avoid using abbreviations in the medical record that are not on the official approved list. Appendix C also lists abbreviations and designations that should be avoided. Given the immense human toll resulting from medical errors, this section should be considered "must" reading for all student learners.

The Casebook also contains some photographs of commercial drug products. These illustrations are provided as examples only and are not intended to imply endorsement of those particular products.

PHARMACEUTICAL CARE AND DRUG THERAPY PROBLEMS

Medication therapy plays a crucial role in improving human health by enhancing quality of life and extending life expectancy. The advent of biotechnology has led to the introduction of unique compounds for the prevention and treatment of disease that were unimagined just a decade ago. Each year the US Food and Drug Administration (FDA) approves approximately two dozen new drug products that contain active substances that have never before been marketed in the United States. Although the cost of new therapeutic agents often receives intense scrutiny, drug therapy actually accounts for a relatively small proportion of overall health care expenditures. Appropriate drug therapy is cost-effective and may actually serve to reduce total expenditures by decreasing the need for surgery, preventing hospital admissions and readmissions, shortening hospital stays, and preventing emergency department and physician visits.

Several studies have indicated that improper use of prescription medications is a frequent and serious problem. Based on a decision analytic model, one study estimated that the cost of drug-related morbidity and mortality was more than $177 billion in 2000.

Hospital admissions accounted for almost 70% ($121.5 billion) of total costs; long-term care admissions were responsible for 18% of costs ($32.8 billion).[5] In 1999, the Institute of Medicine estimated that 7,000 patients die each year from medication errors that occur both within and outside hospitals. A societal need for better use of medications clearly exists. Widespread implementation of pharmaceutical care (or comprehensive medication management) has the potential to positively impact this situation by the design, implementation, and monitoring of rational therapeutic plans to produce defined outcomes that improve the quality of patients' lives.[6]

According to the American Pharmacists Association (APhA), the mission of the pharmacy profession is to serve society as the profession responsible for the appropriate use of medications, devices, and services to achieve optimal therapeutic outcomes.[7] The Joint Commission of Pharmacy Practitioners (JCPP) *Vision of Pharmacy Practice* states that by 2015 pharmacists will be the health care professionals responsible for providing patient care that ensures optimal medication therapy outcomes.[8] Schools and colleges of pharmacy have implemented innovative instructional strategies and curricula that have an increased emphasis on patient-centered care, including more skills-based laboratory exercises and experiential training, especially in ambulatory settings. Most programs are structured to promote self-directed learning, develop problem-solving and communication skills, and instill the desire for lifelong learning.

In its broadest sense, a pharmaceutical care practice involves identification, resolution, and prevention of actual or potential drug therapy problems. A drug therapy problem has been defined as "any undesirable event experienced by a patient that involves, or is suspected to involve, drug therapy and that interferes with achieving the desired goals of therapy and requires professional judgment to resolve."[9] Seven distinct types of drug therapy problems have been identified that may potentially lead to an undesirable event that has physiologic, psychological, social, or economic ramifications.[9] These seven problem types relate to assessment of medication indication, effectiveness, safety, or adherence:

Indication for drug use:

1. The drug therapy is unnecessary because the patient does not have a clinical indication at this time.

2. Additional drug therapy is required to treat or prevent a medical condition.

Effectiveness of therapy:

3. The drug product is not being effective at producing the desired patient response.

4. The dosage is too low to produce the desired patient response.

Safety of therapy:

5. The drug is causing an adverse reaction.

6. The dosage is too high, resulting in undesirable effects.

Medication adherence:

7. The patient is not able or willing to take the drug therapy as intended.

These drug therapy problems are discussed in more detail in **Chapter 4**. Because this Casebook is intended to be used in conjunction with the *Pharmacotherapy* textbook, one of its purposes is to serve as a tool for learning about the pharmacotherapy of disease states. For this reason, the primary problem requiring identification and resolution for many patients in the Casebook is needed for additional drug treatment for a specific medical indication (**problem 2** above). Other actual or potential drug therapy problems may coexist during the initial presentation or may develop during the clinical course of the disease.

PATIENT-FOCUSED APPROACH TO CASE PROBLEMS

In this Casebook, each patient presentation is followed by a set of patient-centered questions that are similar for each case. These questions are applied consistently from case to case to demonstrate that a systematic patient care process can be applied successfully regardless of the underlying disease state(s). The questions are designed to enable students to identify and resolve problems related to pharmacotherapy. They help students recognize what they know and what they do not know, thereby guiding them in determining what information must be learned to satisfactorily resolve the patient's problems.[10] A description of each of the steps involved in solving drug therapy problems is included in the following paragraphs.

1. Identification of real or potential drug therapy problems

The first step in the patient-focused approach is to collect pertinent patient information, interpret it properly, and determine whether drug therapy problems exist. Some authors prefer to divide this process into two or more separate steps because of the difficulty that inexperienced students may have in performing these complex tasks simultaneously.[11] This step is analogous to documenting the subjective and objective patient findings in the *Subjective, Objective, Assessment, Plan* (SOAP) format. It is important to differentiate the process of identifying the patient's drug therapy problems from making a disease-related medical diagnosis. In fact, the medical diagnosis is known for most patients seen by pharmacists. However, pharmacists must be capable of assessing the patient's database to determine whether drug therapy problems exist that warrant a change in drug therapy. In the case of preexisting chronic diseases, such as asthma or rheumatoid arthritis, one must be able to assess information that may indicate a change in severity of the disease. This process involves reviewing the patient's symptoms, the signs of disease present on physical examination, and the results of laboratory and other diagnostic tests. Some of the cases require the learner to develop complete patient problem lists. Potential sources for this information in actual practice include the patient or his or her advocate, the patient's physician or other health care professionals, and the patient's medical record.

After the drug therapy problems are identified, the clinician should determine which ones are amenable to pharmacotherapy. Alternatively, one must also consider whether any of the problems could have been caused by drug therapy. In some cases (both in the Casebook and in real life), not all of the information needed to make these decisions is available. In that situation, providing precise recommendations for obtaining additional information needed to satisfactorily assess the patient's problems can be a valuable contribution to the patient's care.

2. Determination of the desired therapeutic outcome

After pertinent patient-specific information has been gathered and the patient's drug therapy problems have been identified, the next step is to define the specific goals of pharmacotherapy. The primary therapeutic outcomes include:

- Cure of disease (eg, bacterial infection)

- Reduction or elimination of symptoms (eg, pain from cancer)

- Arresting or slowing of the progression of disease (eg, rheumatoid arthritis, HIV infection)

- Preventing a disease or symptom (eg, coronary heart disease)

Other important outcomes of pharmacotherapy include:

- Not complicating or aggravating other existing disease states
- Avoiding or minimizing adverse effects of treatment
- Providing cost-effective therapy
- Maintaining the patient's quality of life

Sources of information for this step may include the patient or his or her advocate, the patient's physician or other health care professionals, medical records, and the *Pharmacotherapy* textbook or other literature references.

3. Determination of therapeutic alternatives

After the intended outcome has been defined, attention can be directed toward identifying the types of treatments that might be beneficial in achieving that outcome. The clinician should ensure that all feasible pharmacotherapeutic alternatives available for achieving the predefined therapeutic outcome(s) are considered before choosing a particular therapeutic regimen. Nondrug therapies (eg, diet, exercise, psychotherapy) that might be useful should be included in the list of therapeutic alternatives when appropriate. Useful sources of information on therapeutic alternatives include the *Pharmacotherapy* textbook and other references, as well as the clinical experience of the health care provider and other health care professionals on the patient care team.

There has been a resurgence of interest in dietary supplements and other alternative therapies in recent years. The public spends billions of dollars each year on supplements to treat diseases for which there is little scientific evidence of efficacy. Furthermore, some products are hazardous, and others may interact with a patient's prescription medications or aggravate concurrent disease states. On the other hand, scientific evidence of efficacy does exist for some dietary supplements (eg, glucosamine for osteoarthritis). Healthcare providers must be knowledgeable about these products and prepared to answer patient questions regarding their efficacy and safety. The Casebook contains a separate section devoted to this important topic (**Section 19**). This portion of the Casebook contains a number of fictitious patient vignettes that are directly related to patient cases that were presented earlier in this Casebook. Each scenario involves the potential use of one or more dietary supplements by the patient. Additional follow-up questions are then asked to help the reader gain the scientific and clinical knowledge required to provide an evidence-based recommendation about use of the supplement in that particular patient. The use of 13 different dietary supplements for 18 different disorders is included in this section: garlic (dyslipidemia), fish oil (diabetes, psoriasis, dyslipidemia), *Ginkgo biloba* (peripheral arterial disease, Alzheimer's disease), St. John's wort (depression), black cohosh (menopausal symptoms), soy (menopausal symptoms), α-lipoic acid (chronic pain, type 2 diabetes), Co-Q10 (Parkinson's disease), kava (anxiety), pygeum (benign prostatic hypertrophy), butterbur (migraine prevention, allergic rhinitis), feverfew (migraine prevention), and cinnamon (diabetes). Current reference sources are provided for all of the supplements.

4. Design of an optimal individualized pharmacotherapeutic plan

The purpose of this decision-making step is to determine the drug, dosage form, dose, route of administration, schedule, and duration of therapy that are best suited for a given patient. Individual patient characteristics should be taken into consideration when weighing the risks and benefits of each therapeutic alternative. For example, an asthma patient who requires new drug therapy for hypertension might better tolerate treatment with a thiazide diuretic rather than a β-blocker. On the other hand, a hypertensive patient with gout may be better served by use of a β-blocker rather than a thiazide diuretic.

Students should state the reasons for avoiding specific drugs in their therapeutic plans. Some potential reasons for drug avoidance include drug allergy, drug–drug or drug–disease interactions, patient age, renal or hepatic impairment, adverse effects, inconvenient dosage schedule, likelihood of poor adherence, pregnancy, and high treatment cost.

The specific dose selected may depend on the indication for the drug. For example, the dose of aspirin used to treat rheumatoid arthritis is much higher than that used to prevent myocardial infarction. The analgesic effects of nonsteroidal anti-inflammatory drugs are achieved at lower doses than are required for anti-inflammatory activity. The likelihood of adherence with the regimen and patient tolerance come into play in the selection of dosage forms. For example, some patients receiving the tumor necrosis factor inhibitor golimumab for rheumatoid arthritis may prefer to self-administer the medication subcutaneously at home; others may require golimumab intravenous infusions because they are either unwilling or unable to use subcutaneous injections. The economic, psychosocial, and ethical factors that are applicable to the patient should also be given due consideration in designing the pharmacotherapeutic regimen. An alternative plan should also be in place that would be appropriate if the initial therapy fails or cannot be used.

5. Identification of parameters to evaluate the outcome

Students must identify the clinical and laboratory parameters necessary to assess the therapy for achievement of the desired therapeutic outcome and for detection and prevention of adverse effects. The outcome parameters selected should be specific, measurable, achievable, directly related to the therapeutic goals, and have a defined end point. As a means of remembering these points, the acronym SMART has been used (Specific, Measurable, Achievable, Related, and Time bound). If the goal is to cure bacterial pneumonia, students should outline the subjective and objective clinical parameters (eg, relief of chest discomfort, cough, and fever), laboratory tests (eg, normalization of white blood cell count and differential), and other procedures (eg, resolution of infiltrate on chest x-ray) that provide sufficient evidence of bacterial eradication and clinical cure of the disease. The intervals at which data should be collected are dependent on the outcome parameters selected and should be established prospectively. It should be noted that expensive or invasive procedures may not be repeated after the initial diagnosis is made.

Adverse effect parameters must also be well defined and measurable. For example, it is insufficient to state that one will monitor for potential drug-induced "blood dyscrasias." Rather, one should identify the likely specific hematologic abnormality (eg, anemia, leukopenia, or thrombocytopenia) and outline a prospective schedule for obtaining the appropriate parameters (eg, obtain monthly hemoglobin/hematocrit, white blood cell count, or platelet count).

Monitoring for adverse events should be directed toward preventing or identifying serious adverse effects that have a reasonable likelihood of occurrence. For example, it is not cost-effective to obtain periodic liver function tests in all patients taking a drug that causes mild abnormalities in liver injury tests only rarely, such as omeprazole. On the other hand, serious patient harm may be averted by outlining a specific screening schedule for drugs associated more frequently with hepatic abnormalities, such as methotrexate for rheumatoid arthritis.

6. Provision of patient education

A direct patient care practice requires the provider to establish a personal relationship with the patient. Patients are our partners in health care, and our efforts may be for naught without their informed participation in the process. For chronic diseases such as diabetes mellitus, hypertension, and asthma, patients may have a greater role in managing their diseases than do health care professionals. Self-care is becoming widespread as increasing numbers of prescription medications receive over-the-counter status. For these reasons, patients must be provided with sufficient information to enhance compliance, ensure successful therapy, and minimize adverse effects. **Chapter 3** describes patient interview techniques that can be used efficiently to determine the patient's level of knowledge. Additional information can then be provided as necessary to fill in knowledge gaps. In the questions posed with individual cases, students are asked to provide the kind of information that should be given to the patient who has limited knowledge of his or her disease. Under the Omnibus Budget Reconciliation Act (OBRA) of 1990, for patients who accept the offer of counseling, pharmacists should consider including the following items:

- Name and description of the medication (which may include the indication)
- Dosage, dosage form, route of administration, and duration of therapy
- Special directions or procedures for preparation, administration, and use
- Common and severe adverse effects, interactions, and contra-indications (with the action required should they occur)
- Techniques for self-monitoring
- Proper storage
- Prescription refill information
- Action to be taken in the event of missed doses

Instructors may wish to have simulated patient-interviewing sessions for new and refill prescriptions during case discussions to practice medication education skills. Factual information should be provided as concisely as possible to enhance memory retention. One source for information on individual drugs is "*Detailed Drug Information for the Consumer™*—*Drug Information in Lay Language.* Available through *Micromedex Healthcare Series*, this subscription-based electronic product provides drug information written for patients at the 12th grade literacy level.[12] MedlinePlus is the National Institute of Health's free Web site for consumers that contains information on prescription and nonprescription drugs, dietary supplements, medical conditions, wellness, diagnostic tests, and other medical information.[13]

7. Communication and implementation of the pharmacotherapeutic plan

The most well-conceived plan is worthless if it languishes without implementation because of inadequate communication with prescribers or other health care providers. Permanent, written documentation of significant recommendations in the medical record is important to ensure accurate communication among practitioners. Oral communication alone can be misinterpreted or transferred inaccurately to others. This is especially true because there are many drugs that sound alike when spoken but have far different therapeutic uses.

The SOAP format has been used by clinicians for many years to assess patient problems and to communicate findings and plans in the medical record. Writing SOAP notes may not be the optimal process for learning to solve drug therapy problems because several important steps taken by experienced clinicians are not always apparent and may be overlooked. For example, the precise therapeutic outcome desired is often unstated in SOAP notes, leaving others to presume what the desired treatment goals are. Health care professionals using the SOAP format also commonly move directly from an assessment of the patient (diagnosis) to outlining a diagnostic or therapeutic plan, without necessarily conveying whether careful consideration has been given to all available feasible diagnostic or therapeutic alternatives. The plan itself as outlined in SOAP notes may also give short shrift to the monitoring parameters that are required to ensure successful therapy and to detect and prevent adverse drug effects. Finally, there is often little suggestion provided as to the treatment information that should be conveyed to the most important individual involved: the patient. If SOAP notes are used for documenting drug therapy problems, consideration should be given to including each of these components.

In **Chapter 5** of this Casebook, the FARM note (*Findings, Assessment, Recommendations, Monitoring*) is presented as a useful method of consistently documenting therapeutic recommendations and implementing plans.[14] This method can be used by students as an alternative to the SOAP note to practice communicating pharmacotherapeutic plans to other members of the health care team. Although preparation of written communication notes is not included in written form with each set of case questions, instructors are encouraged to include the composition of a SOAP or FARM note as one of the requirements for successfully completing each case study assignment.

In addition to communicating with other health care professionals, practitioners of pharmaceutical care must also develop a personal record of each patient's drug therapy problems and the health care provider's plan for resolving them, interventions made, and actual therapeutic outcomes achieved. A pharmaceutical care plan is a well-conceived and scientifically sound method of documenting these activities. **Chapter 4** of this Casebook discusses the philosophy of care planning and describes their creation and use. A sample care plan document is included in that chapter for use by students as they work through the cases in this book.

CLINICAL COURSE

The process of pharmaceutical care entails an assessment of the patient's progress in order to ensure achievement of the desired therapeutic outcomes. A description of the patient's clinical course is included with many of the cases in this book to reflect this process. Some cases follow the progression of the patient's disease over months to years and include both inpatient and outpatient treatment. Follow-up questions directed toward ongoing evaluation and problem solving are included after presentation of the clinical course.

SELF-STUDY ASSIGNMENTS

Each case concludes with several study assignments related to the patient case or the disease state that may be used as independent study projects for students to complete outside class. These assignments generally require students to obtain additional information that is not contained in the corresponding *Pharmacotherapy* textbook chapter.

LITERATURE REFERENCES AND INTERNET SITES

Selected literature references that are specific to the case at hand are included at the end of the cases. References selected for inclusion are those thought to be useful to students for answering the questions posed. The citations are generally limited to major clinical trials or meta-analyses, authoritative review articles, and clinical practice guidelines. The *Pharmacotherapy* textbook contains a more comprehensive list of references pertinent to each disease state.

Some cases list Internet sites as sources of drug therapy information. The sites listed are recognized as authoritative sources of information, such as the FDA (*www.fda.gov*) and the Centers for Disease Control and Prevention (*www.cdc.gov*). Students should be advised to be wary of information posted on the Internet that is not from highly regarded health care organizations or publications. The uniform resource locators (URLs) for Internet sites sometimes change, and it is possible that not all sites listed in the Casebook will remain available for viewing.

DEVELOPING ANSWERS TO CASE QUESTIONS

The use of case studies for independent learning and in-class discussion may be unfamiliar to many students. For this reason, students may find it difficult at first to devise complete answers to the case questions. **Appendix D** contains the answers to three cases in order to demonstrate how case responses might be prepared and presented. The authors of the cases contributed the recommended answers provided in the appendix, but they should not be considered the sole "right" answer. Thoughtful students who have prepared well for the discussion sessions may arrive at additional or alternative answers that are also appropriate.

With diligent self-study, practice, and the guidance of instructors, students will gradually acquire the knowledge, skills, and self-confidence to develop and implement pharmaceutical care plans for their own future patients. The goal of the Casebook is to help students progress along this path of lifelong learning.

REFERENCES

1. Herreid CF. Case studies in science: a novel method of science education. J Coll Sci Teach 1994;23:221–229.
2. DiPiro JT, Talbert RL, Yee GC, et al., eds. Pharmacotherapy: A Pathophysiologic Approach, 8th ed. New York, McGraw-Hill, 2011.
3. Chisholm-Burns MA, Schwinghammer TL, Wells BG, Malone PM, Kolesar JM, DiPiro JT. Pharmacotherapy Principles & Practice, 2nd ed. New York, McGraw-Hill, 2010.
4. Caldwell SH, Popenoe R. Perceptions and misperceptions of skin color. Ann Intern Med 1995;122:614–617.
5. Ernst FR, Grizzle AJ. Drug-related morbidity and mortality: updating the cost-of-illness model. J Am Pharm Assoc 2001;41:192–199.
6. Cipolle RJ, Strand LM, Morley PC. Preface. In: Cipolle RJ, Strand LM, Morley PC, eds. Pharmaceutical Care Practice: The Patient-Centered Approach to Medication Management Services, 3rd ed. New York, McGraw-Hill, 2012.
7. American Pharmacists Association. Vision and Mission for the Pharmacy Profession. Washington, DC, American Pharmacists Association, 2013. Available at: *http://www.pharmacist.com/vision-and-mission-pharmacy-profession*. Accessed July 21, 2013.
8. Joint Commission of Pharmacy Practitioners. Future Vision of Pharmacy Practice. November 10, 2004. Available at: *http://pharmacy.osu.edu/academics/introduction-to-pharmacy/materials/jcpp_vision_for_pharmacy_practice.pdf*. Accessed July 21, 2013.
9. Cipolle RJ, Strand LM, Morley PC. Drug therapy problems. In: Cipolle RJ, Strand LM, Morley PC, eds. Pharmaceutical Care Practice: The Patient-Centered Approach to Medication Management Services, 3rd ed. New York, McGraw-Hill, 2012:chap 5. Available at: *http://www.accesspharmacy.com/content.aspx?aID=56172882*. Accessed July 21, 2013.
10. Delafuente JC, Munyer TO, Angaran DM, et al. A problem-solving active-learning course in pharmacotherapy. Am J Pharm Educ 1994;58:61–64.
11. Winslade N. Large-group problem-based learning: a revision from traditional to pharmaceutical care-based therapeutics. Am J Pharm Educ 1994;58:64–73.
12. Detailed Drug Information for the Consumer. Micromedex® Healthcare Series [Internet database]. Greenwood Village, CO, Thomson Reuters (Healthcare) Inc., 2013. Updated periodically. Available at: *http://www.micromedex.com/products/ddic/*. Accessed July 21, 2013.
13. MedlinePlus: Trusted Health Information for You. A Service of the U.S. National Library of Medicine. Bethesda, MD, National Institutes of Health, 2013. Available at: *http://www.nlm.nih.gov/medlineplus/*. Accessed July 21, 2013.
14. Canaday BR, Yarborough PC. Documenting pharmaceutical care: creating a standard. Ann Pharmacother 1994;28:1292–1296.

CHAPTER

2

Active Learning Strategies

RACHEL W. FLURIE, PharmD, BCPS
GRETCHEN M. BROPHY, PharmD, BCPS, FCCP, FCCM, FNCS
CYNTHIA K. KIRKWOOD, PharmD, BCPP

Healthcare providers are faced with situations every day that require the use of effective problem solving, critical thinking, and communication skills. Therefore, providing students with knowledge alone is insufficient to equip them with the tools needed to be valuable contributors to patient care. Students must understand that it is imperative to provide more than just drug information, which is readily obtained in today's world from Internet sites, smartphone mobile apps, and online reference texts. They must be able to evaluate, analyze, and synthesize information and apply their knowledge to prevent and resolve drug-related problems. As clinicians, they will be required to contribute their expertise to team discussions about patient care, ask appropriate questions, integrate information, and develop action plans.

Students who finish their formal training in health care must also recognize that learning is a lifelong process. Scores of new drugs are approved every year, drug use practices change, and innovative research alters the way that diseases are treated. Students must be prepared to proactively expand their knowledge base and clinical skills to adapt to the changing profession.

Warren identified several traits that prepare students for future careers: analytic thinking, polite assertiveness, tolerance, communication skills, understanding of one's own physical well-being, and the ability to continue to teach oneself after graduation.[1] To prepare students to become healthcare professionals who are essential members of the healthcare team, many healthcare educators are using active learning strategies in the classroom.[2,3]

ACTIVE LEARNING VERSUS TRADITIONAL TEACHING

Active learning has numerous definitions, and various methods are described in the educational literature. Simply put, *active learning is the process of having students engage in activities that require reflection on ideas and how students use them.*[3] Most proponents of active learning strategies agree that compared with passively receiving lectures, active engagement of students promotes deeper learning, enhances critical thinking skills, provides feedback to students and instructors, and promotes social development. Learning is reinforced when students are actively engaged and apply their knowledge to new situations.[3] Active learning is learner-focused and helps students take responsibility for their own learning.[2]

In contrast, traditional teaching involves a teacher-centered approach. At the beginning of the course, students are given a course syllabus packet that contains "everything they need to know" for the semester. In class, the teacher lectures on a predetermined topic that does not require student preparation and allows students to be passive recipients of information. The testing method is usually a written examination that employs a multiple-choice or short-answer format, which focuses on the student's ability to recall isolated facts that the teacher has identified as being important. They do not learn to apply their knowledge to situations that they will ultimately encounter in practice. The reward is an external one (ie, exam or course grade) that may or may not reflect a student's actual ability to use the knowledge they have to improve patient care.

To teach students to be lifelong learners, it is essential to stimulate them to be inquisitive and actively involved with the learning that takes place in the classroom. This requires that teachers move away from more comfortable teaching methods and learn new techniques that will help students "learn to learn." In classes with active learning formats, students are involved in much more than listening. The transmission of information is deemphasized and replaced with the development of skills and application of knowledge. Active learning shifts the control of learning from the teacher to the students; this provides an opportunity for students to become active participants in their own learning.[2]

ACTIVE LEARNING STRATEGIES

Teachers implement active learning exercises into classes in a variety of ways. While some strategies engage individual students with the material, such as giving students the opportunity to pause and recall information, other active learning strategies involve the use of student groups, such as problem-based learning (PBL), team-based learning (TBL), or cooperative or collaborative learning whereby students work together to perform specific tasks in a small group (ie, solve problems, discuss case studies).[2,4-6] Technology is increasingly used in active learning in numerous ways to maximize the use of class time for higher-order thinking tasks such as analysis, synthesis, and evaluation.[7-10] The following are the examples of active learning strategies that involve students in the learning process.

EXERCISES FOR INDIVIDUAL STUDENTS

These exercises can complement lectures and are easily implemented. Quick writing tasks can assess student understanding of (or reaction to) material. Writing helps students to identify knowledge deficits, clarify understanding of the material, and organize thoughts in a logical manner. The "minute paper" or "half-sheet response" has students provide written responses to a question asked in class.[11] Example questions might be, "What was the main point of today's class session?" or "What was the muddiest point of today's class session?" In-class quizzes can be strategically placed to break up lecture time and engage students. Quizzes given at the beginning of class on pre-class readings help stimulate students to review information they did not know and listen for clarification during class. Quizzes can also be given throughout class (eg, using electronic audience response systems [ARS]) and may or may not be graded. ARS can help instructors engage students in lecture content, promote interactivity, identify misconceptions, and stimulate discussion.[8] Quizzes at the end of class allow students to use their problem-solving skills by applying what they have just learned to a patient case or problem.

QUESTIONS AND ANSWERS

Active learning strategies that involve questions and answers can increase student involvement and comprehension. "Wait time" is a method whereby the instructor poses a question and asks students to think about it.[12] After a brief pause, the instructor can ask for volunteers or randomly call on a student to answer the question. This wait time forces every student to think about the question rather than relying on those students who immediately raise their hands to answer questions. With the "fish bowl" method, students are asked to write questions related to the course material for discussion at the end of class or at the beginning of the next class session.[12] Instructors then draw several questions out of the "fish bowl" to discuss or ask the class to answer. In classes that use active learning, much of the learning will come from class discussion. However, many students may not pay attention to their classmates, but rather wait for instructors to either repeat or clarify what one of their classmates has said. To promote active listening, after one student has volunteered to answer a question, instructors could ask another student if they agree with the previous response and why.

THINK–PAIR–SHARE

The "think–pair–share" exercise involves providing students with a question or problem to solve.[13] After working on the assignment individually (think) for 2–5 minutes, they discuss their ideas for 3–5 minutes with the student sitting next to them (pair). Finally, student pairs are chosen to share their ideas with the whole class (share). By sharing ideas with a partner first, students are kept on task and can have a more intimate discussion to work out problems before sharing with others. This method provides immediate feedback and can lead to productive class discussion. Another type of sharing involves small-group discussions. Pre-assigned small groups of three to four students work together throughout the course to complete activities. Groups may have 20–30 minutes for discussion and apply a topic presented in class to a new situation. To create heterogeneity for discussion, one example is to group students with different experiences (eg, community vs hospital IPPE).[14] Assigning functional roles and role-playing can create multiple perspectives.

PROBLEM-BASED LEARNING

Problem-solving skills can be developed during a class period by applying knowledge of pharmacotherapy to a patient case. Application reinforces the previously learned material and helps students understand the importance of the topic in a real-life situation. PBL is a teaching and learning method in which a complex problem is used as the stimulus for developing critical thinking and problem-solving skills, group skills, and investigative techniques. The process of PBL starts with the student identifying the problem in a patient case. The student spends time either alone or in a group exploring and analyzing the case and identifying learning resources needed to solve the problem. After acquiring the knowledge, the student applies it to solve the problem.[15] Small or large groups can be established for case discussions to help students develop communication skills, respect for other students' opinions, satisfaction for contributing to the discussion,

and the ability to give and receive constructive feedback.[15] Interactive PBL computer tools and the use of real patient cases also stimulate learning both outside and inside the classroom.[16,17] Computer-assisted PBL can provide instant feedback throughout the process and incorporate other methods of active learning such as quizzes.[18] Programs that create virtual patients can be used creatively in PBL cases to simulate actual patient outcomes based on student recommendations.[19]

COOPERATIVE OR COLLABORATIVE LEARNING

Cooperative or collaborative learning strategies involve students in the generation of knowledge.[5] Students are randomly assigned to groups of four to six at the beginning of the school term. Several times during the term, each group is given a patient case and a group leader is selected. Each student in the group volunteers to work on a certain portion of the case. The case is discussed in class, and each member receives the same grade. After students have finished working in their small groups or during large-group sessions, the teacher serves as a facilitator of the discussion rather than as a lecturer. The students actively participate in the identification and resolution of the problem. The integration of this technique helps with development of skills in teamwork, interdependency, and communication.[14] Group discussions help students formulate opinions and recommendations, clarify ideas, and develop new strategies for clinical problem solving. These skills are essential for lifelong learning and will be used by the students throughout their careers.

TEAM-BASED LEARNING

TBL is a learner-centered, instructor-directed, small-group learning strategy that can be implemented in large-group educational settings. The course is structured around the activity of teams of five to seven students who work together over an entire semester. TBL focuses on deepening student learning and enhancing team development. This is accomplished by the TBL structure, which involves: (1) pre-class preparation, (2) assurance of readiness to apply learned concepts, and (3) application of content to real-world scenarios through team problem-solving activities in class. A peer review process provides important feedback to help team members develop the attitudes, behaviors, and skills that contribute positively to individual learning and effective teamwork.[6,20–22] A growing number of schools are adopting this strategy, resulting in various combinations and permutations of TBL. Guidance documents describing the core elements of TBL that should be incorporated to maximize student engagement and learning within teams have been published.[22,23]

CASE-BASED LEARNING

Case-based learning (CBL) is used by a number of professional schools to teach pharmacotherapy.[2,16,24,25] CBL involves a written description of a real-world problem or clinical situation. Only the facts are provided, usually in chronologic sequence similar to what would be encountered in a patient care setting. Many times, as in real life, the information given is incomplete, or important details are not available. When working through a case, the student must distinguish between relevant and irrelevant facts and realize that there is no single "correct" answer. CBL promotes self-directed learning because the student is actively involved in the analysis of the facts and details of the case, selection of a solution to the problem, and defense of his or her solution through discussion of the case.[26,27] In CBL, students use their recall of previously learned information to solve clinical cases.[28]

During class, active participation is essential for the maximum learning benefit to be achieved. Because of their various backgrounds, students learn different perspectives when dealing with patient problems. Some general steps proposed by McDade[27] for students when preparing cases for class discussion include:

- Skim the text quickly to establish the broad issues of the case and the types of information presented for analysis.
- Reread the case very carefully, underlining key facts as you go.
- Note on scratch paper the key issues and problems. Next, go through the case again and sort out the relevant considerations and decisions for each problem.
- Prioritize problems and alternatives.
- Develop a set of recommendations to address the problems.
- Evaluate your decisions.

ADVICE ON ACTIVE LEARNING FOR STUDENTS AND INSTRUCTORS

The use of active learning strategies provides students with opportunities to take a dynamic role in the learning process. Willing students, innovative teachers, and administrative support within the school are required for active learning to take place and be successful.[28,29]

ADVICE FOR STUDENTS

Students may have concerns about active learning. Some students may be accustomed to passively receiving information and feel uncomfortable participating in the learning process. Taking initiative is the key to deriving the benefits of active learning. It is crucial to recognize the three largest squelchers of initiative: laziness, fear of change, and force of habit.[30]

Prepare for class. Assigned readings and homework must be completed before class in order to use class time efficiently for questions that are not answered in other reference material. Time management is important. Use time between classes wisely, identify the times of day when you are most productive, and focus on the results rather than the time to complete an activity.[1] When reading assignments, take notes and summarize the information using tables or charts. Alternatively, make lists of questions from class or readings to discuss with your colleagues or faculty or try to answer them on your own.

Seek to understand versus memorize. To develop appropriate therapeutic recommendations or answers to a question, you may have to look beyond the reading materials provided by the teacher. You may need to go back to review notes from previous courses or perform literature searches and use the library or Internet to retrieve additional information. It is important that you understand "why" and "how" and not just memorize "what." Memorizing results in short-term retention of knowledge, whereas understanding results in long-term retention and will enable you to better justify your clinical recommendations. In active learning, much of what you learn you will learn on your own. You will probably find that you read more, but you will gain understanding from reading. At the same time, you are developing a critical lifelong learning skill. Your reading will become more "depth processing" in which you focus on:

- The intent of the reading;
- Actively integrating what you read with previous parts of the text or previous courses;

- Using your own ability to make a logical construction;
- Thinking about the functional role of the different parts of an argument.

During class, take an active role in the learning process. Be an active participant in class or group discussions; lively debates about pharmacotherapy issues allow more therapeutic options to be discussed.[31] Discussing material helps you to apply your knowledge, verbalize the medical and pharmacologic terminology, engage in active listening, think critically, and develop interpersonal skills. When working in groups, all members should participate in problem solving. Teaching others is an excellent way to learn the subject matter.[1] Listen carefully to and be respectful of the thoughts and opinions of classmates. Writing about a topic develops critical thinking, communication, and organization skills. Stopping to write allows you to reflect on the information you have just heard and reinforces learning. Although many options for digital note-taking are available, it is not known whether these enhance or deter learning.[30] By talking about what you are learning, writing about it, relating it to previous patient cases, and applying it to the current case, you repeatedly manipulate the information until it becomes a part of you.

ADVICE FOR INSTRUCTORS

Instructors may also have concerns about incorporating active learning strategies. They may feel as though their class is too large to accommodate active learning, have concerns that they will not be able to cover all the content or that it will take too much time to change their course, or even have fears that students may be resistant to active learning strategies. Some of the hesitation may lie in the belief that active learning is an alternative to lecture. Rather, active learning strategies can be incorporated into didactic lectures to enhance learning sessions. Educators can move some course content online by assigning pre-class mini-lectures, quizzes, or article readings.[2] Several strategies can be used to increase the successful implementation of active learning.

Discuss course expectations. Take time to describe teaching, learning, and assessment methods and how students can be successful in the course. Help students to understand the benefits of active learning.[32]

Consider slowly implementing a change in the classroom. To implement active learning strategies, teachers must overcome the anxiety that change often creates. Experiment with simple active learning methods (ie, the pause technique) and slowly implement active learning approaches.

Consider techniques to maximize student discussion. Allowing students to discuss content in pairs or small groups before asking them to share their ideas with the entire class can help minimize student anxiety about engaging in classroom discussions. Consider moving around the room during discussions, if possible, and make an effort to learn the names of all students.

Take a stepwise approach. Learners become self-directed in stages, not in one single moment of transformation. Sequence activities and assignments that gradually develop all three stages: learning, intellectual development, and interpersonal skills.[33]

Prepare students for group learning. Group learning is not intuitive. Instructors who use group learning should create a workable environment, ensure that expectations of students are understood, and structure the learning sessions to maximize student engagement and learning within teams.

Have a preconceived plan for how the learning session will go and stick to it. Determine what learning objectives you would like to achieve during the session. Consider developing an outline for the learning session, estimating the time that will be spent on each active learning activity.[2]

USING THE CASEBOOK

The Casebook was prepared to assist in the development of each student's understanding of a disease and its management as well as problem-solving skills. It is important for students to realize that learning and understanding the material is guided through problem solving. Students are encouraged to solve each of the cases individually or with others in a study group before discussion of the case and topic in class. These cases can be used as an active learning strategy by allowing time for students to work on the cases during class as an application exercise for TBL.[20] Teams can then report verbally on the questions and debate various treatment options.

SUMMARY

The use of case studies and other active learning strategies will enhance the development of essential skills necessary to practice in any setting, including community, ambulatory care, primary care, health systems, long-term care, home health care, managed care, and the pharmaceutical industry. The role of the healthcare professional is constantly changing; thus, it is important for students to acquire the knowledge, skills, and attitudes to develop the lifetime skills required for continued learning. Teachers who incorporate active learning strategies into the classroom are facilitating the development of lifelong learners who will be able to adapt to change that occurs in their profession.

REFERENCES

1. Warren G. Carpe Diem: A Student Guide to Active Learning. Landover, MD: University Press of America; 1996.
2. Gleason BL, Peeters MJ, Resman-Targoff BH, et al. An active-learning strategies primer for achieving ability-based educational outcomes. Am J Pharm Educ. 2011;75(9):186.
3. Michael J. Where's the evidence that active learning works? Adv Physiol Educ. 2006;30:159–167.
4. Bonwell CC, Eison JA. Active Learning: Creating Excitement in the Classroom. Washington, DC: George Washington University, School of Education and Human Development; 1991. ASHE-ERIC Higher Education Report No. 1.
5. Shakarian DC. Beyond lecture: active learning strategies that work. JOPERD. 1995;May–June:21–24.
6. Michaelsen LK, Parmelee DX, McMahon KK, Levine RE. Team-Based Learning for Health Professions Education: A Guide for Using Small Groups to Improve Learning. Sterling, VA: Stylus Publishing; 2008.
7. Moore AH, Fowler SB, Watson CE. Active learning and technology: designing change for faculty, students, and institutions. EDUCAUSE Rev. 2007;42:42–61.
8. Cain J, Robinson E. A primer on audience response systems: current applications and future considerations. Am J Pharm Educ. 2008:72(4):Article 77; 1–6.
9. DiVall MV, Hayney MS, Marsh W, et al. Perceptions of pharmacy students, faculty members, and administrators on the use of technology in the classroom. Am J Pharm Educ. 2013;77(4):Article 75; 1–7.
10. Poirier TI, O'Neil CK. Use of web technology and active learning strategies in a quality assessment methods course. Am J Pharm Educ. 2000;64:289–298.
11. Stead DR. A review of the one-minute paper. Active Learn Higher Educ. 2005;6(2):118–131.
12. Paulson DR, Faust JL. Active Learning for the College Classroom. http://www.calstatela.edu/dept/chem/chem2/Active/main.htm. Accessed February 21, 2013.
13. Elliot DD. Promoting critical thinking in the classroom. Nurs Educ. 1996;21:49–52.
14. Sylvia LM, Barr JT. Pharmacy Education: What Matters in Learning and Teaching. Sudbury, MA: Jones & Bartlett; 2011.
15. Walton HJ, Matthews MB. Essentials of problem-based learning. Med Educ. 1989;23:542–558.
16. Raman-Wilms L. Innovative enabling strategies in self-directed, problem-based therapeutics: enhancing student preparedness for pharmaceutical care. Am J Pharm Educ. 2001;65:56–64.
17. Dammers J, Spencer J, Thomas M. Using real patients in problem-based learning: students' comments on the value of using real, as opposed to paper cases, in a problem-based learning module in general practice. Med Educ. 2001;35:27–34.
18. McFalls M. Integration of problem-based learning and innovative technology into a self-care course. Am J Pharm Educ. 2013;77(6): Article 127; 1–6.
19. Benedict N. Virtual patients and problem-based learning in advance therapeutics. Am J Pharm Educ. 2010;74(8):Article 143; 1–6.
20. Conway SE, Johnson JL, Ripley TL. Integration of team-based learning strategies into a cardiovascular module. Am J Pharm Educ. 2010;74(2):35.
21. Thompson BM, Schneider VF, Haidet P, et al. Team-based learning at ten medical schools: two years later. Med Educ. 2007;41:250–257.
22. Haidet P, Levine RE, Parmelee DX, et al. Guidelines for reporting team-based learning activities in the medical and health sciences education literature. Acad Med. 2012;87:292–299.
23. Parmelee D, Michaelsen LK, Cook S, Hudes PD. Team-based learning: a practical guide: AMEE guide no. 65. Med Teach. 2012;34:e275–e287.
24. Hartzema AG. Teaching therapeutic reasoning through the case-study approach: adding the probabilistic dimension. Am J Pharm Educ. 1994;58:436–440.
25. Delafuente JC, Munyer TO, Angaran DM, et al. A problem-solving active-learning course in pharmacotherapy. Am J Pharm Educ. 1994;58:61–64.
26. Thistlethwaite JE, Davies D, Ekeocha S, et al. The effectiveness of case-based learning in health professional education. A BEME systematic review: BEME guide no. 23. Med Teach. 2012;34:e421–e444.
27. McDade SA. An Introduction to the Case Study Method: Preparation, Analysis, Participation. New York: Teachers College Press; 1988.
28. Williams B. Case-based learning—a review of the literature: is there scope for this educational paradigm in prehospital education? Emerg Med J. 2005;22:577–581.
29. Stacy EM, Cain J. Note-taking and handouts in the digital age. Am J Pharm Educ. 2015;79(7):Article 107; 1–6.
30. Robbins A. Awaken the Giant Within. New York: Simon & Schuster; 1991.
31. Chickering AW, Gamson ZF, Barsi LM. Seven Principles for Good Practice in Undergraduate Education. Racine, WI: The Johnson Foundation; 1989.
32. Prince M. Does active learning work? A review of the research. J Eng Educ. 2004;93:223–231.
33. Weimer ME. Learner-Centered Teaching. 1st ed. San Francisco, CA: Jossey-Bass; 2002:167–183.

3

Patient Communication: Getting the Most Out of That One-on-One Time

KRISTA D. CAPEHART, PharmD, MSPharm, AE-C

Talking with patients is a crucial component of the medication use process. Regardless of practice area, pharmacists have the opportunity to teach and learn from people they interact with each day. Pharmacists must have superb scientific knowledge and clinical skills to be medication experts, but they must also possess excellent communication skills. This chapter focuses on key elements of communication in various practice settings. The intricacies of interpersonal communication can be found in other resources.[1-3]

PATIENT-CENTERED CARE AND THE ROLE OF COMMUNICATION

With the movement toward value-based, accessible, high-quality care, pharmacist participation on interprofessional teams is vital. The Patient Protection and Affordable Care Act of 2010 fostered development of accountable care organizations (ACOs) and patient-centered medical homes (PCMHs). The National Center for Quality Assurance defines a PCMH as "a way of organizing primary care that emphasizes care coordination and communication to transform primary care into 'what patients want it to be.'"[4] Using medication expertise and communication skills, pharmacists work with the healthcare team to optimize the medication use process and ensure that the patient truly is at the center of care.

In patient-centered care, the patient participates in his/her own health care through shared decision making with healthcare providers. Shared decision making involves decision aids or a process to facilitate patient understanding when multiple treatment options could be used.[5] Shared decision making has been shown to increase knowledge and improve patient understanding of the risks of their care, as well as making patients more likely to receive care that is consistent with their values and beliefs.[6]

Consequently, the patient–pharmacist interaction must involve more than simply collecting information during a medication history interview or conveying verbal or written information about a prescription. Active listening skills must be employed to understand the patient's concerns about medication therapy, engage the patient in his/her care, and develop the trust required for a positive longstanding relationship. Establishing a trusting relationship is necessary for effective communication, but trust does not come quickly or easily. In the community pharmacy, it may result from a caring pharmacist always taking the time to ask how a patient's medications are working. In an ambulatory clinic, it could come from a pharmacist teaching about diabetes care and improving A1C levels. Pathways to a trusting relationship may vary, but the ultimate goal is for patients to feel that they can confide in and rely on their pharmacist about medication-related needs.

Patient interactions vary depending on the practice setting, pharmacist training, the purpose of the interaction, and other factors. In 2015, the Joint Commission of Pharmacy Practitioners (JCPP)

published the Pharmacist's Patient Care Process, which is intended to standardize the patient's experiences in each encounter with the pharmacist.[7] The steps of the Pharmacists' Patient Care Process include: (1) Collect, (2) Assess, (3) Plan, (4) Implement, and (5) Follow-up: Monitor and Evaluate (Fig. 3-1).

Optimal communication is necessary in the *Collect* and *Implement* parts of the process. During the *Collect* portion, the pharmacist gathers information about the patient and the present medical situation. The information available may vary by practice site, but the process remains the same. During the *Implement* stage, the pharmacist has the opportunity to educate the patient about the care plan. This may include new medications, lifestyle modifications, changes in therapy, or referrals to other healthcare providers. The key to the process is collaboration with the patient and healthcare team members.

IMPROVING THE PATIENT ENCOUNTER

Talking with a patient and collecting information require patience, empathy, and the ability to direct the conversation. The pharmacist should use open-ended questions, which start with *who*, *what*, *when*, *where*, *why*, or *how*. Close-ended questions are those that permit the patient to respond with a simple *yes* or *no* and tend to leave much unsaid. With a close-ended question, the patient may not give the pharmacist complete information. For example, if a pharmacist asks, "Have you been taking your warfarin as the doctor prescribed?" the patient may simply respond, "Yes." However, it could be that the patient understood and adhered to the one-tablet-daily directions that were initially prescribed but did not realize that the directions were recently changed to one tablet Monday, Wednesday, Friday, and Saturday, and one-half tablet the other days of the week. An open-ended question such as, "How are you taking your warfarin each day?" requires more explanation from the patient, allowing the pharmacist to collect more accurate information to assess the patient's medication/medical history and status. There is a place for close-ended questions; after most of the information has been collected, close-ended questions can be used to narrow down the details about the patient's situation.

The pharmacist must be an exceptional listener, open to what the patient is sharing and not sharing. Becoming an active listener is not always easy in the pharmacy environment. It includes removing distractions, empathizing with the patient, acknowledging the patient's individuality, and recognizing nonverbal signals from the patient.

Regardless of practice setting, distractions should be minimized to ensure that the patient is the primary focus of the pharmacist's attention. Separate counseling rooms may be used, if available. Attempts to maintain privacy help demonstrate the pharmacist's focus on the patient.

Empathy and sympathy are often confused. Empathy is the ability to understand the patient's feelings and share them, whereas

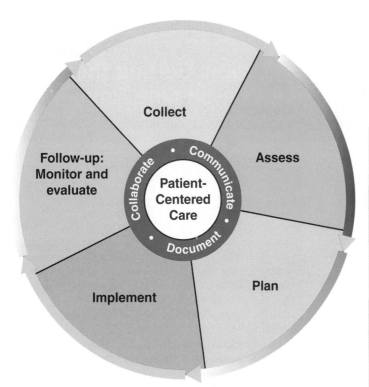

Pharmacists' patient care process
Pharmacists use a patient-centered approach in collaboration with other providers on the health care team to optimize patient health and medication outcomes.

Using principles of evidence-based practice, pharmacists:

Collect
The pharmacist assures the collection of the necessary subjective and objective information about the patient in order to understand the relevant medical/medication history and clinical status of the patient.

Assess
The pharmacist assesses the information collected and analyzes the clinical effects of the patient's therapy in the context of the patient's overall health goals in order to identify and prioritize problems and achieve optimal care.

Plan
The pharmacist develops an individualized patient-centered care plan, in collaboration with other health care professionals and the patient or caregiver that is evidence-based and cost-effective.

Implement
The pharmacist implements the care plan in collaboration with other health care professionals and the patient or caregiver.

Follow-up: Monitor and evaluate
The pharmacist monitors and evaluates the effectiveness of the care plan and modifies the plan in collaboration with other health care professionals and the patient or caregiver as needed.

FIGURE 3-1. The Patient Care Process. (Adapted with permission from the Joint Commission of Pharmacy Practitioners. Pharmacists' Patient Care Process. May 29, 2014. https://www.pharmacist.com/sites/default/files/files/PatientCareProcess.pdf, accessed January 26, 2016.)

sympathy is feeling sorry for the patient. Acknowledging emotions, reassuring the patient, and providing answers to questions helps to improve the interaction and outcomes. Each patient enters the medical encounter with a set of experiences, beliefs, and expectations; understanding them through active listening facilitates creation and implementation of the therapeutic plan.

Nonverbal communication can be as important as what the patient relates verbally, and pharmacists must recognize these as well. Nonverbal cues may include body language, time, tone of voice, touch, distance, and physical environments. Body language clues include crossing the arms (a sign the patient is closing themselves off) or nodding the head (an indication the listener is paying attention or agreeing). Time can be used to delay (as with dramatic pauses) or to rush through situations that may be uncomfortable. Tone of voice is revealing because it includes pitch and intonation and can relate anger, fascination, confusion, and a variety of other emotions. Touch, distance, and physical environment are specific to the individual. Generally, people prefer approximately 2 feet of personal space when having a one-on-one encounter. Some patients are comfortable with a touch on the arm, whereas others require much greater personal space and shy away from physical contact. This concept can sometimes be tricky and may take time to master. The pharmacist must be aware of his or her nonverbal cues as well. Egan developed a mnemonic to assist in demonstrating nonverbal cues for good listening (SOLER), which can help build a trusting patient relationship (see Table 3-1).[8]

EXAMPLES OF COMMUNICATION WITHIN THE PHARMACIST–PATIENT RELATIONSHIP

The opportunities to talk with patients vary with practice settings and expectations. For example, hospital pharmacists may perform counseling on all discharge medications or discuss injectable

TABLE 3-1	Nonverbal Cues to Demonstrate Good Listening
Letter	**Meaning**
S	Squarely face the patient (do not have your body angled in another direction)
O	Open posture (do not cross your legs and arms)
L	Lean toward the patient (not encroaching on personal space) to show interest
E	Eye contact
R	Relax

medications being started with the patient. The community pharmacist may counsel on new or refill medications or help select an over-the-counter (OTC) medication for a particular problem. Pharmacists communicate with patients to undertake medication therapy management, participate in collaborative drug therapy management, and perform medication reconciliation.

MEDICATION/MEDICAL HISTORY

It is important to collect comprehensive information when conducting a patient medication interview. Using the tips presented previously, information can be gathered from the patient to improve patient care and safety.

Initially, collect demographic information about the patient, including name, address, and date of birth. This enables the pharmacy to begin a patient chart and documentation. Use an open-ended question to inquire about the patient's allergies (medication, environmental, and food), such as, "What medication allergies have you experienced in the past?" Be sure to document what happened when the patient experienced the reaction. It may be necessary at some point in the future to evaluate risk versus benefit and determine if a true allergy exists. Query the patient regarding social history, including tobacco use, alcohol consumption, illicit drug use, and caffeine intake. Asking about social history can sometimes make both the pharmacist and the patient uncomfortable. One method to ease tension is to advise the patient that some medications interact with alcohol or tobacco, and that it is important for information to be complete to evaluate drug–drug interactions. Remember to ask about the type of substance, quantity, and frequency of use as well.

When verifying prescription medications, it is helpful to start by asking whether the patient has either brought their medications or a written list to the visit. This is also a good practice in the emergency department or other settings in which the patient was not expecting to meet with a pharmacist. Regardless of whether the patient has a list, ask the patient, "What prescription medications do you take?" For each medication, specifically document the name, strength, route of administration, physician, and how he or she takes the medication. The way the patient actually takes each medication can be compared to the label directions to assess patient adherence. Remember that nonadherence could be due to misunderstanding the correct directions, attempting to save money, or any of a number of reasons other than simply choosing **not** to take the medication as directed. Also, be sure to ask the patient why each medication was prescribed. Remind each patient about nonoral routes of administration also. This could be a close-ended question followed up by an open-ended one, such as, "Do you use any medications that you apply to your skin? What other medications do you use that you don't swallow by mouth?" This may prompt the patient to remember some medications they may have forgotten.[9]

Patients should be asked about nonprescription items used, including OTC medications, herbals, vitamins, and dietary supplements. Patients may have the misconception that OTC or "natural" substances do not interact with prescription medications or medical conditions. This is an opportunity to educate the patient about the potential dangers of incorrect use of these products.

The pharmacist must collect information on diagnosed medical conditions during the medication interview, but there is flexibility in when this occurs. One option is to address medical conditions after asking about allergies and before beginning questions on medications. This gives the interviewer an idea of the therapeutic categories of medications the patient may be taking. The other option is to cover diagnosed medical conditions after collecting the list of prescription and nonprescription medications. Using this order of questioning enables the interviewer to ask the patient "What are you taking X medication for?" if the patient fails to list an indication for a medication named earlier.

The comprehensive medication interview is optimal for pharmacist care and the provision of medication reconciliation, medication therapy management, and collaborative drug therapy management. However, it is not always feasible to perform an interview. Sometimes, the information may need to be collected from the pharmacy dispensing record, a family member, or another source. Information not obtained personally from the patient may need to be reconfirmed later.

COUNSELING ON A NEW PRESCRIPTION

The Omnibus Budget Reconciliation Act of 1990 (OBRA 90) was passed, in part, to help ensure safe medication use for Medicaid patients. While it is often considered to be the law that precipitated the offer to counsel on medications, OBRA 90 also gave rise to new record-keeping requirements and mandated that pharmacists complete a prospective drug utilization review for all Medicaid patients. Requirements vary by state regarding what must be done for drug counseling, but OBRA 90 required an offer to counsel, not that counseling must be completed.[10]

Counseling on medications increases the patient's knowledge and comfort level in using their medication correctly.[11] Part of the patient's comfort can derive from the process as well as from the information. The counseling should occur in a private area, if possible. If a separate room is not available, use a divider or area that makes the counseling space relatively easy to maintain patient confidentiality and privacy. A patient may be uncomfortable receiving counseling on certain types of medication, such as a medication for a vaginal infection; speaking in a confidential tone in a private area will improve patient satisfaction with the encounter.

Educating the patient on new medications should start by assessing what the patient already knows about the medication that has been prescribed. Asking "What did your doctor tell you about the medication you are getting today?" is an excellent way to begin the session. After determining the patient's knowledge about the medication, state medication name (including whether it is generic), strength, route of administration, and schedule. Inquire about the patient's daily activities and attempt to incorporate the schedule into routine daily activities to increase adherence. Explain the medication in terms of what condition it is intended to treat, what the expected action is, and how the patient can self-monitor for efficacy. The patient should realize if and when he/she should "feel different." For example, with medications for hypertension and dyslipidemia, the patient may not notice a difference in how they feel and should be counseled about the importance of laboratory testing or other monitoring. Potential side effects can be discussed by dividing them into two categories: those that are more likely to occur but are not serious, and those that are rare but serious. Provide guidance on how the patient can avoid some of the most common side effects, if possible, and what should be done if a serious one occurs. Also inform the patient about other drugs or conditions that interact with the medication and how to manage the interaction. In finishing this portion of the session, discuss storage information, what to do if a dose is missed, and any pertinent refill information.

As the counseling session is concluding, verify the patient's understanding of the information covered during the session. One of the best methods for this is the "Teach-back Method," which is used to determine what the patient understands and to correct any misunderstandings.[12] To avoid the impression that you are testing the patient, a good approach is to say, "I have covered quite a bit of information about your new medication. Just to make sure that I did not forget anything, how are you going to take the medication when you get home?" This places the appearance of responsibility for remembering everything on the pharmacist and reduces stress for the patient.

COUNSELING ON A REFILL

Counseling on a medication refill is an abbreviated process compared to that described for a new medication. The focus changes from how to take the medication to monitoring of the patient with queries such as, "What side effects have been experienced?" and "Have you followed up with the prescriber?" Counseling on refills is especially important when use of a device is involved. For example, metered-dose inhalers are difficult to use correctly. Correct inhaler use decreases over time, even in as little as 2–3 months, and studies show that pharmacist counseling improves correct inhaler technique and adherence.[13] Additionally, it is important to follow up with the patient to answer any questions that have arisen since the last fill and to provide contact information for any future questions that arise.

OVER-THE-COUNTER SESSIONS

Assisting a patient in the self-care aisle is another common form of patient communication. This communication differs in that the pharmacist has to assess the current symptoms and evaluate whether self-management with OTC medications is appropriate or whether referral is needed. There are a variety of mnemonics to assist pharmacists in asking all necessary questions before recommending a product. These include: CHAPS-FRAPS (Chief complaint, History of present illness, Allergies, Past medical history, Social history, Family history, Review of symptoms, Assessments, Plans, and SOAP); The Basic seven (location, quality, severity, timing, context, modifying factors, and associated symptoms); and PQRST (Palliation and provocation, Quality and quantity, Region and radiation, Signs and symptoms, Temporal relationship).[14-16] The most comprehensive mnemonic is the QuEST/SCHOLAR approach.[17] This method enables the pharmacist to evaluate the patient and most accurately select the best nonprescription product. The QuEST/SCHOLAR process includes:

1. **Qu**ickly and accurately assess the patient

   Ask about the current complaint (SCHOLAR), other medications, and allergies

   - **S**ymptoms
   - **C**haracteristics
   - **H**istory
   - **O**nset
   - **L**ocation
   - **A**ggravating factors
   - **R**emitting factors

2. **E**stablish that the patient is a self-care candidate

   - No severe symptoms, symptoms do not persist or return, patient is not using self-care to avoid medical care

3. **S**uggest appropriate self-care strategies

   - Recommend the medication and nonpharmacologic therapy

4. **T**alk with the patient

   - How the drug is going to work, when it should be taken, expected adverse events

For example, Joe comes into your pharmacy requesting assistance in selecting an OTC product for heartburn. Utilizing the QuEST/SCHOLAR process, you could:

1. **Qu**ickly and accurately assess the patient: "Let's talk a little about the type of problems you have been having."

   Ask about the current complaint (SCHOLAR), other medications, allergies

   - **S**ymptoms: "What symptoms are you having?"
   - **C**haracteristics: "How would you describe the pain...burning, sharp, shooting?"
   - **H**istory: "Have you experienced this before? What have you tried already? Did it work?"
   - **O**nset: "When did the symptoms start?"
   - **L**ocation: "Where is the pain you are describing as heartburn?"
   - **A**ggravating factors: "What makes it worse?"
   - **R**emitting factors: "What makes it better?"

2. **E**stablish that the patient is a self-care candidate

   - "Based on this information, I think that it would (or would not) be appropriate for you to use OTC treatment."

3. **S**uggest appropriate self-care strategies

   - "I would recommend _____ and some non-medication strategies, too."

4. **T**alk with the patient

   - "You can take ___ tablet(s) every ___ hours to help with symptoms. This medication will work by _____. You should start to notice improvement in _____ minutes. Also, try lifestyle modifications like avoiding spicy foods and raising the head of the bed. If your symptoms persist for more than 2 weeks or do not improve, see your doctor. The OTC medications can cover up symptoms that need to be checked out further by your doctor."

The QuEST/SCHOLAR method provides a technique for systematically assessing patients in the OTC aisle and providing a thorough but efficient evaluation. It is vital to maintain the patient's privacy (using a private area, if possible) and be cognizant of topics that make patients uncomfortable. These occur with OTC items, too; recognizing this and being prepared will help put the patient at ease. Try to employ the teach-back method with OTCs and herbals to ensure patient understanding of the information discussed.

BARRIERS TO COMMUNICATION

Patient communication does not always happen the way we plan. There are common barriers to communication, and knowing them can help you to be prepared. The common barriers can be divided into three categories: patient barriers, pharmacist barriers, and pharmacy/corporate barriers. The barriers are summarized in Table 3-2.

Because the patient is ultimately in charge of his/her health care, patient barriers can be some of the most difficult to overcome. These barriers include patient education and health literacy level. The aging patient brings unique challenges to communication, such as changes in physical health, depression, cognitive decline, and changes in hearing, vision, voice, and speech processes.[18] Also, you may be presented with the caregiver and not the patient, and he/she may be in a rush or functioning under the misconception that the pharmacist just "puts the pills in the bottle."

HEALTH LITERACY

Health literacy is defined as the degree to which individuals have the capacity to obtain, process, and understand basic health information and services needed to make appropriate health decisions. It is not enough for patients to simply "understand" information about their health. They must be able to make decisions about what to do—to be able to navigate the healthcare system and be somewhat confident about it. Health literacy may be tied to level of education

TABLE 3-2	Barriers to Communication	
Patient barriers	**Pharmacist barriers**	**Pharmacy/corporate barriers**
Patient education level	Pharmacist attitude toward counseling	Lack of privacy
Health literacy level	Lack of patient communication training	Low financial resources
Misconceptions of pharmacist role		Large number of patients per pharmacist
Patient is in a hurry		
Aging		
Visual difficulties		
Hearing difficulties		

completed, but not necessarily. For example, you may have a woman with an MBA, highly educated and very successful in the corporate world, not realize that it is unsafe to take OTC acetaminophen and an OTC cough and cold product also containing acetaminophen. On the other hand, you may have a woman who only completed the 10th grade and has a young child with a pediatric cancer. She may be well versed in the healthcare system and able to tell you more about her child's medication and medical needs than most of the nurses and other healthcare workers. It is important to realize that you cannot make assumptions about health literacy by looking at the patient and assessing his/her education or social status.

A sense of shame often accompanies a patient's low health literacy. Since patients do not typically volunteer their lack of knowledge, identifying low health literacy is important, especially in light of its association with medication nonadherence.[19] Some indicators that health literacy may be a problem with a given patient are leaving forms partially filled out, referring to medication by their color, opening the bottle to look at the medication rather than the label, making excuses like "I forgot my glasses," postponing appointments, chronic nonadherence, failing to look at written materials, or bringing someone with them.

Once you recognize that a patient presents health literacy concerns, it is vital to remain respectful, considerate, and maintain privacy. Failure to be sensitive to the needs of these patients can result in loss of the relationship that was forming and loss of an opportunity to impact the patient's health outcomes. Recognizing that time is a limitation, there are some tips to help with patient understanding. First, limit the number of main counseling points to two or three. Covering too many topics can be overwhelming. Second, demonstrate the procedure or technique. One example of this is to show the patient how to use an inhaler and spacer device. Then ensure that understanding is complete with the teach-back method discussed previously. Pictures can also be used to convey information about medication instructions and safety. Standard pictograms created by the United States Pharmacopeia are available for download at http://www.usp.org/usp-healthcare-professionals /related-topics-resources/usp-pictograms/download-pictograms. Finally, summarize the information and be positive, communicating in an open manner while maintaining eye contact.

Using plain language is one of the most important tenets for working with patients with low health literacy. This involves using common words instead of medical jargon to improve understanding of complex situations. An example is to use "water pill" instead of "diuretic", "a medication that helps open the airways" instead of "bronchodilator," and "sore" instead of "abscess." Additional examples can be found at http://www.plainlanguage.gov./populartopics /health_literacy/index.cfm under the Plain Language Thesaurus.

AGING

The aging patient experiences many physiological changes such as cognitive decline and dementia that can make communication more difficult. Sensory loss, including both hearing and vision, may also occur with aging.[18] Because these are challenging in their own right, living with them while navigating the healthcare system can be frustrating for patients.

Some general techniques can make the encounter with these patients more effective. Know the patient's strengths and weaknesses and cater to them. Select educational materials that are most appropriate for that patient. Be prepared to take some extra time with the patient to ensure full understanding and buy-in of the information. Use an environment that is conducive to the conversation—a place with minimal distractions. If the patient has difficulty hearing, speaking louder will not help; it will only distort the sound. Speak slowly and simplify your sentences. Use plain language when speaking, making sure to avoid medical jargon that can be confusing and overwhelming. Finally, if the patient has visual difficulties, ensure that they have their glasses and be prepared to provide the materials in a larger font. You may also want to determine whether your prescription filling software can print prescription label information in a larger font for easier reading.

FUTURE OF PHARMACY PRACTICE AND THE ROLE OF COMMUNICATION

With the implementation of electronic medical records and the rise of Medicare Star Ratings (a complex system of using performance measures to evaluate prescription drug plans and community pharmacy performance), the pharmacist's ability to develop masterful patient communication skills is becoming essential. The pharmacist can use the tips for patient communication to develop new and expected pharmacy services. In some settings, this may be collaborative drug therapy management working with the team to optimize medication therapy. In the community pharmacy, the pharmacist will complete comprehensive medication reviews (CMRs) to improve Star Ratings and medication adherence. Managed care pharmacists will optimize medications and counseling for avoidance of adverse events.

CONCLUSION

Talking with the patient is the cornerstone of pharmacy practice. Communication starts with developing a pharmacist–patient relationship and results in the professional satisfaction that most pharmacists start their careers desiring. Recognize the special needs of patients and those patients do not come to the pharmacy because they "feel good." A patient with a chronic condition may need someone to take the time to express an interest in his/her health. That one person can be you. When you do show that needed interest, the patient may be more willing to work with you to reach their own healthcare goals. Simply stated, communication is key.

REFERENCES

1. Patterson K, Grenny J, McMillan R, Switzler A. Crucial Conversations. 2nd ed. New York, NY: McGraw Hill; 2012.
2. Rantucci M. Pharmacists Talking With Patients: A Guide to Patient Counseling. 2nd ed. Philadelphia, PA: Lippincott, Williams, & Wilkins; 2007.
3. Berger B. Communication Skills for Pharmacists: Building Relationships, Improving Patient Care. 3rd ed. Washington, DC: American Pharmacists Association; 2009.
4. Ncqa.org. Patient-Centered Medical Home (PCMH). 2014. *http://www .ncqa.org/Programs/Recognition/Practices/PatientCenteredMedical-HomePCMH.aspx.* Accessed September 15, 2015.
5. Shafir A, Rosenthal J. Shared-Decision Making: Advancing Patient-Centered Care through State and Federal Implementation. 1st ed. Washington, DC: National Academy for State Health Policy; 2012. *http://www.nashp.org/sites/default/files/shared.decision.making.report .pdf.* Accessed September 15, 2015.
6. Stacey D, Bennett C, Barry M. Decision aids for people facing health treatment or screening decisions. Cochrane Database Syst Rev. 2011;10:CD001431.
7. Bennett M, Kliethermes M. How to Implement the Pharmacists' Patient Care Process. Washington, DC: American Pharmacist Association; 2015.
8. Egan G. The Skilled Helper. Belmont, CA: Brooks Cole, Cengage Learning; 2010.
9. Ahrq.gov. Figure 9: Tips for Conducting a Patient Medication Interview | Agency for Healthcare Research & Quality. 2012. *http://www .ahrq.gov/professionals/quality-patient-safety/patient-safety-resources /resources/match/matchfig9.html.* Accessed September 15, 2015.

10. Drug Diversion Toolkit. Patient Counseling—A Pharmacists Responsibility to Ensure Compliance. 1st ed. Baltimore, MD: Center for Medicare and Medicaid Services; 2014. *https://www.cms.gov/Medicare-Medicaid-Coordination/Fraud-Prevention/Medicaid-Integrity-Education/Provider-Education-Toolkits/Downloads/drugdiversion-patientcounseling-111414.pdf*. Accessed September 15, 2015.

11. Erickson S, Kirking D, Sandusky M. Michigan Medicaid recipients perceptions of medication counseling as required by OBRA 90. J Am Pharm Assoc. 1998;38(3):333–338.

12. Schillinger D, Piette J, Grumbach K, et al. Closing the loop. Arch Intern Med. 2003;163(1):83. doi:10.1001/archinte.163.1.83.

13. Mehuys E, Van Bortel L, De Bolle L, et al. Effectiveness of pharmacist intervention for asthma control improvement. Eur Respir J. 2008;31(4):790–799. doi:10.1183/09031936.00112007.

14. The pharmacist's role in self-care. J Am Pharm Assoc. 2002;42(5s1):S40. doi:10.1331/108658002764653743.

15. Boyce R, Herrier R. Obtaining and using patient data. Am Pharm. 1991;31:65–71.

16. Bates B, Bates B, Northway D. PQRST: a mnemonic to communicate a change in condition. J Am Med Direct Assoc. 2002;3(1):23–25. doi:10.1016/s1525-8610(04)70239-x.

17. Leibowitz K, Ginsburg D. Counseling self-treating patients quickly and effectively. In: APhA Inaugural Self-Care Institute. Washington, DC: American Pharmacist Association; 2002.

18. Yorkston K, Bourgeois M, Baylor C. Communication and aging. Phys Med Rehab Clin North Am. 2010;21(2):309–319. doi:10.1016/j.pmr.2009.12.011.

19. Ngoh L. Health literacy: a barrier to pharmacist–patient communication and medication adherence. J Am Pharm Assoc. 2009;49(5):e132–e149. doi:10.1331/japha.2009.07075.

4

The Patient Care Plan

TERRY L. SCHWINGHAMMER, PharmD, FCCP, FASHP, FAPhA, BCPS

THE PATIENT CARE PROCESS

The *patient care process* is a systematic and comprehensive method for interacting with patients that is applied consistently to every patient seen by the healthcare provider. The process may vary among healthcare practitioners who have different purposes and goals. For pharmacists, the primary purpose of the patient care process is to identify, solve, and prevent drug therapy problems.[1] A drug therapy problem is "any undesirable event experienced by a patient which involves, or is suspected to involve, drug therapy and that interferes with achieving the desired goals of therapy and requires professional judgment to resolve."[1] The pharmacist's patient care process includes three essential elements: (1) assessment of the patient's drug-related needs; (2) creation of a care plan to meet those needs; and (3) follow-up evaluation to determine whether positive outcomes were achieved. Consequently, development of a care plan is only one component of the overall patient care process. Before developing a patient-specific care plan, it is important for the clinician to understand the comprehensive nature of the patient care process. This process offers a logical and consistent framework that can be most useful in care planning and serves as the framework for this chapter.

ASSESSMENT OF DRUG-RELATED NEEDS

The first step in assessment is to identify the patient's drug-related needs by collecting, organizing, and integrating pertinent patient, drug, and disease information. In the patient care process, as with all direct patient care services, the patient is the primary source of information. This involves asking patients what they *want* (expectations) and what they *do not want* (concerns) and determining how well they understand their drug therapies. For example, the clinician may ask, "How may I help you today?" or "What concerns do you have that I may address for you today?" In addition to speaking with the patient, data can also be obtained from: (1) family members or caretakers when appropriate; (2) the patient's current and past medical records; and (3) discussions with other healthcare providers. The types of information that may be relevant are described below.[1,2]

Patient Information

- Demographics and background information: age, gender, race, height, and weight.
- Social history: living arrangements, occupation, and special needs (eg, physical abilities, cultural traits, drug administration devices).
- Family history: relevant health histories of parents and siblings.
- Insurance/administrative information: name of health plan and primary care physician.

Disease Information

- Past medical history.
- Current medical problems.
- History of present illness.
- Pertinent information from the review of systems, physical examination, laboratory results, and x-ray/imaging results.
- Medical diagnoses.

Drug Information

- Allergies and side effects (include the name of the medication and the reaction that occurred).
- Current prescription medications:
  ✓ How the medication was prescribed.
  ✓ How the patient is actually taking the medication.
  ✓ Effectiveness and side effects of current medications.
  ✓ Questions or concerns about current medications.
- Current nonprescription medications, vitamins, dietary supplements, and other alternative/complementary therapies.
- Past prescription and nonprescription medications (ie, those discontinued within the past 6 months).

The information obtained is then organized, analyzed, and integrated to: (1) determine whether the patient's drug therapy is appropriate, effective, safe, and convenient for the patient; (2) identify drug therapy problems that may interfere with goals of therapy; and (3) identify potential drug therapy problems that require prevention. One method of organizing and integrating this information with appropriate pharmacotherapeutic knowledge has been described as the Pharmacotherapy Workup© (copyright 2003–2012, Cipolle et al.).[1]

Drug therapy problems are uncovered through careful assessment of the patient, drug, and disease information to determine the appropriateness of each medication regimen. This process involves a logical sequence of steps. It begins with evaluating each medication regimen for appropriateness of indication, then optimizing the drug and dosage regimen to ensure maximum effectiveness, and finally, individualizing drug therapy to make it as safe as possible for the patient. After completing these three steps, the practitioner considers other issues such as cost, compliance, and convenience.

TABLE 4-1 Drug Therapy Problems to Be Resolved or Prevented

Assessment	Drug Therapy Problem
Indication	**Unnecessary drug therapy**
	No medical indication
	Duplicate therapy
	Nondrug therapy indicated
	Treating avoidable adverse drug reaction
	Addictive/recreational use
	Needs additional drug therapy
	Untreated condition
	Preventive/prophylactic
	Synergistic/potentiating
Effectiveness	**Needs different drug product**
	More effective drug available
	Condition refractory to drug
	Dosage form inappropriate
	Not effective for condition
	Dosage too low
	Wrong dose
	Frequency too long
	Duration too short
	Drug interaction
	Incorrect administration
Safety	**Adverse drug reaction**
	Undesirable effect
	Unsafe drug for patient
	Drug interaction
	Dose administered or changed too rapidly
	Allergic reaction
	Contraindications present
	Dosage too high
	Wrong dose
	Frequency too short
	Duration too long
	Drug interaction
	Incorrect administration
Compliance	**Nonadherence**
	Directions not understood
	Patient prefers not to take
	Patient forgets to take
	Drug product too expensive
	Cannot swallow or administer
	Drug product not available

Adapted with permission from Cipolle RJ, Strand LM, Morley PC. Pharmaceutical Care Practice: A Clinician's Guide, 2nd ed. New York, McGraw-Hill, 2004:168.

TABLE 4-2 Causes of Drug Therapy Problems

Drug Therapy Problem	Possible Causes of Drug Therapy Problems
Unnecessary drug therapy	No valid medication indication for the drug at this time
	Multiple drug products are used when only single-drug therapy is required
	The condition is better treated with nondrug therapy
	Drug therapy is used to treat an avoidable adverse drug reaction associated with another medication
	The medical problem is caused by drug abuse, alcohol use, or smoking
Need for additional drug therapy	A medical condition exists that requires initiation of new drug therapy
	Preventive therapy is needed to reduce the risk of developing a new condition
	A medical condition requires combination therapy to achieve synergism or additive effects
Ineffective drug	The drug is not the most effective one for the medical problem
	The drug product is not effective for the medical condition
	The condition is refractory to the drug product being used
	The dosage form is inappropriate
Dosage too low	The dose is too low to produce the desired outcome
	The dosage interval is too infrequent
	A drug interaction reduces the amount of active drug available
	The duration of therapy is too short
Adverse drug reaction	The drug product causes an undesirable reaction that is not dose related
	A safer drug is needed because of patient risk factors
	A drug interaction causes an undesirable reaction that is not dose related
	The regimen was administered or changed too rapidly
	The product causes an allergic reaction
	The drug is contraindicated because of patient risk factors
Dosage too high	The dose is too high for the patient
	The dosing frequency is too short. The duration of therapy is too long
	A drug interaction causes a toxic reaction to the drug product
	The dose was administered too rapidly
Nonadherence	The patient does not understand the instructions
	The patient prefers not to take the medication
	The patient forgets to take the medication
	Drug product is too expensive
	The patient cannot swallow or self-administer the medication properly
	The drug product is not available for the patient

Adapted with permission from Cipolle RJ, Strand LM, Morley PC. Pharmaceutical Care Practice: A Clinician's Guide, 2nd ed. New York, McGraw-Hill, 2004:178–179.

Drug therapy problems can be placed into distinct categories, as summarized below. See Table 4-1 for a checklist that can be used in actual practice situations.[1]

Indication for drug use:

1. The drug therapy is unnecessary because the patient does not have a clinical indication at this time.

2. Additional drug therapy is required to treat or prevent a medical condition.

Effectiveness of therapy:

3. The drug product is not being effective at producing the desired patient response.

4. The dosage is too low to produce the desired patient response.

Safety of therapy:

5. The drug is causing an adverse reaction.

6. The dosage is too high, resulting in undesirable effects.

Medication adherence:

7. The patient is not able or willing to take the drug therapy as intended.

A drug therapy problem can be resolved or prevented only when the cause of the problem is clearly understood. Therefore, it is necessary to identify and categorize both the drug therapy problem and its cause (Table 4-2).[1]

CREATION OF A PATIENT CARE PLAN

Care plan development is a cooperative effort that should involve the patient as an active participant. It may also involve an interprofessional team of care providers and the patient's family. Care planning involves establishing therapeutic goals and determining appropriate interventions to:

1. Resolve all existing drug therapy problems.

2. Achieve the goals of therapy intended for each active medical problem.

3. Prevent future drug therapy problems that have a potential to develop.

Although care plans have been a standard component of the practice of other health professionals (eg, nurses, physical therapists, respiratory therapists) for many years, there is no standard method of care planning in pharmacy. In 1995, the Joint Commission on Accreditation of Healthcare Organizations (JCAHO) made pharmaceutical care planning a requirement for accreditation in all settings that it accredits. This requirement mandates that pharmaceutical care planning be included in the overall plan of care for the patient.[3] Implementation of a systematic care planning process serves to organize the pharmacist's practice, to communicate activities to other healthcare professionals, and to provide a record of drug therapy interventions in the event that questions arise regarding the standard of care provided to a patient.

A plan of care is not merely a document; rather, it is a systematic, ongoing process of planning, action, and documentation. It is a dynamic instrument that reflects the continuing care that is modified according to the patient's changing needs.[4] The most essential element to remember is that the needs of the patient drive the plan, regardless of the care planning format used. In short, the plan must be tailored to the needs of each unique patient. All care providers and the patient should agree on the care plan because each participant has a responsibility for implementing a portion of the plan. In the ambulatory care setting, the patient often assumes much of the responsibility for plan implementation.

Organization of a care plan is important, and each medical problem should be addressed separately and in its entirety so that the drug therapy problems associated with each condition and the plans for intervention are logically organized and implemented. The elements of a care plan include:

- *Medical condition:* List the disease state for which the patient has drug-related needs.

- *Drug therapy problems:* State the drug therapy problems by including the patient's problem or condition, the drug therapy involved, and the association between the drug(s) and the patient's condition(s).

- *Goals of therapy:* State the goals in the future tense. Goals should be realistic, measurable and/or observable, specific, and associated with a definite time frame.

- *Interventions:* In collaboration with the patient, the practitioner develops and prioritizes a list of activities to address the patient's drug-related needs. The patient's input is important because the plan should adequately address the patient's unique concerns, needs, and preferences. The list of activities may be stated in the past, present, or future tense. Include the recommendations made to the patient, the caregiver on the patient's behalf, or the prescriber to resolve (or prevent) the patient's drug therapy problems.

- *Follow-up plan:* Determine when the patient should return for follow-up and what will occur at that subsequent visit.

An example of how each of these components might be incorporated into a care plan is given in the following case vignette:

Patrick Murphy is a 73-year-old man who underwent coronary artery bypass grafting 2 months ago and was started on simvastatin 10 mg by mouth (po) once daily 6 weeks ago for dyslipidemia. The results of this week's fasting lipid profile revealed total cholesterol 230 mg/dL, low-density lipoprotein (LDL) cholesterol 141 mg/dL,

high-density lipoprotein cholesterol 45 mg/dL, and triglycerides 220 mg/dL. He continues to smoke 1.5 packs of cigarettes per day.

- *Medical condition:* Dyslipidemia.

- *Drug therapy problems:* Dyslipidemia treated with an inadequate dose of a lipid-lowering agent.

- *Goals of therapy:* The patient's LDL cholesterol will be lowered to <100 mg/dL within 6 weeks. (*Note:* Because the patient has known coronary artery disease, his goal LDL cholesterol is <100 mg/dL, with an optional goal of 70 mg/dL.[5])

- *Interventions:* The maximum dose of simvastatin is 80 mg, so the dose should be increased in an attempt to achieve the target LDL level. Increase simvastatin to 20 mg po once daily; #30 dispensed. Reviewed possible side effects of simvastatin with patient (constipation, rare muscle weakness). Recommended that the patient consider stopping smoking—advised to keep a log of smoking habits, including number of cigarettes, time of day, and trigger events.

- *Follow-up plan:* Patient will return to clinic in 6 weeks for a repeat fasting lipid profile, questioning about potential adverse effects, and discussion of a plan for smoking cessation.

FOLLOW-UP EVALUATION

The purpose of a follow-up evaluation is to evaluate the positive and negative impact of the care plan on the patient, to identify new drug therapy problems, and to take appropriate action to address new problems or adjust previous therapies as needed. Follow-up evaluation requires direct contact with the patient to obtain feedback about the benefits of therapy achieved, the occurrence of problems such as side effects, and patient concerns about the treatment. Additionally, relevant data are gathered from current clinical assessments, laboratory tests, radiographs, and other procedures. The practitioner evaluates and documents the patient's progress in achieving the goals of therapy.

The evaluation involves comparing goals of therapy with the patient's current status. Cipolle et al. developed terminology to describe the patient's status, the medical conditions, and the comparative evaluation of that status with the previously determined therapeutic goals.[1] These terms also describe the actions taken as a result of the follow-up evaluation:

Status	Definition
Resolved	Therapeutic goals achieved for the acute condition; discontinue therapy
Stable	Therapeutic goals achieved; continue the same therapy for chronic disease management
Improved	Progress is being made in achieving goals; continue the same therapy because more time is required to assess the full benefit of therapy
Partial improvement	Progress is being made, but minor adjustments in therapy are required to fully achieve the therapeutic goals before the next assessment
Unimproved	Little or no progress has been made, but continue the same therapy to allow additional time for benefit to be observed
Worsened	A decline in health is observed despite an adequate duration using the optimal drug; modify drug therapy (eg, increase the dose of the current medication, add a second agent with additive or synergistic effects)
Failure	Therapeutic goals have not been achieved despite an adequate dose and duration of therapy; discontinue current medication(s) and start new therapy
Expired	The patient died while receiving drug therapy; document possible contributing factors, especially if they may be drug related

Example: If the patient Mr Murphy described above returns in 6 weeks with a repeat fasting LDL cholesterol of 120 mg/dL without complaints of side effects, the outcome status of this patient would be partial improvement. Another adjustment in therapy is indicated to further reduce his LDL cholesterol (eg, increase the simvastatin dose to 40 mg po once daily).

EXAMPLE OF CARE PLAN DOCUMENTATION

Each step in the patient care process must be documented. Documentation should take place on an ongoing basis to provide an updated record of the patient's current and changing needs, care activities in response to those needs, the patient's progress, and plans for future care and follow-up evaluation. This document provides a means for communication among healthcare providers and should reflect the systematic and dynamic process of patient care. The example provided in Figure 4-1 is intended to demonstrate to students how a patient care plan might be created.

A blank care plan form is also included at the end of this chapter for use by students who are completing the cases for this Casebook (see Appendix A). Students may practice using this form when completing the case studies in this Casebook. The vast amount of medical information available and the widespread computerization of patient records make the use of electronic patient care records virtually mandatory. Consequently, use of this relatively simple hard-copy form should be considered only the first step in developing the student's ability to electronically organize and manage large volumes of complex medical information.

Example Case Vignette: Donald Bennett is a 64-year-old man with osteoarthritis currently treated with nabumetone. He has been diagnosed with hypertension based on the average of two blood pressure (BP) readings taken at three previous clinic visits.[6] *The hypertension is presently untreated. What information must be included in the patient's pharmaceutical care plan?*

PATIENT INFORMATION

- *The patient's name* is essential to identify the patient to whom the record belongs. The name, Donald Bennett, should be the first information placed on the chart. Although this guideline seems logical, it sometimes does not happen. When in a hurry, a care provider may grab a blank form and begin to make notes with the intention of placing the patient's personal information on it later, and in the midst of distractions, the name is not recorded.

- *Current address and phone number* are necessary for future contact and follow-up evaluation. The information should be complete (621 E. Greene Street, Washington, PA 15301), and the telephone number should include the area code (412-555-1950).

- *Insurance* information should include the name of the insurance plan and policy number (Metro United Health Plan #1234789) to ensure accurate billing of services.

- *Demographic* information including *age (birth date), gender, race, height, and weight* should be recorded for the purpose of individualizing drug therapy. Mr Bennett is a 64-year-old Caucasian man who is 5'11" tall and weighs 177 lb. Include weight information in both pounds and kilograms. The equation for converting pounds to kilograms is as follows: weight in pounds/2.2 = weight in kilograms. Mr Bennett weighs 177 lb or 80.4 kg (177/2.2 = 80.4). This information is used to determine the appropriate drug and dosage regimens

for treatment. *Ideal body weight (IBW)* is necessary for calculating appropriate dosage for medications that do not distribute into fatty tissues. IBW is calculated as follows: for men, IBW = 50 kg + (2.3 × [height in inches above 5 ft]); for women, IBW = 45.5 kg + (2.3 × [height in inches above 5 ft]). For Mr Bennett, 50 kg + (2.3 × 11) = 75.3 kg.

- *Allergies and adverse drug reactions* should be documented with specific descriptions of the reactions that occurred. Reactions should be clearly identified as allergies or side effects. Mr Bennett has an allergic reaction to penicillin that resulted in hives. He also has experienced dyspepsia, a well-documented side effect of ibuprofen. This information is critical to avoiding patient harm. Allergies are distinct from side effects. An allergy is an immune-mediated reaction that often precludes future use of the medication except in rare cases in which the benefit of using the drug outweighs the risk of the reaction. However, a side effect may sometimes be self-limiting with continued use, or it may be successfully managed with adjustments in the dosage regimen or administration. For example, a drug that is taken once daily and causes drowsiness may be administered at bedtime. A drug that causes GI upset may be successfully managed by taking it with meals.

- *Tobacco/alcohol/substance use* information is important for appropriate drug selection, dosing calculation, and patient education. Include the name of the substance, the amount, and frequency, when possible. Mr Bennett occasionally smokes approximately three cigars each week and drinks 1 oz of whiskey with each cigar. It is important to record pertinent negatives for substance use. For example, caffeine may increase BP acutely, although tolerance to this effect develops quickly. Nevertheless, caffeine use may be relevant to this patient and should be recorded. Alcohol and tobacco may affect the metabolism of certain drugs and potentiate or counteract the benefits of other drugs. For example, tobacco enhances the metabolism of theophylline. Therefore, smokers generally require higher doses of theophylline to achieve therapeutic benefits. Substances such as cocaine, caffeine, or tobacco may enhance the sympathomimetic effect of some drugs while counteracting the sympatholytic effects of others, such as some antihypertensive medications.

- *Medical conditions* should be listed to offer a general overview of the patient's medical problems. The care plan is also organized according to the medical condition whereby all drug therapy problems associated with each medical condition are addressed separately and in their entirety.

MEDICATION RECORD

- The list of medications should include the date each was started; the indication for use; and the drug name, strength, and regimen that the patient is actually taking. The *actual* regimen may differ from the *prescribed* regimen because patients do not always take medications as directed. Assessment of therapy must be made based on the actual therapy the patient is receiving. Mr Bennett is currently taking nabumetone two 750-mg tablets po daily. A stop date should be recorded for medications that have been discontinued.

- Relevant clinical impressions or comments can also be recorded, for example: "Discontinued ibuprofen secondary to dyspepsia that occurred even when taken with food." Also note the antihypertensive regimen, which was initiated with hydrochlorothiazide 25 mg po once daily and subsequently

PHARMACEUTICAL CARE PATIENT RECORD

Patient Name: Donald Benferardo	**Gender:** M
Address: 621 E. Greene St., Washington PA 15301	**Race:** W
Telephone: 412-555-1950 **Age:** 64	**Actual Weight:** 177 lb (80 kg)
Insurance: Metro United Health Plan #1234789	**Ideal Weight:** 166 lb (75.3 kg)
Medical Conditions: Osteoarthritis left knee (stable)	**Allergies:** Penicillin ⟶ hives
Tobacco/Alcohol/Substance Use: Occasional cigar 3×/wk; EtOH 3×/wk; no caffeine	**Adverse Reactions:** Ibuprofen ⟶ dyspepsia

Medication Record

Start Date	Stop Date	Indication	Drug Name	Actual Strength	Regimen	Clinical Impressions
12/14/15		Osteoarthritis	Nabumetone	750 mg	2 tablet po once daily	Tolerating well minor knee pain
5/03/16	5/17/16	HTN	Hydrochlorothiazide	25 mg	1 tablet po once daily	5/17/16: D/C due to hypokalemia
5/17/16		HTN	Triamterene/ Hydrochlorothiazide	37.25/25 mg	1 tablet po once daily	5/31/16: K^+ WNL; HTN partially improved
5/31/16		HTN	Atenolol	50 mg	1 tablet po once daily	

Assessment, Plan, and Follow-Up Evaluation

Date	Medical Condition	Drug-Therapy Problem	Goal	Current Status	Interventions	Follow-Up Plan
5/3/16	HTN	Untreated HTN	Lower BP to 110–138/70–88 within 4 wks	Untreated (BP 160/104)	Start hydrochlorothiazide 25 mg po once daily × 4 wks	Return for BP check & serum K^+ in 2 wks
5/17/16	HTN	Hypokalemia secondary to hydrochlorothiazide	K^+ 3.5–5.0 mEq/L	Untreated (K^+ 3.2 mEq/L)	Discontinue HCT Start triamterene/HCT 3.75/25 mg po once daily	Recheck K^+ in 2 wks
5/17/16	HTN	HTN inadequately treated with hydrochlorothiazide	BP 110–138/70–88	Partial improvement (BP 150/92)	Change to triamterene/HCT as above	Return in 2 wks for BP & K^+ check
5/31/16	HTN	Hypokalemia requiring drug therapy	K^+ 3.5–5.0 mEq/L	Stable (K^+ 3.6 mEq/L)	Continue current therapy	Check symptoms of ↓K^+ in 1 mo
5/31/16	HTN	HTN inadequately treated with hydrochlorothiazide	Same as above	Partial improvement (BP 146/92)	Add atenolol 50 mg po once daily × 4 wks	Return for BP check in 1 mo

FIGURE 4-1. Sample patient care record. (BP, blood pressure; HTN, hypertension; WNL, within normal limits; K^+, potassium; HCT, hydrochlorothiazide.)

changed to triamterene/hydrochlorothiazide 37.5/25 mg po once daily. Atenolol 50 mg po once daily was added later because only partial improvement in hypertension was achieved with diuretic therapy.

ASSESSMENT, PLAN, AND FOLLOW-UP EVALUATION

This section of the patient's record provides a record of therapeutic interventions and the patient's responses to them. Information is documented as events occur, providing a "flowchart" of the patient's progress to date. The historical information contained in this chart is important to incorporate in therapeutic decision making.

- *The date* should be recorded in the far left column to document when each encounter occurred. Mr Bennett's chart shows that he has been seen three times: on May 3, May 17, and May 31, 2016.

- The next column, *medical condition*, specifies the medical diagnosis for which the medications are indicated. On May 3, Mr Bennett was diagnosed with hypertension; his subsequent visits also were for evaluation of hypertension.

- The *drug therapy problem* is recorded in the next column to indicate the drug therapy problem(s) associated with each medical diagnosis. Each medical diagnosis may have one or more drug therapy problems associated with it. On May 3, Mr Bennett had one drug therapy problem—untreated hypertension. That is, he had an indication for drug therapy but was not receiving treatment. On May 17 and May 31, the dates were recorded twice because on these days he had two drug therapy problems that were being addressed. Each drug therapy problem should be recorded in a separate row. Although he had only one active diagnosis (hypertension), he had two drug therapy problems associated with that diagnosis as shown on May 17 and May 31. He had hypokalemia possibly secondary to hydrochlorothiazide and hypertension inadequately treated with hydrochlorothiazide.

- The *goal* of therapy is recorded in the next column. Using the SMART acronym, therapy goals should be *Specific*, *Measurable* (or observable), and *Achievable*. The goal should also be directly *Related* to the drug therapy problem. In this case, the systolic BP goal should be less than 140 mm Hg with a diastolic pressure of less than 90 mm Hg. Treatment to lower levels may be useful if tolerated by the patient. For example, the clinician may establish an acceptable range of BP control, such as systolic BP between 110 and 138 mm Hg and diastolic BP between 70 and 88 mm Hg. The *Timeline* to achieve the goal should also be specified. For example, his BP should be reduced to within the indicated range within 4 weeks of therapy.

- The *current status* includes the patient's actual BP at each encounter. In this case, Mr Bennett's BP was 160/104 mm Hg on May 3 prior to starting drug therapy. Notice that his BP continues to decline with treatment. On May 17 and May 31, his BPs were 150/92 and 146/92 mm Hg, respectively. The status on May 31 (4 weeks after treatment) is considered partially improved because the BP did decrease with treatment, but an adjustment in treatment is still required to achieve the BP goal.

- *Interventions* that were implemented must be recorded. The drug name, dose, route, frequency, and duration of therapy should be documented. On May 3, hydrochlorothiazide was started at a dose of 25 mg orally once a day. As you look down this column, you can see that the therapy was adjusted on May 17 and May 31. These interventions were made in response to the patient's BP as recorded in the previous column. By looking across the row, you can see the supportive evidence for the intervention: a clearly documented problem (hypertension) and the patient's status measured objectively (BP). Looking down the columns, one can see what interventions have been made and also how the patient has responded over time.

- The *follow-up plan* specifies details of how the outcome of therapy will be assessed. This column should contain information about who will do what and when they will do it. The plan made on May 3 indicated that Mr Bennett was to return to the clinic in 2 weeks to have his BP and serum potassium level measured. This flowchart provides an easy way to see whether the patient is appearing for the follow-up visits. Mr Bennett did return for follow-up in 2 weeks (May 17) according to the plan. There should continue to be a follow-up plan as long as a person is receiving drug therapy. After the patient's condition is stabilized, the follow-up intervals may be much longer, such as every 6 months or once a year. However, the assessment, plan, and follow-up must continue for the duration of drug therapy. In this case, after Mr Bennett's BP is stabilized, he may be responsible for monitoring his own BP and assessing the side effects by self-monitoring while keeping a twice-yearly appointments for a more formal evaluation at the clinic. The patient's care plan remains active and represents the ongoing and dynamic process of providing pharmaceutical care.

PATIENT SUMMARY

Based on the information documented in the care plan, the practitioner providing care to this patient and other healthcare professionals who have access to this information should be able to extract the following summary of this patient's past and present status regarding hypertension treatment and response:

Mr Bennett is a 64-year-old man diagnosed with osteoarthritis and hypertension. He was seen on May 3, 2016, at which time his BP was 160/104 mm Hg. His goal BP range was set as systolic BP of 110–138 mm Hg and diastolic BP of 70–88 mm Hg. This was the standard against which future BP measurements would be compared. He was started on hydrochlorothiazide 25 mg orally once daily for 2 weeks and was to return to clinic for a follow-up BP check and serum potassium level 2 weeks later. He returned according to the plan, but the BP reading of 152/98 mm Hg indicated only a partial improvement. The BP reduction had not yet reached the goal level; it may take 4 weeks for the full effect of diuretic therapy to be manifested. Consequently, no adjustment in therapy was made pending an adequate trial of single-agent diuretic therapy. However, the low serum potassium value of 3.2 mEq/L (reference range 3.5–5.0 mEq/L) indicated hypokalemia that required treatment. Because the hypokalemia may have resulted from the thiazide diuretic, hydrochlorothiazide 25 mg was discontinued and a combination product containing triamterene 37.5 mg + hydrochlorothiazide 25 mg, one tablet orally once daily, was begun. He returned 2 weeks later as planned and his BP continued to show improvement (148/96 mm Hg), but it was not at the therapeutic goal that had been established 4 weeks earlier. This indicated partial improvement requiring further adjustment of his antihypertensive therapy. However, his potassium level had risen to within the normal range. Therefore, atenolol 50 mg orally once daily was added to the regimen. The patient was scheduled to return for a follow-up visit in 1 month.

CONCLUSIONS

Implementation of a care planning process is necessary for providing consistent pharmaceutical care and for documenting the outcomes of that care. It is also essential for obtaining compensation for care provided. Care planning captures past and current events occurring in a dynamic patient care process that is provided in response to changing patient needs. This process should be incorporated into the practice of each pharmacy provider of direct patient care, regardless of the practice setting.

REFERENCES

1. Cipolle RJ, Strand LM, Morley PC. Pharmaceutical Care Practice: The Patient-Centered Approach to Medication Management Services, 3rd ed. New York, McGraw-Hill, 2012.
2. ASHP Council on Professional Affairs. ASHP guidelines on a standard method for pharmaceutical care. Am J Hosp Pharm 1996;53:1713–1716.
3. Rich DS. JCAHO's pharmaceutical care plan requirements. Hosp Pharm 1995;30(4):315–319.
4. McCallian DJ, Carlstedt BC, Rupp MT. Elements of a pharmaceutical care plan. Am J Pharm Assoc 1999;39(1):82–83.
5. Expert Panel on Detection, Evaluation, and Treatment of High Blood Cholesterol in Adults. Executive summary of the third report of the National Cholesterol Education Program (NCEP) Expert Panel on Detection, Evaluation, and Treatment of High Blood Cholesterol in Adults (Adult Treatment Panel III). JAMA 2001;285:2486–2497.
6. Chobaman AV, Bakris GL, Black HR, et al. The seventh report of the Joint National Committee on Prevention, Detection, Evaluation, and Treatment of High Blood Pressure: the JNC 7 report. JAMA 2003;289(19):2560–2572.

APPENDIX A

Sample Patient Care Plan Template

PHARMACEUTICAL CARE PATIENT RECORD

Patient Name:	**Gender:**
Address:	**Race:**
Telephone: **Age:**	**Actual Weight:**
Insurance:	**Ideal Weight:**
Medical Conditions:	**Allergies:**
Tobacco/Alcohol/Substance Use:	**Adverse Reactions:**

Medication Record

Start Date	Stop Date	Indication	Drug Name	Actual Strength	Regimen	Clinical Impressions

Assessment, Plan, and Follow-Up Evaluation

Date	Medical Condition	Drug-Therapy Problem	Goal	Current Status	Interventions	Follow-Up Plan

5

Documentation of Pharmacist Encounters and Interventions

TIMOTHY J. IVES, PharmD, MPH, FCCP, CPP

LORI T. ARMISTEAD, PharmD

If you didn't document it, then it hasn't been done. This adage is the standard in all healthcare settings because all providers must generate and maintain clear and concise records of each patient's health and medical conditions for enhancing workflow, usability, and patient safety, all critical components of quality patient care.[1] Further, documentation is required for providers to receive accurate and timely payment for services. Documentation outlines the care the patient received in a chronological and organized manner, and serves as a form of communication among practitioners, which is an important element that contributes to the quality of care provided. Each practitioner involved knows what evaluation has occurred, what the patient's treatment plan is, and who will provide it. Furthermore, third-party payers may require documentation from practitioners that assures that the services provided are consistent with the insurance coverage.[1,2] General components of documentation include:

- A complete and legible record;
- Date of service, site of service, and identity of the practitioner;
- Documentation for each encounter with a rationale for the encounter, physical findings, prior test results, and identified health risk factors;
- An easily inferred rationale for ordering diagnostic tests or ancillary services, assessment, clinical impression (or diagnosis), and plan for care; and
- Patient progress, response to and changes in treatment, and revision of the original diagnosis/assessment.

Traditionally, this documentation was paper based; however, such records are often inaccessible at the point of care, not easily transferable or transportable, illegible, poorly organized, and missing key information. Due to these limitations, many academic centers and healthcare systems have developed and implemented electronic health records (EHRs). Further, the 2001 Institute of Medicine report *Crossing the Quality Chasm* identified the EHR as a key component in improving provider access to medical information, facilitating decision support and data collection, and reducing medical errors and associated costs.[3] The EHR may also improve documentation with reduced clinical variation, better provision of quality preventative and chronic care, and increased security of confidential patient information.[4-7] Furthermore, EHRs are associated with higher performance on certain quality measures.[8-10]

PRINCIPLES OF DOCUMENTATION

Documentation includes pertinent facts, findings, and observations about a patient's health history, including past and present illnesses, examinations, tests, treatments, and outcomes. With the growth of EHRs, other benefits have been identified:[6,9]

- Enhanced ability of providers to evaluate care, plan immediate treatment, and monitor care over time;
- Easier communication and continuity of care among providers involved in the patient's care;
- More accurate and timely claims review and payment;
- Improvement in the quality of care provided;
- Increased time efficiency;
- Greater adherence to practice guidelines;
- Fewer medication errors and adverse drug events;
- More appropriate utilization review and quality of care evaluations; and
- Greater clarity of coding (ie, Current Procedural Terminology [CPT] and International Statistical Classification of Diseases and Related Health Problems, Tenth Revision, Clinical Modification [ICD-10-CM], from the World Health Organization) on health insurance claim forms, which must be supported by documentation in the patient record.

Much of this documentation is derived from a systematic patient care process that is standardized within each discipline. For example, physicians perform a history and physical examination based on a standardized review of body systems and document their results using a universally accepted, standardized, and systematic process.

Several evaluation/documentation systems have been suggested for healthcare professionals. More than 45 years ago, the use of a Problem-Oriented Medical Record was proposed,[11] and most physicians, nurse practitioners, physician associates, and other healthcare practitioners write progress notes using the Subjective, Objective, Assessment, Plan (SOAP) format. The elements of SOAP are as follows:

S = Subjective: Chief complaint; history of present illness; why the patient is being seen;

O = Objective: Physical findings and measurable data such as laboratory values, drug levels, and imaging studies;

A = Assessment: Analysis or conclusion about the patient's current status/behavior, evidence of progress, response to intervention or medication, and change in functional status;

P = Plan: Interventions or actions taken in response to assessment, collaboration with others, plan for follow-up, change in diagnosis, and documentation that the patient was informed of changes in interventions and/or medications.

Institutional consultant notes often use an abbreviated version of the SOAP format. This abbreviated version usually includes Findings (ie, subjective and objective information), Assessment (or Impression), and Diagnosis (or Recommendations). In most cases, the EHR has embraced many of the key components of the above formats.

EHR documentation is tailored to documenting medical encounters and history, and also to maximize billing by meeting requirements established by the U.S. Centers for Medicare & Medicaid Services. Traditionally, this documentation was performed by dictation and transcription. Most EHRs use predetermined templates to accept automated insertion of clinical data to facilitate the documentation process.

DOCUMENTING PHARMACIST-PROVIDED PATIENT CARE

The provision of health care is evolving into team-based, patient-centered care, with the pharmacist serving as an accountable and integral member of that team.[12] As one example, pharmacists have been shown to identify drug therapy problems with greater confidence when having access to patients' primary care health records, and such access can help community pharmacists to build an efficient and comprehensive medication management practice.[13] Growth in pharmacists' clinical acumen has resulted in the need for a standardized patient care process by pharmacists that is applicable to all pharmacy practice settings.[14] In 2013, the Joint Commission of Pharmacy Practitioners (JCPP) adopted a vision for pharmacy practice in which patients achieve optimal health and medication outcomes with pharmacists as essential and accountable providers within patient-centered, team-based health care.[15] In 2014, the JCPP promulgated a process of care for the delivery of patient care services provided by pharmacists in any practice setting.[16] Collaboration, communication, and documentation are key components in that process. The need for interoperable information technology systems to facilitate efficient documentation and effective communication among all healthcare practitioners also has been identified.

As described in **Chapter 1**, a systematic approach is used in this Casebook to identify and resolve the medication-related problems of patients. The steps can be summarized as follows:

1. Identification of real or potential medication therapy problems;
2. Determination of desired therapeutic outcomes and therapeutic end points;
3. Determination of therapeutic alternatives;
4. Design of an optimal pharmacotherapeutic plan for the patient;
5. Identification of parameters to evaluate the outcome;
6. Provision of patient education;
7. Communication and implementation of the pharmacotherapeutic plan.

Step 7 is crucial; at the very least, pharmacists should document the actual or potential drug therapy problems identified, as well as the associated interventions that they desire to implement or have implemented. Pharmacists must adequately communicate their recommendations and actions to nonpharmacy healthcare practitioners (eg, physicians, nurses), the patient or caregiver (eg, parents), or other pharmacists. The goal is to provide a clear, concise record of the actual/potential problem,[17,18] the thought process that led the pharmacist to select an intervention, and the intervention itself. Additionally, the ability to receive remuneration for services provided also necessitates an acceptable documentation strategy.

MEDICATION THERAPY MANAGEMENT (MTM)

MTM has been defined as a distinct service or group of services that optimize therapeutic outcomes for individual patients.[19] Pharmacists are the largest provider of MTM services,[20] which are independent of, but can occur in conjunction with, provision of a medication product. MTM encompasses a broad range of professional activities and responsibilities within the scope of practice of the licensed pharmacist or other qualified healthcare providers. MTM interventions include, but are not limited to, the following patient-focused activities:[21]

- Performing or obtaining necessary assessments of the patient's health status;
- Formulating a medication treatment plan;
- Selecting, initiating, modifying, or administering medication therapy;
- Monitoring and evaluating the patient's response to therapy, including safety and effectiveness;
- Performing a comprehensive medication review to identify, resolve, and prevent medication-related problems, including adverse drug events;
- Documenting the care delivered and communicating essential information to the patient's other primary care providers;
- Providing verbal education and training designed to enhance patient understanding and appropriate use of his or her medications;
- Providing information, support services, and resources designed to enhance patient adherence with his or her therapeutic regimens;
- Coordinating and integrating MTM services within the broader healthcare management services being provided to the patient.

In this process, the pharmacist is responsible for documenting services in a manner appropriate for evaluating patient progress and sufficient for billing purposes. The use of core documentation elements helps create consistency in documentation and information sharing among members of the healthcare team, while facilitating practitioner, organization, and regional variations.[19] Documentation of MTM services includes the following information categories:

- Patient demographics;
- Known allergies, diseases (eg, heart failure), or conditions (eg, pregnancy);
- A record of all medications, including prescription, nonprescription, herbal, and other dietary supplement products;
- Assessment of medication therapy problems and plans for resolution;
- Therapeutic monitoring performed;
- Interventions or referrals made;
- Education provided to the patient;
- Feedback provided to providers or patients;
- Schedule and plan for follow-up appointment;
- Amount of time spent with the patient;
- Appropriate billing codes.

Similarly, the American Society of Health-System Pharmacists (ASHP) has suggested the following categories of information that a pharmacist may need to document in the patient medical record (PMR):[22]

- A summary of the patient's medication history on admission, including medication allergies and their manifestations;
- Oral and written consultations provided to other healthcare professionals regarding the patient's drug therapy selection and management;
- Physicians' oral orders received directly by the pharmacist;

- Clarification of drug orders;
- Adjustments made to drug dosage, dosage frequency, dosage form, or route of administration;
- Drugs, including investigational drugs, administered;
- Actual and potential drug-related problems that warrant surveillance;
- Pharmacotherapy monitoring findings, including:
  - ✓ Therapeutic appropriateness of the patient's drug regimen, including the route and method of administration;
  - ✓ Therapeutic duplication in the patient's drug regimen;
  - ✓ The degree of patient compliance with the prescribed drug regimen;
  - ✓ Actual and potential drug–drug, drug–food, drug–laboratory test, and drug–disease interactions;
  - ✓ Clinical and pharmacokinetic laboratory data pertinent to the drug regimen;
  - ✓ Actual and potential drug toxicity and adverse effects;
  - ✓ Physical signs and clinical symptoms relevant to the patient's pharmacotherapy.
- Drug-related patient education and counseling provided.

THE SOAP NOTE FORMAT FOR DOCUMENTATION

As discussed previously, in the SOAP note format subjective (S) and objective (O) data are recorded and then assessed (A) to formulate a plan (P). Subjective data include patient symptoms (eg, pain), clinician observations (eg, agitation), or information obtained about the patient (eg, history of smoking). By its nature, subjective information is descriptive and generally cannot be confirmed by diagnostic tests or procedures. Much of the subjective information is obtained by speaking with the patient while obtaining the medical history, as described in **Chapter 1** (ie, chief complaint, history of present illness, past medical history, family history, social history, medications, allergies, and review of systems). Important subjective information may also be obtained by direct interview with the patient after the initial medical history has been performed (eg, a description of an adverse drug effect, rating of pain severity using standard scales).

A primary source of objective information (O) is the physical examination. Other relevant objective information includes laboratory values, serum drug concentrations (along with the target therapeutic range for each level), and the results of other diagnostic tests (eg, electrocardiogram [ECG], X-rays, culture, and sensitivity tests). Risk factors that may predispose the patient to a particular problem should also be considered for inclusion. The communication note should include only the pertinent positive and negative findings. Pertinent negative findings are signs and symptoms of the disease or problem that are not present in the particular patient being evaluated.

The assessment (A) section outlines what the practitioner thinks the patient's problem is, based on the subjective and objective information acquired. This assessment often takes the form of a diagnosis or differential diagnosis. This portion of the SOAP note should include all of the reasons for the clinician's assessment. This helps other healthcare providers reading the note to understand how the clinician arrived at his or her particular assessment of the problem.

The plan (P) may include ordering additional diagnostic tests or initiating, revising, or discontinuing treatment. If the plan includes changes in pharmacotherapy, the rationale for the specific changes recommended should be described. The drug, dose, dosage form, schedule, route of administration, and duration of therapy should be included. The plan should be directed toward achieving a specific, measurable goal or end point, which should be clearly stated in the note. The plan should also outline the efficacy and toxicity parameters that will be used to determine whether the desired therapeutic outcome is being achieved and to detect or prevent drug-related adverse events. Ideally, information about the therapy that should be communicated to the patient should also be included in the plan. The plan should be reviewed and referred to in the note as often as necessary.

FARM NOTE FOR DOCUMENTING PHARMACOTHERAPY PROBLEMS AND PLANS

While there is no current, uniform documentation system specific to pharmacy, a pharmacist's equivalent of a physician's progress note, differing somewhat in approach, has been proposed for the construction and maintenance of a record reflecting the pharmacist's contributions to care.[23] This process includes provisions for the identification and assessment of actual or potential medication-related problems, description of a therapeutic plan, and appropriate follow-up monitoring of the problems. In this system, medication-related problems that have been identified are addressed systematically in a pharmacist's note under the headings Findings, Assessment, Resolution/Recommendation, and Monitoring. The sections of the pharmacist's note can be easily recalled with the mnemonic F-A-R-M.

IDENTIFICATION OF DRUG THERAPY PROBLEMS

The first step in the construction of a FARM note is to clearly state the nature of the drug-related problem(s). Each problem in the FARM note should be addressed separately and assigned a sequential number. Understanding the types of problems that may occur facilitates identification of pharmacotherapy problems. Several classifications of medication-related problems have been suggested, and include:[24,25]

- Unnecessary or suboptimal drug therapy
- Ineffective drug
- Dosage too low or too high
- Adverse drug events
- Noncompliance
- Suboptimal duration of treatment
- Noncost effective medication use
- Inadequate or lack of medication monitoring

Use of classification systems such as these for the various types of medication-related problems offers at least two advantages. First, it presents a framework, applicable in any practice setting, to assure that the pharmacist has considered each possible type of problem. Second, categorization allows optimal data analysis and retrieval capabilities. Thus, problems as well as the interventions to resolve them can be stored in a standardized format in a computer. When an analysis of this information is needed at a later date, such as determining how much money was saved through an intervention, how outcomes were improved by the pharmacist, or how many problems of a certain type have occurred, the problems and interventions can be reviewed by groups rather than individually.

DOCUMENTATION OF FINDINGS

Each statement of a drug-related problem should be followed by documentation of the pertinent findings (F) indicating that the problem may or does exist. Information included in this section should include a summary of the pertinent information obtained after collection and thorough assessment of the available patient information. Demographic data that may be reported include a patient identifier (eg, name, initials, or medical record number), age, race (if pertinent), and gender. As noted earlier in the section "The SOAP Note Format for Documentation," medical information included in the note should include both subjective and objective findings that indicate a drug-related problem.

ASSESSMENT OF PROBLEMS

The assessment (A) section of the FARM note includes the pharmacist's evaluation of the current situation (ie, the nature, extent, type, and clinical significance of the problem). This part of the note should delineate the thought process that led to the conclusion that a problem did or did not exist and that an active intervention either was or was not necessary. If additional information is required to satisfactorily assess the problem and make recommendations, then these data should be stated along with their source (eg, the patient, pharmacist, or physician). The severity or urgency of the problem should be indicated by stating whether the interventions that follow should be made immediately or within 1 day, 1 week, 1 month, or longer. The desired therapeutic end point or outcome should be stated. This may include both short-term goals (eg, lower blood pressure [BP] to <140/90 mm Hg in a patient with primary hypertension [HTN] [therapeutic endpoint]) and long-term goals (eg, prevent cardiovascular complications in that patient [therapeutic outcome]).

PROBLEM RESOLUTION

The resolution (R) section should reflect the actions proposed (or already performed) to resolve the drug-related problem based on the preceding analysis. The note should convey that, after consideration of all appropriate therapeutic options, the option(s) considered to be the most beneficial was either carried out or suggested to someone else (eg, the primary care provider, patient, or caregiver). Recommendations may include nonpharmacologic therapy, such as dietary modification or assistive devices (eg, cane, walker, and wheelchair); the rationale for this method of treatment should be described. If pharmacotherapy is recommended, a specific drug, dose, route, schedule, and duration of therapy should be specified. It is not sufficient to simply provide a list of choices for the prescriber. Importantly, the rationale for selecting the particular regimen(s) should be stated. It is reasonable to include alternative regimens that would be satisfactory if the patient is unable to complete treatment with the initial regimen because of adverse effects, allergy, cost, or other reasons. If patient education is recommended, the information that will be included in the session should be described. Conversely, if certain types of information will be withheld from the patient, the reasons for doing so should be stated. If no action is recommended or was taken, that should be documented as well. In this situation, the note serves as a record of the pharmacist's involvement in the patient's care. The pharmacist then has documentation that patient care activities were performed.

MONITORING FOR ENDPOINTS AND OUTCOMES

It is not enough to only provide a clear, concise record of the nature of a problem, the assessment that led to the conclusion that a problem exists, and the selection of a plan for resolution of the problem. To truly "close the loop" of patient care, follow-up on the plan must occur to assure that the intended outcome was achieved. A plan for follow-up monitoring (M) of the patient must be documented and adequately implemented. This process should include questioning the patient, gathering laboratory data, and performing the ongoing physical assessments necessary to determine the effect of the plan that was implemented to assure that it results in an optimal outcome for the patient.

Monitoring parameters to assess efficacy generally include improvement in or resolution of the signs, symptoms, and laboratory abnormalities that were initially assessed. The monitoring parameters used to detect or prevent adverse reactions are determined by the most common and most serious events known to be associated with the therapeutic intervention. Potential adverse reactions should be precisely described along with the method of monitoring. For example, rather than stating "monitor for gastrointestinal (GI) complaints," the recommendation may be to "question the patient about the presence of dyspepsia, diarrhea, or constipation." The frequency, duration, and target endpoint for each monitoring parameter should be identified. The points at which changes in the plan may be warranted should be included. For example, in the case of a patient with type 2 diabetes mellitus (DM), one may recommend to "return to clinic (RTC) in 2 weeks to check blood glucose (BG) levels; recheck lipids in 4–6 weeks and recheck A1C in 3 months. If the goal A1C < 7% is not achieved with good adherence at 3 months, increase metformin from 500 mg by mouth twice daily to metformin 1000 mg by mouth twice daily. If goal A1C is achieved, maintain metformin 500 mg by mouth twice daily and repeat A1C in 6 months."

SUMMARY

A SOAP or FARM progress note constructed in the manner described identifies each drug-related problem and states the pharmacist's Findings observed, an Assessment of the findings, the actual or proposed Resolution of the problem based on the analysis, and the parameters and timing of follow-up Monitoring. Either form of note should provide a clear, concise record of process, activity, and projected follow-up. When written for each medication-related problem, these notes should provide data in a standardized, logical system.

Based on recommendations from organizations such as the Institute of Medicine, Centers for Medicare & Medicaid Services, and researchers involved in the provision of quality of care, EHRs will continue to proliferate and change the way pharmacists and other healthcare providers document patient care encounters. Although the format of the documentation may not strictly follow the SOAP or FARM format, the common principles of documentation will remain.

SAMPLE CASE PRESENTATION

The following case presentation illustrates how such a system can be used in practice.

Julia Stevens is a 71-year-old woman seen Monday morning in clinic for her first visit.

CHIEF COMPLAINT

"I get a little short of breath working around the house sometimes, and my feet have been bothering me recently."

HISTORY OF PRESENT ILLNESS

She states that she has mild heart failure and had a heart attack 4 years ago. She lives alone and has generally maintained a good level of activity and self care; however, she reports watching a lot of television and not getting out very much. She complains of some fatigue and shortness of breath while cleaning her house or when climbing stairs. She also complains of occasional pain and tingling in her feet, which she says has become bothersome over the past few months.

PAST MEDICAL HISTORY

She has just moved to town to be near her son following the death of her husband. In addition to her CHF and MI history, she has a history of atrial fibrillation and type 2 DM. She is maintained on metformin 500 mg PO BID, omeprazole 20 mg PO daily, digoxin 0.125 mg PO Q AM, warfarin 5 mg PO Q AM, enteric-coated (EC) aspirin 81 mg PO Q AM, furosemide 40 mg PO daily, and metoprolol XL 100 mg PO Q AM.

FAMILY HISTORY

Her husband died recently. She has one son alive and well living in the area and had one son who committed suicide 8 years ago.

SOCIAL HISTORY

She denies illicit drugs and quit smoking 15 years ago. She has a 35 pack-year history. She drinks alcohol rarely on social occasions and denies excessive use.

MEDICATIONS

Metformin 500 mg PO BID

Omeprazole 20 mg PO daily

Digoxin 0.125 mg PO Q AM

Warfarin 5 mg PO Q AM

EC aspirin 81 mg PO Q AM

Furosemide 40 mg PO Q AM

Metoprolol XL 100 mg PO Q AM

ALLERGIES

Penicillins (rash)

REVIEW OF SYSTEMS

General: Denies weight loss, fevers, or chills. Complains of occasional fatigue/SOB upon exertion.

HEENT: Last eye exam was less than 2 years ago, no hearing loss, tinnitus, mouth sores, sees dentist regularly, no voice change, sinus congestion.

Pulmonary: No cough, pneumonia, tuberculosis exposure, orthopnea, paroxysmal nocturnal dyspnea.

Cardiac: No known murmur, rheumatic fever, palpitations, chest pressure/pain.

GI: No dysphagia, odynophagia, nausea, vomiting, abdominal pain, diarrhea, constipation, melena, hematochezia, or change in stool caliber.

Genitourinary: No h/o STI; no urinary pain, burning, blood, or nocturia; no sexual dysfunction/dissatisfaction.

Hematologic: No bruising, bleeding problems.

Endocrine: No thyroid disease, hot/cold intolerance, polyuria/polydipsia.

Vascular: No leg pain with walking.

Neurologic: Pain/tingling in feet. Denies dizziness, weakness, balance, or gait problems.

Dermatologic: No rashes, skin lesions.

Psychiatric: No anxiety or depression, notes she had a difficult time adjusting to her husband's untimely death, but now feels she is doing fine.

PHYSICAL EXAMINATION

General

The patient is a 71-year-old Caucasian female whose appearance is consistent with her stated age. She appears well developed, well nourished, and in no acute distress.

Vital Signs

BP 169/88, P68 and regular, RR 13, T 99°F; Weight 184 lb, Height 5′4″

Skin

Unremarkable

HEENT

Slight arteriovenous (AV) nicking, otherwise unremarkable

Neck/Lymph Nodes

Neck supple, thyroid normal with no mass, nodules, or tenderness; JVP 6 cm; normal carotid pulsations; no carotid bruits

No cervical, supraclavicular, axillary, or inguinal lymphadenopathy

Chest/Lungs

Slight crackles at the right and left bases; no rales, e-to-a changes, or tactile fremitus

Breasts

Normal breasts without pain, swelling, discharge, or masses

Cardiovascular

No murmurs or rubs. (+) S_3 gallop; PMI in the fifth intercostal space 3 cm to the left of the midclavicular line. (+) Hepatojugular reflux. Mild neck vein distention at 45°.

Abdomen

Soft, nontender, nondistended, bowel sounds normal. No hepatosplenomegaly.

Genital/Rectal

Unremarkable

Musculoskeletal/Extremities

1–2+ pedal edema bilaterally. Ankle brachial index (ABI) 1.02 (negative). Strength 5/5.

Neurologic

Cranial nerves II–XII grossly intact bilaterally

Semmes–Weinstein monofilament is unremarkable

Deep tendon reflexes brisk and 3/4 bilaterally

Laboratory Values Are Unremarkable with the Following Exceptions

INR 3.5

FBG 198 mg/dL

A1C 9.5% = eAG 226 mg/dL

Serum creatinine 1.3 mg/dL

TC 183 mg/dL, LDL 128 mg/dL, HDL 38 mg/dL, TG 150 mg/dL

Digoxin level 1.0 ng/mL

Imaging

Chest X-ray demonstrates some diffuse patchiness at the bases. Enlarged cardiac silhouette.

Echo reveals no valvular abnormalities with an ejection fraction of 40%.

Electrocardiogram

Normal sinus rhythm. Changes are consistent with left ventricular hypertrophy.

Medical Assessment

1. Mild, Class II–III heart failure with pedal edema and mild pulmonary congestion; taking digoxin, furosemide, and metoprolol.

2. Type 2 diabetes mellitus, not optimally controlled on metformin.

3. Peripheral neuropathy symptoms, currently untreated.

4. Atrial fibrillation, currently rate-controlled on digoxin and metoprolol. Warfarin anticoagulation per guidelines above target (target INR 2–3).

5. Hypertension not optimally managed on metoprolol.

6. Clinical ASCVD (S/P MI) on aspirin and metoprolol; no statin therapy.

7. Moderate renal insufficiency stage 3: SCr 1.3, estimated ClCr 29 mL/min, glomerular filtration rate (GFR) Michigan Disability Resource Directory (MDRD)[26] 43 mL/min.

8. Obesity: BMI 31.6 kg/m^2.

9. Medication with no indication: Omeprazole.

10. Adverse medication effects associated with β-blocker use.

11. Patient nonadherence/noncompliance with medication use.

MEDICAL PLAN

1. CHF: Increase furosemide to 40 mg PO BID. Consult Cardiology for evaluation of CHF.

2. Type 2 diabetes mellitus: Increase metformin to 1000 mg PO BID, Consult diabetes teaching nurse for education and review of injection technique should insulin become necessary.

3. Peripheral neuropathy: Initiate gabapentin therapy at 100 mg PO QHS.

4. Atrial fibrillation: Decrease warfarin dose. Continue digoxin and metoprolol.

5. Hypertension: Add ACE inhibitor or an ARB for BP reduction and renal protection.

6. Clinical ASCVD (S/P MI): Continue metoprolol and aspirin, add a high-intensity statin.

7. Consult nephrology for evaluation of renal insufficiency.

8. Obesity: Counsel on lifestyle modifications for weight reduction.

9. Discontinue omeprazole.

10. Clinic appointment for follow-up in 2 weeks. Will reassess medication adherence at that time, and offer recommendations to enhance medication use.

CONSTRUCTION OF A SOAP OR FARM NOTE

Note: The Subjective and Objective findings of the SOAP note are combined into Findings for a FARM note. The Plan of the SOAP note is split into Recommendations/Resolution and Monitoring/Follow-Up in the FARM note.

Findings

Subjective A 71-year-old woman recently moved here after the death of her husband. Patient complains of slight shortness of breath when walking up stairs and long distances as well as occasional pain and tingling in her feet. She has a history of atrial fibrillation, type 2 diabetes mellitus, mild–moderate heart failure, and S/P MI 4 years ago. She lives alone and maintains a good level of self care but reports few outings and a lot of television watching at home. She reports that she takes metformin, omeprazole, digoxin, warfarin, aspirin, furosemide, and metoprolol. She states that she takes her medications as prescribed, but she has some difficulty describing precisely how she takes them and is not certain what each medication does for her.

Objective

VS: BP 169/88, P 68 and regular, RR 13, T 99.0°F; Weight 184 lbs, Height = 5′4″

Cardiac: S$_3$ gallop, PMI in the fifth intercostal space 3 cm to the left of the midclavicular line

Chest: Slight crackles at the right and left bases

Extremities: 1–2+ pedal edema bilaterally, ABI negative

HEENT: Slight AV nicking, otherwise unremarkable

Medications (per labels on vials):

   Metformin 500 mg PO BID

   Omeprazole 20 mg PO daily

   Digoxin 0.125 mg PO Q AM

   Warfarin 5 mg PO Q AM

   EC aspirin 81 mg PO Q AM

   Furosemide 40 mg PO Q AM

   Metoprolol XL 100 mg PO Q AM

Labs:

   INR 3.5

   Fasting blood glucose 198 mg/dL

   A1C 9.5% (eAG 226 mg/dL)

   Serum creatinine 1.3 mg/dL

   TC 183 mg/dL, LDL 128 mg/dL, HDL 38 mg/dL, TG 150 mg/dL

   Serum digoxin 1.0 ng/mL

Chest X-ray: Diffuse patchiness at the bases. Enlarged cardiac silhouette.

ECG: LVH

Assessment

1. Mild heart failure, Class II, as suggested by pedal edema, DOE, symptoms on engaging in ordinary activities, cardiomegaly on chest X-ray, and diminished EF. Maintained on a β-blocker and digoxin (level within target range) and is not currently prescribed an ACE inhibitor.

2. Type 2 diabetes mellitus, not well controlled on current metformin dose. A1C above goal of <7%. Not prescribed either an ACE inhibitor or an ARB for renal protective effects.

3. Patient experiencing symptoms of peripheral neuropathy: Pain and tingling in her feet.

4. Atrial fibrillation:

   a. Rate control: Rate currently under control with metoprolol and digoxin. Digoxin level acceptable. No adjustment indicated.

   b. Anticoagulation: INR above target range of 2.0–3.0, without clinical complications at this time. No cause could be identified; although a change in diet associated with recent life events is possible, the patient provides no information to substantiate that idea. Decreased warfarin dose may be appropriate.

5. Hypertension, not optimally controlled on metoprolol, as suggested by increased BP, elevated serum creatinine, and AV nicking. The renal and ophthalmic findings are suggestive of significant, sustained hypertension. Repeated measurements will be necessary to confirm this assessment. Addition of ACE inhibitor may improve control as well.

6. Clinical ASCVD (S/P MI): On low-dose aspirin and metoprolol; no statin therapy.

7. Possible moderate renal insufficiency as indicated by increased SCr/decreased GFR by MDRD. Renal dose adjustments evaluated. No changes necessary at this time. Addition of ACE inhibitor therapy may be beneficial to slow rate of GFR decline.

8. Obesity: Classified as obese with BMI 31.6 kg/m^2.

9. Medication without indication (omeprazole 20 mg): On further questioning, the patient recalls being started on it while hospitalized for MI 4 years ago. She was given a prescription upon discharge. She has no complaints related to GERD or PUD. No need for omeprazole can be identified.

10. Adverse medication effects: Although metoprolol may be considered appropriate for both the post-MI and CHF indications and is a β$_1$-selective β-blocker, its β$_2$-blocking properties may contribute to worsening CHF due to negative inotropic effects.

11. Possible nonadherence/nonconcordance and lack of knowledge about medications.

Plan (Recommendations/Resolution)

1. Mild heart failure: Continue both the β-blocker metoprolol and digoxin, pending evaluation by the Cardiology Service to determine appropriateness. Suggest initiation of an ACE inhibitor: Lisinopril 10 mg daily titrating to 40 mg daily as tolerated. Increase furosemide to 40 mg PO BID because of persistent pedal edema and pulmonary congestion. No added dietary salt. Reassess medications at follow-up in 2 weeks.

2. Type 2 diabetes mellitus:

   a. Medication: Start lisinopril 10 mg daily as above per current ADA guidelines. Suggest increasing metformin to 1000 mg PO BID to improve blood glucose control. Continue to follow serum creatinine. Monitor blood glucose readings and, if indicated, supplement with insulin lispro for elevated pre-meal BG, based on an estimated insulin sensitivity of 1 unit per 30–40 mg/dL.

   b. Diet: Encourage three meals and bedtime snack, with no concentrated carbohydrate (CHO) choices. Limit CHO intake per meal to 60 g; snacks 15–20 g of CHO. No added salt. Check blood glucose AC and HS. Refer to dietitian.

3. Peripheral neuropathy: Start gabapentin 100 mg PO Q HS. If necessary, titrate dose over several weeks to 300 mg PO BID for better symptom control, as tolerated.

4. Atrial fibrillation:

   a. Rate control: Suggest continuing metoprolol and digoxin unless Cardiology recommends otherwise. No adjustment indicated at this time.

   b. Anticoagulation: INR is above target range of 2.0–3.0. Recommend warfarin 2.5 mg today and then resume 5 mg PO daily Monday–Saturday and 2.5 mg on Sunday (decrease in total weekly dose by 7.1%). Recheck INR in 2 weeks; adjust dose as needed to maintain INR between 2.0 and 3.0.

5. Hypertension: Present BP is ≥ 160/100 mm Hg; goal is < 140/90 mm Hg per ADA 2015 Standards of Medical Care in Diabetes. Start lisinopril 10 mg daily as recommended above. If repeated measurements confirm HTN diagnosis, titrate dose to maintain BP control (and improve CHF symptoms); target dose 40 mg daily.

6. Clinical ASCVD (S/PMI): Recommend continuation of EC aspirin 81 mg PO Q AM. Suggest initiation of lisinopril as noted above and a high-intensity statin (atorvastatin 40 mg PO daily). Continue metoprolol, if acceptable to Cardiology.

7. Renal insufficiency: Repeat serum creatinine. No medication dosage adjustments are indicated currently. Begin low-dose ACE inhibitor (lisinopril 10 mg daily as above) for renal protective effects with diabetes to slow rate of GFR decline.

8. Obesity: Counsel on lifestyle modifications for weight reduction.

9. Medication without indication: Discontinue omeprazole 20 mg.

10. Adverse medication effects: As noted above, will await Cardiology opinion on need for/appropriateness of β-blocker and digoxin to manage CHF.

11. Assess and reinforce adherence/concordance with recommended therapy. Educate on purpose of each medication. Recommend a pill-box organizer to improve adherence.

Monitoring/Follow-Up

1. RTC in 2 weeks.

2. Prior to RTC:

   Labtests (orders entered):

   a. Baseline electrolytes today (K, Na, Ca, and Mg levels in light of unopposed furosemide therapy of unknown duration and use of digoxin)

   b. Serum creatinine today

   c. INR at next clinic visit

3. Consultation:

   a. Cardiology consultation/education. Appointment made with Dr Welford's office.

   b. Dietary consultation. Appointment made with Mary Ann Stamos, RD.

4. Patient was instructed to monitor blood glucose before meals and at bedtime and to bring information on RTC.

5. Prescribed medication after this visit:

- Lisinopril 10 mg PO daily for CHF, hypertension, and type 2 DM

- Metformin 1000 mg PO BID for type 2 DM

- Insulin lispro, as indicated

- Gabapentin 100 mg PO QHS for peripheral neuropathy, with a 2-week titration to 300 mg PO BID

- Digoxin 0.125 mg PO Q AM for CHF symptoms and rate control

- Furosemide 40 mg PO BID for CHF

- Warfarin 5 mg PO Q AM Monday–Saturday, 2.5 mg on Sunday for S/P MI and CVA prevention

- EC aspirin 81 mg PO daily for secondary cardiovascular prevention

- Metoprolol XL 100 mg PO Q AM for S/P MI and rate control

- Atorvastatin 40 mg PO daily for secondary ASCVD prevention

- D/C omeprazole

REFERENCES

1. Patterson ES, Lowry SZ, Ramaiah M, et al. Improving clinical workflow in ambulatory care: implemented recommendations in an innovation prototype for the Veteran's Health Administration. EGEMS (Washington, DC). 2015;3(2):1149.

2. Evaluation and Management Services Guide. Washington, DC: Centers for Medicare & Medicaid Services; November 2014. www.cms.gov/Outreach-and-Education/Medicare-Learning-Network-MLN/MLNProducts/downloads/eval_mgmt_serv_guide-ICN006764.pdf. Accessed October 25, 2015.

3. Institute of Medicine. Crossing the Quality Chasm: A New Health System for the 21st Century. Washington, DC: National Academy Press; 2001.

4. Bates DW, Gawande AA. Improving safety with information technology. N Engl J Med. 2003;348:2526–2534.

5. Andel C, Davidow SL, Hollander M, et al. The economics of health care quality and medical errors. J Health Care Finance. 2012;39:39–50.

6. Wright A, McCoy AB, Hickman TT, et al. Problem list completeness in electronic health records: a multi-site study and assessment of success factors. Int J Med Inform. 2015;84(10):784–790.

7. Jamoom E, Beatty P, Bercovitz A, et al. Physician Adoption of Electronic Health Record Systems: United States, 2011. NCHS Data Brief, No. 98. Hyattsville, MD: National Center for Health Statistics; 2012.

8. Poon EG, Wright A, Simon SR, et al. Relationship between use of electronic health record features and health care quality: results of a statewide survey. Med Care. 2010;48:203–209.

9. Campanella P, Lovato E, Marone C, et al. The impact of electronic health records on healthcare quality: a systematic review and meta-analysis. Eur J Public Health. 2015;Jun 30. pii:ckv122. http://dx.doi.org/10.1093/eurpub/ckv122.

10. McNally ME. The importance of detailed documentation in ICD-10. Bull Am Coll Surg. 2015;100(8):63–64.

11. Weed LL. Medical records that guide and teach. N Engl J Med. 1968;278:593–600, 652–657.

12. Adams AJ, Clark DR, DeLander GE, et al. Report of the AACP task force on patient-centered medical homes and accountable care organizations. Am J Pharm Educ. 2013;77(7):Article 142.

13. van Lint JA, Sorge LA, Sorensen TD. Access to patients' health records for drug therapy problem determination by pharmacists. J Am Pharm Assoc. 2015;55:278–281.

14. American College of Clinical Pharmacy. Standards of practice for clinical pharmacists. Pharmacotherapy. 2014;34(8):792–795.

15. Bennett MS, Kliethermes MA, Derr S, Irwin A. APhA academies reflect on the pharmacists' patient care process of the joint commission of pharmacy practitioners. J Am Pharm Assoc. 2015;55:230–236.

16. Joint Commission of Pharmacy Practitioners. Pharmacists' patient care process. http://www.pharmacist.com/sites/default/files/files/PatientCareProcess.pdf. Accessed October 27, 2015.

17. Donnelly WJ. The language of medical case histories. Ann Intern Med. 1997;127:1045–1048.

18. Voytovich AE. Reduction of medical verbiage. Ann Intern Med. 1999;131:146–147.

19. Bluml BM. Definition of medication therapy management: development of professionwide consensus. J Am Pharm Assoc. 2005;45:566–572.

20. Center for Medicare and Medicaid Services. 2015. Medication Therapy Management (MTM) Fact Sheet. https://www.cms.gov/medicare/prescription-drug-coverage/prescriptiondrugcovcontra/mtm.html. Accessed November 8, 2015.

21. American Pharmacists Association, National Association of Chain Drug Stores Foundation. Medication therapy management in pharmacy practice: core elements of an MTM service model (version 2.0). J Am Pharm Assoc. 2008;48(3):341–353.

22. American Society of Health-System Pharmacists. ASHP guidelines on documenting pharmaceutical care in patient medical records. Am J Health Syst Pharm. 2003;60:705–707.

23. Canaday BR, Yarborough PC. Documenting pharmaceutical care: creating a standard. Ann Pharmacother. 1994;28:1292–1296.

24. Cipolle RJ, Strand LM, Morley PC. Pharmaceutical Care Practice: The Clinician's Guide. 3rd ed. New York, NY: McGraw-Hill; 2012.

25. Roth MT, Moore CG, Ivey JL, et al. The quality of medication use in older adults: methods of a longitudinal study. Am J Geriatr Pharmacother. 2008;6:220–233.

26. Levey AS, Bosch JP, Lewis JB, et al. A more accurate method to estimate glomerular filtration rate from serum creatinine: a new prediction equation. Modification of Diet in Renal Disease Study Group. Ann Intern Med. 1999;130:461–470.

6

PEDIATRICS

Children Are Not Just Little Adults . . . . Level III

Amanda Geist, PharmD

LEARNING OBJECTIVES

After completing this case study, the reader should be able to:

- Determine the role that the rate and extent of organ development plays in the variation of absorption, distribution, metabolism, and elimination of medications in the pediatric population.

- Compare and contrast the pharmacokinetic and pharmacodynamic differences between pediatric and adult patients, as well as among various pediatric age groups.

- Identify and manage challenges in pediatric pain management.

- Identify and manage challenges in pediatric drug formulation and administration.

PATIENT PRESENTATION

■ Chief Complaint

Nursing reports of new-onset fever and hypotension, increased number of apnea episodes, and "infant acting different."

■ HPI

Alexander Halstrom is a premature 730-g male infant born at 25 4/7 weeks, now day of life 22, who is currently intubated, sedated, on vasopressors and parenteral nutrition with new-onset fever, increased number of apnea episodes, and a 1-day history of "acting different" according to nursing reports.

■ PMH

Prematurity: born at 25 4/7 weeks with APGARs of 1, 4, and 6
Extremely low birth weight (ELBW) = 760 g
Respiratory distress syndrome (RDS)
Anemia
Apnea of prematurity
At risk for retinopathy of prematurity
Cholestasis
Diaper dermatitis
Grade II intraventricular hemorrhage (IVH)
Hypotension
Microcephaly, head circumference below 10th percentile
Newborn sepsis
NPO, receiving nutritional support
Patent ductus arteriosus (PDA)—small with left-to-right shunt
Pulmonary hemorrhage
Immunizations up-to-date

■ FH

Infant born to a 24-year-old Gravida 2 Para 0 Abortion 1 (G2 P0 AB1) mother secondary to polyhydramnios, nonreassuring fetal status, and premature onset of labor

Maternal labs: HBsAg (–), rubella (–), VDRL (–), and HIV (–) with unknown GBS status who received partial penicillin prophylaxis prior to delivery and indomethacin for tocolysis.
Mother denies drug and alcohol use during pregnancy.

■ SH

Noncontributory

■ Current Meds

Ampicillin 73 mg IV every 12 hours (200 mg/kg per day)
Gentamicin 1.8 mg IV every 8 hours (7.5 mg/kg per day)
Caffeine 3.7 mg IV every 24 hours (5 mg/kg per day)
Phenobarbital 3.7 mg IV every 24 hours (5 mg/kg per day; off-label use for cholestasis)
Morphine continuous infusion 10 mcg/kg/hour
Midazolam continuous infusion 0.05 mg/kg/hour
Dopamine continuous IV infusion 10 mcg/kg/min
TPN at total fluid volume of 150 mL/kg per day
Nystatin 100,000 U/g cream one application to affected area PRN
Aquaphor, one application to affected area PRN
Glycerin suppository, one PR every 24 hours PRN constipation
Acetaminophen 7.3 mg PO/PR every 6 hours PRN pain/fever (10 mg/kg/dose)

■ All

NKDA

■ Physical Examination

Gen

Intubated, sedated, premature infant in an isolette with hypotension who requires intensive cardiac and respiratory monitoring and continuous vital sign assessment.

VS

BP 43/23, HR 178, RR 73, current temperature: 38.7°C, O_2 saturation: 92%

HEENT

Anterior fontanelle soft, open, flat

Neck

Supple, nontender, no masses, no lymphadenopathy

Lungs

Tachypneic; positive crackles and rhonchi; equal breath sounds

CV

Tachycardic, regular rhythm, 3/6 systolic murmur; normal pulses

Abd

Soft, nontender, nondistended; no masses or organomegaly; (+) bowel sounds

Genit

Normal male external genitalia; rectal exam deferred

Ext

No deformities noted; normal range of motion in all extremities

Skin

Skin is thin and vascular; no rashes, vesicles, or other lesions are noted

Neuro

Sedated on morphine and midazolam; normal tone and activity for gestational age

Laboratory Values

Na 138 mEq/L	Hgb 11.5 g/dL	Calcium 9.8 mg/dL
K 3.5 mEq/L	Hct 35%	Magnesium 2 mEq/L
Cl 99 mEq/L	Plt 170 × 10³/mm³	Albumin 1.9 g/dL
CO₂ 28 mEq/L	WBC 22.5 × 10³/mm³	Triglyceride 103 mg/dL
BUN 12 mg/dL	Neutrophils 73%	T. bili 13.1 mg/dL
SCr 0.2 mg/dL	Bands 17%	D. bili 9.1 mg/dL
Glu 87 mg/dL	Lymphs 6%	CRP 14.8 mg/dL
	Monos 4%	Meconium drug screen at birth (MDS) (−)

Culture and Sensitivity Data

Source	Sensitivities
Blood, central line	Pending
Blood, peripheral	Pending
Urine, catheter	No growth to date
Tracheal aspirate	Gram-negative bacilli
CSF	No growth to date
HSV PCR	Pending

■ Assessment

Premature infant in an isolette with a history of microcephaly, RDS, apnea of prematurity, grade II IVH, cholestasis, anemia, and PDA; currently intubated and sedated, receiving nutritional and hemodynamic support, now with new late-onset sepsis.

QUESTIONS

Problem Identification

1.a. What is Alexander's gestational age, postnatal age, and postmenstrual age?

1.b. What influence, if any, do gestational and postmenstrual ages have on pediatric pharmacotherapy?

1.c. What information indicates the presence of infection in this neonate?

1.d. Compare and contrast the clinical findings required to make the diagnosis of sepsis in a child with those required to make the diagnosis in an adult.

■ CLINICAL COURSE

Several days later, the final culture and sensitivity data were reported as follows:

Source	Organism(s)/Sensitivity
Blood, central line	**Staphylococcus aureus**
	Ampicillin—R
	Ampicillin/sulbactam—R
	Cefuroxime—R

(continued)

Source	Organism(s)/Sensitivity
	Ceftazidime—R
	Cefepime—R
	Clindamycin—S
	Erythromycin—R
	Levofloxacin—S
	Oxacillin—R
	Linezolid—S
	Sulfamethoxazole/trimethoprim—S
	Vancomycin—S
Blood, peripheral	**Staphylococcus aureus**
	Ampicillin—R
	Ampicillin/sulbactam—R
	Cefuroxime—R
	Ceftazidime—R
	Cefepime—R
	Clindamycin—S
	Erythromycin—R
	Levofloxacin—S
	Oxacillin—R
	Linezolid—S
	Sulfamethoxazole/trimethoprim—S
	Vancomycin—S
Urine, catheter	**No growth**
Tracheal aspirate	**Stenotrophomonas maltophilia**
	Aztreonam—S
	Ceftazidime—R
	Levofloxacin—S
	Sulfamethoxazole/trimethoprim—S
CSF	**No growth**
HSV PCR	**Negative**

R, resistant; S, sensitive; I, intermediate; HSV, herpes simplex virus.

The medical resident on the NICU team asks you for the appropriate dose of sulfamethoxazole/trimethoprim because he is unable to find it in any of the drug information sources he has used. He plans to start the patient on sulfamethoxazole/trimethoprim for the treatment of both *Stenotrophomonas maltophilia* and methicillin-resistant *Staphylococcus aureus* (MRSA).

Desired Outcome

2. What are the goals of pharmacotherapy for this infant?

Therapeutic Alternatives

3.a. What therapeutic alternatives are available for the empiric treatment of neonatal sepsis?

3.b. Was the empiric gentamicin dose appropriate for this patient? If not, recommend an alternative dose and frequency and provide the rationale for your choice.

3.c. What therapeutic alternatives are available for the treatment of *S. maltophilia* in this neonate?

3.d. What therapeutic alternatives are available for the treatment of MRSA bacteremia in this neonate?

Optimal Plan

4.a. Recommend an appropriate pharmacotherapy regimen for the empiric treatment of neonatal sepsis in this patient based on his initial presentation.

4.b. Based on the final culture results, provide an appropriate pharmacotherapy regimen for subsequent treatment of this neonate's infections.

Outcome Evaluation

5. What clinical and laboratory parameters should be monitored to evaluate efficacy and to prevent adverse drug effects for the therapeutic regimen you recommended?

Patient Education

6. Alexander's mother is concerned about her child receiving a morphine drip. She has read on the Internet that babies his size are too small and underdeveloped to feel pain, and she is concerned that the physicians are prescribing a medication that is unnecessary and will cause him to be "addicted to drugs." What information and counseling would you provide to this mother to explain the use of morphine in this patient?

■ ADDITIONAL CASE QUESTION

1. What pharmaceutical concerns must be considered when using sulfamethoxazole/trimethoprim in neonates?

■ SELF-STUDY ASSIGNMENTS

1. In addition to sulfamethoxazole/trimethoprim, what other medications can cause neonatal gasping syndrome?

2. Which patient populations are most likely to be affected by infection with *S. maltophilia*?

3. In addition to sulfamethoxazole/trimethoprim, what other medications have the potential to cause Stevens–Johnson syndrome?

4. Compare and contrast the differences in morphine metabolism between neonates and adults.

CLINICAL PEARL

Term and preterm infants can experience alterations in the function of cells involved in the response to infection, which can decrease their ability to fight infection and increase their risk for sepsis. For example, chemotaxis is abnormal at birth, premature infants can have decreased amounts of immunoglobulin, and stressors such as respiratory distress can lead to decreased ability to phagocytose gram-negative bacteria.

REFERENCES

1. Kearns GL, Abdel-Rahman SM, Alander SE, Blowey DL, Leeder JS, Kauffman RE. Developmental pharmacology: drug disposition, action, and therapy in infants and children. N Engl J Med. 2003;349:1157–1167.
2. Goldstein B, Giroir B, Randolph A, et al. International pediatric sepsis consensus conference: definitions for sepsis and organ dysfunction in pediatrics. Pediatr Crit Care Med. 2005;6:2–8.
3. Dellinger RP, Levy MM, Rhodes A, et al. Surviving Sepsis Campaign: international guidelines for management of sever sepsis and septic shock, 2012. Intensive Care Med. 2013;39(2):165–228.
4. Pacifici GM. Clinical pharmacokinetics of aminoglycosides in the neonate: a review. Eur J Clin Pharmacol. 2009;65:419–427.
5. Anand KJS, Aranda JV, Berde CB, et al. Summary proceedings from the neonatal pain-control group. Pediatrics. 2006;117:S9–S22.
6. Anand KJS. Consensus statement for the prevention and management of pain in the newborn. Arch Pediatr Adolesc Med. 2001;155:173–180.

7

GERIATRICS

Falling Frannie.................................. Level II

Amy M. Lugo, PharmD, BCPS, BC-ADM, FAPhA

LEARNING OBJECTIVES

After completing this case study, the reader should be able to:

- Identify medications listed as Beers List drugs, and describe the reason they may be inappropriate in older adults.

- Discuss common geriatric syndromes, including falls, dizziness, syncope, and urinary incontinence, and identify ways to prevent exacerbations of these conditions.

- Establish goals for the treatment of pain, urinary incontinence, and allergic rhinitis in older adults based on patient-specific characteristics and comorbid disease states.

- Describe ways to prevent falls in older adults.

- Provide appropriate patient counseling to help seniors minimize the cost of their medications.

PATIENT PRESENTATION

■ Chief Complaint

"I get so dizzy when I stand up, and I don't have control of my bladder."

■ HPI

Fran Jones is an 87-year-old woman who presents to your pharmacotherapy clinic today reporting dizziness and urinary incontinence. She was referred by her PCP for a polypharmacy consult and an adverse drug event review. She reports having fallen last night after getting out of the bed to use the bathroom. She states that her hip is hurting where she fell on it. She admits to being "very blue" often and has crying spells when she discusses her husband who passed away last year.

■ PMH

Osteoporosis
Nonvalvular atrial fibrillation, no h/o VTE
Seasonal allergic rhinitis
Early onset Alzheimer's dementia diagnosed 2 years ago

■ PSH

One cesarean section

■ FH

Noncontributory

■ SH

Mrs Jones reports having just started taking *Ginkgo biloba* to help with memory and taking "lots" of Tylenol since her fall. She does not remember the other meds she is taking, and her daughter fills her pill box. She denies using any tobacco or alcohol. She has lived alone since her husband passed away 6 months ago. She is very concerned about paying for medications. She says the last time she was at the pharmacy, the pharmacist said something about being in a "donut hole." She has a Medicare Part D plan.

■ Meds

Warfarin 2 mg Mon–Wed–Fri–Sun and 4 mg Tue–Thu–Sat
Alendronate 70 mg PO once weekly
Diphenhydramine 25 mg PO TID for allergies
Acetaminophen OTC Extra Strength 1–2 PO PRN pain
Metoprolol succinate 50 mg PO every morning
Donepezil 5 mg PO every morning
G. biloba PO every morning

■ All

NKDA

■ ROS

Reports occasional bladder incontinence and hip pain where she fell as well as a runny nose from allergies; denies heartburn, chest pain, or shortness of breath

■ Physical Examination

Gen

WDWN Caucasian female who appears her stated age; NAD

VS

BP 118/72 mm Hg sitting, 100/60 mm Hg standing; HR 76 bpm (irregularly irregular), RR 18/min, T 98.4°F, Ht 5′4″, Wt 55 kg, G3P3

HEENT

NCAT; PERRL, EOMI, fundi benign; TMs intact; mild sinus drainage

Neck

Neck supple without thyromegaly or LAD

Lungs

Lung fields CTA bilaterally

Heart

Rhythm is irregularly irregular; no murmurs or bruits

Abd

Soft, NT/ND; no masses, bruits, or organomegaly; normal BS

Genit/Rect

Deferred

Ext

No CCE, normal ROM

Neuro

Motor, sensory, CNs, cerebellar, and gait normal. Folstein MMSE score 17/30, compared with a score of 17/30 and 19/30 last year and at the initial diagnosis, respectively. Disoriented to month, date, and day of week. Good registration but impaired attention and very poor short-term memory. Able to remember only one of three items after 3 minutes. Able to follow commands. Displayed apathy during MMSE.

■ Labs

Na 139 mEq/L	Hgb 13.5 g/dL	T. bili 0.9 mg/dL	Ca 9.7 mg/dL
K 3.7 mEq/L	Hct 39.0%	D. bili 0.3 mg/dL	Phos 4.5 mg/dL
Cl 108 mEq/L	AST 25 IU/L	T. prot 7.5 g/dL	TSH 3.8 mIU/L
CO_2 25.5 mEq/L	ALT 24 IU/L	Alb 4.5 g/dL	T4 5.9 ng/dL
BUN 16 mg/dL	Alk phos 81 IU/L	Chol 212 mg/dL	UA 6.8 mg/dL
SCr 1.1 mg/dL	GGT 22 IU/L	INR 3.1	25-OH vitamin
Glu 78 mg/dL	LDH 85 IU/L	A1C 5.8%	D 21 ng/mL

■ Radiology

CT scan (head, 2 years ago): Mild-to-moderate generalized cerebral atrophy

Bone mineral density (last year): T-score –2.6

■ ECG

Atrial fibrillation, rate controlled

■ Assessment

1. Falls, secondary to multiple factors including medications
2. Urinary incontinence
3. Atrial fibrillation, rate controlled
4. Allergic rhinitis
5. Osteoporosis
6. Self-pay for medications, Medicare Part D "donut hole"

QUESTIONS

Problem Identification

1.a. Create a list of this patient's drug-related problems, including any medications that may be contributing to the patient's falls and incontinence. Which of her medications are Beers Criteria drugs?

1.b. What are the patient's known risk factors for falls?

Desired Outcome

2. List the goals of treatment for this patient.

Therapeutic Alternatives

3.a. What nonpharmacologic therapies should be implemented to prevent falls and other adverse drug events?

3.b. What pharmacotherapeutic options are available for controlling this patient's pain, allergic rhinitis, and urinary incontinence?

3.c. What comorbidities and patient considerations should be taken into account when selecting pharmacologic therapy for her?

Optimal Plan

4.a. Outline specific lifestyle modifications for this patient as well as preventive health measures.

4.b. Outline a specific and appropriate pharmacotherapeutic regimen for this patient including drug(s), dose(s), dosage form(s), and schedule(s). Consider her out-of-pocket costs for medications.

Outcome Evaluation

5. Based on your recommendations, what parameters should be monitored after initiating this regimen and throughout the treatment course? At what time intervals should these parameters be monitored?

Patient Education

6. Based on your recommendations, provide appropriate education to this patient.

■ SELF-STUDY ASSIGNMENTS

1. Review the Beers Criteria for potentially inappropriate use of medications in older adults, and consider your first-line recommendations for optimal treatment of depression, insomnia, and diabetes in the older adult.

2. Outline the changes that you would make to the pharmacotherapeutic regimen for this patient if she had a history of each of the following comorbidities or characteristics:

   • Creatinine clearance <30 mL/min

   • Major depression

   • Moderate to severe Alzheimer's disease

3. What is Mrs Jones' CHA_2DS_2-VASc score for atrial fibrillation? What is her risk for VTE? Should she receive warfarin or aspirin? Why or why not? Would she be a candidate for dabigatran, rivaroxaban, apixaban, or edoxaban? Why or why not?

4. Assume that Mrs Jones exhibits further cognitive decline at her next neurological follow-up appointment. What would you consider the next step in treatment of her worsening Alzheimer's dementia?

CLINICAL PEARL

Each year, an estimated one-third of older adults fall, and the likelihood of falling increases substantially with advancing age. In 2005, a total of 15,802 persons aged ≥65 years died as a result of injuries from falls.[5]

REFERENCES

1. The American Geriatrics Society 2012 Beers Criteria Update Expert Panel. American Geriatrics Society updated Beers Criteria for potentially inappropriate medication use in older adults. J Am Geriatr Soc. 2012;60(4):616–631.

2. National Osteoporosis Foundation. Clinician's Guide to Prevention and Treatment of Osteoporosis. Washington, DC, National Osteoporosis Foundation, 2013.

3. Anon. Acetaminophen Overdose and Liver Injury—Background and Options for Reducing Injury. Food and Drug Administration. Available at: *http://www.fda.gov/downloads/AdvisoryCommittees /.../UCM164897.pdf*. Accessed November 4, 2015.

4. Centers for Medicare and Medicaid Services. Bridging the coverage gap in 2011. Available at: *www.medicare.gov/Publications/Pubs/pdf/11213. pdf*. Accessed November 4, 2015.

5. Gillespie LD, Robertson MC, Gillespie WJ, et al. Interventions for preventing falls in older people living in the community. Cochrane Database Syst Rev. 2012 Sep 12;9:CD007146.

6. Inouye SK, Studenski S, Tinetti ME, Kuchel GA. Geriatric syndromes: clinical, research, and policy implications of a core geriatric concept. J Am Geriatr Soc. 2007;55:780–791.

7. Centers for Disease Control and Prevention (CDC). Self-reported falls and fall-related injuries among persons aged 65 years—United States, 2006. MMWR Wkly Rep. 2008;57(9):225–229.

8. Granziera S, Cohen AT, Nante G, Manzato E, Sergi G. Thromboembolic prevention in frail elderly patients with atrial fibrillation: a practical algorithm. J Am Med Dir Assoc. 2015;16(5):358–364.

9. Winslow B, Onysko MK, Stob CM, Hazlewood KA. Treatment of Alzheimer disease. Am Fam Physician. 2011;15;83(12):1403–1412.

10. U.S. Preventive Services Task Force. Screening for depression in adults: U.S. Preventive Services Task Force recommendation statement. Ann Intern Med. 2009;151:784–792.

8

PALLIATIVE CARE

Helpful Hospice . . . . Level III

Jennifer L. Swank, PharmD, BCOP

LEARNING OBJECTIVES

After completing this case study, the reader should be able to:

• Define the goals for pain management in a patient with chronic malignant pain with hospice services.

• Define a pharmacotherapeutic pain management plan.

• Differentiate between palliative care and hospice care.

• Select or recommend medication options for management of nausea in a hospice setting.

• Define the role of continuation of nutritional support and antibiotic therapy in a hospice setting.

PATIENT PRESENTATION

■ Chief Complaint

"I have been having fevers up to 102°F and chills for two days. I have also noticed that my skin is orange in color."

■ HPI

Jamie Park is a 48-year-old woman with a history of metastatic gastric adenocarcinoma originally diagnosed 3 years ago. At that time, she had a subtotal gastrectomy with 16 out of 16 positive lymph nodes. She received adjuvant chemoradiation with 6 months of 5-fluorouracil. Two years ago, she developed gastric outlet obstruction and underwent laparotomy with extensive lysis of adhesions and revision of the gastrojejunostomy. She had no evidence of malignancy after this surgery. Three months later, she presented with symptoms of obstruction and underwent a sigmoid colectomy with pathology, revealing metastatic gastric adenocarcinoma. She was then started on chemotherapy with epirubicin, cisplatin, and capecitabine × 6 cycles. Her chemotherapy course was complicated by neutropenia requiring significant dose reduction. After completing six cycles, she had worsening small bowel obstruction and underwent surgery, where recurrent metastases to the small intestine were found. The metastases were resected, but several other malignant peritoneal nodules were seen during surgery. Four months after the surgery, she underwent colonoscopy due to further obstruction at the level of the colon. The procedure was complicated by cecal dilatation, requiring an urgent percutaneous cecostomy. A week later, she underwent a repeat exploratory laparotomy with jejunojejunal bypass and ileosigmoid bypass. After the last surgery, the patient did not recover any intestinal function and was started on chronic TPN therapy. Four months ago, the patient underwent elective percutaneous biliary drain placement for biliary obstruction due to tumor. She was recently enrolled in supportive hospice services but continues on TPN for treatment of chronic small bowel obstruction.

Mrs Park presents today with a 2-day history of fevers and chills, abdominal pain, and recurrent jaundice. She had been using Tylenol suppositories for the fevers at home without relief. Her abdominal pain has worsened over the past 2 days, and she currently rates the pain as 8 out of 10. This pain is not relieved by the use of as-needed oxycodone liquid.

■ PMH

Cholangitis
Gastric outlet obstruction and small bowel obstruction
Subtotal gastrectomy 5 years ago
Sigmoid colectomy 2 years ago

■ FH

Mother—cervical cancer
Maternal aunt—laryngeal cancer
Maternal uncle—liver cancer

■ SH

Mrs Park is from Korea and has lived in the United States for 10 years. She is married and has two children. She denies the use of alcohol or tobacco.

■ Meds

Total parental nutrition
Fentanyl 200-mcg patch, change every 72 hours
Oxycodone concentrated liquid 20 mg/mL, 1 mL PO every 3 hours PRN pain
Ondansetron 8 mg ODT, one tablet PO every 8 hours PRN nausea or vomiting
Acetaminophen suppository 650 mg, one rectally every 6 hours PRN fever

■ All

NKDA

■ ROS

Ten organ systems were reviewed. The patient reports fever, chills, nausea, vomiting, headache, and abdominal pain rated 8 out of 10. She denies chest pain, sore throat, cough, increased urinary frequency, rash, hematuria, hemoptysis, hematemesis, or black stool.

■ Physical Examination

Gen

The patient is a 48-year-old woman in acute distress holding her abdomen

VS

BP 77/50, P 90, RR 16, T 100.9°F; Wt 45.8 kg, Ht 5′2″; pain 8/10 sharp, and stabbing in nature

Skin

Warm; dry; jaundice is appreciated

HEENT

PERRLA; EOMI; TMs intact; moist mucous membranes

Neck

No JVD; full range of motion; no masses

Resp

CTA; no crackles, rhonchi, or wheezes

CV

Normal S_1, S_2; RRR; no murmurs

Abd

Soft and distended; (+) BS; moderate RUQ pain with deep palpation and mild guarding; biliary drain is in place and noted to be draining appropriately but with a foul-smelling, greenish liquid

Genit/Rect

Deferred

MS/Ext

Negative lower extremity edema; palpable pedal and radial pulsations

Neuro

CN II–XII intact, A & O × 3; no sensory or focal deficits apparent

■ Labs

Na 147 mEq/L	WBC 27.71 × 10³/mm³	T. Prot 8 g/dL
K 4.5 mEq/L	Neutros 65%	Alb 2.4 g/dL
Cl 115 mEq/L	Bands 12%	T. bili 13.5 mg/dL
CO₂ 19 mEq/L	Lymphs 22%	D. bili 11.2 mg/dL
BUN 50 mg/dL	Eos 0%	AST 402 IU/L
SCr 1.7 mg/dL	Monos 1%	ALT 400 IU/L
Glu 101 mg/dL	Hgb 10 g/dL	Alk phos 321 IU/L
Ca 8.8 mg/dL	Hct 31.1%	Cortisol 39.8 mcg/dL
Phos 3.9 mg/dL	Plt 158 × 10³/mm³	Lactic acid 0.7 mmol/L
Mg 3.0 mg/dL		

■ Chest X-Ray

Mild increased interstitial lung markings; bilateral nonspecific changes that can be seen with pulmonary edema; no consolidation to suggest pneumonia

■ RUQ Ultrasound

Sonographically abnormal appearance of the gallbladder, which is ill defined on this examination; no intrahepatic or extrahepatic biliary ductal dilatation; however, cholangitis cannot be excluded based on these findings

■ Blood Cultures × 2 Sets

Pending

■ Urine Culture

Pending

■ Biliary Drainage Culture

Pending

■ Assessment

Acute-on-chronic abdominal pain due to peritoneal metastases from gastric cancer

Hypotension and probable cholangitis due to biliary obstruction

Chronic bowel obstruction requiring TPN for nutrition

Nausea due to pain medications and chronic small bowel obstruction

QUESTIONS

Problem Identification

1.a. Create a list of the patient's drug therapy problems.

1.b. What clinical information indicates the presence of an acute-on-chronic pain syndrome?

1.c. What additional information is needed to satisfactorily assess this patient's pain?

1.d. What subjective and objective data support the diagnosis of cholangitis in this patient?

1.e. How does the role of hospice services affect the treatment plan for this patient's care?

Desired Outcome

2. What are the goals of pharmacotherapy in this case?

Therapeutic Alternatives

3.a. What nondrug therapies might be useful for this patient?

3.b. Compare the pharmacotherapeutic alternatives available for treatment of this patient's pain.

3.c. Compare the pharmacotherapeutic alternatives available for treatment of this patient's nausea and vomiting.

Optimal Plan

4.a. What drug, dosage form, and schedule are best for treating this patient's pain?

4.b. What alternatives would be appropriate if the initial therapy fails or cannot be used?

4.c. Outline a drug regimen for the treatment of the patient's nausea.

Outcome Evaluation

5. What clinical and laboratory parameters are necessary to evaluate the therapy for the achievement of the desired therapeutic outcome and to detect or prevent adverse effects?

Patient Education

6. What information should be provided to the patient to enhance compliance, ensure successful therapy, and minimize adverse effects?

■ CLINICAL COURSE

The patient was given IV fluids and started on empiric antibiotic therapy with meropenem 1 g IV Q 12 H, vancomycin 750 mg IV daily, and fluconazole 100 mg IV daily. The patient's blood pressure normalized to 105/75 mm Hg, and SCr improved to 1.5 mg/dL with NS @ 150 mL/hour. The blood and urine cultures were negative, but the biliary drainage cultures were positive for *Enterococcus faecalis* sensitive to vancomycin and *Pseudomonas stutzeri* sensitive to cefepime, ciprofloxacin, piperacillin/tazobactam, and tigecycline. The empiric antibiotic therapy was continued due to appropriate sensitivities to the antibiotics. Interventional radiology was consulted to evaluate the biliary drain for possible obstruction due to poor output. The internal/external catheter was exchanged with an external drain. The patient's bilirubin did not improve after the new external biliary drain was placed and remained in the range of 8–10 mg/dL. The patient was started on a fentanyl PCA pump at a basal rate of 30 mcg/hour with on-demand dosing of 10 mcg every 8 minutes with an hourly lockout of 100 mcg/hour, which resulted in adequate pain control rated 2 out of 10. The patient's overall prognosis is poor due to chronic jaundice from biliary obstruction, worsening renal function, and infection. She has metastatic gastric adenocarcinoma of the colon and small bowel and is not a candidate for further chemotherapy or surgery. The patient and her husband discussed her overall prognosis and made the choice to transition to full hospice services. The patient did choose to continue the 14-day course of IV antibiotic therapy. She was discharged home with home health services on IV meropenem 1 g IV Q 12 H, vancomycin 750 mg IV daily, and fluconazole 100 mg IV daily × 14 days, fentanyl PCA basal rate 30 mcg/hour on demand 10 mcg Q 8 minutes, and TPN. After the patient completes the IV antibiotics, she will choose to stop the TPN and just continue with comfort measures only and enroll in full hospice services.

■ FOLLOW-UP QUESTIONS

1. Based on this new information of the patient discontinuing TPN and being discharged to hospice, are there any other supportive medications that may benefit the patient?

2. If the patient reports her pain to be 7 out of 10 at the time of discharge, how would you alter your treatment plan?

■ SELF-STUDY ASSIGNMENTS

1. Prepare a list of opioids and their corresponding equianalgesic dosing.

2. Prepare a set of guidelines for managing chronic malignant cancer pain.

3. Prepare a list of antiemetics and dosing regimens useful in palliative care.

CLINICAL PEARL

Hospice is a specific type of palliative care team dedicated to managing patients with advanced illness, who have a life expectancy of less than 6 months. Hospice has various levels of service and covers different therapies/services depending on the area in which the patient lives. Some hospice services will allow palliative therapy (ie, chemotherapy), IV antibiotics, and IV nutrition, whereas other hospice agencies require the patient to stop all such therapies prior to enrolling in their services.

REFERENCES

1. Cherny N. Cancer pain: principles of assessment and syndromes. In: Berger A, Shuster J, Roenn J, eds. Principles and Practice of Palliative Care & Supportive Oncology. 3rd ed. Philadelphia, PA, Lippincott Williams & Wilkins, 2007.

2. Williamson A, Hoggart B. Pain: a review of three commonly used pain rating scales. J Clin Nurs 2005;14:798–804.

3. Cassileth B. Psychiatric benefits of integrative therapies in patients with cancer. Int Rev Psychiatry 2014;26:114–127.

4. World Health Organization. WHO definition of palliative care. Available at: *http://www.who.int/cancer/palliative/definition/en/*. Accessed November 10, 2015.

5. Asch DA, Faber-Langendoen K, Shea JA, Christakis NA. The sequence of withdrawing life-sustaining treatment from patients. Am J Med 1999;107:153–156.

6. McCarberg BH, Barkin RL. Long-acting opioids for chronic pain: pharmacotherapeutic opportunities to enhance compliance, quality of life, and analgesia. Am J Ther 2001;8:181–186.

7. Trescot AM, Datta S, Lee M, Hansen H. Opioid pharmacology. Pain Physician 2008;11(2 Suppl):S133–S153.

8. Davis M, Walsh D. Treatment of nausea and vomiting in advanced cancer. Support Care Cancer 2000;8:444–452.

9. Kress H, Von der Laage D, Hoerauf K, et al. A randomized, open, parallel group, multicenter trial to investigate analgesic efficacy and safety of a new transdermal fentanyl patch compared to standard opioid treatment in cancer pain. J Pain Symptom Manage 2008;36:268–279.

9

CLINICAL TOXICOLOGY: ACETAMINOPHEN TOXICITY

If One Is Good, More Is Better... .... Level II

Elizabeth J. Scharman, PharmD, DABAT, BCPS, FAACT

LEARNING OBJECTIVES

After completing this case study, the reader should be able to:

- Determine when a potentially toxic acetaminophen exposure exists.

- Monitor a patient for signs and symptoms associated with acetaminophen toxicity.

- Recommend appropriate antidotal therapy for acetaminophen poisoning, and monitor its use for effectiveness and adverse effects.

- Describe the appropriate management of adverse drug reactions related to *N*-acetylcysteine.

PATIENT PRESENTATION

Chief Complaint

The patient is uncooperative and states that he just wants to be left alone.

HPI

The poison center receives a telephone call at 1:40 AM from a physician in a local ED regarding a 54-year-old man named Steven Marks. Mr Marks was brought to the ED via ambulance accompanied by police because the patient had been belligerent and was refusing referral. According to his wife, he took a handful of pills following a heated argument she had with him that evening. She estimates the time of the fight was about 6:00 PM. She left the house and came back 2 hours later. When she returned, she found him lying on the bed and saw two empty bottles in the bathroom wastepaper basket that were not there before. The wife thinks he was trying to kill himself. He states that he took a few extra pills because he had a backache and did not think one or two pills would work. The ambulance crew brings in the two empty bottles of medicine. The wife cannot remember how much, if any, was remaining in the bottles prior to today. According to the wife, all other medications in the house are accounted for. One of the bottles originally contained sixty 500-mg acetaminophen tablets, and the other bottle originally contained thirty 300-mg acetaminophen/5-mg hydrocodone tablets. The physician reports that Mr Marks vomited twice in the ambulance and an additional four times since his arrival in the ED. He has not received any antiemetics.

PMH

Patient states that he is healthy. He has not seen a physician "in years" according to his wife.

FH

Father died of a heart attack when the patient was 12 years old. Mother is living. He has no sisters. He has one younger brother with "a bad heart."

SH

Smokes two packs of cigarettes a day. Drinks "about as much as anybody else" according to his wife.

Meds

No prescription medications
Often takes nonprescription diphenhydramine because of insomnia

All

None

Physical Examination

Gen

The patient appears drowsy. There are no external signs of trauma. The patient has vomited a total of six times. The vomitus has not been bloody. His estimated height is 5'10".

VS

BP 142/98, HR 72, RR 14, O_2 sat 98% on room air, T 37°C; Wt 98 kg

Skin

Mucous membranes are moist

HEENT

Pupil size is normal; pupils are equal and reactive to light; retinal exam is unremarkable

Lungs/Thorax

Occasional cough is noted

CV

No murmurs or gallops heard

Abd

Bowel sounds are present. No guarding or tenderness.

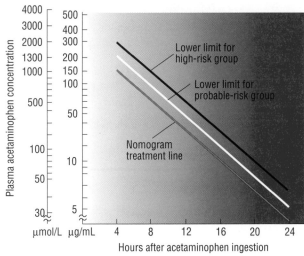

FIGURE 9-1. Nomogram for assessing hepatotoxic risk following acute ingestion of acetaminophen. (*Reprinted with permission from DiPiro JT, Talbert RL, Yee GC, et al., eds. Pharmacotherapy: A Pathophysiologic Approach, 8th ed. New York, McGraw-Hill, 2011.*)

Neuro

The patient is noticeably drowsy and uncooperative but is oriented to time and place; no tremors noted. The patient states that his headache has resolved.

■ Labs (Drawn at 01:00)

Na 142 mEq/L	Glucose 225 mg/dL	T. bili 0.8 mg/dL
K 3.1 mEq/L	Urine: (+) PCP	INR 1.2
Cl 96 mEq/L	Hgb 15.7 g/dL	Salicylates (–)
CO_2 23 mEq/L	Hct 48.2%	Acetaminophen 124 mcg/mL
BUN 24 mg/dL	AST 38 IU/L	Ethanol (EtOH) 138 mg/dL
SCr 1.1 mg/dL	ALT 42 IU/L	

■ ECG

Normal sinus rhythm

■ Assessment

The physician asks the poison center if acetaminophen toxicity is present (Fig. 9-1)

QUESTIONS

Problem Identification

1.a. Is determining the amount of acetaminophen the patient ingested an important factor in determining whether acetaminophen toxicity is present? Why or why not?

1.b. Which signs, symptoms, and laboratory values indicate that acetaminophen toxicity is present?

1.c. What are possible causes of vomiting in this patient?

1.d. Does toxicity from any other drug(s)/toxin(s) need to be considered in this patient? If so, which one(s) and why?

1.e. Develop a problem list for this patient. Identify the problem(s) that need to be addressed first. For the other problems, describe the rationale behind whether they need to be managed now or whether they just need to be addressed prior to discharge.

Desired Outcome

2. What are the goals of pharmacotherapy for managing acetaminophen toxicity in this case?

Therapeutic Alternatives

3. What feasible pharmacotherapeutic alternatives are available for treating acetaminophen toxicity in this patient?

Optimal Plan

4.a. What antidote route, dose, schedule, and duration of therapy for acetaminophen toxicity are best for this patient, and when should therapy be initiated for optimal results?

4.b. If the physician asks the pharmacy to make an IV containing the exact dose of IV *N*-acetylcysteine (Acetadote) for this patient, instead of rounding to the nearest dose designated in the prescribing information dosing table, how many milliliters of *N*-acetylcysteine should this patient receive? Show all calculations, including how the total dose needed was obtained and how the amount of *N*-acetylcysteine in each milliliter of Acetadote was calculated.

4.c. Will administration of *N*-acetylcysteine have any influence on the pharmacologic management of the patient's other problems as identified in his problem list? Why or why not?

4.d. If this patient had been a female who was human chorionic gonadotropin (β-hCG) (+), would recommendations for *N*-acetylcysteine therapy change? Why or why not?

Outcome Evaluation

5. What clinical and laboratory parameters are necessary to evaluate the therapy for achievement of the desired therapeutic outcome for acetaminophen toxicity and to detect adverse effects?

Patient Education

6. What should the patient be told about the effectiveness of *N*-acetylcysteine therapy?

■ CLINICAL COURSE

At 02:20 the same day, the poison center gets a call from the patient's treating physician. He states that Mr Marks developed flushing and urticaria at the end of the loading dose; some faint wheezes were heard, and the baseline cough is unchanged. The physician thinks the patient may be having an anaphylactic reaction and has stopped the IV *N*-acetylcysteine. He wants poison center recommendations for an alternative antidote. The poison specialist determines that the correct mg/kg dosage was administered, although the loading dose was administered over 15 minutes. Vital signs are BP 138/99, HR 68, RR 14, and nonlabored. Blood chemistries are scheduled to be repeated at 08:00. Administration of ondansetron has controlled the vomiting.

■ FOLLOW-UP QUESTIONS

1. Do you agree that this is an anaphylactic reaction? If not, what type of reaction is this and how is it different from an anaphylactic reaction?

2. What are the appropriate management options for this reaction and for continued management of acetaminophen toxicity in this patient?

3. The prescribing information for IV *N*-acetylcysteine lists one contraindication. Do you agree with this contraindication? Why or why not?

4. If this patient is discharged from the hospital on medications to treat other medical problems, how will his history of an overdose affect the health care provider's decision on which medication(s) to select?

■ SELF-STUDY ASSIGNMENTS

1. Defend the argument that all patients with an intentional drug overdose, no matter what their stated history, should have an acetaminophen level drawn to rule out acetaminophen toxicity.

2. If this patient had been 104 kg instead of 98 kg, the dose given would have been the same as that of a person weighing 100 kg. Why do patients weighing over 100 kg not receive an IV *N*-acetylcysteine dose calculated on an mg/kg basis, and what is the rationale for this maximum dose being clinically effective?

CLINICAL PEARL

The FDA Modernization Act of 1997 states that acceptable compounding practice excludes the extemporaneous compounding of commercially available products (eg, Acetadote). Therefore, pharmacists should not prepare IV *N*-acetylcysteine extemporaneously using the oral formulation. Although compounding IV *N*-acetylcysteine in an emergency could be justified (as in this case), a pharmacy could not decide in advance to prepare IV *N*-acetylcysteine extemporaneously in lieu of purchasing the commercially available product. USP Chapter 797, which some state pharmacy boards have adopted, identifies the sterility conditions that would need to be met during the compounding process. Due to the frequency of acetaminophen toxicity, and the potential for hepatotoxicity leading to the need for liver transplantation and/or death, all hospital pharmacies should stock IV *N*-acetylcysteine for use when oral *N*-acetylcysteine is not appropriate or not tolerated.

REFERENCES

1. Dart RC, Erdman AR, Olson KR, et al. Acetaminophen poisoning: an evidence-based consensus guideline for out-of-hospital management. Clin Toxicol (Phila) 2006;44:1–18.

2. Payen C, Dachraoui A, Pulce C, et al. Prothrombin time prolongation in paracetamol poisoning: a relevant marker of hepatic failure? Hum Exp Toxicol 2003;22:617–621.

3. Rowden AK, Norvell J, Eldridge DL, et al. Acetaminophen poisoning. Clin Lab Med 2006;26:49–65.

4. Betten DP, Burner EE, Thomas SC, Tomaszewski C, Clark RF. A retrospective evaluation of shortened-duration oral *N*-acetylcysteine for the treatment of acetaminophen poisoning. J Med Toxicol 2009;5:183–190.

5. Dribben WH, Porto SM, Jeffords BK. Stability and microbiology of inhalant *N*-acetylcysteine used as an intravenous solution for the treatment of acetaminophen poisoning. Ann Emerg Med 2003;42:9–13.

6. Acetadote Package Insert. Nashville, TN, Cumberland Pharmaceuticals Inc., June 2013.

7. Waring WS. Novel acetylcysteine regimens for treatment of paracetamol overdose. Ther Adv Drug Saf 2012;3:305–315.

8. Wilkes JM, Clark LE, Herrera JL. Acetaminophen overdose in pregnancy. South Med J 2005;98:1118–1122.

9. Curtis RM, Sivilotti ML. A descriptive analysis of aspartate and alanine aminotransferase rise and fall following acetaminophen overdose. Clin Toxicol (Phila) 2015;53:849–855.

10. Sandilands EA, Bateman DN. Adverse reactions associated with acetylcysteine. Clin Toxicol (Phila) 2009;47:81–88.

10

CYANIDE EXPOSURE

Expect the Unexpected........................ Level II

Elizabeth J. Scharman, PharmD, DABAT, BCPS, FAACT

LEARNING OBJECTIVES

After completing this case study, the reader should be able to:

• Identify which signs, symptoms, and laboratory data indicate a possible cyanide exposure.

• Compare and contrast the two different antidotes for cyanide exposure.

• Recommend specific dosing regimens for antidotes and supportive care for children and adults.

• State monitoring parameters and management of antidote side effects.

• Explain the factors involved in determining the amount of cyanide antidote a hospital should stock for immediate availability.

PRESENTATION OF PATIENTS

A 60-year-old laboratory worker with a history of major depressive disorder has stayed after normal laboratory hours on the pretense of completing a project. Once his coworkers have left, he ingests a bottle containing a toxic chemical. His biochemistry laboratory is on the fifth (top) floor of a university building containing eight other offices occupying the four floors below, all of which are faculty and staff offices for the biochemistry department. He loses consciousness. Meanwhile, the heating unit in the basement of the office building catches fire that quickly spreads through the first three floors of the building. At least 10 other individuals were in the other building's offices working late. They were not able to evacuate before being overcome by smoke.

■ HPI

Firefighters and Emergency Medical Services (EMS) personnel are at the scene. Ambulances are bringing the 11 victims from the fire to your hospital's ED; some are comatose, and others present with a variety of signs/symptoms including confusion, coughing, wheezing, and minor burns. One of the victims brought in is a man who appears to be in his sixties. He has profound cyanosis and seizure activity. Unlike the other victims, he has no soot on his clothing. The ambulance worker reports that he was found on a floor receiving very little smoke damage and no fire damage. This victim has been tagged John Doe (JD).

■ PMH, PSH, FH, and SH

Not available. The hospital is initially overwhelmed because the ED was nearly full before the arrival of these patients.

■ ROS

Patients are presenting with a variety of symptoms and illness severity. ED nurses and doctors are only able to do brief physical exams. Ages and weights are being estimated as needed. JD is the most critically ill patient.

■ **Physical Examination (Victims Excluding JD)**

Gen

Four of the 10 patients appear weak and are breathing rapidly. Two additional victims are unconscious and required intubation to support breathing. All six of these patients have soot in their nares and around their mouths. The remaining four patients have mild coughing, wheezing, and burning eyes; soot is not present in their nares or inside their mouths, and systemic signs and symptoms are absent. Facial burns are not evident on any of these 10 individuals.

VS

BP: The 6 sickest patients are hypotensive.
HR: The 6 sickest patients have rates between 110 and 120 bpm.
RR: The 6 sickest patients have rates between 22 and 26.
T: All have normal temperatures.
Pain: Patients not intubated are anxious but are not in obvious pain.
O$_2$ sat: Normal for all.

Skin

No notable contusions, abrasions; second-and third-degree burns are absent. Two of the 10 have some mild blistering on their hands.

HEENT

Mydriasis observed in some patients

Neck/Lymph Nodes

No lymphadenopathy

Lungs/Thorax

Rapid respiratory rate; patients complain of some chest tightness and dyspnea

CV

Bradycardia for the six sickest patients, too noisy in ED to listen for heart sounds

Abd

Bowel sounds presents in all; the six sickest patients have nausea and some vomiting

Genital/Rect

Deferred

MS/Ext

No abnormal movements noted

Neuro

Two of the six sickest victims are ventilated. No convulsions are observed. The six sickest patients are confused. The remaining four fire victims are neurologically intact.

■ **Pertinent Physical Findings for JD**

Gen

Unconscious; generalized convulsions are present. Oxygen saturation via pulse oximetry was 98%. An almond smell was noted by one of the medical care providers after the patient vomited. JD has been intubated.

VS: HR 22 bpm, RR 8, BP 60/35 mm Hg, T 37.0°C

■ **Lab**

Ranges for the Six Sickest Fire Victims: HCO$_3^-$ 13–15 mEq/L from the metabolic panel; CBC within normal limits; lactate 14 mmol/L; carboxyhemoglobin 12–15%
Reported for JD: HCO$_3^-$ 8 mEq/L from the metabolic panel; CBC normal; lactate 22 mmol/L; carboxyhemoglobin 1%
Four Remaining Fire Victims: Labs are within normal limits

■ **Other**

Example initial blood gas for an intubated patient: pH 7.2, PaCO$_2$ 40 mm Hg, PaO$_2$ 110 mm Hg, HCO$_3$ 13 mEq/L
Blood gas for JD: pH 7.1, PaCO$_2$ 40 mm Hg, PaO$_2$ 240 mm Hg, HCO$_3$ 9 mEq/L
Blood gases were not obtained for the four fire victims without systemic symptoms
Chest X-rays for JD and the six sickest fire victims are pending

■ **Follow-Up**

The ED clinical pharmacist contacts the Poison Center after overhearing one of the EMS workers mention that JD was found in his laboratory next to an opened and empty chemical bottle. The Poison Center will check with the on-scene Incident Commander (IC) and follow-up with the clinical pharmacist as quickly as possible. Based on the presenting toxidrome the most likely chemical ingested by JD is cyanide. There is agreement that products of combustion and toxic gases from smoke inhalation are causing toxicity in the six sickest patients.

QUESTIONS

Problem Identification

1.a. JD and the six sickest fire victims share a similar toxidrome pattern. How is this possible when only JD ingested chemical from the bottle? Compare the signs and symptoms of severe cyanide poisoning with less severe intoxication.

1.b. List the laboratory tests that may be abnormal in patients exposed to cyanide. Explain the pathophysiology underlying these abnormalities.

1.c. What are the potential short- and long-term sequelae from these cyanide exposures?

Desired Outcome

2. What are the goals of pharmacotherapy in these cases?

Therapeutic Alternatives

3.a. What nonpharmacologic measures are available to treat cyanide poisoning in these victims?

3.b. What feasible pharmacotherapeutic alternatives are available for treating cyanide poisoning (see Fig. 10-1)?

Optimal Plan

4.a. Outline your pharmacotherapeutic plan for treating cyanide poisoning in these patients.

4.b. What supportive care measures may be necessary for optimal management in these patients?

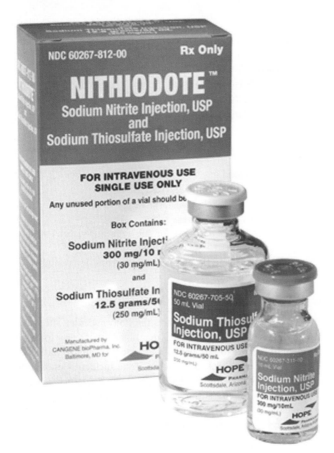

FIGURE 10-1. Nithiodote® (sodium nitrite injection and sodium thiosulfate injection for intravenous infusion). Individual ingredients may also be purchased separately. Photo courtesy of Hope Pharmaceuticals.

Outcome Evaluation

5.a. Describe the clinical and laboratory parameters required to determine whether the treatment for these patients has been successful.

5.b. How often should these patients be monitored to assess for treatment efficacy?

Patient Education

6.a. For patients who are alert and oriented, what information would you share with them about the possible immediate side effects of each of the antidotes?

6.b. How long might it take for the patients to recover from potential long-term effects of acute cyanide exposure?

■ CLINICAL COURSE

The bottle from the laboratory is confirmed to have contained cyanide. JD went into cardiac arrest shortly after being intubated. He was given the cyanide antidote during the resuscitation efforts. Catastrophic hypoxic brain injury became evident, and his family requested that life-support be withdrawn. Five of the six sickest patients survived; the sixth victim died of complications from cardiac arrest and acute respiratory distress syndrome. The four ambulatory patients were discharged to home from the ED. Legal charges were brought against the building's landlord because of the faulty heating unit and the fact that over one-quarter of the emergency exits were blocked.

■ FOLLOW-UP QUESTIONS

1. For how many patients should a hospital stock the cyanide antidotes? Consider the cost of the antidotes in your answer.

2. Suppose there are 100 patients in your hospital's ED needing a cyanide antidote and you only have enough antidote to treat four patients. Who may be involved in making these ethical treatment decisions, and how would these decisions be made?

■ SELF-STUDY ASSIGNMENTS

1. Cyanide is usually obtained for suicidal exposures by persons who have access to it in a workplace setting. Other exposures to pure cyanide are the result of unintentional occupational exposures in industrial settings. The public might be exposed after a cyanide transportation accident that spills cyanide into sources of drinking water, leads to direct physical contact with the spilled cyanide, or results in the inhalation of cyanide fumes emanating from the spill. There is also the possibility that terrorists might obtain cyanide from manufacturing locations or transportation vehicles (chemical trucks, train cars). Describe which specific occupational settings utilize cyanide on a regular basis.

2. Describe why amyl nitrite is not required for the management of cyanide toxicity.

CLINICAL PEARL

Hydrogen cyanide is a colorless gas; however, cyanide has an odor that has been described as that of "bitter almonds." Unfortunately, it is estimated that only 10% of the population is genetically able to detect cyanide's smell.

REFERENCES

1. Thompson JP, Marrs TC. Hydroxocobalamin in cyanide poisoning. Clin Toxicol (Phila) 2012;50:875–885.

2. Leybell I, Borron SW, Roldan CJ, Rivers CM. Emedicine [Internet]. New York, Web MD Inc, © 1994–2013 [updated July 21, 2014; cited January 23, 2013]. Cyanide toxicity. Available at: *http://emedicine.medscape.com/article/814287-overview*.

3. Centers for Disease Control (CDC) Emergency Preparedness and Response [Internet]. Atlanta, GA [updated June 27, 2013; cited November 15, 2015]. Facts about cyanide. Available at: *www.bt.cdc.gov/agent/cyanide*.

4. Baud FJ. Cyanide: critical issues in diagnosis and treatment. Hum Exp Toxicol 2007;26:191–201.

5. Borron SW, Baud FJ. Antidotes for acute cyanide poisoning. Curr Pharm Biotechnol 2012;13:1940–1948.

6. Baud FJ, Borron SW, Mégarbane B, et al. Value of lactic acidosis in the assessment of the severity of acute cyanide poisoning. Crit Care Med 2002;30:2044–2050.

7. Howland MA. Antidotes in depth: sodium thiosulfate. In: Flomenbaum NE, Hoffman RS, Howland MA, Lewin N, Nelson LS, Goldfrank LR, eds. Goldfrank's Toxicologic Emergencies, 10th ed. New York, McGraw-Hill, 2014:1614–1618.

8. Cyanokit Package Insert. Nashville, TN, Columbia, MD; Meridian Medical Technologies™, Inc., April 2011.

9. Dal Ponte ST, Dornelles CF, Arquilla B, Bloem C, Roblin P. Mass-casualty response to the Kiss Nightclub in Santa Maria, Brazil. Prehosp Disaster Med 2015;30:93–96.

11

CHEMICAL THREAT AGENT EXPOSURE

Name That Poison . . . . Level II

Elizabeth J. Scharman, PharmD, BCPS, DABAT, FAACT

LEARNING OBJECTIVES

After completing this case study, the reader should be able to:

- Identify one of the toxidromes associated with a chemical threat agent attack.

- Determine the indications for antidotes and supportive care options based on patient signs and symptoms.

- State the difference between the utilization of a medical model and a mass care model during a public health emergency.

- Identify antidote and drug treatment stockpile sources and when state or national stockpiles options may be utilized.

PATIENT PRESENTATION

■ Patient Scenario

Via the disaster response radio in the ED, hospital staff learn that attendees at an outdoor concert have suddenly become ill. A series of four loud popping sounds had been heard immediately prior. EMS personnel are on scene donning personal protective equipment (PPE) and setting up decontamination stations. Some concert attendees have been fleeing the scene despite orders from law enforcement to stay on site for decontamination. At least four backpacks have been observed in the area via binoculars but have not yet been examined. They are suspicious because backpacks were not allowed at the concert venue and attendees were checked for large bags prior to entry. Due to the large number of attendees, it is suspected that security measures were imperfect.

■ HPI

The on-scene incident commander ensures that the communication chief notifies all local emergency departments (total of four) to stand up their emergency operation centers (EOC).The concert venue held 1,000 and seats had been sold out. Hospital #1 is the largest of the four and is also a Level I trauma center. Within 20 minutes of the notification, patients begin arriving at that hospital's outdoor staging and decontamination areas via car, by foot, and via ambulance. Hospital security personnel have donned full PPE and are working to ensure that those not arriving via ambulance (and therefore lacking prior decontamination) do not enter the ED until they have been through the hospital's decontamination stations, which are in the final stages of being set up. Security personnel are also directing friends and family members of the victims to a waiting area across the street so those needing care are not lost in the crowd.

An emergency triage center is established just outside Hospital #1's ED entrance. It is staffed by a lead physician, three nurses, two nursing aides, two medical residents, and the ED clinical pharmacist.

Dozens of victims are in the staging area awaiting decontamination, and they appear to be in various states of illness and anxiety levels. Victims arriving in the triage area via ambulance are unconscious.

In the triage area, the large number of victims and mass panic are creating chaos, making thorough individual assessment impossible. After ensuring that triage staff are properly gowned and double gloved, the ED lead physician at Hospital #1 instructs the nursing aides to obtain patient vital signs on those arriving via ambulance. Nurses are directed to establish an IV line in each comatose patient. The medical residents are assigned to triage patients into four groups based on need for immediate threats to life, focusing on prominent findings observed with a brief physical exam. The clinical pharmacist is instructed to call the Poison Center for information on what the chemical threat agent is likely to be based on the cluster of symptoms being observed and to obtain antidote information.

■ PMH, PSH, FH, and SH

Not obtained

■ ROS

At Hospital #1, at least 300 victims are waiting for care. In the triage area, patients are tagged with color-coded bracelets into one of four groups:

- *Red*—Unconscious and having immediate life-threatening symptoms.

- *Yellow*—Severe but not immediately life-threatening symptoms; awake but not ambulatory and not conversing well.

- *Black*—Distressing symptoms, but ambulatory and conversing well.

- *Green*—Ambulatory without obvious symptoms, or mild symptoms not impairing function.

■ Physical Examination

Triage has been completed for an estimated 75% of those waiting for care at Hospital #1. Physical findings observed on each patient category are as follows:

- *Red*—45 patients, and all are unconscious; 11 are having multiple convulsions; 43 are having large- and small-muscle fasciculations. Breathing is labored, and rhonchi are present throughout the lung fields in all 45 victims; respiratory paralysis appears to be imminent in 28 cyanotic patients. CPR is being performed on one patient by an anesthesiologist who was called in for assistance. In the other victims, HR's are less than 40 bpm. Profuse diaphoresis is present, and bowel sounds are hyperactive; vomitus and fecal staining are present on the clothing of some of the victims. Miosis is present in approximately half of the patients.

- *Yellow*—36 patients; these victims have a decreased level of consciousness and severe muscle weakness but respond somewhat to stimuli. All are unable to communicate except for brief responses and sometimes not at all. Facial fasciculations are present in six, but none have experienced a witnessed convulsion. Wheezing is heard on auscultation, and patients complain of shortness of breath. None appear cyanotic. HR's are not less than 40 bpm, but it has been too chaotic to record individual rates consistently. Vomiting, hyperactive bowel sounds, and fecal incontinence are common. Moderate diaphoresis is noted. Miosis is present in 10 patients; communication difficulties make it impossible to assess if visual changes are present.

- *Black*—86 patients; victims are ambulating and conversing. Wheezing and rhonchi are absent and only four complain of chest tightness. Nausea is present in all, but no one has had more than one or two episodes of vomiting. Ten victims have miosis and are complaining of blurry vision. Tearing, runny noses, and mild–moderate diaphoresis are noted. Vital signs were not obtained at this time because nurses are overwhelmed.

- *Green*—75 patients; victims are ambulating and conversing, although many are visibly distraught. 52 patients are asymptomatic but are extremely concerned and demand to receive an antidote because they are sure they are going to die. 25 victims complain of nausea, headache, and dizziness. Diaphoresis, tearing, runny noses are absent. No vomiting or fecal incontinence has occurred in this group.

Next Steps

The clinical pharmacist at Hospital #1 contacted the Poison Center to report patient numbers and the signs and symptoms being observed. The Poison Center relates that victims from all four hospitals are showing a similar toxidrome pattern. The Poison Center has been in communication with the on-scene incident commander to review additional information from the concert venue. The category of chemical threat agent most likely involved and antidote and treatment recommendations are reviewed with the clinical pharmacist, who then reports this information to the lead physician. The Poison Center faxes information to the hospital ED and pharmacy to ensure that the antidote and dosing information are readily available.

The lead physician prioritized the Red group for entry into the ED for immediate care. He assigned the Yellow group to be managed in a medical tent sent up near the ED entrance approximately 50 yards away from the triage area. The Black group was assigned to be managed as health care professionals become free. Those in the Green group are moved to a location 200 yards from the triage area with a portable curtain erected to put them out of the line of sight of the other victims. The lead physician called for the behavioral health disaster response team to provide supportive mental health services to the Green group. A clinical pharmacist will be there to answer questions about the incident. A nurse will be with the Green group to observe for the onset of any new symptoms.

The ED clinical pharmacist contacted the clinical pharmacist in charge of the pharmacy's disaster plan to report the number of victims requiring antidotal and supportive therapies. The initial supply of pharmaceuticals is transported to the ED. Another cart of pharmaceuticals is on its way to the area serving the Yellow group. The pharmaceutical cart for the Black group will be ready in the next five minutes. Hospital #1's disaster plan has been activated and will be used to obtain additional antidotes, supportive therapies, and supplies. The ED clinical pharmacist and the clinical pharmacist in the pharmacy department will communicate with each other to coordinate antidote needs and availability.

Laboratory Findings

Immediate resuscitative measures on the 45 victims is taking precedence at this time. A team of phlebotomists has been called to the ED to begin drawing blood samples. Hand-printed labels are used to mark the vials to save time. Physicians use clinical judgment to monitor patient status.

Radiology Findings

Diffuse pulmonary edema is observed on plain film chest X-rays obtained on the victim who was receiving CPR and has now been intubated.

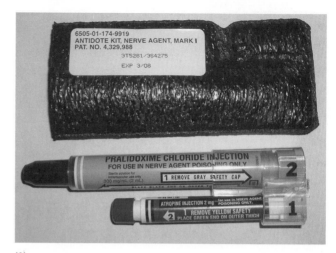

(A)

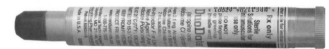

(B)

FIGURE 11-1. (A) The Mark I™ autoinjector, consisting of two antidotes to be used after exposures to a nerve or organophosphate agent in a disaster situation. The kit contains an atropine autoinjector (2 mg/0.7 mL) and a pralidoxime chloride (2-PAM) autoinjector (600 mg/2 mL). (B) The DuoDote™ autoinjector (replacing the Mark I™ autoinjector) contains 2.1 mg atropine and 600 mg of pralidoxime chloride in one syringe.

QUESTIONS

Problem Identification

1.a. Which category of chemical threat agent is most likely to be involved? Describe how you made this decision.

1.b. To initiate antidotal therapies, is it important to know which specific chemical agent in this chemical agent category is involved? Why or why not?

Desired Outcome

2.a. What are the goals of pharmacotherapy for each group (Red, Yellow, Black, and Green)?

2.b. How would your goals change if there were 5 victims instead of 300 victims presenting to your hospital with an exposure to a chemical threat agent?

Therapeutic Alternatives

3.a. What nonpharmacologic measures are required and available to manage these patients?

3.b. What feasible pharmacotherapeutic alternatives are available for treating these patients? (See Figs. 11-1 and 11-2.)

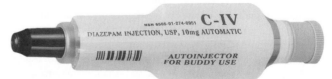

FIGURE 11-2. Diazepam provided as a 10-mg dose in a military designed autoinjector.

CHAPTER 11

Optimal Plan

4.a. Provide adult and pediatric doses by route for each chemical threat agent antidote required in this case scenario.

4.b. If a patient's condition worsens and seizure activity occurs, what class of medications should be used for this chemical-induced seizure?

4.c. Which clinical and/or laboratory findings determine whether or not an individual will require the antidote(s)?

4.d. Suppose there are 100 patients in your hospital's emergency department meeting the criteria for the antidote(s), and you only have enough antidote(s) to treat 25 patients. How do you decide who receives the antidote?

Outcome Evaluation

5. Outline a monitoring plan to assess whether the pharmaco-therapy treatment for these patients is successful.

Patient Education

6.a. What information would you share with the patients about immediate side effects of each of the antidotes?

6.b. How long might it take for patients to recover from the ocular effects of the chemical exposure? Incorporate this information into your educational efforts.

■ CLINICAL COURSE

At Hospital #1, 21 patients die from the exposure and 24 remain in critical condition. The critically-ill patients are transferred to the ICU's, and half of the telemetry floor beds have been temporarily converted into additional ICU beds.

■ FOLLOW-UP QUESTION

1. What is the initial and ongoing source of antidotes for use after a chemical terrorist event at hospital pharmacies in the United States?

■ SELF-STUDY ASSIGNMENTS

1. Research information on the Strategic National Stockpile Program and the CHEMPACK program. Evaluate the difference in response times and focus for both programs.

2. Research information on your county and state threat preparedness plan. Review the expectations of health care professionals according to the plans. Identify gaps in the plan that you may be able to assist in correcting by working with your local health department or state threat preparedness planning agency.

CLINICAL PEARL

Most chemical agents that could be used for a terrorist attack would likely be exploded or released as a gas or vapor in order to increase the extent of the exposure and allow for rapid systemic entry into victims. A general rule of thumb for chemical exposures is that the higher the concentration (or total dose) the faster the onset of symptoms; the lower the concentration (or total dose), the slower the onset of symptoms.

REFERENCES

1. US Army Medical Research Institute of Chemical Defense (USAMRICD). Field Management of Chemical Casualties Handbook, 2nd ed. [Internet]. Aberdeen Proving Ground, MD, Chemical Casualty Care Division, July 2000 [cited November 15, 2015]. Available at: https://www.rke.vaems.org/wvems/Libraryfiles/Dis/E_04.pdf.

2. Centers for Disease Control and Prevention. Emergency Preparedness and Response; Chemical Emergencies [Internet]. Atlanta, GA [updated November 25, 2014; cited November 15, 2015. Available at: http://emergency.cdc.gov/chemical/index.asp.

3. Leikin JB, Thomas RG, Walter FG, Klein R, Meislin HW. A review of nerve agent exposure for the critical care physician. Crit Care Med 2002;30:2346–2354.

4. Bartlett JG, Sifton DW, Gwynned LK. PDR Guide to Biological and Chemical Warfare Response. 1st ed. Montvale, NJ, Thomson Healthcare, 2002:79–86, 101–102, 126–127.

5. Jones TF. Mass psychogenic illness: role of the individual physician. Am Fam Physician 2000;62:2649–2653.

6. Atropen Auto-Injector [package insert]. Columbia, MD, Meridian Technologies Inc, November 2005 [cited November 15, 2015]. Available at: http://www.meridianmeds.com/pdf/Atropen_PI.pdf.

7. Pralidoxime Chloride Injection Auto-Injector [package insert]. Columbia, MD, Meridian Technologies Inc, October 2003 [cited November 15, 2015]. Available at: http://www.meridianmeds.com/pdf/Pralidoxime_Chloride_PI.pdf.

8. DuoDote [package insert]. Columbia, MD, Meridian Technologies Inc, September 2006 [cited November 15, 2015]. Available at: http://www.meridianmeds.com/pdf/DuoDote_PI.pdf.

9. Diazepam Autoinjector [package insert]. Columbia, MD, Meridian Technologies Inc, July 2005 [cited November 15, 2015]. Available at: http://www.meridianmeds.com/pdf/diazepam_PI.pdf.

12

CARDIAC ARREST

Staying Alive .... Level II

Jennifer McCann, PharmD, BCPS, BCCCP

Sarah Hittle, PharmD, BCPS, BCCCP

LEARNING OBJECTIVES

After completing this case study, the reader should be able to:

- Discuss possible causes for cardiac arrest.

- Outline medications used to treat cardiac arrest.

- List the pharmacologic actions of medications used in cardioversion.

- Outline the Advanced Cardiac Life Support (ACLS) guidelines.

- Identify appropriate parameters to monitor a patient who has been returned to spontaneous circulation.

PATIENT PRESENTATION

■ Chief Complaint

"I feel like I can't breathe."

■ HPI

Beatrice ("Bee") A. Hart is a 68-year-old female who presented to the emergency department Monday morning with shortness of breath and weakness. She reports these symptoms along with a decreased oral intake beginning Thursday last week, which ultimately led to her missing her scheduled dialysis session prior to the weekend.

■ PMH

ESRD requiring hemodialysis Monday, Wednesday and Friday
Endometriosis
HTN
Dyslipidemia
Type 2 DM

■ PSH

Hysterectomy in 1985

■ FH

Mother had HTN and died of an AMI at age 69; no information available for father; one brother is alive with HTN and DM at age 73.

■ SH

Smoker; quit 8 years ago; previously 1.5 ppd

■ Meds PTA

Atorvastatin 20 mg PO daily
Metoprolol 50 mg PO twice daily
Sevelamer 800 mg PO TID with meals
Lisinopril 20 mg PO daily
Epoetin Alfa 10,000 units SC three times a week
Insulin glargine 40 units SC daily
Insulin lispro 5 units SC with meals

■ All

Sulfa

■ ROS

Difficulty breathing

■ Physical Examination

Gen

White woman

VS

BP 98/60, P 112, RR 24, O_2 saturation 81% on 4L NC; T 37.9°C; dry weight 90 kg; height 162.5 cm

Skin

Cold

HEENT

PERRLA; EOMI; arteriolar narrowing on funduscopic exam; no hemorrhages, exudates, or papilledema; oral mucosa clear

Neck/Lymph Nodes

Supple with no JVD or bruits; no lymphadenopathy or thyromegaly

Chest

Mild bibasilar rales with decreased breath sounds

CV

Tachycardic; S_1, S_2 normal; no S_3 or S_4; no murmurs or rubs

Abd

Obese, soft, nontender; (+) BS

Genit/Rect

Stool heme (−)

MS/Ext

3+ pitting edema, age-appropriate strength and ROM

Neuro

A & O × 3, GCS 15

■ Labs

Na 130 mEq/L	Mg 4 mg/dL	Hgb 8.3 g/dL
K 6.3 mEq/L	Phos 6.5 mg/dL	Hct 28%
Cl 106 mEq/L	Alb 1.8 g/dL	Plt 229 × 10³/mm³
CO₂ 20 mEq/L		WBC 9.9 × 10³/mm³
BUN 55 mg/dL		PMNs 79%
SCr 4.6 mg/dL		Bands 1%
Glu 55 mg/dL		Lymphs 17%
Ca 6.7 mg/dL		Monos 3%

■ ECG

Sinus tachycardia at a rate of 112 bpm

CLINICAL COURSE

The patient's clinical condition deteriorated shortly after presentation to the ED, at which time she was subsequently intubated for respiratory failure. The patient was noted to have multifocal PVCs with a disorganized rhythm on the monitor and no pulse was detected. A code was called.

■ Assessment

68-Year-old patient with a complex medical history presents to the ED and develops cardiac arrest after missing a hemodialysis session.

QUESTIONS

Problem Identification

1.a. What actual and potential drug-therapy problems does this patient have just prior to the development of pulseless electrical activity (PEA)?

1.b. Discuss the possible causes for the development of PEA.

Desired Outcome

2. What are the short-term goals of pharmacotherapy for this patient?

Therapeutic Alternatives

3.a. What nonpharmacologic maneuvers should be taken immediately in a patient with PEA?

3.b. What pharmacotherapeutic agents are available for the acute therapy of this patient's condition?

■ CLINICAL COURSE

See Table 12-1 for a record of cardiopulmonary resuscitation (CPR) events and orders.

Optimal Plan

4.a. A pharmacist was not available to participate in this resuscitation effort. Assess the appropriateness of the treatment used to obtain a cardiac conversion in this patient (see Table 12-1).

4.b. After achieving return of spontaneous circulation (ROSC), what is your pharmacotherapeutic plan to maintain the patient's stability and optimize neurological function?

Outcome Evaluation

5. How should the patient be monitored to prevent or detect adverse effects?

■ SELF-STUDY ASSIGNMENTS

1. Search the Internet for commercially available automated external defibrillator (AED) devices. Explain how such a device would be used by a layperson during a cardiac arrest that occurred in the home or workplace.

2. Perform a literature search to determine the odds of surviving a cardiac arrest while hospitalized.

3. List medications that can be administered via the intraosseous route in an emergent situation.

4. Investigate the effects of induced hypothermia following cardiac arrest on patient outcomes.

CLINICAL PEARL

During a cardiac arrest, it is important to identify the underlying cause of the arrest through a rapid assessment of the H's (hypovolemia,

TABLE 12-1	Cardiopulmonary Resuscitation Record of Events and Orders				
Time	**BP**	**Rhythm**	**Pulse**	**Defib. (J)**	**Treatment given**
0220	56/?	PEA	No pulse Chest compressions	None	Epi 1 mg IVP IO placement Labs ordered: Potassium, ABG, Lactate
0221	46/?	PEA	No pulse	None	Resume compressions Regular insulin 10 units IVP Sodium bicarbonate 50 mEq IVP Calcium chloride 1 gram IVP
0223	73/?	Bradycardia (see Fig. 12-1)	Pulse detected HR 50	None	Epi 1 mg IVP D50 1 amp
0225	88/?	VF (see Fig. 12-2)	No pulse Chest compressions	360	Vasopressin 40 units IVP
0227	?/133	SVT (see Fig. 12-3)	No pulse Chest compressions	360	Chest compressions resumed
0229	160/84	Sinus Tach	Pulse detected HR 180	None	

Key: ?, not recorded; ABG, arterial blood gas; BP, blood pressure; Defib., defibrillation; D50, dextrose 50%; Epi, epinephrine; HR, heart rate; IO, intraosseous; IVP, intravenous push; PEA, pulseless electrical activity; Sinus tach, sinus tachycardia; SVT, supraventricular tachycardia; VF, ventricular fibrillation; .

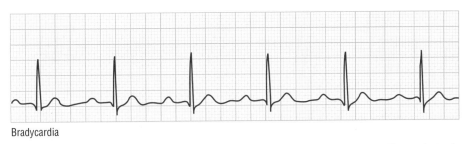

Bradycardia

FIGURE 12-1. Electrocardiogram showing bradycardia. (Reproduced with permission from acls-algorithms.com, Jeffery Media Productions, LLC.)

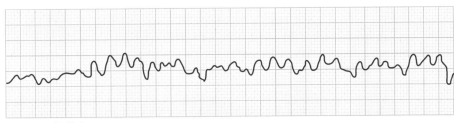

Ventricular fibrillation

FIGURE 12-2. Electrocardiogram showing ventricular fibrillation. (Reproduced with permission from acls-algorithms.com, Jeffery Media Productions, LLC.)

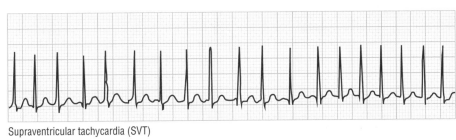

Supraventricular tachycardia (SVT)

FIGURE 12-3. Electrocardiogram showing supraventricular tachycardia. (Reproduced with permission from acls-algorithms.com, Jeffery Media Productions, LLC.)

hypoxia, hydrogen ion, hyper-/hypokalemia, hypothermia) and T's (toxins, tamponade, tension pneumothorax, thrombosis).

REFERENCES

1. Link MS, Berkow LC, Kudenchuk PJ, et al., 2015 American Heart Association update for cardiopulmonary resuscitation and emergency cardiovascular care. Circulation 2015;132(Suppl 2):S444–S464.

2. Vanden Hoek TL, Morrison LJ, Shuster M, et al. Part 12: Cardiac Arrest in Special Situations: 2010 American Heart Association guidelines for cardiopulmonary resuscitation and emergency cardiovascular care. Circulation 2010;122:S829–S861.

3. Neumar RW, Otto CW, Link MS, et al. Part 8: Advanced Life Support: 2010 American Heart Association guidelines for cardiopulmonary resuscitation and emergency cardiovascular care. Circulation 2010;122:S729–S767.

4. Ong ME, Tiah L, Leong BS, et al. A randomized, double-blind, multicentre trial comparing vasopressin and adrenaline in patients with cardiac arrest presenting to or in the Emergency Department. Resuscitation 2012;83:953–960.

5. Gueugniaud PY, David JS, Chanzy E, et al. Vasopressin and epinephrine vs. epinephrine alone in cardiopulmonary resuscitation. N Engl J Med 2008;359:21–30.

6. Mukoyama T, Kinoshita K, Nagao K, et al. Reduced effectiveness of vasopressin in repeated doses for patients undergoing prolonged cardiopulmonary resuscitation. Resuscitation 2009;80:755–761.

7. Mentzelopoulos SD, Malachias S, Chamos C, et al. Vasopressin, steroids, and epinephrine and neurologically favorable survival after in-hospital cardiac arrest: a randomized clinical trial. JAMA 2013;310:270–279.

8. Barr J, Fraser GL, Puntillo K, et al. Clinical practice guidelines for the management of pain, agitation, and delirium in adult patients in the intensive care unit. Crit Care Med 2013;41:263–306.

13

HYPERTENSION

Pass the Salt, Please . . . . Level II

Julia M. Koehler, PharmD, FCCP

James E. Tisdale, PharmD, BCPS, FCCP, FAPhA, FAHA

LEARNING OBJECTIVES

After completing this case study, the reader should be able to:

- Classify blood pressure according to current hypertension guidelines, and discuss the correlation between blood pressure and risk for cardiovascular morbidity and mortality.

- Identify medications that may cause or worsen HTN.

- Discuss complications (eg, target organ damage) that may occur as a result of uncontrolled and/or long-standing HTN.

- Establish goals for the treatment of HTN, and choose appropriate lifestyle modifications and antihypertensive regimens based on patient-specific characteristics, comorbid disease states, and current HTN guidelines.

- Provide appropriate patient counseling for antihypertensive drug regimens.

PATIENT PRESENTATION

■ Chief Complaint

"I'm here to see my new doctor for a checkup. I'm just getting over a cold. Overall, I'm feeling fine, except for occasional headaches and some dizziness in the morning. My other doctor prescribed a low-salt diet for me, but I don't like it!"

■ HPI

James Frank is a 64-year-old black man who presents to his new family medicine physician for evaluation and follow-up of his medical problems. He generally has no complaints, except for occasional mild headaches and some dizziness after he takes his morning medications. He states that he is dissatisfied with being placed on a low-sodium diet by his former primary care physician.

■ PMH

HTN × 14 years
Type 2 diabetes mellitus × 16 years
COPD, GOLD 3/Group C
BPH
CKD
Gout

■ FH

Father died of acute MI at age 73. Mother died of lung cancer at age 65. Father had HTN and dyslipidemia. Mother had HTN and diabetes mellitus.

■ SH

Former smoker (quit 6 years ago; 35 pack-year history); reports moderate amount of alcohol intake. He admits he has been nonadherent to his low-sodium diet (states, "I eat whatever I want"). He does not exercise regularly and is limited somewhat functionally by his COPD. He is retired and lives alone. He works at Wal-Mart and has healthcare insurance through his employer.

■ Meds

Triamterene/hydrochlorothiazide 37.5 mg/25 mg PO Q AM
Insulin glargine 36 units SC daily
Insulin lispro 12 units SC TID with meals
Doxazosin 2 mg PO Q AM
Carvedilol 12.5 mg PO BID
Albuterol HFA MDI, two inhalations Q 4–6 H PRN shortness of breath
Tiotropium DPI 18 mcg, one capsule inhaled daily
Fluticasone/salmeterol DPI 250/50, one inhalation BID
Mucinex D® two tablets Q 12 H PRN cough/congestion
Naproxen 220 mg PO Q 8 H PRN pain/HA
Allopurinol 200 mg PO daily

■ All

PCN—rash.

■ ROS

Patient states that overall he is doing well and recovering from a cold. He has noticed no major weight changes over the past few years. He complains of occasional headaches, which are usually relieved by naproxen, and he denies blurred vision and chest pain. He states that shortness of breath is "usual" for him, and that his albuterol helps. He reports having had two COPD exacerbations within the past 12 months. He denies experiencing any hemoptysis or epistaxis; he also denies nausea, vomiting, abdominal pain, cramping, diarrhea, constipation, or blood in stool. He denies urinary frequency, but states that he used to have difficulty urinating until his physician started him on doxazosin a few months ago. He has no prior history of arthritic symptoms and states that his occasional gout pain is also relieved with naproxen.

■ Physical Examination

Gen

WDWN, black male; moderately overweight; in no acute distress

VS

BP 162/90 mm Hg (sitting; repeat 164/92 mm Hg), HR 76 bpm (regular), RR 16/min, T 37°C; Wt 95 kg, Ht 6'2"

HEENT

TMs clear; mild sinus drainage; AV nicking noted; no hemorrhages, exudates, or papilledema

Neck

Supple without masses or bruits, no thyroid enlargement or lymphadenopathy

Lungs

Lung fields CTA bilaterally. Few basilar crackles, mild expiratory wheezing.

Heart

RRR; normal S_1 and S_2. No S_3 or S_4

Abd

Soft, NTND; no masses, bruits, or organomegaly. Normal BS

Genit/Rect

Enlarged prostate

Ext

No CCE; no apparent joint swelling or signs of tophi

Neuro

No gross motor-sensory deficits present. CN II–XII intact. A & O × 3

■ Labs

Na 138 mEq/L	Ca 9.7 mg/dL	*Fasting lipid panel*	*Spirometry (6 months ago)*
K 4.7 mEq/L	Mg 2.3 mEq/L		
Cl 99 mEq/L	A1C 6.1%	Total Chol 161 mg/dL	FVC 2.38 L (54% pred)
CO₂ 27 mEq/L	Alb 3.4 g/dL	LDL 79 mg/dL	FEV₁ 1.21 L (38% pred)
BUN 22 mg/dL	Hgb 13 g/dL	HDL 53 mg/dL	
SCr 2.2 mg/dL	Hct 40%	TG 144 mg/dL	FEV₁/FVC 51%
Glucose 110 mg/dL	WBC 9.0 × 10³/mm³		
Uric acid 6.7 mg/dL	Plts 189 × 10³/mm³		

UA

Yellow, clear, SG 1.007, pH 5.5, (+) protein, (–) glucose, (–) ketones, (–) bilirubin, (–) blood, (–) nitrite, RBC 0/hpf, WBC 1–2/hpf, neg bacteria, 1–5 epithelial cells.

ECG

Abnormal ECG: normal sinus rhythm; left atrial enlargement; left axis deviation; LVH

ECHO (6 Months Ago)

Mild LVH, estimated EF 45%

Assessment

1. HTN, uncontrolled
2. Type 2 DM, controlled on current insulin regimen
3. COPD, stable on current regimen
4. BPH, symptoms improved on doxazosin
5. Gout, controlled on current regimen

QUESTIONS

Problem Identification

1.a. Create a list of this patient's drug-related problems, including any medications that may be contributing to his uncontrolled HTN.

1.b. How would you classify this patient's HTN, according to current HTN guidelines?

1.c. What evidence of target organ damage or clinical cardiovascular disease does this patient have?

Desired Outcome

2. List the goals of treatment for this patient (including his goal blood pressure).

Therapeutic Alternatives

3.a. What lifestyle modifications should be encouraged for this patient to help achieve and maintain adequate blood pressure reduction?

3.b. What reasonable pharmacotherapeutic options are available for controlling this patient's blood pressure, and what comorbidities and individual patient considerations should be taken into account when selecting pharmacologic therapy for his HTN? How might Mr Frank's HTN medications potentially affect his other medical problems?

Optimal Plan

4.a. Recommend specific lifestyle modifications for this patient.

4.b. Outline a specific and appropriate pharmacotherapeutic regimen for this patient's uncontrolled HTN, including drug(s), dose(s), dosage form(s), and schedule(s).

Outcome Evaluation

5. Based on your recommendations, what parameters should be monitored after initiating this regimen and throughout the treatment course? At what time intervals should these parameters be monitored?

Patient Education

6. Based on your recommendations, provide appropriate education to this patient.

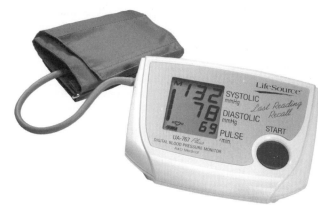

FIGURE 13-1. The LifeSource UA-767 Plus—One-Step Plus Memory digital home blood pressure monitor. (*Photo courtesy of A&D Medical, Milpitas, California.*)

■ SELF-STUDY ASSIGNMENTS

1. Describe the major causes of secondary HTN and the methods by which those could be ruled out in this patient.

2. Outline the changes, if any, that you would make to the pharmacotherapeutic regimen for this patient if he had a history of each of the following comorbidities or characteristics:
   - Severe persistent asthma
   - Major depression
   - Ischemic heart disease with a history of MI
   - Cerebrovascular accident
   - Peripheral arterial disease
   - Isolated systolic HTN
   - Migraine headache disorder
   - Liver disease
   - Renovascular disease (bilateral or unilateral renal artery stenosis)
   - Heart failure with reduced EF

3. Describe how you would explain to a patient how to use a digital home blood pressure monitor such as the one shown in Fig. 13-1.

CLINICAL PEARLS

1. The risk of hemorrhagic stroke may be increased by the use of aspirin therapy in patients with uncontrolled HTN (eg, BP > 150/90 mm Hg).

2. The majority of hypertensive patients will require two or more blood pressuring-lowering medications to achieve recommended blood pressure goals.

REFERENCES

1. Salerno SM, Jackson JL, Berbano EP. Effect of oral pseudoephedrine on blood pressure and heart rate: a meta-analysis. Arch Intern Med 2005;165:1686–1694.

2. Weber MA, Schiffrin EL, White WB, et al. Clinical practice guidelines for the 3 management of hypertension in the community: a statement by the American Society of Hypertension and the International Society of Hypertension. J Clin Hypertension 2014;16:14–26. doi:10.1111/jch.12237.

3. James PA, Oparil S, Carter BL, et al. 2014 Evidence-based guideline for the management of high blood pressure in adults: report from the panel members appointed to the Eighth Joint National Committee (JNC 8). JAMA 2013. doi:10.1001/jama2013.284427.

4. American Diabetes Association. Standards of medical care in diabetes—2016. Diabetes Care 2016;39(1 Suppl):S1–S112.

5. KDIGO clinical practice guideline for the management of blood pressure in kidney disease. Kidney Int Suppl 2012; 2: 337–414. doi:10.1038/kisup.2012.46.

6. Eckel RH, Jakicic JM, Ard JD, et al. 2013 AHA/ACC guideline on lifestyle management to reduce cardiovascular risk: a report of the American College of Cardiology/American Heart Association Task Force on practice guidelines. Circulation 2013. doi:10.1161/01.cir.0000437740.48606.d1.

7. Douglas JG, Bakris GL, Epstein M, et al. Management of high blood pressure in African Americans: consensus statement of the Hypertension in African Americans Working Group of the International Society on Hypertension in Blacks. Arch Intern Med 2003;163:525–541.

8. Heart Outcomes Prevention Evaluation Study Investigators. Effects of an angiotensin-converting enzyme inhibitor, ramipril, on cardiovascular events in high-risk patients. N Engl J Med 2000;342:145–153.

9. Heart Outcomes Prevention Evaluation Study Investigators. Effects of ramipril on cardiovascular and microvascular outcomes in people with diabetes mellitus: results of the HOPE study and the MICRO-HOPE substudy. Lancet 2000;355:253–259.

10. The ALLHAT Officers and Coordinators for the ALLHAT Collaborative Research Group. Major cardiovascular events in hypertensive patients randomized to doxazosin vs chlorthalidone: the Antihypertensive and Lipid-Lowering Treatment to Prevent Heart Attack Trial (ALLHAT). JAMA 2000;283:1967–1975.

11. Hou FF, Zhang X, Xie D, et al. Efficacy and safety of benazepril for advanced chronic renal insufficiency. N Engl J Med 2006;354:131–140.

14

HYPERTENSIVE CRISIS

I Don't Really Need Those Pills . . . . Level I

James J. Nawarskas, PharmD, BCPS

LEARNING OBJECTIVES

After completing this case study, the reader should be able to:

- Distinguish a hypertensive urgency from a hypertensive emergency.

- Identify treatment goals for a patient with a hypertensive crisis.

- Develop an appropriate treatment plan for a patient with a hypertensive crisis.

- Describe how a pharmacist can educate a patient about hypertension (HTN) and the importance of providing this education.

PATIENT PRESENTATION

■ Chief Complaint

"I'm having trouble seeing, and my chest feels tight."

■ HPI

Brenda Flores is a 63-year-old Hispanic woman who was admitted to the emergency department with a chief complaint of difficulty seeing and chest tightness. She describes "blurry vision" that has been happening off and on for the last few days. At first, it would just last for a second or two and then go away, but it has become progressively more lingering. She initially attributed this to her eyes "just getting old" but now is more concerned that it may be something else. The chest tightness started yesterday and was initially very mild, occurring when she would walk her dog outside and resolving readily with rest. However, it has since gotten more troublesome and is limiting her daily activities. While the chest discomfort still improves with rest, it no longer completely resolves. She tried to self-medicate by taking a double dose of ranitidine last night and another dose this morning, but she says that didn't help. She also states that this discomfort is very different from her gastroesophageal reflux. While seated in the emergency department she describes the chest discomfort as a 2 on a scale of 1–10 (highest). She has a past medical history significant for HTN and gastroesophageal reflux. She had been taking lisinopril and hydrochlorothiazide for several years with good blood pressure control, but about 6 months ago she stopped taking both medicines, because she had to make an urgent trip to visit her daughter out of state and ended up staying with her for a couple of months. Since her daughter lives in a rural area with no pharmacy nearby, she never got the medications refilled when she ran out. After several days, Ms Flores noticed that she felt just fine despite not taking the medicines. Consequently, she never resumed them and has not seen her provider since.

■ PMH

HTN × 9 years
Gastroesophageal reflux × 11 years

■ FH

Both parents had HTN. Father had a heart attack in his early 60s and died in his late 70s of a second heart attack; mother died a few years later from a stroke. Two brothers, 59 and 62 years old, are both alive; the elder has HTN and hypercholesterolemia and underwent CABG surgery 3 years ago; the younger has no chronic diseases. One sister who is 55 years old is in fairly good health.

■ SH

Married for 38 years with four children (two boys, two girls all over 25 years of age with no notable medical problems); she works part time (2–3 days per week) as a cashier at a large department store. She smoked cigarettes rather heavily when she was younger, but cut back to 1–2 per day when she was raising her children. As her children got older, she gradually increased her cigarette use and is now smoking about one pack per day and has been doing so for about the past 10 years. She drinks alcohol infrequently (maybe once or twice a month), when she is at a social gathering. She denies ever using recreational drugs. She does not exercise and leads a rather sedentary lifestyle. In terms of diet, for breakfast she typically has a cup of coffee, toast with butter, and two eggs. For lunch, she usually eats a cold cut sandwich, although on days she works, she typically does not eat lunch at all and compensates by eating a large breakfast. She does munch on snack cakes and chips on breaks during her work shift, however. For dinner, she likes to eat baked chicken and prepares some canned vegetables as a side dish along with a dinner salad with Italian dressing. She admits to the liberal use of salt during breakfast and dinner. She has a high school education. Her husband is alive and well and works as an accountant.

Her household income is average middle class. She has good health insurance through her husband's employer.

■ Meds

Ranitidine 75 mg PO once daily in the evening (over the counter); she has taken extra doses over the last 24 hours as mentioned above

Lisinopril/hydrocholorthiazide 20/12.5 mg PO once daily—stopped approximately 6 months ago

■ All

NKDA

■ ROS

Ms Flores complains of vision trouble as mentioned above; no hearing problems. She complains of chest discomfort as mentioned above but denies palpitations and dizziness. She admits to becoming short of breath more easily in the last few weeks and has felt a loss of energy over this same time period, although she never has been very active. She denies nausea, vomiting, or abdominal pain. She denies any swelling in her extremities or weight gain. She denies mental status changes.

■ Physical Examination

Gen

The patient is a middle-aged Hispanic woman appearing to be in moderate distress

VS

BP 240/130 mm Hg right arm, 232/128 mm Hg left arm (manual readings performed in the emergency department). A repeat measurement in the right arm after several minutes yields a BP of 236/134 mm Hg.

P 74, RR 24, T 36.8°C; Wt 80 kg, Ht 5′5″

Skin

Normal tone and temperature, good turgor

HEENT

PERRLA; EOMI; funduscopic exam revealed arterial tortuosity with A/V nicking and papilledema

Neck/Lymph Nodes

Neck supple, no JVD, no bruits, no thyromegaly, or lymphadenopathy

Chest

CTA

CV

PMI shifted laterally, RRR, no murmurs or rubs appreciated; +S_4 heard at apex

Abd

Soft, NT/ND, no guarding, (+) BS, no abdominal bruits appreciated, liver span about 12 cm

Genit/Rect

Normal female genitalia, heme-negative stool

MS/Ext

Normal ROM, no CCE, pulses 2+ radial; 1+ to 2+ in the rest of her upper and lower extremities

Neuro

A & O × 3, CN II–XII intact, motor/sensory normal, DTRs 2+

■ Labs

Na 140 mEq/L	Hgb 13.2 g/dL	AST 27 IU/L
K 4.9 mEq/L	Hct 43%	ALT 45 IU/L
Cl 100 mEq/L	WBC 6.6 × 10³/mm³	Cholesterol 196 mg/dL
CO₂ 28 mEq/L	Plt 222 × 10³/mm³	HDL 42 mg/dL
BUN 30 mg/dL		Triglycerides 142 mg/dL
SCr 1.6 mg/dL		LDL 126 mg/dL
Glu 122 mg/dL		Troponin-I normal

■ UA

Specific gravity 1.010; pH 5.8; negative for blood or protein; negative for recreational drugs

■ Chest X-Ray

Enlarged heart, no infiltrates

■ ECG

Normal sinus rhythm; LVH by voltage criteria. There are no ST-segment changes, although there does appear to be some T-wave flattening in the anterior leads. No old ECGs are available for comparison.

■ Assessment

A 63-year-old woman with a long-standing history of HTN and gastroesophageal reflux presents with an extremely elevated blood pressure and signs and symptoms of target organ damage. She admits to not taking any antihypertensive drug therapy for 6 months which was initially due to difficulty in getting her medications refilled, and then later due to feeling just fine despite not taking the medications.

QUESTIONS

Problem Identification

1.a. Did this patient's situation result from a drug-related problem? Why or why not?

1.b. What signs and symptoms are present that may be related to the severity of this patient's hypertension?

1.c. Is this a hypertensive urgency or an emergency? Explain your answer.

Desired Outcome

2.a. What are the goals of pharmacotherapy for this patient's hypertension?

2.b. How would the treatment goals differ if this patient presented with the same blood pressure, but was asymptomatic with normal laboratory findings and no acute changes on ECG or physical examination?

Therapeutic Alternatives

3.a. What nondrug therapies might be useful for this patient?

3.b. What feasible pharmacotherapeutic alternatives are available for the treatment of this patient's acute hypertension?

Optimal Plan

4.a. What drug and dosage form are best for treating this patient's acute hypertension?

4.b. How would your treatment recommendations differ if this patient presented with the same blood pressure, but was asymptomatic with normal laboratory findings and no acute changes on physical examination?

Outcome Evaluation

5. Which clinical and laboratory parameters are necessary to evaluate your therapy for reducing this patient's blood pressure and monitoring for adverse events?

Patient Education

6. What information can you provide to Ms Flores to enhance adherence, ensure successful therapy, and minimize adverse effects?

Clinical Course

Once Ms Flores's blood pressure is lowered to an acceptable level, her inpatient provider consults with you regarding chronic antihypertensive therapy for Ms Flores.

7.a. Do you recommend Ms Flores resume her lisinopril/HCTZ as prescribed, or would you recommend alternative drug therapy? Rationalize your answer. If you would recommend alternative drug therapy, which drug(s) would you recommend and why?

7.b. What nonpharmacologic measures can Ms Flores incorporate as part of an overall treatment plan for her chronic hypertension?

■ SELF-STUDY ASSIGNMENTS

1. You are a pharmacist working in a community pharmacy that has a designated patient care center equipped with a manual blood pressure cuff. Describe your approach in dealing with a patient who reports that the automated blood pressure monitor in the waiting area of the pharmacy provided him or her with extremely high blood pressure measurements.

2. Describe any ethnic and racial differences in response to antihypertensive medications and the impact these differences may have on drug selection.

3. Use an algorithm or flow diagram to illustrate your approach to dealing with a patient who is nonadherent to antihypertensive therapy. After you do so, read the article: Can drugs work in patients who do not take them? The problem of nonadherence in resistant hypertension (Curr Hypertens Rep 2015;17:69). Then redesign your approach if necessary.

CLINICAL PEARL

Of patients presenting to the emergency department with a hypertensive emergency, the vast majority of them have been diagnosed with hypertension and have been prescribed antihypertensive medication. Only 8% of hypertensive emergencies presenting to the emergency department involve patients unaware of having a diagnosis of hypertension.

REFERENCES

1. Chobanian AV, Bakris GL, Black HR, et al. Seventh report of the Joint National Committee on Prevention, Detection, Evaluation, and Treatment of High Blood Pressure. Hypertension 2003;42:1206–1252.

2. Rodriguez MA, Kumar SK, De Caro M. Hypertensive crisis. Cardiol Rev 2010;18:102–107.

3. Hebert CJ, Vidt DG. Hypertensive crises. Prim Care Office Pract 2008;35:475–487.

4. Ramos AP, Varon J. Current and newer agents for hypertensive emergencies. Curr Hypertens Rep 2014;16:450.

5. Mansoor GA, Frishman WH. Comprehensive management of hypertensive emergencies and urgencies. Heart Dis 2002;4:358–371.

6. Varon J. Treatment of acute severe hypertension: current and newer agents. Drugs 2008;68:283–297.

7. James PA, Oparil S, Carter BL, et al. 2014 Evidence-based guideline for the management of high blood pressure in adults. Report from the Panel Members Appointed to the Eighth Joint National Committee (JNC 8). JAMA 2014;311(5):507–520.

8. Aggarwal M, Khan I. Hypertensive crisis: hypertensive emergencies and urgencies. Cardiol Clin 2006;24:135–146.

9. Thach AM, Schultz PJ. Nonemergent hypertension: new perspectives for the emergency medicine physician. Emerg Med Clin North Am 1995;13:1009–1035.

10. Gales MA. Oral antihypertensives for hypertensive urgencies. Ann Pharmacother 1994;28:274–284.

15

HEART FAILURE WITH REDUCED EJECTION FRACTION

Cross My Heart and Hope to Live . . . . Level III

Julia M. Koehler, PharmD, FCCP

Alison M. Walton, PharmD, BCPS

LEARNING OBJECTIVES

After completing this case study, the reader should be able to:

- Recognize the signs and symptoms of heart failure.

- Develop a pharmacotherapeutic plan for treatment of heart failure with reduced ejection fraction (HFrEF).

- Outline a monitoring plan for heart failure that includes both clinical and laboratory parameters.

PATIENT PRESENTATION

■ Chief Complaint

"I've been more short of breath lately. I can't seem to walk as far as I used to, and either my feet are growing or my shoes are shrinking!"

■ HPI

Rosemary Quincy is a 68-year-old African-American female who presents to her family medicine physician for evaluation of her shortness of breath and increased swelling in her lower extremities. She reports that her shortness of breath has been gradually increasing over the past 4 days. She has noticed that her shortness of breath is particularly worse when she is lying in bed at night, and she has to prop her head up with three pillows in order to sleep. She also reports exertional dyspnea that is usual for her, but especially worse over the past couple of days.

CHAPTER 15

PMH

Hypertension × 20 years
CHD with history of MI in 2005 (PCI performed and bare metal stents placed in LAD and RCA)
Heart failure (NYHA FC III)
Type 2 DM × 25 years
Atrial fibrillation
COPD (GOLD 3, Group D)
CKD (Stage 4)

FH

Father died of lung cancer at age 71, mother died of MI at age 73.

SH

Reports occasional alcohol intake. States she has been trying to follow her low-cholesterol and low-sodium diet. Former smoker (35 pack-year history; quit approximately 10 years ago).

Meds

Valsartan 160 mg PO BID
Furosemide 40 mg PO BID
Warfarin 2.5 mg PO once daily
Carvedilol 3.125 mg PO BID
Pioglitazone 30 mg PO once daily
Glimepiride 2 mg PO once daily
Potassium chloride 20 mEq PO once daily
Atorvastatin 40 mg PO once daily
Aspirin 81 mg PO once daily
Albuterol MDI, two inhalations by mouth q 4–6 hours PRN shortness of breath
Tiotropium DPI 18 mcg, one inhalation by mouth daily
Fluticasone/salmeterol DPI 250 mcg/50 mcg, one inhalation by mouth BID

All

Lisinopril (cough).

ROS

Approximate 7-kg weight gain over the past week. No fever or chills. Denies any recent chest pain, palpitations, or dizziness. Reports worsening shortness of breath with exertion and three-pillow orthopnea. Describes a chronic, dry (nonproductive), hacking cough, which she describes as usual without recent worsening. No abdominal pain, nausea, constipation, or change in bowel habits. Denies joint pain or weakness.

Physical Examination

Gen

African-American female in moderate respiratory distress

VS

BP 134/76 (sitting; repeat 138/78), HR 65 (irreg irreg), RR 24, T 37°C, O_2 sat 90% RA, Ht 5′5″, Wt 79 kg (Wt 1 week ago: 72 kg)

Skin

Color pale and diaphoretic; no unusual lesions noted

HEENT

PERRLA; lips mildly cyanotic; dentures

Neck

(+) JVD at 30° (7 cm); no lymphadenopathy or thyromegaly

Lungs/Thorax

Crackles bilaterally, 2/3 of the way up; no expiratory wheezing

Heart

Irregularly irregular; (+) S_3; displaced PMI

Abd

Soft, mildly tender, nondistended; (+) HJR; no masses, mild hepatosplenomegaly; normal BS

Genit/Rect

Guaiac (–), genital examination not performed

MS/Ext

3+ pitting pedal edema bilaterally; radial and pedal pulses are of poor intensity bilaterally

Neuro

A & O × 3, CNs intact. No motor deficits

Labs

Na 131 mEq/L	Hgb 13 g/dL	Mg 1.9 mEq/L	INR 2.3
K 3.5 mEq/L	Hct 40%	Ca 9.3 mg/dL	A1C 6.1%
Cl 99 mEq/L	Plt 192 × 10³/mm³	Phos 4.3 mg/dL	
CO_2 28 mEq/L	WBC 9.1 × 10³/mm³	AST 34 IU/L	
BUN 32 mg/dL		ALT 27 IU/L	
SCr 2.3 mg/dL (baseline SCr 2.1 mg/dL)			
Glucose 124 mg/dL			
BNP 776 pg/mL (BNP drawn 2 months prior: 474 pg/mL)			

ECG

Atrial fibrillation, LVH.

Chest X-Ray

PA and lateral views (Fig. 15-1) show evidence of congestive failure with cardiomegaly, interstitial edema, and some early alveolar edema. There is a small right pleural effusion.

No evidence of infiltrates; evidence of pulmonary edema suggestive of congestive heart failure; enlarged cardiac silhouette.

Echocardiogram

LVH, reduced global left ventricular systolic function, estimated EF 20%; evidence of impaired ventricular relaxation, Stage 1 diastolic dysfunction.

Assessment

Admit to hospital for acute exacerbation of heart failure

QUESTIONS

Problem Identification

1.a. Create a list of this patient's drug-related problems.

1.b. What signs, symptoms, and other information indicate the presence and type of heart failure in this patient?

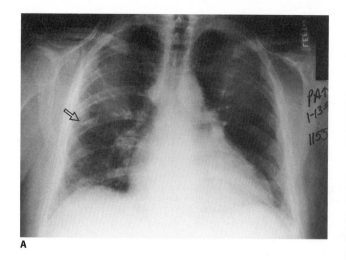

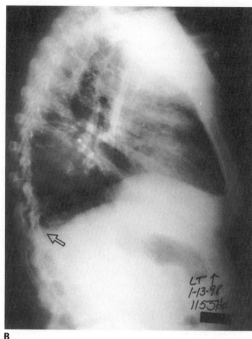

FIGURE 15-1. *A.* PA CXR demonstrates increased vascular markings representative of interstitial edema, with some early alveolar edema. The *arrow* points out fluid lying in the fissure of the right lung. Note the presence of cardiomegaly. *B.* Lateral view of CXR. *Arrow* points out the presence of pulmonary effusion.

1.c. What is the classification and staging of chronic heart failure for this patient?

1.d. Could any of this patient's problems have been caused by drug therapy?

Desired Outcome

2. What are the goals for the pharmacologic management of heart failure in this patient?

Therapeutic Alternatives

3.a. What diuretic therapy should be recommended for this patient initially for acute treatment of her heart failure exacerbation?

3.b. How should this patient's pharmacotherapy be adjusted for chronic management of her heart failure?

3.c. What nonpharmacologic therapy should be recommended for this patient with respect to her heart failure?

Optimal Plan

4. What drugs, doses, schedules, and duration are best suited for the management of this patient?

Outcome Evaluation

5. What clinical and laboratory parameters are needed to evaluate the therapy for achievement of the desired therapeutic outcome and to detect and prevent adverse events?

Patient Education

6. What information should be provided to the patient about the medications used to treat her heart failure?

■ SELF-STUDY ASSIGNMENTS

1. Develop a table illustrating the recommended target doses for ACE inhibitors, angiotensin II receptor blockers, and β-blockers in patients with heart failure with reduced EF.

2. Research the topic of diuretic resistance, and write a report describing the phenomenon and methods used to overcome it.

3. Review the guidelines and evidence describing the role of routine BNP monitoring in patients with heart failure.

CLINICAL PEARL

The presence of pitting edema is associated with a substantial increase in body weight; it typically takes a weight gain of 10 lb to result in the development of pitting edema.

REFERENCES

1. Nesto RW, Bell D, Bonow RO, et al. AHA/ADA consensus statement for thiazolidinedione use, fluid retention, and congestive heart failure. Circulation 2003;108:2941–2948.

2. Yancy CW, Jessup M, Bozkurt B, et al. 2013 ACCF/AHA guideline for the management of heart failure: a report of the American College of Cardiology Foundation/American Heart Association Task Force on Practice Guidelines. J Am Coll Cardiol 2013;62:e147–e239. doi: 10.1016/j.jacc.2013.05.019.

3. Cohn JN, Tognoni G; Valsartan Heart Failure Trial Investigators. A randomized trial of the angiotensin-receptor blocker valsartan in chronic heart failure. N Engl J Med 2001;345:1667–1675.

4. Mentz RJ, Wojdyla D, Fiuzat M, Chiswell K, Fonarow GC, O'Connor CM. Association of beta-blocker use and selectivity with outcomes in patients with heart failure and chronic obstructive pulmonary disease (from OPTIMIZE-HF). Am J Cardiol 2013;111:582–587.

5. Pitt B, Zannad F, Remme WJ. The effect of spironolactone on morbidity and mortality in patients with severe heart failure. Randomized Aldactone Evaluation Study Investigators. N Engl J Med 1999;341:709–717.

6. Pitt B, Remme W, Zannad F, et al. Eplerenone, a selective aldosterone blocker, in patients with left ventricular dysfunction after myocardial infarction. N Engl J Med 2003;348:1309–1321.

7. Zannad F, McMurray JJV, Krum H, et al.; for the EMPHASIS-HF Study Group. Eplerenone in patients with systolic heart failure and mild symptoms. N Engl J Med 2011;364:11–21.

8. Butler J, Ezekowitz JA, Collins JP, et al. Update on aldosterone antagonists use in heart failure with reduced left ventricular ejection fraction. Heart Failure Society of America Guidelines Committee. J Card Fail 2012;18:265–281.

9. Taylor AL, Ziesche S, Yancy C, et al.; for the African-American Heart Failure Trial Investigators. Combination of isosorbide dinitrate and hydralazine in blacks with heart failure. N Engl J Med 2004;351:2049–2057.

10. Swedberg K, Komajda M, Bohm M, et al. Ivabradine and outcomes in chronic heart failure (SHIFT): a randomised placebo-controlled study. Lancet 2010;367:875–885.

11. Yancy CW, Jessup M, Bozkurt B, et al. 2016 ACC/AHA/HFSA Focused Update on New Pharmacological Therapy for Heart Failure: An Update of the 2013 ACCF/AHA Guideline for the Management of Heart Failure: A Report of the American College of Cardiology Foundation/American Heart Association Task Force on Clinical Practice Guidelines and the Heart Failure Society of America. Circulation 2016;134. DOI:10.1161/CIR0000000000000435.

12. McMurray JV, Packer M, Desai AS, et al. Angiotensin-neprilysin inhibition versus enalapril in heart failure. N Engl J Med 2014;371:993–1004.

13. Moe GW, Ezekowitz JA, O'Meara E, et al. The 2014 Canadian Cardiovascular Society Heart Failure Management Guidelines Focus Update: anemia, biomarkers and recent therapeutic trial implications. Can J Cardiol 2015;15:3–16.

16

HEART FAILURE WITH PRESERVED EJECTION FRACTION

A Balancing Act .... Level II

Joel C. Marrs, PharmD, FASHP, FCCP, FNLA, BCPS-AQ Cardiology, BCACP, CLS

Joseph P. Vande Griend, PharmD, FCCP, BCPS, CGP

LEARNING OBJECTIVES

After completing this case study, the reader should be able to:

• Recognize the signs and symptoms of heart failure with preserved ejection fraction (HFpEF).

• Develop a pharmacotherapeutic plan for treatment of HFpEF.

• Outline a monitoring plan for HFpEF that includes both clinical and laboratory parameters.

• Initiate, titrate, and monitor β-adrenergic blocker, calcium channel blocker, angiotensin-converting enzyme inhibitor, angiotensin receptor blocker, aldosterone antagonist and diuretic therapy in HFpEF when indicated.

PATIENT PRESENTATION

■ Chief Complaint

"Why do I keep gaining all this weight?"

■ HPI

Lawrence Smith is a 62-year-old man who presents to the ED with shortness of breath and lower extremity edema. He reports his symptoms started approximately 1–1.5 weeks ago. He noted that he was gaining about 2 lb daily and gained approximately 15 lb of weight over the week prior to admission. He attempted to use his albuterol/ipratropium MDI for relief of symptoms at home without improvement. As his symptoms worsened, he called his primary care physician, who increased his furosemide dose over the phone to 80 mg twice daily. In the ED he was noted to be hypoxic with an increased oxygen need from 2 to 4 L by nasal cannula. He was given one dose of IV furosemide 80 mg with improvement and then admitted to the medicine service for further evaluation and management.

■ PMH

CAD (s/p STEMI 6 years ago)
COPD × 3 years
HFpEF × 4 years (last hospitalization 6 months ago)
Dyslipidemia × 10 years
HTN × 20 years
Type 2 DM × 3 years

■ FH

Father is alive at age 86 with type 2 DM; mother is alive at age 84 and has HTN and dyslipidemia; two brothers (age 56 and 60) alive and both have type 2 DM and HTN.

■ SH

History of tobacco use (30 pack-year history), but quit 3 years ago. Denies any alcohol or substance abuse. Lives alone.

■ Meds

Albuterol/ipratropium MDI, two puffs inhaled Q 6 H PRN
Aspirin 81 mg PO daily
Lisinopril 40 mg PO daily
Carvedilol 12.5 mg PO BID
Furosemide 80 mg PO BID (previously 40 mg PO BID)
Isosorbide mononitrate ER 30 mg PO Q AM
Metformin 500 mg PO BID
Nitroglycerin 0.4 mg SL q 5 minutes PRN chest pain
Potassium chloride 20 mEq PO BID
Rosuvastatin 20 mg PO daily

■ All

NKDA

■ ROS

Gen

Patient reports a recent 15-lb weight gain over the past week

CV

No complaints of chest pain but reports dyspnea on exertion

Resp

Reports an increase in shortness of breath from baseline

GI

No recent changes noted in bowel habits

GU

No complaints

MS

No complaints of MS pain or weakness

Neuro

No complaints

■ Physical Examination

Gen

Patient with 15-lb weight gain over past week with increased short-ness of breath

VS

BP 150/92, P 68 (regular), RR 24, T 36.9°C; Wt 100 kg (usual weight 93 kg), Ht 5′8″, oxygen saturation of 95% on 4-L nasal cannula

Skin

Chronic venous stasis changes on bilateral lower extremities and 2+ edema to the knees bilaterally

HEENT

PERRLA, EOMI, fundi were not examined. Normocephalic, atrau-matic. Nasal cannula in place

Neck

(+) JVD at 30° (4 cm). Carotid bruit is not appreciated. No lymph-adenopathy or thyromegaly

Lungs/Thorax

Respirations are even. Crackles noted in the right lung base

Heart

RRR. No murmurs, rubs, or gallops

Abd

Obese with a nontender, nondistended abdomen; hypoactive bowel sounds

Genit/Rect

Guaiac (–), genital examination not performed

MS/Ext

2+ pitting pedal edema bilaterally; radial and pedal pulses are of poor intensity bilaterally; grip strength even

Neuro

A & O × 3; CNs intact; DTR intact

■ Labs

Na 140 mEq/L	Hgb 15.3 g/dL	Mg 1.7 mEq/L	CK 20 IU/L
K 4.2 mEq/L	Hct 47.2%	Ca 9.1 mg/dL	CK-MB 0.8 IU/L
Cl 103 mEq/L	Plt 298 × 10³/mm³	AST 50 IU/L	PT 12.6 s
CO_2 26 mEq/L	WBC 6.4 × 10³/mm³	ALT 43 IU/L	INR 1.1
BUN 20 mg/dL	Troponin I 0.5 ng/mL	Alk phos 80 IU/L	TSH 2.01 mIU/L
SCr 0.9 mg/dL		GGT 24 IU/L	A1C 7.2%
Glucose 108 mg/dL		T. bili 0.2 mg/dL	
BNP 900 pg/mL			

■ ECG

Sinus rate of 70; QRS 0.08; no ST–T wave changes; low voltage.

■ CXR

PA and lateral views show evidence of interstitial edema and some early alveolar edema.

■ Assessment

Decompensated heart failure with pulmonary and lower extremity edema.

CLINICAL COURSE

The patient was admitted to a telemetry unit. The patient has a known history of heart failure with preserved systolic function (EF 55%) per an echocardiogram from 1 year ago. A 2D echocar-diogram was obtained today to evaluate the patient's current LV and valvular function. Results revealed evidence of impaired ven-tricular relaxation and elevated left atrial filling pressures consistent with grade II diastolic dysfunction. EF was estimated at 53%; there was no evidence of mitral stenosis or pericardial disease. A dilated inferior vena cava suggests increased right atrial pressure. Moderate pulmonary HTN is evident.

QUESTIONS

Problem Identification

1.a. Create a list of this patient's drug-related problems.

1.b. What signs, symptoms, and other information indicate the presence and severity of the patient's heart failure?

1.c. What are the classification and staging of this patient's heart failure on presentation?

1.d. Could any of this patient's problems have been caused by drug therapy or lack of optimal drug therapy?

Desired Outcome

2.a. What are the goals for the pharmacologic management of HFpEF in this patient?

2.b. Considering this patient's other medical problems, what other treatment goals should be established?

Therapeutic Alternatives

3. What medications are indicated in the long-term management of this patient's HFpEF based on his stage of heart failure?

Optimal Plan

4. What drugs, doses, schedules, and duration are best suited for the management of this patient?

Outcome Evaluation

5. What clinical and laboratory parameters are needed to evaluate the therapy for achievement of the desired therapeutic outcome and to detect and prevent adverse events?

■ CLINICAL COURSE (PART 1)

Over the next 3 days, the patient received maximal drug therapy, and his condition improved. He was discharged on spironolactone 12.5 mg PO daily, lisinopril 40 mg PO daily, carvedilol 25 mg PO BID, furosemide 80 mg PO twice daily, metformin 500 mg PO twice daily, rosuvastatin 20 mg PO daily, albuterol/ipratropium MDI two puffs four times a day, and aspirin 81 mg PO daily. On the day of discharge his serum potassium was 4.0 mEq/L, creatinine 1.1 mg/dL, and BUN 18 mg/dL, and he had a blood pressure of 140/88 mm Hg with a heart rate of 70 bpm.

Patient Education

6. What information should be provided to the patient about the medications used to treat his HF*p*EF?

■ CLINICAL COURSE (PART 2)

On follow-up with his primary care physician, the patient is noted to have sustained a 5-lb weight gain from baseline dry weight at discharge. He feels much better than prior to coming to the hospital and is back to most of his daily living activities.

■ FOLLOW-UP QUESTIONS

1. Outline a plan for maximizing the patient's current medication regimen for HF*p*EF.

2. Would you consider titrating up his carvedilol to a higher dose? If so, why? Is switching the patient to a long-acting, once-daily carvedilol product indicated?

■ SELF-STUDY ASSIGNMENTS

1. Describe the common causes of HF*p*EF.

2. Describe how you would evaluate and monitor this patient's quality of life.

3. Evaluate whether evidence exists to support the role of eplerenone in HF*p*EF.

CLINICAL PEARL

Patients with heart failure who require chronic diuretic therapy with furosemide and still struggle to maintain fluid balance (eg, multiple hospitalizations for fluid overload despite maximized furosemide as an outpatient) may need their diuretic therapy optimized by switching to another loop diuretic with better oral bioavailability (eg, torsemide or bumetanide).

REFERENCES

1. Tang WH, Francis GS, Morrow DA, et al. National Academy of Clinical Biochemistry Laboratory Medicine Practice Guidelines: clinical utilization of cardiac biomarker testing in heart failure. Circulation 2007;116:e99–e109.

2. Yancy C, Jessup M, Bozkurt B, et al. 2013 ACCF/AHA guideline for the management of heart failure: a report of the American College of Cardiology Foundation/American Heart Association Task Force on Practice Guidelines. Circulation 2013;128:eh240–e327.

3. Lindenfeld J, Albert NM, Boehmery JP, et al. Executive summary: HFSA 2010 comprehensive heart failure practice guideline. J Card Fail 2010;16:475–539.

4. Stone NJ, Robinson J, Lichtenstein AH, et al. 2013 ACC/AHA guideline on the treatment of blood cholesterol to reduce atherosclerotic cardiovascular risk in adults: a report of the American College of Cardiology/American Heart Association Task Force on Practice Guidelines. Circulation 2014;129(25 Suppl 2):S1–S45.

5. The Digitalis Investigation Group. The effect of digoxin on mortality and morbidity in patients with heart failure. N Engl J Med 1997;336:525–533.

6. Basaraba JE, Barry AR. Pharmacotherapy of heart failure with preserved ejection fraction. Pharmacotherapy 2015;35:351–360.

7. Nanaykkara S, Kaye DM. Management of heart failure with preserved ejection fraction: a review. Clin Ther 2015;37:2186–2198.

8. Hernandez AF, Hammill BG, O'Connor CM, Schulman KA, Curtis LH, Fonarow GC. Clinical effectiveness of beta-blockers in heart failure: findings from the OPTIMIZE-HF (organized program to initiate life-saving treatment in hospitalized patients with heart failure) registry. J Am Coll Cardiol 2009;53:184–192.

9. Nichols GA, Reynolds K, Kimes TM, Rosales AG, Chan WW. Comparison of risk of re-hospitalization, all-cause mortality, and medical care resource utilization in patients with heart failure and preserved versus reduced ejection fraction. Am J Cardiol 2015;116:1088–1092.

10. Pitt B, Pfeffer MA, Assmann SF, et al. Spironolactone for heart failure with preserved ejection fraction. N Engl J Med 2014;370:1383–1392.

11. Pfeffer MA, Claggett B, Assmann SF, et al. Regional variation in patients and outcomes in the Treatment of Preserved Cardiac Function Heart Failure With an Aldosterone Antagonist (TOPCAT) trial. Circulation 2015;131:34–42.

12. Mentz RJ, Wojdyla D, Fiuzat M, et al. Association of beta-blocker use and selectivity with outcomes in patients with heart failure and chronic obstructive pulmonary disease (from OPTIMIZE-HF). Am J Cardiol 2013;111:582–587.

17

ACUTE DECOMPENSATED HEART FAILURE

Don't Be Such a Busy Body . . . . Level II

Kena J. Lanham, PharmD, BCPS

LEARNING OBJECTIVES

After completing this case study, the reader should be able to:

- Identify the signs and symptoms of acute decompensated heart failure (ADHF).

- Classify a patient into the appropriate hemodynamic subset based on symptoms and clinical presentation.

- List goals of therapy for treating ADHF.

- Develop a pharmacotherapeutic plan for treating a patient with ADHF in the hemodynamic subset presented.

- Outline a monitoring plan for treating a patient with ADHF in the hospital.

PATIENT PRESENTATION

■ Chief Complaint

"I can no longer lie down flat because I can't breathe and I've gained 3 pounds in 3 days."

■ HPI

Bizzy Fuller is a 64-year-old female with a history of ischemic cardiomyopathy with last known EF 25% (ECHO 1.5 years ago). She presents to the emergency department with approximately 2–3 days of increasing shortness of breath, and she reports having gained approximately 3 lb over the past 3 days. She also notes that she has had increasing leg swelling over the same time period. Over the past week, the patient has noted increasing bloating in her abdomen and has felt slightly nauseated. She has had problems with diarrhea and constipation since her cholecystectomy several months ago. She has been on a fiber supplement, from which she has derived some benefit. She states that she had been on torsemide many years ago but for an unknown reason was switched to furosemide.

■ PMH

CAD (status postmyocardial infarction × 2 in early 2000s; CABG in 2000, PCI in May 2002)
Paroxysmal ventricular tachycardia (status post-ICD placement in 2011)
Obstructive sleep apnea
Diabetes mellitus type 2
Depression
Dyslipidemia
Mild osteoarthritis
GERD
Seasonal allergies

■ FH

Both her mother and father died of MI in their 60s

■ SH

Patient is a happily married, retired school teacher and is fully functional with ADLs. She is an occasional alcohol drinker (two to three drinks per week) and has a 30 pack-year history, but quit smoking approximately 12 years ago.

■ Meds

Fexofenadine 60 mg orally BID
Insulin detemir 40 units SC at bedtime
Insulin aspart 7 units SC before each meal
Aspirin 81 mg orally once daily
Carvedilol 12.5 mg orally BID
Duloxetine 30 mg orally once daily
Fluticasone nasal spray 50 mcg/inh one spray BID
Lasix 80 mg orally BID
Lisinopril 20 mg orally once daily
Meloxicam 15 mg orally daily PRN joint pain
Nitroglycerin 0.4 mg sublingually PRN chest pain
Simvastatin 20 mg orally QHS
Ranitidine 150 mg orally BID

■ All

NKDA

■ ROS

She denies any fevers, chills, sweats, or coughs. She states that her diet has not changed recently, and she tries to watch her salt intake, but she states that she has been nonadherent to her medication regimen for the last 2 days, stating, "I have been too busy to take my medicine." She denies any significant chest pain and also denies any history of additional coronary intervention procedures since 2002. All others negative.

■ Physical Examination

Gen

A 64-year-old obese, Caucasian female in mild respiratory distress

VS

BP 186/92 mm Hg, P 71 bpm, RR 32 on admission (16 currently), oxygen saturation 86–92%; T 97.5°F; Ht 5′3″; Wt 87.4 kg

Skin

Warm and diaphoretic

HEENT

NC/AT with trachea midline

Neck/Lymph Nodes

Neck supple, (+) JVD, no bruits, no thyromegaly

Lungs/Thorax

Crackles in the bases bilaterally

Breasts

Normal

CV

Regular rate and rhythm without any murmurs, gallops, or rubs

Abd

Soft, nondistended, nontender

Genit/Rect

Deferred

MS/Ext

Extremities reveal 2+ pitting edema; all pulses palpable

Neuro

A & O × 3, CNs intact, history of depression but no apparent symptoms at present

■ Labs

Na 131 mEq/L	BNP 2867 pg/mL
K 3.7 mEq/L	Troponin 0.03 ng/mL
Cl 101 mEq/L	WBC 8.7 × 10³/mm³
CO_2 20 mEq/L	Hgb 14.1 g/dL
BUN 24 mg/dL	Hct 42.3%
SCr 1.7 mg/dL	Plt 226 × 10³/mm³
Glu 96 mg/dL	A1C 6.5%
Ca 9.6 mg/dL	

■ Chest X-Ray

Interstitial infiltrates throughout, tiny pleural effusions bilaterally; mild cardiomegaly; implanted defibrillator leads are at the right atrial appendage and right ventricular apex. No focal pneumonia, pneumothorax, or evidence of frank pulmonary edema.

■ ECG

Sinus rhythm with occasional premature ventricular complexes; no acute ischemia indicated

■ Assessment

Congestive heart failure exacerbation due to medication nonadherence; poorly controlled hypertension. Admit for medical management.

QUESTIONS

Problem Identification

1.a. What signs and symptoms indicate the presence of ADHF in this patient?

1.b. Create a list of BF's drug-related problems, including those that may have led to ADHF.

1.c. Which complaints and clinical findings characterize the patient's volume status (wet or dry)? Which complaints and clinical findings characterize the patient's perfusion status (warm or cold)?

Desired Outcome

2. What are the short-term goals of pharmacotherapy regarding treatment of ADHF?

Therapeutic Alternatives

3.a. What nondrug therapies might be useful for alleviating this patient's symptoms and preventing a recurrence of ADHF?

3.b. What pharmacotherapeutic options are available for treatment of this patient's ADHF?

Optimal Plan

4 What drugs, doses, schedule, and duration are best for achieving the pharmacotherapeutic goals for this patient?

Outcome Evaluation

5. What clinical and laboratory parameters are necessary to evaluate your chosen therapy for achievement of the desired therapeutic outcome and to detect or prevent adverse effects?

Patient Education

6. What discharge education should be provided in order to enhance adherence, ensure successful therapy, minimize adverse effects, and prevent an unplanned readmission?

■ SELF-STUDY ASSIGNMENTS

1. Review the current heart failure treatment guidelines, and create a table highlighting the patient characteristics that necessitate hospital admission versus those that are conducive to treatment in the outpatient setting.

2. List all Heart Failure National Hospital Inpatient Quality Measures (core measures) that must be fulfilled prior to BF's discharge.

3. Review the available literature on prognostic indicators in heart failure, and create a list of prognostic indicators for readmission or mortality in patients with heart failure.

4. Contrast the pharmacotherapeutic plan developed in this case with that of a pharmacotherapeutic plan for a patient presenting with heart failure with preserved EF.

CLINICAL PEARL

Patients with heart failure are at a high risk of mortality and morbidity and thus have increasingly high costs of care. Due to our aging population, among other factors, total costs for heart failure are estimated to reach almost $70 billion by 2030, with 80% of these costs directed at treatment of the hospitalized patient with ADHF.

REFERENCES

1. Yancy CW, Jessup M, Bozkurt B, et al. 2013 ACCF/AHA guideline for the management of heart failure: a report of the American College of Cardiology Foundation/American Heart Association Task Force on Practice Guidelines. Circulation 2013;128:e240–e327.

2. Bumetanide Package Insert. Deerfield, IL, Baxter Healthcare, 2009.

3. Furosemide Package Insert. Lake Forest, IL, Hospira Incorporated, 2004.

4. Torsemide Package Insert. Somerset, NJ, Meda Pharmaceuticals, 2009.

5. Felker GM, Lee KL, Bull DA, et al. Diuretic strategies in patients with acute decompensated heart failure. N Engl J Med 2011;364:797–805.

6. Jentzer JC, DeWald TA, Hernandez AF. Combination of loop diuretics with thiazide-type diuretics in heart failure. J Am Coll Cardiol 2010;56:1527–1534.

7. Lindenfeld JA, Albert NM, Boehmer JP, et al. HFSA 2010 comprehensive heart failure practice guidelines. J Card Fail 2010;16:e1–e194.

8. O'Connor CM, Startling RC, Hernandez AF, et al. Effect of nesiritide in patients with acute decompensated heart failure. N Engl J Med 2011;365:32–43.

9. Sinusas K. Osteoarthritis: diagnosis and treatment. Am Fam Physician 2012;85:49–56.

18

ISCHEMIC HEART DISEASE: CHRONIC STABLE ANGINA

An Uphill Battle.................................Level III

Alexander J. Ansara, PharmD, BCPS-AQ Cardiology

Dane L. Shiltz, PharmD, BCPS

TuTran T. Nguyen, PharmD, BCPS

LEARNING OBJECTIVES

After completing this case study, the reader should be able to:

- Identify modifiable risk factors for ischemic heart disease (IHD), and discuss the potential benefit to be gained by their modification in an individual patient.

- Optimize medical therapy in a patient with persistent angina considering response to current therapy and the presence of comorbidities.

- Assess clinical response to antianginal therapy by identifying relevant monitoring parameters for efficacy and adverse effects.

PATIENT PRESENTATION

■ Chief Complaint

"Doc, these drugs just aren't working for my chest pain anymore."

■ HPI

Jack Palmer is a 72-year-old man with coronary artery disease. He is an avid golfer and prefers to walk the course, but this is becoming progressively more difficult for him due to frequent angina. He has had two coronary artery bypass operations in the past. A coronary angiogram performed 1 month ago revealed significant disease in the RCA proximal to his graft, but this was considered high risk for angioplasty. His dose of isosorbide mononitrate was increased at that time from 60 to 120 mg once daily. This had no effect on his angina. He is still using about 30 nitroglycerin tablets a week, and these do relieve his chest pain. He reports that most often the chest discomfort comes on with activity, such as walking up slight inclines on the golf course. The discomfort is located in the center of his chest and rated 3–4/10 on average. He reports that the chest discomfort slowly fades as he slows his activity. He also complains of occasional lightheadedness with a pulse around 50 bpm and SBP near 100 mm Hg.

▓ PMH

1. Acute anterior wall MI with CABG surgery in 2009
2. Posterior lateral MI in 1990 and PTCA to the circumflex at that time
3. Dyslipidemia
4. Chronic low back pain
5. Depression

▓ FH

Noncontributory for premature CAD.

▓ SH

Retired dairy farmer, lives with wife, drinks occasionally, previous smoker—quit in 1998

▓ Meds

Carvedilol 6.25 mg PO twice daily
Lisinopril 5 mg PO once daily
Aspirin 325 mg PO once daily
Isosorbide mononitrate, extended release 120 mg PO once daily
Diltiazem, extended release 240 mg PO once daily
St. John's wort 300 mg PO three times daily
Celecoxib 200 mg PO once daily
Simvastatin 40 mg PO once daily
Nitroglycerin 0.4 mg SL PRN

▓ All

NKDA

▓ ROS

No fever, chills, or night sweats. No recent viral illnesses. No shortness of breath; occasional cough with cold weather. No nausea, vomiting, diarrhea, constipation, melena, or hematochezia. No dysuria or hematuria. No myalgias or arthralgias.

▓ Physical Examination

Gen

Pleasant, cooperative man in no acute distress

VS

BP 105/68, P 50, RR 22, T 36.4°C, Ht 5'11", Wt 93 kg, waist circumference 43 in

Skin

Intact, no rashes or ulcers

HEENT

PERRL; EOMI; oropharynx is clear

Neck

Supple, no masses; no JVD, lymphadenopathy, or thyromegaly

Lungs

Bilateral air entry is clear. No wheezes

CV

RRR, S_1, S_2 normal; no murmurs or gallops; PMI palpated at left fifth ICS, MCL

Abd

Soft, NT/ND; bowel sounds normoactive

Genit/Rect

Heme (–) stool

Ext

No CCE; pulses 2+ throughout

Neuro

A & O × 3, CN II–XII intact; speech is fluent; no motor or sensory deficit; no facial asymmetry; tongue midline

▓ Labs

Na 137 mEq/L	Hgb 11.8 g/dL	*Fasting lipid profile*
K 4.8 mEq/L	Hct 35.1%	Chol 202 mg/dL
Cl 103 mEq/L	Plt 187 × 10³/mm³	LDL 121 mg/dL
CO_2 21 mEq/L	WBC 7.9 × 10³/mm³	HDL 38 mg/dL
BUN 24 mg/dL	MCV 77 μm³	Trig 215 mg/dL
SCr 1.2 mg/dL	MCHC 29 g/dL	
Glu 98 mg/dL	Trop I 0.02 ng/mL × 2	

▓ ECG

Sinus rhythm, first-degree AVB, 50 bpm, old AWMI, no ST–T wave changes noted, QT 406 milliseconds

▓ Assessment

A 72-year-old man with poorly controlled angina on multiple medications, who is a poor candidate for angioplasty

QUESTIONS

Problem Identification

1.a. What drug-related problems appear to be present in this patient?

1.b. Could any of these problems potentially be caused or exacerbated by his current therapy?

Desired Outcome

2. What are the goals of pharmacotherapy for IHD in this case?

Therapeutic Alternatives

3.a. Does this patient possess any modifiable risk factors for IHD?

3.b. What pharmacotherapeutic options are available for treating this patient's IHD? Discuss the agents in each class with respect to their relative utility in his care.

CHAPTER 19

Optimal Plan

4. Given the patient information provided, construct a complete pharmacotherapeutic plan for optimizing management of his IHD.

Outcome Evaluation

5. When the patient returns to the clinic in 2 weeks for a follow-up visit, how will you evaluate the response to his new antianginal regimen for efficacy and adverse effects?

■ CLINICAL COURSE

Mr Palmer improved hemodynamically following a switch from diltiazem to amlodipine. However, due to continued frequent episodes of angina, his amlodipine was titrated to 10 mg once daily. He returned to cardiology clinic today stating that his angina frequency has improved somewhat on the maximum dose of amlodipine but is still bothersome to him. His cardiologist decided to add ranolazine 500 mg twice daily to his regimen in an attempt to further decrease his angina frequency.

Patient Education

6. What information will you communicate to the patient about his antianginal regimen to help him experience the greatest benefit and fewest adverse effects?

■ FOLLOW-UP QUESTION

1. What drug therapy changes would you recommend to avoid or minimize drug interactions with ranolazine?

■ SELF-STUDY ASSIGNMENTS

1. Summarize the potential role of L-arginine in the treatment of chronic angina.

2. Describe the potential role of allopurinol in the treatment of chronic angina.

CLINICAL PEARL

The COURAGE trial made major headlines in 2007 by showing that coronary stenting with optimal medical therapy is no better at preventing future coronary events than optimal medical therapy alone in patients with stable coronary disease, potentially saving the US health care system $5 billion a year.

REFERENCES

1. Fihn SD, Gardin JM, Abrams J, et al. 2012 ACCF/AHA/ACP/AATS/PCNA/SCAI/STS guideline for the diagnosis and management of patients with stable ischemic heart disease. J Am Coll Cardiol 2012;60:e44–e164.

2. Stone NJ, Robinson J, Lichtenstein A H, et al. 2013 ACC/AHA Guideline on the Treatment of Blood Cholesterol to Reduce Atherosclerotic Cardiovascular Risk in Adults. J Am Coll Cardiol 2014;63:2889–2934.

3. The SPRINT Research Group, Wright JT, et al. A randomized trial of intensive versus standard blood-pressure control. N Engl J Med 2015;373:2103–2116.

4. Smith SC, Benjamin EJ, Bonow RO, et al. AHA/ACCF secondary prevention and risk reduction therapy for patients with coronary and other atherosclerotic vascular disease: 2011 update. J Am Coll Cardiol 2011;58:2432–2446.

5. Boden WE, Finn AV, Patel D, et al. Nitrates as an integral part of optimal medical therapy and cardiac rehabilitation for stable angina: review of current concepts and therapeutics. Clin Cardiol 2012;35:263–271.

6. Bangalore S, Steg PG, Deedwania P, et al. β-Blocker use and clinical outcomes in stable outpatients with and without coronary artery disease. JAMA 2012;308:1340–1349.

7. Chaitman BR. Ranolazine for the treatment of chronic angina and potential use in other cardiovascular conditions. Circulation 2006;113:2462–2472.

8. Antithrombotic Trialists' Collaboration. Collaborative meta-analysis of randomised trials of antiplatelet therapy for prevention of death, myocardial infarction, and stroke in high risk patients. BMJ 2002;324:71–86.

9. CAPRIE Steering Committee. A randomised, blinded, trial of clopidogrel versus aspirin in patients at risk of ischaemic events (CAPRIE). Lancet 1996;348:1329–1339.

10. Heart Outcomes Prevention Evaluation Study Investigators. Effects of an angiotensin-converting-enzyme inhibitor, ramipril, on cardiovascular events in high risk patients. N Engl J Med 2000;342:145–153.

19

ACUTE CORONARY SYNDROME: ST-ELEVATION MYOCARDIAL INFARCTION

I Can't Handle the Pressure . . . . Level III

Kelly C. Rogers, PharmD, FCCP

Robert B. Parker, PharmD, FCCP

LEARNING OBJECTIVES

After completing this case study, the reader should be able to:

• Determine the goals of pharmacotherapy for patients with ST-segment elevation myocardial infarction (STEMI).

• Discuss interventional strategies for patients with STEMI, and understand the pharmacotherapeutic agents used with interventions.

• Design an optimal therapeutic plan for the management of STEMI, and describe how the selected drug therapy achieves the therapeutic goals.

• Identify appropriate parameters to assess the recommended drug therapy for both efficacy and adverse effects.

• Provide appropriate education to a patient who has suffered STEMI.

PATIENT PRESENTATION

■ Chief Complaint

"This is the worst pain I have ever felt in my life."

■ HPI

Gary Roberts is a 68-year-old man admitted to the ED complaining of chest pressure/pain lasting 20–30 minutes occurring at rest.

He describes the pain as substernal, crushing, and pressure-like that radiates to his jaw and is accompanied by nausea and diaphoresis. The pain first started approximately 6 hours ago after he ate breakfast and was unrelieved by antacids or SL NTG × 3. He also states that he has been experiencing intermittent chest pain over the past 3–4 weeks with minimal exertion.

▨ PMH

HTN
Type 2 DM
Dyslipidemia
CAD with PCI with a drug eluting stent (DES) 3 years ago

▨ FH

Father died from heart failure at age 75 and mother is alive at age 88 with HTN and type 2 DM.

▨ SH

(+) Tobacco × 20 years but quit when he received his DES 3 years ago; drinks beer usually on weekends; denies illicit drug use.

▨ Meds

Aspirin 81 mg PO daily
Metoprolol tartrate 25 mg PO BID
Simvastatin 40 mg PO QHS
Metformin 500 mg PO BID
SL NTG PRN CP

▨ All

NKDA

▨ ROS

Positive for some baseline CP on exertion for the past 3–4 weeks, now with CP at rest

▨ Physical Examination

Gen

WDWN man, A & O × 3, still with ongoing chest pain, somewhat anxious

VS

BP 145/92, P 89, RR 18, T 37.1°C; Wt 95 kg, Ht 5′10″

HEENT

PERRLA, EOMI, fundi benign; TMs intact

Neck

No bruits; mild JVD; no thyromegaly

Lungs

Few dependent inspiratory crackles; bibasilar rales; no wheezes

CV

Normal S_1 and S_2, no MRG

Abd

Soft, nontender; liver span 10–12 cm; no bruits

Genit/Rect

Deferred

MS/Ext

Normal ROM; muscle strength on right 5/5 UE/LE; on left 4/5 UE/LE; pulses 2+; no femoral bruits or peripheral edema

Neuro

CNs II–XII intact; DTRs decreased on left; negative Babinski's sign

▨ Labs

			Fasting lipid profile
Na 134 mEq/L	Ca 9.8 mg/dL	Hgb 14.0 g/dL	
K 4.4 mEq/L	Mg 2.0 mg/dL	Hct 44%	T. chol 159 mg/dL
Cl 102 mEq/L	PO_4 2.4 mg/dL	WBC $5.0 \times 10^3/mm^3$	Trig 92 mg/dL
CO_2 23 mEq/L	AST 22 units/L	Plt $268 \times 10^3/mm^3$	LDL 105 mg/dL
BUN 15 mg/dL	ALT 30 units/L	PT 12.5 s	HDL 36 mg/dL
SCr 1.0 mg/dL	Alk Phos 75 units/L	aPTT 32.4 s	A1C 7.6%
Glu 140 mg/dL	Troponin I 8.6 ng/mL	INR 1.0	

▨ ECG

2- to 3-mm ST-segment elevation in leads II, III, and aVF (Fig. 19-1).

▨ Assessment

Acute inferior STEMI.

QUESTIONS

Problem Identification

1.a. Which findings in this patient's case history are consistent with acute STEMI?

1.b. What risk factors for the development of coronary artery disease are present in this patient?

Desired Outcome

2.a. What is the immediate goal of therapy in this patient?

2.b. How can this goal be achieved using pharmacotherapy?

Therapeutic Alternatives

3.a. What nonpharmacologic therapeutic alternative can also achieve the immediate goal in this patient?

3.b. What is the role of adjunctive anticoagulant therapy during PCI, and how should these therapies be monitored?

3.c. What is the role of adjunctive antiplatelet therapy before, during, and after PCI, and how should these therapies be monitored?

Optimal Plan

4.a. What are other important goals of therapy in this patient?

4.b. Based on the history and presentation, what initial drug therapy is indicated in this patient?

Outcome Evaluation

5. How should the recommended therapy be monitored for efficacy and adverse effects?

▪ CLINICAL COURSE

The patient received aspirin, morphine, oxygen, IV unfractionated heparin (UFH), IV nitroglycerin, and oral metoprolol.

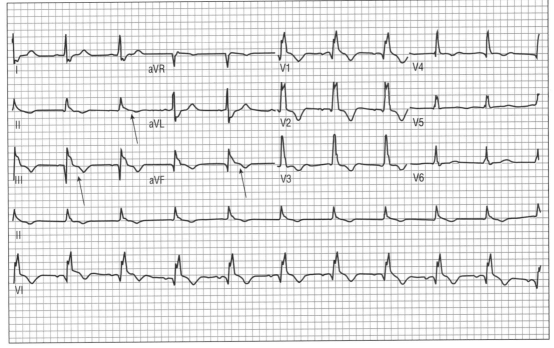

FIGURE 19-1. ECG taken on arrival in the emergency department showing ST-segment elevation (arrows) in leads II, III, and aVF, consistent with acute inferior myocardial infarction. Right bundle branch block is also present in leads V₁–V₃.

An interventional cardiologist was consulted and discussed with the patient the need for primary PCI to restore blood flow to the heart. Within 1 hour of his arrival to the ED, the patient was transported to the cardiac catheterization lab. The catheterization revealed a 60–70% proximal stenosis in the RCA with thrombus. Additionally, there was a 40% mid-LAD obstruction and 20–30% distal circumflex disease, neither of which was amenable to PCI. In the catheterization lab, the patient was loaded with oral clopidogrel 600 mg, anticoagulation was continued with UFH, and an eptifibatide infusion was started. The LVEF by echocardiogram was 35%. The remainder of the patient's hospital stay was uncomplicated, and he was discharged 4 days post-MI.

Patient Education

6.a. Based on his hospital course, which discharge medications would be most appropriate for this patient?

6.b. What education should you provide to this patient?

■ SELF-STUDY ASSIGNMENTS

1. A patient comes into your pharmacy and states that he has heard on the news that you should not take clopidogrel and stomach medicine together. He tells you that he takes omeprazole for his GERD and recently started taking clopidogrel because of a stent in his heart. Review the potential drug–drug interaction between clopidogrel and PPIs. How should you respond to him?

2. Perform a literature search and evaluate the use of vorapaxar in a patient post-MI. What are the clinical risks and benefits with this agent?

3. Whether UFH or bivalirudin is the optimal anticoagulant in patients undergoing PCI remains controversial. Review recent clinical trials comparing these two agents and describe the benefits and risks of each in patients undergoing primary PCI.

CLINICAL PEARL

The FDA recently issued an announcement strengthening the warning that NSAIDs increase the chance of MI or stroke in patients with or without heart disease or risk factors for heart disease. After an MI, patients should not be prescribed NSAIDs as they are more likely to die in the first year compared to those who do not use NSAIDs.

REFERENCES

1. O'Gara PT, Kushner FG, Ascheim DD, et al. 2013 ACCF/AHA guideline for the management of ST-elevation myocardial infarction: a report of the American College of Cardiology Foundation/American Heart Association Task Force on Practice Guidelines. Circulation 2013;127:e362–e425.

2. Levine GN, Bates ER, Blankenship JC, et al. 2011 ACCF/AHA/SCAI guideline for percutaneous coronary intervention: a report of the American College of Cardiology Foundation/American Heart Association Task Force on Practice Guidelines and the Society for Cardiovascular Angiography and Interventions. Circulation 2011;124:e574–e651.

3. Fleg JL, Forman DE, Berra K, et al. Secondary prevention of atherosclerotic cardiovascular disease in older adults: a scientific statement from the American Heart Association. Circulation 2013;128:2422–2473.

4. Guimarães PO, Tricoci P. Ticagrelor, prasugrel, or clopidogrel in ST-segment elevation myocardial infarction: which one to choose? Expert Opin Pharmacother 2015;16(13):1983–1995. doi: 10.1517/14656566.2015.1074180. Epub 2015 Jul 29.

5. Wiviott SD, Braunwald E, McCabe CH, et al. Prasugrel versus clopidogrel in patients with acute coronary syndromes. N Engl J Med 2007;357:2001–2015.

6. Wallentin L, Becker RC, Budaj A, et al. Ticagrelor versus clopidogrel in patients with acute coronary syndromes. N Engl J Med 2009;361:1045–1057.

7. Stone NJ, Robinson JG, Lichtenstein AH, et al. 2013 ACC/AHA guideline on the treatment of blood cholesterol to reduce atherosclerotic

cardiovascular risk in adults: a report of the American College of Cardiology/American Heart Association Task Force on Practice Guidelines. Circulation 2014;129(25 Suppl 2):S1–S45. doi:10.1161/01.cir.0000437738.63853.7a.

8. American Diabetes Association. Standards of medical care in diabetes-2016. Diabetes Care 2016;39(Suppl.1):S1–S112. Available at: *http://care.diabetesjournals.org/site/misc/2016-Standards-of-Care.pdf*.

9. FDA Drug Safety Communication: FDA Strengthens Warning that Non-aspirin Nonsteroidal Anti-inflammatory Drugs (NSAIDs) Can Cause Heart Attacks or Strokes. Silver Spring, MD, US FDA. Available at: *http://www.fda.gov/Drugs/DrugSafety/ucm451800.htm*. Accessed December 10, 2015.

20

VENTRICULAR ARRHYTHMIA

Nyagon's Parking Lot Accident.................Level III

Kwadwo Amankwa, PharmD, BCPS

LEARNING OBJECTIVES

After completing this case study, the reader should be able to:

- Understand the risk factors for the development of drug-induced torsades de pointes (TdP).

- Differentiate TdP from other cardiac arrhythmias.

- Select appropriate first-line therapy for acute treatment of TdP.

- Identify appropriate dosing, common adverse effects, and monitoring parameters for pharmacologic agents used to treat TdP.

- Discuss long-term approaches for the prevention of drug-induced TdP.

PATIENT PRESENTATION

■ Chief Complaint

"I was not feeling well, and I think I passed out."

■ HPI

Nyagon Doellefeld is a 55-year-old woman who experienced syncope while parking her car in the parking lot of the neighborhood grocery store. There were no injuries from the accident, and she was brought to the ED for evaluation. She reports being in her usual state of relatively good health until she developed a "cold" approximately 4 days before admission. She called her primary care physician complaining of her upper respiratory tract symptoms, and the physician called in a prescription for erythromycin 500 mg QID for 10 days to her pharmacy. She took the first dose on the morning of admission. She started feeling that something was wrong on her way to the grocery store approximately 1 hour after taking the second dose of erythromycin. She reports symptoms of lightheadedness, shortness of breath, as well as palpitations while driving. She passed out while parking, and her car collided with another car with minimal impact, damage, or injury. On medic arrival, she was awake and alert but looked shaken. She was transported to the ED without

further events. While being evaluated in the ED, she had another syncopal episode. ACLS protocol was initiated, and a rhythm strip showed TdP.

■ PMH

CAD S/P PTCA
Heart failure (EF 30%)
Dyslipidemia
Paroxysmal atrial fibrillation

■ SH

She lives with her husband and does not smoke or drink alcohol.

■ Meds

Carvedilol 3.125 mg PO BID
Pravastatin 40 mg PO once daily
Furosemide 40 mg PO BID (recently increased from 40 mg PO once a day due to increased edema)
Warfarin 4 mg PO once daily
Amiodarone 200 mg PO BID
Centrum Silver PO once daily
Ranitidine 150 mg PO once daily
Candesartan 8 mg PO once daily
Aspirin 325 mg PO once daily
Erythromycin 500 mg PO QID (started on the day of admission)

■ All

NKDA

■ ROS

The patient has no complaints other than those mentioned in the HPI

■ Physical Examination

Gen

The patient is awake on an ED bed in moderate distress

VS

BP 104/50, P 98 (200 during syncope), RR 30, T 36.3°C; Ht 5'7", Wt 90 kg

Skin

Warm and dry; no rashes seen

HEENT

NC/AT. PERRLA. EOMI. Oropharynx is clear

Neck/Lymph Nodes

Supple; no JVD or bruits; no lymph nodes palpated

Lungs/Thorax

CTA bilaterally

Breasts

Deferred

CV

RRR with no murmurs or gallops

Abd

NTND; no rebound or guarding; (+) bowel sounds

Genit/Rect

Deferred

MS/Ext

Trace edema in the lower extremities; pulses intact

Neuro

A & O × 3

■ Labs

Na 140 mEq/L	Hgb 12.1 g/dL	WBC 12 × 10³/mm³
K 2.8 mEq/L	Hct 35%	
Cl 100 mEq/L	RBC 3.88 × 10⁶/mm³	
CO₂ 29 mEq/L	Plt 200 × 10³/mm³	
BUN 36 mg/dL	MCV 90.5 μm³	
SCr 1.4 mg/dL	MCHC 34.4 g/dL	
Glu 110 mg/dL	INR 2.3	
Mg 1.2 mg/dL		

■ ECG

NSR, QTc 605 milliseconds; rhythm strip from oscilloscope during syncope: TdP (Fig. 20-1).

■ Assessment

A 55-year-old white woman S/P syncopal episodes from drug-induced TdP; upper respiratory tract symptoms; drug-induced electrolyte imbalance.

QUESTIONS

Problem Identification

1.a. What risk factors predisposed the patient to drug-induced arrhythmia?

1.b. What features of the patient's ECG are characteristic of TdP?

1.c. Discuss pharmacologic and nonpharmacologic factors that may have contributed to drug-induced TdP in this patient.

Desired Outcome

2. What are the short-term goals of pharmacotherapy for this patient?

Therapeutic Alternatives

3.a. What nonpharmacologic therapies may be useful for this patient?

3.b. What pharmacotherapy options are available for acute treatment of TdP?

Optimal Plan

4. Design a pharmacotherapeutic plan for the treatment of acute drug-induced TdP for this patient.

Outcome Evaluation

5. What monitoring parameters should be used to assess the efficacy and toxicity of treatment?

Patient Education

6. What medication counseling should be provided for the patient to prevent recurrence?

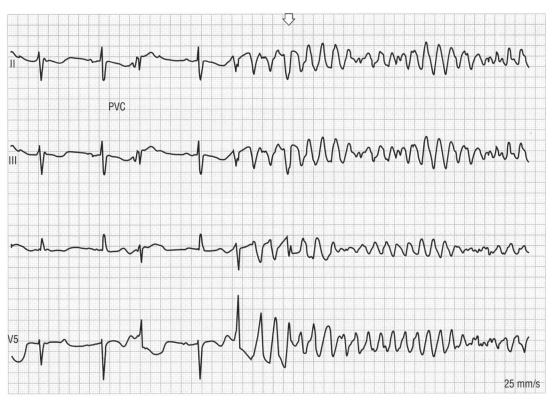

FIGURE 20-1. Electrocardiogram showing torsades de pointes.

■ CLINICAL COURSE

The patient was treated with a magnesium infusion, and she converted to normal sinus rhythm. The erythromycin was stopped. Potassium and magnesium were replaced, and the patient was admitted for further electrophysiology workup.

■ SELF-STUDY ASSIGNMENTS

1. List the most common drug classes associated with TdP.
2. List 10 commonly used medications that have a potential to cause TdP.

CLINICAL PEARL

There is a need for increased pharmacovigilance regarding drug-induced arrhythmias in the outpatient setting because a large number of pharmacologic agents and/or conditions that cause QT prolongation and TdP are present in the outpatient population.

REFERENCES

1. Gowda RM, Khan IA, Wilbur SL, Vasavada BC, Sacchi TJ. Torsades de pointes: the clinical considerations. Int J Cardiol 2004;95:219–222.
2. Arizona CERT—Center for Education and Research on Therapeutics. Available at: *http://www.azcert.org/*. Accessed May 1, 2013.
3. Yee GY, Camm AJ. Drug induced QT prolongation and torsades de pointes. Heart 2003;89:1363–1372.
4. Owens RC, Nolin TD. Antimicrobial-associated QT interval prolongation: pointes of interest. Clin Infect Dis 2006;43:1603–1611.
5. Tisdale JT. Torsades de pointes. In: Tisdale JE, Miller DA, eds. Drug-Induced Diseases: Prevention, Detection and Management. Bethesda, MD, American Society of Health-Systems Pharmacists, 2010:485–515.
6. European Heart Rhythm Association, Heart Rhythm Society, Zipes DP, et al. ACC/AHA/ESC 2006 guidelines for management of patients with ventricular arrhythmias and the prevention of sudden cardiac death: a report of the American College of Cardiology/American Heart Association Task Force and the European Society of Cardiology Committee for Practice Guidelines (Writing Committee to Develop Guidelines for Management of Patients With Ventricular Arrhythmias and the Prevention of Sudden Cardiac Death): developed in collaboration with the European Heart Rhythm Association and the Heart Rhythm Society. J Am Coll Cardiol 2006;48:e247–e346.
7. Berul CI, Seslar SP, Zimetbaum PJ, et al. Acquired QT syndrome. In: Triedman J, Levy S, eds. UpToDate. Waltham, MA. Available at: *http://www.uptodateonline.com*. Accessed May 4, 2013.

21

ATRIAL FIBRILLATION

Go Easy on My Beating Heart . . . . Level III

Virginia H. Fleming, PharmD, BCPS

Bradley G. Phillips, PharmD, BCPS, FCCP

LEARNING OBJECTIVES

After completing this case study, the reader should be able to:

- Describe the cornerstones of atrial fibrillation (AF) treatment.
- Determine therapeutic goals for managing AF in patients with heart failure.
- Recommend an optimal agent for anticoagulation in AF patients with heart failure.

PATIENT PRESENTATION

■ Chief Complaint

"Lately, I feel like my heart has been racing a bit. It really doesn't bother me that much, but I wanted to have it checked out to be sure."

■ HPI

Cooper Riley is a 64-year-old man with heart failure and a history of persistent AF who presents to his primary care physician complaining of palpitations that he first noticed 7 days ago. He reports that he is aware of the palpitations but that he has remained relatively asymptomatic. There has not been a noticeable change in his level of fatigue or exercise capacity during his normal daily activities. Mr Riley has had congestive heart failure for 6 years. For the past few years, his baseline exercise capacity would be described as slight limitation of physical activity with some symptoms during normal daily activities but asymptomatic at rest. He has a history of AF that was cardioverted to NSR and he has been on amiodarone to maintain NSR for the past 8 months. In the office today, Mr Riley's ECG shows that he is in AF (see Fig. 21-1).

■ PMH

Hypertension
Persistent AF (previously in NSR with amiodarone therapy)
Heart failure with reduced ejection fraction (LVEF 35%)
Obstructive sleep apnea (AHI 28 events/hour), alleviated with CPAP therapy

■ FH

Both parents are deceased. Father died from AMI at age 64. Mother died of breast cancer at age 70 years.

■ SH

Mr Riley works as an accountant. He is married with two healthy children. He does not smoke but occasionally "drinks a few beers on the weekend."

■ Medications

Carvedilol 6.25 mg PO BID
Digoxin 0.0625 mg PO once daily
Amiodarone 400 mg PO once daily
Furosemide 40 mg PO once daily
KCl 20 mEq PO once daily
Lisinopril 10 mg PO once daily
Warfarin 5 mg PO once daily
CPAP therapy (8 cm H_2O) at night

■ Allergies

NKDA

■ ROS

Reports no change in level of fatigue, some exercise intolerance; no headache, lightheadedness, chest pain, angina, or fainting spells; 2+ pitting edema.

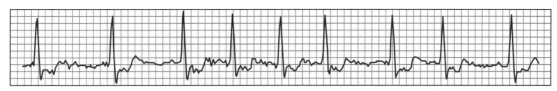

FIGURE 21-1. Rhythm recorded in Mr Riley's physician's office that depicts AF with a ventricular response rate of 110 bpm. AF is characterized by the absence of atrial "p" waves with varying distances between QRS complexes. AF is sometimes referred to as an irregularly irregular rhythm: irregular because it is not NSR; irregular because it produces an irregular ventricular response rate or peripheral pulse.

■ Physical Examination

Gen

Cooperative overweight man in no apparent distress

VS

BP 158/92, P 110 (irregular), RR 20, T 36.3°C, Wt 108.3 kg, Ht 5'11"

Skin

Cool to touch, normal turgor and color

HEENT

PEERLA, EOMI, fundoscopic exam reveals mild arteriolar narrowing but no hemorrhages, exudates, or papilledema

Neck

Large and supple, no carotid bruits; no lymphadenopathy or thyromegaly, (–) JVD

Lungs/Thorax

Inspiratory and expiratory rales bilaterally, no rhonchi

CV

Pulse 110 bpm and irregular; normal S_1, S_2, (+) S_3, no S_4

Abd

NT/ND, (+) BS; no organomegaly, (–) HJR

Genit/Rect

Normal male anatomy; stool heme (–)

MS/Ext

Pulses 1+ weak, full ROM, no clubbing or cyanosis; mild edema (2+)

Neuro

A & O × 3; CN II–XII intact; DTR 2+, negative Babinski

■ Labs

Na 140 mEq/L	Hgb 12.0 g/dL	Ca 8.5 mg/dL
K 4.0 mEq/L	Hct 35.8%	Mg 2.1 mEq/L
Cl 105 mEq/L	Plt 212 × 10³/mm³	Dig 0.8 ng/mL
CO_2 24 mEq/L	WBC 9.5 × 10³/mm³	
BUN 22 mg/dL	Polys 65%	
SCr 1.1 mg/dL	Bands 2%	
Glu 109 mg/dL	Lymphs 30%	
INR 2.3	Mono 3%	

■ ECG

Persistent AF, ventricular rate 110 bpm (see Fig. 21-1).

■ Echo

Evidence of systolic dysfunction (LVEF 35%) and moderate left atrial enlargement (5.2 cm). No thrombus seen.

■ Chest X-Ray

Enlarged cardiac silhouette; no evidence of acute pulmonary infection or edema.

■ Assessment

Persistent AF, previously in NSR on amiodarone therapy: mildly symptomatic, appropriately anticoagulated with warfarin therapy. Ventricular response rate not controlled.
HF: mildly symptomatic, standard meds not at target doses.
HTN: not controlled; optimize therapy for blood pressure control.
OSA: controlled on CPAP therapy.

QUESTIONS

Problem Identification

1.a. List and prioritize the patient's drug therapy problems.

1.b. How effective is amiodarone therapy in maintaining NSR long-term in patients with AF?

1.c. What factors may hinder preservation of NSR in Mr Riley?

1.d. Mr Riley has persistent AF. How is this different than permanent AF?

Desired Outcomes

2.a. What are the goals for pharmacotherapy in patients with AF?

2.b. What are the goals for pharmacotherapy for this patient's comorbid disease states or conditions?

Therapeutic Alternatives

3.a. What therapeutic rhythm-control alternatives exist for patients with AF and heart failure?

3.b. What are therapeutic options for rate control?

3.c. What nondrug therapies might be options for Mr Riley's AF?

Optimal Plan

4. How would you manage Mr Riley's AF at this time?

Outcome Evaluation

5. How would you monitor and adjust Mr Riley's drug therapies for AF?

Patient Education

6. What patient education would you provide Mr Riley about his AF and heart failure at this time to explain choice of management strategy, ensure adherence, and minimize risk of side effects?

■ SELF-STUDY ASSIGNMENTS

1. Recommend a management strategy/plan for Mr Riley if he returned in 2 weeks with a therapeutic INR, a heart rate of 95 bpm, and no symptoms of tachycardia but with 2+ pitting edema and a 1.2-kg gain in body weight.

2. List the drugs that have been demonstrated to improve mortality in the setting of heart failure and AF.

CLINICAL PEARL

In treating AF with concomitant systolic heart failure, lenient ventricular rate control (<110 bpm) plus anticoagulation is a viable treatment option over maintaining NSR with antiarrhythmic therapy.

REFERENCES

1. January CT, Wann LS, Alpert JS, et al. 2014 AHA/ACC/HRS Guideline for the management of patients with atrial fibrillation: executive summary. A report of the American College of Cardiology/American Heart Association Task Force on Practice Guidelines and the Heart Rhythm Society. JACC 2014;64(21):2246–2280.

2. Fuster V, Ryden LE, Cannom DS, et al. 2011 ACCF/AHA/HRS focused update incorporated into the ACC/AHA/EHC 2006 Guidelines for management of patients with atrial fibrillation: a report of the American College of Cardiology Foundation/American Heart Association Task Force on practice guidelines. Circulation 2011;123:e269–e367.

3. Shelton RJ, Clark AL, Goode K, et al. A randomized, controlled study of rate versus rhythm control in patients with chronic atrial fibrillation and heart failure: (CAFE-II Study). Heart 2009;95(11):924–930.

4. Roy D, Talajic M, Nattel S, et al. Rhythm control versus rate control for atrial fibrillation and heart failure. N Engl J Med 2008;358:2667–2677.

5. Hunt SA, Abraham WT, Chin MH, et al. 2009 focused update incorporated into the ACC/AHA 2005 guidelines for the diagnosis and management of heart failure in adults: a report of the American College of Cardiology Foundation/American Heart Association Task Force on Practice Guidelines: developed in collaboration with the International Society for Heart and Lung Transplantation. Circulation 2009;199:e391–e479.

6. Yancy CW, Jessup M, Bozkurt B, et al. 2013 ACCF/AHA guideline for the management of heart failure: a report of the American College of Cardiology Foundation/American Heart Association Task Force on Practice Guidelines. Circulation 2013;128:e240–e327.

7. Van Gelder IC, Groenveld HF, Crijns HJ, et al. RACE II Investigators. Lenient versus strict rate control in patients with atrial fibrillation. N Engl J Med 2010;362(15):1363–1373.

8. Wann LS, Curtis AB, Ellenbogen KA, et al. 2011 ACCF/AHA/HRS focused update on the management of patients with atrial fibrillation (update on dabigatran): a report of the American College of Cardiology Foundation/American Heart Association Task Force on practice guidelines. Circulation 2011;123:1144–1150.

9. Giugliano RP, Ruff CT, Braunwald E, et al. Edoxaban versus warfarin in patients with atrial fibrillation (ENGAGE AF-TIMI 48). N Engl J Med 2013;369:2093–2104.

22

DEEP VEIN THROMBOSIS

Trouble from Deep Within . . . . Level II

Sally A. Arif, PharmD, BCPS-AQ Cardiology

Tran Tran, PharmD, BCPS

LEARNING OBJECTIVES

After completing this case study, the reader should be able to:

• Define acute deep vein thrombosis (DVT), and discuss its pathophysiology.

• Discuss the clinical presentation of patients with a DVT.

• Develop a pharmacotherapeutic care plan for the management of a patient with a DVT.

• Educate a patient receiving anticoagulation therapy for the treatment of a DVT.

PATIENT PRESENTATION

■ Chief Complaint

"I'm having pain in my leg."

■ HPI

Rodney Cross is a 51-year-old Caucasian man who presents to his primary care physician because of pain in his right leg. He states that he awoke with the pain 3 days ago and that it has been continuous, although it hurts more when he walks. The pain is located behind his right knee and extends down into his calf. He rates the pain intensity as 3/10 at this time. The patient denies CP and SOB. He denies recent travel, immobility, and leg injury. The patient did start atorvastatin 40 mg daily for treatment of dyslipidemia approximately 3 months prior to this visit. He stopped the atorvastatin 3 days ago because he thought it might be causing his leg pain, but the pain has continued.

■ PMH

Hypertension
Dyslipidemia
Graves' disease with thyroid ablation
Gout
Left ankle fracture 9 years ago that required a cast but no surgery
Remote history of depression

■ PSH

Left herniorrhaphy about 10 years ago. Pilonidal cyst excision in remote past.

■ FH

Father died at age 81 of liver failure. Mother, one brother, and son all alive and well. No family history of venous thromboembolism or clotting disorders.

SH

Married, one adult child. Drinks one to two alcoholic beverages daily. Smokes ½ pack per day of cigarettes but trying to quit. Denies illicit drug use.

Meds

Allopurinol 300 mg PO once daily
Lisinopril 10 mg PO once daily
Levothyroxine 150 mcg PO once daily
Aspirin 81 mg PO daily
Atorvastatin 40 mg PO once daily (discontinued 3 days ago)

All

NKDA

ROS

Constitutional: No chills, no fatigue.
Eyes: No eye pain or changes in vision.
ENT: No sore throat.
Skin: No pigmentation changes, no nail changes.
Cardiovascular: No CP, palpitations, or syncope.
Respiratory: No cough, SOB, wheezing, or stridor.
GI: No abdominal pain, nausea, diarrhea, or vomiting.
Musculoskeletal: No neck pain, back pain, or injury.
Neurologic: No dizziness, headache, or focal weakness.
Psychiatric/behavioral: Remote history of depression. Not a current problem.

Physical Examination

Gen

Somewhat overweight, Caucasian man who appears comfortable. Cooperative, A & O × 3, normal affect

VS

BP 132/76, P 75 regular, RR 16, T 98.3°F, O_2 sat 97%/RA; Wt 194 lb, Ht 6'0"

Skin

Warm, dry, normal color. No rash or induration

HEENT

Pupils equal and reactive to light. EOM intact. Mucous membranes moist and pink

Neck

Normal range of motion with no meningeal signs

Lungs/Thorax

Breath sounds normal, no respiratory distress

CV

RRR, no rubs, murmurs, or gallops

Abd

Nontender, no masses, no distension, no peritoneal signs

MS/Ext

Upper extremities: Normal by inspection, no CCE, normal ROM.

Lower extremities: Right calf tight, warm to touch, and tender with 1+ pretibial pitting edema. LLE without redness, warmth, and swelling. Lower extremity pulses and sensation are normal bilaterally. Normal ROM

Neuro

Glasgow coma scale of 15, no focal motor deficits, no focal sensory deficits

Labs

Na 140 mEq/L	WBC 5.9 × 10³/μL	AST 16 IU/L
K 3.9 mEq/L	RBC 4.28 × 10⁶/μL	ALT 20 IU/L
Cl 103 mEq/L	Hgb 13.5 g/dL	Alk Phos 67 IU/L
CO_2 27 mEq/L	Hct 39.3%	GGT 20 IU/L
BUN 10 mg/dL	Platelets 175 × 10³/μL	Lipid panel (fasting)
SCr 0.84 mg/dL	CK 117 IU/L	TC 180 mg/dL
Glucose 88 mg/dL	INR 1.0	HDL 30 mg/dL
Uric acid 5.0 mg/dL	PT 11.4 seconds	Trig 250 mg/dL
	aPTT 34.8 seconds	LDL 100 mg/dL

Lower extremity venous duplex ultrasonography: Acute DVT of right distal superficial femoral, popliteal, and peroneal veins. No compression or flow in these vessels.

(**Note to reader:** *The "superficial femoral vein" is actually a deep vein, in spite of its name. Use of the name "femoral vein" is preferred because it is less confusing. However, the name "superficial femoral vein" is still encountered, as it is in this patient's venous duplex report.*)

Assessment

Acute DVT in right distal femoral, popliteal, and peroneal veins.

QUESTIONS

Problem Identification

1.a. Create a list of this patient's medication-related problems.

1.b. What subjective and objective findings support the diagnosis of a lower extremity DVT?

Desired Outcome

2. What are the short- and long-term goals of pharmacotherapy for this patient's DVT?

Therapeutic Alternatives

3. What therapeutic alternatives are available for the pharmacologic management of this patient's DVT?

Optimal Plan

4. In order to keep medication costs low, the clinician and patient agree to start warfarin therapy to manage the patient's DVT. Design a treatment plan for the initial management of this patient's DVT and be sure to include dosage form, dose, schedule, and duration of therapy for each drug that is part of the plan.

Outcome Evaluation

5. Design a monitoring plan for this patient's DVT therapy. Be sure to include monitoring for both safety and efficacy.

Patient Education

6. What education should be provided for this patient to optimize the probability of therapeutic success while minimizing the risk of adverse events?

■ CLINICAL COURSE (PART 1)

Mr Cross presents to his PCP 3 days after his first visit. He has been administering his injections and taking warfarin 5 mg daily, as instructed. He continues to experience RLE pain and swelling, but these symptoms are somewhat improved. He denies new CP or SOB. He reports no missed warfarin doses, no changes in his other medications, a diet with consistent vitamin K intake, no change in his alcohol intake, and no acute health problems. He denies bruising and bleeding, other than minor bruising related to his injections. His INR is 1.7.

■ FOLLOW-UP QUESTION

1.a. Identify the patient's anticoagulation therapy-related problem(s), and design treatment and monitoring plans for managing each problem you identify.

■ CLINICAL COURSE (PART 2)

Mr Cross presents to his PCP's office approximately 2 months after his acute DVT episode. He reports that he experienced an episode of very dark brown, "cola"-colored urine 2 days before this visit. He has had no recurrences. The patient denies dysuria, back or groin pain, and blood in his bowel movements. His current dose of warfarin is 2.5 mg on Monday, Wednesday, Friday, and Saturday and 5 mg on Tuesday, Thursday, and Sunday. Physical examination reveals no CVA tenderness. His INR is 2.3.

■ FOLLOW-UP QUESTION

1.b. Identify the patient's anticoagulation therapy-related drug problem(s), and design treatment and monitoring plans for managing each problem you identify.

■ CLINICAL COURSE (PART 3)

Three months after his initial presentation, you see Mr Cross in the new anticoagulation clinic at his primary care physician's office. He is currently taking warfarin 2.5 mg on Monday, Wednesday, Friday, and Saturday and 5 mg on Tuesday, Thursday, and Sunday. His INR is 4.3. The patient's INR 4 weeks ago was 2.3 on the same warfarin dose. Mr Cross has not experienced any symptoms suggesting DVT recurrence or PE occurrence. He states that he has not had any problem with bleeding, has not missed doses or taken extra doses of warfarin in the last month, and has not changed his diet or alcohol intake. His medications have been unchanged, except for a switch from atorvastatin 40 mg daily to rosuvastatin 20 mg daily for the treatment of his dyslipidemia approximately 2–3 weeks ago. You note that the thrombophilia tests given in Table 22-1 were completed prior to the initiation of anticoagulation therapy.

The laboratory summarizes the results in Table 22-1 as consistent with the presence of lupus anticoagulants.

TABLE 22-1 Thrombophilia Test Results		
Test	**Result**	**Reference interval**
Antithrombin III (% activity)	101	85–118
Protein C (% activity)	122	72–220
Protein S (% activity)	111	50–168
Factor V Leiden mutation	Negative	Normal: negative
Prothrombin G-20210-A mutation	Negative	Normal: negative
Anticardiolipin antibodies IgG (GPL units)	5.0	0.0–15.0
Anticardiolipin antibodies IgM (MPL units)	<4.7	0.0–12.5
Thrombin time (s)	15.5	13.0–20.0
DRVVT (s)	63.2	35.0–47.0
DRVVT confirm (s)	36.3	–
DRVVT ratio	1.74	1.10–1.41
StaClot LA	Positive	Normal: negative
Homocysteine, plasma (μmol/L)	10.0	3.7–13.9

■ FOLLOW-UP QUESTION

1.c. Identify this patient's anticoagulation therapy-related problem(s), and design a treatment and monitoring plan for each problem that you identify. Be sure to specify the anticipated duration of his anticoagulation therapy.

■ SELF-STUDY ASSIGNMENTS

1. Create a summary of antiphospholipid syndrome, including its definition, clinical presentation, and management.

2. Summarize the existing literature regarding the effects of various statins on response to warfarin. Does warfarin alter the effect of statins?

CLINICAL PEARL

Current guidelines propose long-term anticoagulation (up to 3 months) over anticoagulation for a shorter period of time. Longer treatment courses (eg, 6, 12, or 24 months) or extended therapy (no scheduled stop date) are recommended for patients with a proximal DVT, isolated distal DVT or PE provoked by surgery/nonsurgical transient risk factors. Extended therapy is recommended in patients with an unprovoked proximal DVT of the leg or PE, or second unprovoked VTE with a low or moderate risk of bleed. Use of anticoagulation should be reassessed annually in all patients who receive extended anticoagulation therapy.

REFERENCES

1. Kearon C, Akl EA, Ornelas J, et al. Antithrombotic therapy for VTE disease: CHEST Guideline and Expert Panel Report. Chest 2016 Feb;149(2):315–352.

2. Robertson L, Kesteven P, McCaslin JE. Oral direct thrombin inhibitors or oral factor Xa inhibitors for the treatment of deep vein thrombosis. Cochrane Database Syst Rev 2015;6:CD010956.

3. Schulman S, Kearon C, Kakkar AK; for the RE-COVER Study Group. Dabigatran versus warfarin in the treatment of acute venous thromboembolism. N Engl J Med 2009;361(24):2342–2352.

4. Schulman S, Kakkar AK, Goldhaber SZ; for the RE-COVER II Trial Investigators. Treatment of acute venous thromboembolism with dabigatran or warfarin and pooled analysis. Circulation 2014;129(7):764–772.

5. Garcia DA, Baglin TP, Weitz JI, Samama MM. Parenteral anticoagulants: Antithrombotic Therapy and Prevention of Thrombosis, 9th ed: American College of Chest Physicians Evidence-Based Clinical Practice Guidelines. Chest 2012;141(Suppl):e24S–e43S.

6. Van Dongen CJ, MacGillavry MR, Prins MH. Once versus twice daily LMWH for the initial treatment of venous thromboembolism. Cochrane Database Syst Rev 2005;3:CD003074.

7. Stern A, Abel R, Gibson GL, et al. Atorvastatin does not alter the anticoagulant activity of warfarin. J Clin Pharamcol 1997;37:1062–1064.

8. Simonson SG, Martin PD, Mitchell PD, et al. Effect of rosuvastatin on warfarin pharmacodynamics and pharmacokinetics. J Clin Pharmacol 2005;45(8):927–934.

9. Miyakis S, Lockshin MD, Atsumi T, et al. International consensus statement on an update of the classification criteria for definite antiphospholipid syndrome (APA). J Thromb Haemost 2006;4:295–306.

23

PULMONARY EMBOLISM

HIT Can Happen.............................. Level II

Kristen L. Longstreth, PharmD, BCPS

Mary E. Fredrickson, PharmD, BCPS

LEARNING OBJECTIVES

After completing this case study, the reader should be able to:

- Identify the signs, symptoms, and risk factors associated with pulmonary embolism (PE).

- Evaluate a patient for heparin-induced thrombocytopenia (HIT).

- Select an appropriate anticoagulant for the treatment of PE complicated by HIT.

- Recommend a pharmacotherapeutic plan to initiate and monitor anticoagulation for the treatment of PE complicated by HIT.

- Provide patient education on anticoagulation therapy.

PATIENT PRESENTATION

■ Chief Complaint

"I'm having chest pain, and I can't catch my breath."

■ HPI

Mary Anton is a 70-year-old woman who arrives at the hospital's emergency department by ambulance transfer from her home. The patient is S/P right TKR (postoperative day #10) for severe osteoarthritis. She was discharged from the hospital's orthopedic nursing unit 4 days ago with a prescription for enoxaparin for DVT prophylaxis. The patient was scheduled to receive physical therapy at a local rehabilitation center; however, she canceled therapy due to pain. She has been inactive at home with the exception of completing her activities of daily living with the assistance of her husband. This morning, the patient developed sharp chest pain and shortness of breath while watching television. She denies nausea, vomiting, and diaphoresis. The patient has a nonproductive cough. She is anxious and also complains of pain in her right knee and right lower extremity.

■ PMH

HTN × 30 years

Dyslipidemia × 25 years

Chronic stable angina × 2 years (negative regadenoson stress test 2 months ago)

CKD secondary to previously uncontrolled HTN, stage 4 (baseline creatinine 1.8–2.0 mg/dL)

Osteoarthritis

Obesity

S/P TKR right leg (postoperative day #10)

■ FH

Father died at age 74 (lung CA)

Mother died at age 89 (MI)

No siblings

■ SH

The patient is retired. She lives at home with her husband. Prior to surgery, she avoided most physical activity due to severe osteoarthritis. Negative for tobacco abuse. Denies alcohol use.

■ Meds

Home medications:

Aspirin 81 mg PO once daily

Metoprolol tartrate 50 mg PO BID

Amlodipine 10 mg PO once daily

Hydralazine 25 mg PO TID

Atorvastatin 20 mg PO once daily

Nitroglycerin 0.4 mg sublingually PRN chest pain

Calcium acetate 1334 mg PO TID with meals

Enoxaparin 30 mg SC Q 24 hours

Oxycodone sustained release 20 mg PO Q 12 hours

Oxycodone immediate release 5 mg PO Q 6 hours PRN pain

Docusate 100 mg PO QHS

Sennosides 17.2 mg PO QHS

■ All

Lisinopril (angioedema).

■ ROS

Positive for shortness of breath and nonproductive cough. Positive for sharp chest pain at rest. The pain does not radiate and is not reproducible by touch. No palpitations, diaphoresis, nausea, vomiting, or diarrhea. The patient denies headache, fever, and chills. Pain rated by patient as 9/10 in chest and 7/10 in right knee and lower extremity.

■ Physical Examination

Gen

Moderate respiratory distress

VS

BP 128/68, P 101, RR 21, T 36.9°C; Wt 85 kg, Ht 5′4″, O$_2$ sat 88% on RA

Skin

Warm and dry; no rashes

HEENT

Head: atraumatic; PERRLA; EOMI

Neck/Lymph Nodes

No carotid bruits; no lymphadenopathy; no thyromegaly

Lungs/Thorax

CTA; no wheezing or crackles

CV

Tachycardia with regular rhythm; normal heart sounds; no MRG

Abd

Obese, soft; NT/ND; +BS; no organomegaly

Genit/Rect

WNL

MS/Ext

S/P TKR right leg; right lower extremity ROM limited with slight redness, warmth, and edema; pain in right knee and lower extremity

Neuro

A&O × 3; no focal deficits noted; cranial nerves intact

◼ Labs (Nonfasting)

Na 144 mEq/L	Mg 1.9 mEq/L	T. chol 165 mg/dL	D-dimer 975 ng/mL
K 4.5 mEq/L	Phos 4.4 mg/dL	LDL 97 mg/dL	Cardiac Enzymes, time 1245
Cl 108 mEq/L	Ca 8.9 mg/dL	HDL 42 mg/dL	CK 67 IU/L
CO_2 26 mEq/L	Alb 3.5 g/dL	TG 130 mg/dL	CK-MB 1.1 IU/L
BUN 35 mg/dL	AST 21 IU/L	Hgb 11.5 g/dL	
SCr 1.8 mg/dL	ALT 15 IU/L	Hct 34.7%	Troponin I 0.03 ng/mL
Glu 106 mg/dL	Alk Phos 57 IU/L	Plt 86 × 10³/mm³	
A1C 6.0%		WBC 6 × 10³/mm³	

◼ ECG

Sinus tachycardia. No T wave or ST changes present.

◼ Venous Doppler Ultrasound of Right Lower Extremity

Occlusive DVT from the right popliteal vein to the right common femoral vein.

◼ CXR

No evidence of acute cardiopulmonary disease.

◼ Assessment

1. Chest pain, SOB—history of chronic stable angina; R/O ACS, R/O PE

2. Right lower extremity DVT

3. Thrombocytopenia—R/O HIT

4. S/P TKR right leg for severe osteoarthritis (postoperative day #10)—not infected, pain not controlled

5. CKD—stage 4, creatinine at patient's baseline

6. HTN—stable on current regimen

7. Dyslipidemia—stable on current regimen

TABLE 23-1	Cardiac Enzymes (Second Set; Time: 1905)

CK 45 IU/L
CK-MB 0.7 IU/L
Troponin I 0.02 ng/mL

TABLE 23-2	Pertinent Medication and Laboratory History from the Previous Admission		
TKR	Plt 239 × 10³/mm³	Hgb 11.8 g/dL	
Postoperative day #1	Plt 233 × 10³/mm³	Hgb 11.5 g/dL	Enoxaparin 30 mg subcutaneously Q 24 hours started
Postoperative day #2	Plt 227 × 10³/mm³	Hgb 11.7 g/dL	
Postoperative day #3	Plt 229 × 10³/mm³	Hgb 11.7 g/dL	
Postoperative day #4	Plt 221 × 10³/mm³	Hgb 11.6 g/dL	
Postoperative day #5	Plt 234 × 10³/mm³	Hgb 11.8 g/dL	
Postoperative day #6	Plt 141 × 10³/mm³	Hgb 11.6 g/dL	Discharged from hospital on enoxaparin 30 mg subcutaneously Q 24 hours

CLINICAL COURSE

The patient is admitted to a telemetry nursing unit within the hospital for treatment of the DVT and further workup for chest pain and shortness of breath (Table 23-1). A V/Q scan is ordered. The patient's medical chart from the previous admission is reviewed to obtain a more complete medication and laboratory history (Table 23-2).

An internal medicine resident physician discontinues enoxaparin and restarts the patient's other home medications. The resident physician also orders the following: consult clinical pharmacist to dose and monitor fondaparinux and warfarin; morphine 2 mg IV or IM Q 4 hours PRN pain; ibuprofen 600 mg PO Q 8 hours PRN pain.

◼ V/Q Scan

Multiple segmental perfusion defects, indicating a ventilation–perfusion mismatch and high probability of PE (see Fig. 23-1).

QUESTIONS

Problem Identification

1.a. What subjective and objective information is consistent with a diagnosis of PE for this patient?

1.b. What risk factors for PE are present for this patient?

1.c. Discuss the process to confirm or rule out a suspected diagnosis of HIT for this patient.

1.d. Develop a list of the potential drug therapy problems for this patient.

Desired Outcome

2.a. What are the goals of therapy for the treatment of PE?

2.b. What additional goals of therapy exist for a patient with HIT?

◼ CLINICAL COURSE (PART 1)

A heparin-induced platelet antibody ELISA is drawn and sent to an outside laboratory. An order is written to avoid all heparin

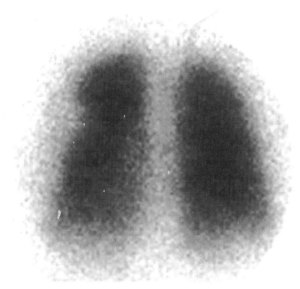

A   1ST Breath

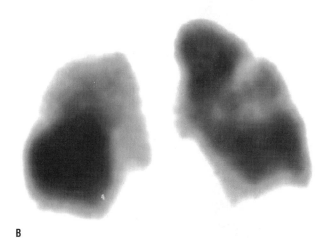

B

FIGURE 23-1. Ventilation–perfusion lung scan. (*A*) Normal ventilation; (*B*) multiple segmental perfusion defects, indicating a ventilation–perfusion mismatch and high probability of PE. *(Reproduced with permission from Rao RK. Pulmonary embolic disease. In: Crawford MH, ed. Current Diagnosis and Treatment in Cardiology, 3rd ed. New York, NY, McGraw-Hill Education, 2009:339.)*

(including heparin catheter flushes). Prior to initiating anticoagulation, a baseline aPTT (29.5 seconds; hospital laboratory's normal range is 25–40 seconds), PT (10.8 seconds), and INR (1.0) are obtained to assist with anticoagulation dosing. The nursing unit notifies the clinical pharmacist of the consultation order to dose and monitor fondaparinux and warfarin.

Therapeutic Alternatives

3.a. Which agents are available to initiate anticoagulation for the treatment of PE in this patient?

3.b. What nonanticoagulant therapies (pharmacologic and non-pharmacologic) are available? Is this patient an appropriate candidate for any of these therapeutic options?

Optimal Plan

4.a. Select an appropriate parenteral anticoagulant to begin therapy and calculate the initial dose for this patient.

4.b. Design a pharmacotherapeutic plan to transition the patient to warfarin and discontinue the parenteral anticoagulant.

4.c. Determine the appropriate length of warfarin therapy for this patient.

Outcome Evaluation

5.a. Choose an appropriate therapeutic monitoring parameter and calculate a therapeutic range for the anticoagulant selected for this patient.

5.b. In addition to the therapeutic monitoring parameter selected above, what clinical and laboratory parameters will you use to monitor the efficacy and safety of anticoagulation in this patient?

■ CLINICAL COURSE (PART 2)

The results of the heparin-induced platelet antibody ELISA were reported as positive with an optical density (OD) of 1.20 (the hospital's laboratory reports OD values greater than 0.40 as positive for heparin-induced antibodies). The patient's INR has been therapeutic for 72 hours on warfarin. The parenteral anticoagulant was discontinued yesterday, and the patient will be discharged home today.

Patient Education

6.a. Prior to discharge, what information should be provided to this patient about warfarin therapy to enhance adherence and ensure efficacy and safety?

6.b. Discuss the information that you will provide to this patient with HIT regarding the future use of heparin and low-molecular-weight heparin therapy.

■ SELF-STUDY ASSIGNMENTS

1. Determine the appropriate frequency of platelet count monitoring when therapeutic or prophylactic unfractionated heparin, low-molecular-weight heparin, or fondaparinux is used in medical or postoperative patients.

2. Investigate the sensitivity and specificity of the various activation and antigen assays available to confirm the diagnosis of HIT.

3. Compare the effects of bivalirudin and argatroban on INR measurement and warfarin monitoring.

4. Review the literature for available options to reverse the effects of the direct thrombin inhibitors if excessive anticoagulation occurs.

CLINICAL PEARL

The optimal duration of anticoagulation in a patient with HIT who does not have evidence of thrombosis (isolated HIT) is unknown. Anticoagulation with a direct thrombin inhibitor should be continued until the platelet count has recovered (to at least $150 \times 10^3/mm^3$) and stabilized; however, evidence-based guidelines also suggest initiating warfarin therapy for 4 weeks to prevent HIT-related thrombosis.[2]

REFERENCES

1. Witt DM, Clark NP, Vazquez SR. Venous thromboembolism. In: DiPiro JT, Talbert RL, Yee GC, et al., eds. Pharmacotherapy: A Pathophysiologic Approach, 10th ed. New York, NY, McGraw-Hill, 2017:231–260.

2. Linkins LA, Dans AL, Moores LK, et al. Treatment and prevention of heparin-induced thrombocytopenia: Antithrombotic Therapy and Prevention of Thrombosis, 9th ed: American College of

Chest Physicians Evidence-Based Clinical Practice Guidelines. Chest 2012;141(2 Suppl):e495S–e530S.

3. Lexi-Comp Online, Lexi-Drugs Online. Hudson, OH, Lexi-Comp Inc, October 20, 2015.

4. Badger NO. Fondaparinux (Arixtra), a safe alternative for the treatment of patients with heparin-induced thrombocytopenia? J Pharm Pract 2010;23(3):235–238.

5. Kang M, Alahmadi M, Sawh S, Kovacs MJ, Lazo-Langner A. Fondaparinux for the treatment of suspected heparin-induced thrombocytopenia: a propensity score-matched study. Blood 2015;125(6):924–929.

6. Miyares MA, Davis KA. Direct-acting oral anticoagulants as emerging treatment options for heparin-induced thrombocytopenia. Ann Pharmacother 2015;49(6):735–739.

7. Linkins LA, Warkentin TE, Pai M, et al. Design of the rivaroxaban for heparin-induced thrombocytopenia study. J Thromb Thrombolysis 2014;38:485–492.

8. Garcia DA, Baglin TP, Weitz JI, Samama MM. Parenteral anticoagulants: Antithrombotic Therapy and Prevention of Thrombosis, 9th ed: American College of Chest Physicians Evidence-Based Clinical Practice Guidelines. Chest 2012;141(2 Suppl):e24S–e43S.

9. Kearon C, Akl EA, Ornelas J, et al. Antithrombotic therapy for VTE disease: CHEST Guideline and Expert Panel Report. Chest 2016;149(2):315–352.

10. Bristol-Myers Squibb. Coumadin medication guide. Food and Drug Administration. Available at: *http://www.fda.gov/downloads/Drugs/DrugSafety/ucm088578.pdf*. Published 2011. Accessed May 1, 2016.

24

CHRONIC ANTICOAGULATION

To Bridge or Not to Bridge,
That Is the Question . . . . Level III

Mikayla L. Spangler, PharmD, BCPS

Beth Bryles Phillips, PharmD, FCCP, BCPS

LEARNING OBJECTIVES

After completing this case study, the reader should be able to:

- List the goals of anticoagulant therapy for periprocedural management of anticoagulation.

- Appropriately assess a patient's response to chronic warfarin therapy.

- Evaluate thromboembolic risk for patients receiving warfarin therapy and determine the need for bridging therapy.

- Develop a patient-specific pharmacotherapeutic plan for warfarin therapy and periprocedural management of anticoagulation.

- Educate patients appropriately about administration of low-molecular-weight heparins (LMWH) and chronic warfarin therapy.

PATIENT PRESENTATION

▤ Chief Complaint

"I am scheduled to have a colonoscopy and my physician said to talk to you about what to do with my warfarin."

▤ HPI

Elizabeth Heartly is a 53-year-old woman with a past medical history of a DVT × 2 and antiphospholipid syndrome. After the first DVT, she was treated for 1 year and then tested for thrombophilias. A diagnosis of antiphospholipid syndrome was made at that time. She recently experienced another DVT 4 months ago when her INR was subtherapeutic for an extended period of time. Treatment options were discussed at that time for treatment of her DVT, and she chose to continue warfarin therapy, because it was working well for her. Today, she presents to the anticoagulation clinic for a follow-up appointment. She also reports that she is scheduled for a colonoscopy 2 weeks from today. She states her physician has been recommending the colonoscopy for routine screening since she turned 50. However, she has been reluctant to schedule it. She realized the need for the procedure after a friend was diagnosed with colon cancer. Although no biopsy is planned, her physician explained that she should be off warfarin in case a biopsy is needed. Ms Heartly states she uses a medication box and has not missed any of her warfarin doses during the last month. She denies any bleeding, excessive bruising, severe headaches, abdominal pain, chest pain, shortness of breath, or pain or swelling in the lower extremities. She states that her arthritis has been really flaring up and therefore has been taking ibuprofen 800 mg TID for the last 2.5 weeks. She has one glass of red wine with dinner each evening. She has had no medication changes over the past month.

▤ PMH

Recurrent DVT × 2, 5 years ago and 4 months ago
Antiphospholipid syndrome
Hypothyroidism
Osteoarthritis of the knee

▤ FH

Father—colon polyps removed when he was in his 50s but is currently alive and well in his 80s.
Mother—hypertension and is 79 years of age.
Brother—healthy.
She has two children who are alive and well.

▤ SH

(+) ETOH—one glass of red wine each evening with supper; (–) smoking.

▤ Meds

Ibuprofen 200 mg one to two tablets PO TID PRN for osteoarthritis pain
Calcium carbonate 600 mg PO BID with meals
Levothyroxine 125 mcg PO once daily
Warfarin 2.5 mg PO Tuesday, Saturday; 5 mg 5 days per week

▤ All

Penicillin—bumps, rash/hives.

▤ ROS

(–) For CP, SOB, severe headaches, abdominal pain, leg pain, bruises, or change in color of stool or urine.

▤ Physical Examination

Gen

Pleasant obese woman in NAD

VS

BP 116/78, HR 76, RR 14, T 36.5°C; Wt 96.3 kg, Ht 5′6″

TABLE 24-1	Thromboembolic Risk After Interruption of Warfarin Therapy[2,3]		
	Warfarin indication		
Risk stratum	**Mechanical heart valve**	**Atrial fibrillation**	**Venous thromboembolism**
High	Any mitral valve prosthesis Any caged ball or tilting disk aortic valve prosthesis Multiple mechanical heart valves Stroke, TIA, or cardioembolic event[a]	CHADS$_2$ score 5–6 Recent (<3 mo) stroke or TIA Severe valvular heart disease	Recent (<3 mo) VTE Severe thrombophilia (eg, protein C, S, or antithrombin deficiency, antiphospholipid syndrome, homozygous for factor V Leiden or prothrombin gene mutation, or multiple abnormalities)
Moderate	Bileaflet aortic valve + AF, prior stroke or TIA, HTN, DM, CHF, age >75	CHADS$_2$ score 3–4	VTE within past 3–12 mo Nonsevere thrombophilia (eg, heterozygous factor V Leiden or prothrombin gene mutation) Recurrent VTE Active cancer (treated <6 mo or palliative)[b]
Low	Bileaflet aortic valve without AF, prior stroke or thromboembolic event, or known intracardiac thrombus	CHADS$_2$ score 0–2 (assuming no prior stroke or TIA)	Single VTE occurred >12 mo ago and no other RF

AF, atrial fibrillation; CHF, chronic heart failure; DM, diabetes mellitus; HTN, hypertension; mo, months; RF, risk factor; TIA, transient ischemic attack; VTE, venous thromboembolism.
[a]The 2012 Chest guidelines specify "recent" stroke or TIA as having occurred within the past 6 months.
[b]A recent review article lists active cancer in the high-risk category.[3]

Skin

Normal turgor and color; warm

HEENT

PERRLA, EOMI; disks flat; fundi with no hemorrhages or exudates

Neck/Lymph Nodes

No lymphadenopathy, thyromegaly, or carotid bruits

Lungs

CTA bilaterally

CV

RRR; normal S$_1$ and S$_2$; no S$_3$ or S$_4$; no M/R/G

Abd

Obese, soft, nontender, nondistended, (+) BS

Genit/Rect

Deferred

Ext

Warm with no clubbing, cyanosis, or edema

Neuro

A & O × 3; CN II–XII intact; DTR 2+; Babinski negative

■ Labs

Date	INR	Warfarin dose
Today	2.8	2.5 mg Tuesday, Saturday; 5 mg 5 days per week
1 month ago	2.7	2.5 mg Tuesday, Saturday; 5 mg 5 days per week
2 months ago	2.8	2.5 mg Tuesday, Saturday; 5 mg 5 days per week
3 months ago	2.4	2.5 mg Tuesday, Saturday; 5 mg 5 days per week

One month ago TSH 1.93 mIU/L.
Six months ago 25(OH)D 45 ng/mL.

■ Assessment

History of recurrent DVT and antiphospholipid syndrome requiring chronic anticoagulation with target INR 2.5 (range, 2.0–3.0)

Therapeutic INR (target 2.5; range, 2.0–3.0)
Periprocedural management of anticoagulation needed
Euthyroid with current dose of levothyroxine
High-dose ibuprofen use for recent osteoarthritis flare

QUESTIONS

Problem Identification

1.a. Create a list of this patient's drug-related problems.

1.b. What questions would you ask this patient to assess her current warfarin therapy?

1.c. What signs or symptoms might she experience if she developed a venous thromboembolism?

1.d. What is her risk of thromboembolism during interruption of warfarin therapy (see Table 24-1)?

1.e. What are the risks of using nonsteroidal anti-inflammatory drugs (NSAIDs) in combination with warfarin?

Desired Outcome

2. What are the goals of anticoagulation therapy in this patient?

Therapeutic Alternatives

3a. What are the options for extended therapy of venous thromboembolism?

3b. What are the options for periprocedural management of anticoagulation?

Optimal Plan

4.a. Based on today's laboratory result, what is your recommendation for this patient's warfarin therapy?

4.b. How should the plan for periprocedural management of anticoagulation be implemented?

Outcome Evaluation

5. How will you monitor this patient's warfarin therapy?

Patient Education

6.a. What information should this patient know regarding her upcoming bridging therapy for her colonoscopy procedure?

6.b. What information should this patient know about her warfarin therapy, especially to minimize subtherapeutic or supratherapeutic INRs and potential hemorrhagic and thromboembolic complications?

■ CLINICAL COURSE

On return to clinic 1 week after the colonoscopy, Ms Heartly reports that the procedure went well, and she has taken her usual weekly dose of warfarin therapy and continues on her bridging therapy. Her INR is 2.0, and she is in need of further instructions regarding her warfarin and bridging therapy.

■ FOLLOW-UP QUESTION

1. Based on this information, what are your recommendations for her warfarin and LMWH therapy?

■ ADDITIONAL CASE QUESTION

1. Ms Heartly has been diagnosed with hypothyroidism. Although her TSH is within normal range at this time, how would untreated hypothyroidism affect the INR?

■ SELF-STUDY ASSIGNMENTS

1. Research the options for bridging in patients with a history of heparin-induced thrombocytopenia, and create a table highlighting the various management options.

2. Research the data on LMWH dosing in morbidly obese patients, and write a one-page paper summarizing how LMWH should be dosed in such patients.

CLINICAL PEARL

Dosing LMWH in obese patients can present challenges due to product availability of dosage strengths. Doses may need to be rounded up or down to the nearest available syringe. The availability of dosage forms may also determine whether enoxaparin may be administered once or twice daily.

REFERENCES

1. Holbrook A, Schulman S, Witt DM, et al. Evidence-based management of anticoagulant therapy. Chest 2012;141:e152S–e184S.
2. Douketis JD, Spyropoulos AC, Spencer FA, et al. Perioperative management of antithrombotic therapy. Chest 2012;141:e326S–e350S.
3. Kearon C, Akl EA, Omelas J, et al. Antithrombotic therapy for VTE disease: CHEST Guideline and Expert Panel Report. Chest 2016;149:315–352.
4. Ageno W, Gallus AS, Wittkowsky A, et al. Oral anticoagulant therapy: antithrombotic therapy and prevention of thrombosis, 9th ed: American College of Chest Physicians Evidence-Based Clinical Practice Guidelines. Chest 2012;141:e44S–e88S.
5. Baron TH, Kamath PS, McBane RD. Management of antithrombotic therapy in patients undergoing invasive procedures. N Engl J Med 2013;368:2113–2124.
6. Douketis JD, Spyropoulos AC, Kaatz S, et al. for the BRIDGE investigators. Perioperative bridging anticoagulation in patients with atrial fibrillation. N Engl J Med 2015;373:823–833. doi:10.1056/NEJMoa1501035.
7. Linkins L, Dans AL, Moores LK, et al. Treatment and prevention of heparin-induced thrombocytopenia. Chest 2012;141:e495S–e530S.
8. Garcia DA, Baglin TP, Weitz JI, Samama MM. Parenteral anticoagulants. Chest 2012;141:e24S–e43S.
9. Garwood CL, Gortney JS, Corbett TL. Is there a role for fondaparinux in perioperative bridging? Am J Health Syst Pharm 2011;68:36–42.
10. ASGE Standards of Practice Committee, Anderson MA, Ben-Menachem T, et al. Management of antithrombotic agents for endoscopic procedures. Gastrointest Endosc 2009;70:1060–1070.

25

STROKE

One Stroke Off Par . . . . Level II

Alexander J. Ansara, PharmD, BCPS AQ-Cardiology

LEARNING OBJECTIVES

After completing this case study, the reader should be able to:

- Identify risk factors for ischemic stroke.

- Discuss the role of thrombolytics in the management of acute ischemic stroke.

- Formulate an appropriate patient-specific drug regimen for the treatment of an acute ischemic stroke.

- Discuss the approach to multidisease state management for the secondary prevention of ischemic stroke, including the management of hypertension, dyslipidemia, and the use of antiplatelet agents.

- Educate a patient regarding secondary stroke prevention strategies.

PATIENT PRESENTATION

■ Chief Complaint

"My dad is having trouble talking and seems to be losing feeling in his left arm and leg."

■ HPI

Marvin Palmer is a 57-year-old man who was brought to the ED by his son at 10 AM after experiencing left arm numbness, slurred speech, and dizziness. His son states that the two of them were enjoying their typical Saturday morning golf outing at the country club when Mr Palmer, on teeing off on hole 6 at 9:30 AM, dropped his golf club and went down on one knee. Mr Palmer's words were "slow and disjointed" according to his son who immediately called 9-1-1. While in the ED, Mr Palmer began to have a left-sided facial droop. He admitted noticing minor dizziness and slight tingling in his left hand at 8 AM, both of which resolved soon thereafter. He assumed these were symptoms due to low blood pressure and therefore opted not to take his blood pressure medications this morning.

■ PMH

HTN, diagnosed 10 years ago
Dyslipidemia

■ FH

Both parents alive and relatively healthy. Sister, age 62, also has HTN. Son, age 31, has type 1 DM.

■ SH

Married, lives with wife and three children. Occasional recreational beer or wine consumption. Denies tobacco use.

■ Meds

Amlodipine 2.5 mg PO daily
Simvastatin 10 mg PO daily
Chlorthalidone 25 mg PO daily

■ All

Shellfish (hives).

■ ROS

Mild blurry vision, but no double vision, loss of vision, or oscillopsia.

■ Physical Examination

Gen

Slender Caucasian man lying in bed in no acute distress, responsive with occasionally slurred speech

VS

BP 192/98, P 70, RR 19, T 98.6°F, O$_2$ sat 97% on RA; Wt 80 kg, Ht 6'0"

Skin

Warm, dry

HEENT

PERRLA, EOMI; no nystagmus, exudates, hemorrhages, or papilledema; mild left-sided facial droop. Normal hearing acuity bilaterally

Neck

(–) Carotid bruits, (–) lymphadenopathy

Chest

Lungs clear to auscultation bilaterally

CV

RRR, S$_1$ and S$_2$ normal, no S$_3$ or S$_4$

Abd

Soft, nontender, nondistended, (+) BS

GU

Deferred

MS/Ext

RUE: 5/5; RLE 4/5; LUE: 2/5; LLE: 3/5. No abnormal or involuntary movements. Strong peripheral pulses and brisk capillary refill; no CCE; DTR: 2+ throughout, normal Babinski reflex

Neuro

Awake, A & O × 3. No aphasia, agnosia, or apraxia. Attention, concentration, and vocabulary are all excellent. No impairment of facial

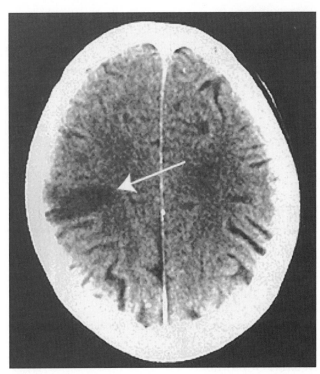

FIGURE 25-1. Head CT scan without contrast negative for hemorrhage and showing right-sided middle cerebral artery infarct.

sensation noted with light touch bilaterally. Moderate left facial weakness, as noted by the presence of left-sided facial droop. Mild dysarthria. Shoulder shrug is symmetrical, and tongue is midline on protrusion. Can easily touch chin to chest, and there are no other signs of meningismus

■ Labs

Na 140 mEq/L	WBC 5.9 × 10^3/mm^3	*Fasting lipid profile*
K 4.2 mEq/L	Hgb 16.4 g/dL	Total cholesterol 200 mg/dL
Cl 103 mEq/L	Hct 49.6%	LDL-C 118 mg/dL
CO$_2$ 28 mEq/L	Plt 310 × 10^3/mm^3	Triglycerides 160 mg/dL
BUN 10 mg/dL	aPTT 25.3 s	HDL-C 50 mg/dL
SCr 0.6 mg/dL		
Glu 98 mg/dL		

Head CT scan: right-sided middle cerebral artery infarct; no evidence of hemorrhage (Fig. 25-1)
Carotid Dopplers: normal blood flow bilaterally, no appreciable ischemia or stenosis
Angiogram: not performed
Echocardiogram: no evidence of LV thrombus, ejection fraction 55–60%; overall unremarkable
EKG: normal sinus rhythm (Fig. 25-2)

■ Assessment

Acute ischemic stroke secondary to atherosclerosis and ischemic disease in a patient with HTN, dyslipidemia, and no prior history of stroke or transient ischemic attack

CLINICAL COURSE

It is now 11:00 AM, and you are seeing the patient with the rest of the neurology team.

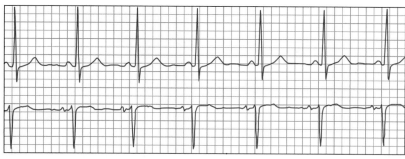

FIGURE 25-2. EKG showing normal sinus rhythm.

QUESTIONS

Problem Identification

1.a. Create a list of the patient's drug therapy problems.

1.b. Identify the nonmodifiable, modifiable, and Framingham risk factors for CHD present in this patient.

1.c. Which signs, symptoms, and other tests indicate the presence of an acute ischemic stroke?

Desired Outcome

2.a. What are the initial goals of pharmacotherapy in this patient?

2.b. What are the long-term goals of pharmacotherapy in this patient?

Therapeutic Alternatives

3.a. What nondrug therapies might be useful for this patient?

3.b. What feasible pharmacotherapeutic alternatives are available for the treatment of acute ischemic stroke?

Optimal Plan

4.a. What is your recommendation for the acute use of antihypertensives in this patient?

4.b. What pharmacotherapeutic regimen would you recommend for the acute treatment of stroke in this patient (include drug, dose, route, frequency, and duration)?

Outcome Evaluation

5. What clinical and laboratory parameters are necessary to evaluate the therapy for achievement of the desired therapeutic outcome(s) and to detect or prevent adverse effects?

Patient Education

6. What information should be provided to Mr Palmer to enhance adherence, ensure successful therapy, and minimize adverse effects?

■ CLINICAL COURSE

Mr Palmer is currently 4 days poststroke and will be discharged home today. He has regained motor coordination and strength in his extremities, and his speech has improved significantly. A mild facial droop is still noted to be present when he is prompted to smile and show his teeth.

■ FOLLOW-UP QUESTIONS

1. What antiplatelet regimen would you recommend for the secondary prevention of acute ischemic stroke in Mr Palmer (include drugs, dose and dosage form, schedule, and duration)?

2. Which parameters related to Mr Palmer's treatment should be monitored to ensure optimal secondary prevention?

3. What recommendations would you make to Mr Palmer's home drug regimen to optimally manage his HTN and dyslipidemia?

■ SELF-STUDY ASSIGNMENTS

1. Explain which patients are candidates to receive aspirin instead of warfarin for the prevention of stroke in the setting of atrial fibrillation.

2. Summarize the role of HMG Co-A reductase inhibitors in the primary and secondary prevention of ischemic stroke.

3. Read the CURE and MATCH trials, and explain when and why patients should be treated with the combination of aspirin and clopidogrel. Explain what the MATCH results tell us about the use of combination antiplatelet therapy for the prevention of ischemic stroke.

4. Write a one-page report summarizing the findings of the NINDS and ECASS III trials pertaining to the use of thrombolytics for the treatment of acute ischemic stroke.

5. Read the PRoFESS trial, and explain the clinical implications of this trial pertaining to the use of clopidogrel and extended-release aspirin and dipyridamole for secondary stroke prevention.

CLINICAL PEARLS

1. Hypoglycemia results in a clinical presentation similar to ischemic stroke and therefore should be ruled out as a diagnosis before treatment for an acute stroke is initiated.

2. Initially elevated blood pressures often decrease, without the use of antihypertensive therapy, within the first few days after an ischemic stroke. When initiating antihypertensive therapy after an acute ischemic stroke, caution should be used to not reduce blood pressures too aggressively unless clinically indicated.

REFERENCES

1. Chaturvedi S, Bruno A, Feasby T, et al. Carotid endarterectomy—an evidence-based review. Report of the American Academy of Neurology. Neurology 2005;65:794–801.

2. Furie KL, Kasner SE, Adams RJ, et al., American Heart Association Stroke Council, Council on Cardiovascular Nursing, Council on Clinical Cardiology, Interdisciplinary Council on Quality of Care and Outcomes Research. Guidelines for the prevention of stroke in patients with stroke or transient ischemic attack: a guideline for healthcare

professionals from the American Heart Association/American Stroke Association. Stroke 2011;42(1):227–276.

3. National Institute of Neurological Disorders and Stroke rt-PA Stroke Study Group. Tissue plasminogen activator for acute ischemic stroke. N Engl J Med 1995;333:1581–1587.

4. Hacke W, Kaste M, Bluhmki E, et al., ECASS III Investigators. Thrombolysis with alteplase 3 to 4.5 hours after acute ischemic stroke. N Eng J Med 2008;359:1317–1329.

5. Parsons M, Spratt N, Bivard A, et al. A randomized trial of tenecteplase versus alteplase for acute ischemic stroke. N Engl J Med 2012;366(12):1099–1107.

6. Jauch EC, Saver JL, Adams HP, et al. Guidelines for the early management of patients with acute ischemic stroke: a guideline for healthcare professionals from the American Heart Association/ American Association. Stroke 2013;44:870–947. doi:10.1161/?STR. 0b013e318284056a.

7. Chinese Acute Stroke Trial Collaborative Group (CAST). Randomized placebo-controlled trial of early aspirin use in 20,000 patients with acute ischemic stroke. Lancet 1997;349:1641–1649.

8. International Stroke Trial Collaborative Group (IST). A randomized trial of aspirin, subcutaneous heparin, both, or neither among 19435 patients with acute ischaemic stroke. Lancet 1997;349:1569–1581.

9. 2014 AHA/ASA guidelines for the prevention of stroke in patients with stroke and transient ischemic attack. Stroke 2014;45:2160–2236.

10. Kennedy J, Hill MD, Ryckborst BA, et al., FASTER Investigators. Fast assessment of stroke and transient ischaemic attack to prevent early recurrence (FASTER): a randomised controlled pilot trial. Lancet Neurol 2007;6:961–969.

11. Diener HC, Cunha L, Forbes C, et al. European Stroke Prevention Study 2: dipyridamole and acetylsalicylic acid in the secondary prevention of stroke. J Neurol Sci 1996;143:1–13.

12. Sacco RL, Diener HC, Yusuf S, et al. Aspirin and extended-release dipyridamole versus clopidogrel for recurrent stroke. N Engl J Med 2008;359:1238–1251.

13. Shinohara Y, Katayama Y, Uchiyama S, et al. Cilostazol for prevention of secondary stroke (CSPS 2): an aspirin-controlled, double-blind, randomized non-inferiority trial. Lancet Neurol 2010;9:959–968.

14. Stone NJ, Robinson J, Lichtenstein AH, et al. 2013 ACC/AHA guideline on the treatment of blood cholesterol to reduce atherosclerotic cardiovascular risk in adults. J Am Coll Cardiol 2014;63:2889–2934.

26

DYSLIPIDEMIA

I Need Refills . . . . Level II

Laurajo Ryan, PharmD, MSc, BCPS, CDE

LEARNING OBJECTIVES

After completing this case study, the reader should be able to:

- Identify patients who require treatment for dyslipidemia.

- Stratify individual patients for risk of coronary heart disease (CHD) and stroke.

- Determine appropriate LDL and non-HDL goals based on individual risk factors.

- Recommend a cholesterol management strategy that includes therapeutic lifestyle changes (TLC), drug therapy, patient education, and monitoring parameters.

PATIENT PRESENTATION

■ Chief Complaint

"I need refills."

■ HPI

Felecia A. Thorngrass is a 56-year-old woman who presents to pharmacotherapy clinic for intake. She has recently moved to your area, and states she has not seen her primary care provider for the last 11 months. Her prescriptions have expired, and she is coming to you for "refills."

■ PMH

Obesity (BMI 31.5 kg/m^2)
Dyslipidemia × 4 years
HTN × 15 years
Postmenopausal—has not had GYN screening since onset of menopause (14 years ago)

■ FH

Father: age 74 with extensive cardiovascular history, most notably first MI at age 42.
Mother: died at age 61 from MVA, medical history unknown.
Patient has one older sister with HTN and history of "mini-strokes" and one younger sister with HTN only.
Her children's medical conditions are noncontributory.

■ SH

Patient is married with three children, all of whom live out of state.
College graduate, works as librarian.
Admits to "social" alcohol and tobacco use, and to previous marijuana use when she visited her children.
Began sporadic exercise regimen when diagnosed with dyslipidemia.

■ Meds (Per Patient History; She Did Not Bring Records)

Metoprolol tartrate 50 mg PO BID
Ezetimibe 10 mg PO once daily
Aspirin 81 mg PO once daily
Ibuprofen 200 mg, four tablets PO PRN leg cramps
Naproxen 220 mg, two tablets PO PRN leg cramps
Garlic capsules

■ All

"Statin" drugs—states she had occasional leg cramps after starting atorvastatin.

■ ROS

Patient states that she just needs refills. She is argumentative about getting labs done and cannot understand why you would not just refill her medications. She denies any acute changes in health. She denies unilateral weakness, numbness/tingling, or changes in vision. She denies CP, and only has SOB when she walks in the park. With further questioning you find that she rarely exercises, but when she does go for a walk she typically overdoes it. She denies changes in bowel or urinary habits and states she does not need to have GYN follow-ups anymore, because she has gone through "the change." She denies any lower extremity edema.

■ Physical Examination

Gen

Obese, somewhat agitated Caucasian woman

VS

BP 162/92, P 89, RR 18, T 37.2°C; Wt 94 kg, Ht 5′8″

Skin

Warm and dry to touch, normal turgor, (−) for acanthosis nigricans

HEENT

PERRLA; EOMI; funduscopic exam deferred; TMs intact; oral mucosa clear

Neck/Lymph Nodes

Neck supple, no lymphadenopathy, thyroid smooth and firm without nodules

Chest

CTA bilaterally, no wheezes, crackles, or rhonchi

Breasts

Normal, slightly fibrotic, no lumps or discharge

CV

RRR, no MRG, normal S_1 and S_2; no S_3 or S_4

Abd

(+) BS, no hepatosplenomegaly

Genit/Rect

Deferred

Ext

No pedal edema, pulses 2+ throughout

Neuro

No gross motor-sensory deficits present

■ Labs (Fasting)

Na 142 mEq/L	Ca 8.2 mg/dL	*Fasting lipid profile*
K 4.9 mEq/L	Mg 2.0 mEq/L	TC 240 mg/dL
Cl 103 mEq/L	AST 28 units/L	HDL 41 mg/dL
CO_2 23 mEq/L	ALT 31 units/L	LDL 163 mg/dL
BUN 16 mg/dL	T. bili 0.5 mg/dL	TG 183 mg/dL
SCr 0.9 mg/dL	T. prot 7.1 g/dL	hsCRP 4.6 mg/L
Glucose 105 mg/dL		
Hgb 11.6 mg/dL		
Hct 34%		

■ Assessment

Mrs Thorngrass is an obese Caucasian woman who presents to pharmacotherapy clinic for intake. She has a significant family history of cardiovascular disease. She has uncontrolled HTN, treated with metoprolol tartrate, and dyslipidemia, treated only with ezetimibe and garlic. She reports an allergy to atorvastatin, but admits that her leg cramps have not improved since discontinuing the drug and coincide with her rare bouts of exercise. She reports liberal use of ibuprofen and naproxen to relieve the cramps. She also has previously undiagnosed anemia.

QUESTIONS

Problem Identification

1.a. What drug-related problems does this patient have?

1.b. What laboratory values indicate the presence and severity of dyslipidemia in this patient?

1.c. What are the patient's risk factors (both modifiable and non-modifiable) for cardiovascular disease?

1.d. What is this patient's risk classification for cardiovascular disease, and how does this relate to her individual therapy?

Desired Outcome

2. What are the pharmacologic and nonpharmacologic treatment goals for this patient?

Therapeutic Alternatives

3.a. What nonpharmacologic therapies are necessary for this patient to achieve and maintain target cholesterol values?

3.b. What pharmacotherapeutic options are available for controlling this patient's dyslipidemia and preventing future CVD events?

Optimal Plan

4.a. Design a plan that details specific lifestyle modifications for this patient.

4.b. Develop a specific pharmacotherapeutic regimen for this patient's dyslipidemia and uncontrolled HTN.

4.c. What options are available if the pharmacotherapy regimen you chose fails, or if she develops an adverse drug reaction?

Outcome Evaluation

5. Based on your treatment regimen, what are the monitoring parameters for each pharmacologic agent selected?

Patient Education

6.a. Based on your recommendations, provide appropriate education to this patient regarding pharmacologic and nonpharmacologic treatments.

6.b. What steps can you take to ensure that patient is successful in implementing nonpharmacologic measures?

■ CLINICAL COURSE: ALTERNATIVE THERAPY

Mrs Thorngrass is already taking garlic capsules, but she is not sure about the type or dose. Because you are making changes to her current prescription regimen, you need to investigate the advisability of continuing the garlic. If Mrs Thorngrass does begin a statin drug as indicated, she would not be able to take red yeast rice, a common supplement used for dyslipidemia, because it contains mevacolin K, a lovastatin analog, and would be duplicative therapy. Would fish oil be a possible option for her? See Section 19 in this Casebook for questions about the use of garlic and fish oil for treatment of dyslipidemia.

■ SELF-STUDY ASSIGNMENTS

1. Describe how this patient's other drug/disease interaction issues that are unrelated to dyslipidemia should be managed.

2. What changes, if any, would you make to the pharmacotherapy regimen for this patient if she had presented at the initial visit with each of the following characteristics:

   • Childbearing age
   • Cirrhosis of the liver

- Renal disease
- Significant alcohol use

CLINICAL PEARL

Rosuvastatin is FDA-approved to decrease risk of stroke, MI, and need for revascularization procedures in men and women without evidence of CHD and normal LDL, if they are considered to be at increased risk based on age, elevated hsCRP, and one or more additional risk factors.

REFERENCES

1. Stone NJ, Robinson J, Lichtenstein AH, et al. 2013 ACC/AHA guideline on the treatment of blood cholesterol to reduce atherosclerotic cardiovascular risk in adults: a report of the American College Cardiology/ American Heart Association Task Force on Practice Guidelines. J Am Coll Cardiol 2014;63:2889–2934.

2. Jacobson TA, Maki KC, Orringer C, et al. National Lipid Association recommendations for patient-centered management of dyslipidemia: part 2. J Clin Lipidol 2015;9:129–169.

3. Ridker PM, Danielson E, Fonseca FA, et al. Rosuvastatin to prevent vascular events in men and women with elevated C-reactive protein. N Engl J Med 2008;359:2195–2207.

4. Eckel RH, Jakicic JM, Ard JD, et al. 2013 AHA/ACC guideline on lifestyle management to reduce cardiovascular risk: a report of the American College of Cardiology American/Heart Association Task Force on Practice Guidelines. Circulation 2014;129:S76–S99.

5. James PA, Oparil S, Carter BL. 2014 evidence-based guideline for the management of high blood pressure in adults: report from the panel members appointed to the Eighth Joint National Committee (JNC 8). JAMA 2014;311(5):507–520.

6. Jensen MD, Ryan DH, Apovian CM, et al. 2013 ACC/AHA/TOS guideline for the management of overweight and obesity in adults: a report of the American College of Cardiology/American Heart Association Task Force on Practice Guidelines, and The Obesity Society. J Am Coll Cardiol 2014:63;2985–3023.

7. Bibbins-Domingo K; U.S. Preventive Services Task Force. Aspirin use for the primary prevention of cardiovascular disease and colorectal cancer: U.S. Preventive Services Task Force Recommendation Statement. Ann Intern Med doi:10.7326/M16-0577. Published online 12 April 2016 ahead of print.

27

PERIPHERAL ARTERY DISEASE

Cold Feet?.....................................Level III

Tracy J. Costello, PharmD, BCPS

Tracy L. Sprunger, PharmD, BCPS

LEARNING OBJECTIVES

After completing this case study, the reader should be able to:

- Identify risk factors for peripheral artery disease (PAD).
- Describe the symptoms and diagnosis of PAD.
- Recommend appropriate nonpharmacologic treatment strategies for PAD, including risk factor modification, exercise, and revascularization.
- Design an appropriate pharmacologic treatment plan for a patient with PAD.
- Provide appropriate education to a patient with PAD.

PATIENT PRESENTATION

◼ Chief Complaint

"I am having pain in both legs and in my left foot."

◼ HPI

Angie Belden is a 47-year-old woman with a history of hypertension, diabetes, stroke, hypothyroidism, dyslipidemia, and a history of bilateral leg weakness for the previous year. She reports to her primary care provider today with increased numbness and weakness when she walks. She reports that it is painful to walk even for 4–5 minutes and that her legs are often weak and "give out." She is concerned because she lives alone and is responsible for walking her beloved Labrador retriever, Jules. Her symptoms tend to get better when she is able to rest and prop her feet up. She would also like a "checkup" on her other chronic conditions as well.

◼ PMH

HTN
Diabetes
Stroke
Hypothyroidism
Dyslipidemia

◼ FH

Mother died of a stroke at the age of 67; father died of pneumonia at the age of 62

◼ SH

Works as a biller in a dentist's office; has one child; lives alone; smokes 1 ppd × 25 years; denies ETOH and illicit drug use; has one dog at home

◼ Meds

Atenolol 50 mg PO daily
Clopidogrel 75 mg PO daily
Gabapentin 600 mg PO TID
Hydrocodone/acetaminophen 7.5/500 mg q 6 hours PRN pain
Levothyroxine 75 mcg PO daily
Metformin 1000 mg PO BID
Simvastatin 20 mg PO daily
Hydrochlorothiazide 25 mg PO daily

◼ All

NKDA

◼ ROS

Complains of dyspnea on exertion, lower extremity muscle aches, and muscle weakness. Denies chest pains, palpitations, syncope, and orthopnea. Denies nausea, vomiting, diarrhea, constipation, change in bowel habits, abdominal pain, or melena. Denies transient paralysis, seizures, syncope, and tremors.

■ Physical Examination

Gen

The patient is a Caucasian woman in NAD. She appears older than her stated age

VS

BP 149/87, P 73, RR 17, T 98.2°F; Wt 85 kg, Ht 5′4″

Skin

Distal to midshin with shiny-appearing skin, skin atrophy, and lack of hair growth. No evidence of skin breakdown or ulceration

HEENT

PERRLA; conjunctivae and lids normal; TM intact; normal dentition, no gingival inflammation, no labial lesions; tongue normal, posterior pharynx without erythema or exudate

Neck/Lymph Nodes

Supple, no masses, trachea midline; no carotid bruit; no lymphadenopathy or thyromegaly

Lungs/Thorax

No rales, rhonchi, or wheezes; no intercostal retractions or use of accessory muscles

CV

RRR, S_1, S_2 normal; no murmurs, rubs, or gallops; no thrill or palpable murmurs, no displacement of PMI

Abd

Soft, nontender, no masses, bowel sounds normal; no enlargement or nodularity of liver or spleen

Genit/Rect

Deferred

MS/Ext

Normal gait; no clubbing, cyanosis, petechiae, or nodes; normal ROM and strength, good stability, and no joint enlargement or tenderness; pedal pulses 1+, symmetric

Neuro

CN II–XII grossly intact; DTRs 2+, no pathologic reflexes; sensory and motor levels intact

■ Labs

Na 137 mEq/L	Hgb 12.7 g/dL	WBC 6.3 × 10³/mm³
K 3.9 mEq/L	Hct 34.4%	CPK 71 IU/L
Cl 97 mEq/L	Plt 313 × 10³/mm³	AST 22 IU/L
CO₂ 24 mEq/L	TSH 1.12 mIU/L	ALT 30 IU/L
BUN 12 mg/dL	TC 224 mg/dL	
SCr 1.0 mg/dL	TG 220 mg/dL	
Glu 99 mg/dL	LDL 140 mg/dL	
A1C 6.3%	HDL 40 mg/dL	

■ Lower Extremity Arterial Doppler

Ankle–brachial index (ABI)—right: 0.53; left: 0.62.

■ Assessment

A 47-year-old woman with a significant smoking history presents with uncontrolled hypertension, dyslipidemia, and new symptoms of intermittent claudication (IC).

Problem Identification

1.a. Create a list of this patient's drug-related problems.

1.b. What information (signs, symptoms, laboratory values) indicates the presence or severity of IC?

1.c. Identify this patient's risk factors for PAD.

Desired Outcome

2. What are the goals of therapy for IC in this case?

Therapeutic Alternatives

3.a. What nondrug therapies might be useful for this patient?

3.b. What feasible pharmacotherapeutic alternatives are available for the treatment of the disease or drug therapy problem?

Optimal Plan

4.a. What drug, dosage form, dose, schedule, and duration of therapy are best for this patient's IC and concomitant disease states?

4.b. What alternatives would be appropriate if the initial therapy fails or cannot be used?

Outcome Evaluation

5. Based on your recommendations, what clinical and laboratory parameters are necessary to evaluate the therapy for the achievement of the desired therapeutic outcome and to detect or prevent adverse effects?

Patient Education

6. What information should be provided to the patient to enhance adherence, ensure successful therapy, and minimize adverse effects?

■ SELF-STUDY ASSIGNMENTS

1. Review the recommendations for dual antiplatelet therapy for the treatment of PAD. Would a patient benefit from combination therapy?

2. Perform a literature search to determine the role of warfarin and nonvitamin K oral anticoagulant agents for the management of PAD.

CLINICAL PEARL

Although cilostazol has antiplatelet effects, it is currently not recommended for the prevention of atherosclerotic events or the treatment of atherosclerotic disease.

REFERENCES

1. Weber MA, Schiffrin EL, White WB, et al. Clinical practice guidelines for the management of hypertension in the community: a statement by the American Society of Hypertension and the International Society of Hypertension. J Clin Hypertens 2013;16(1):14–26.

2. James PA, Oparil S, Carter BL, et al. 2014 evidence-based guideline for the management of high blood pressure in adults: report from the panel members appointed to the Eighth Joint National Committee (JNC 8). JAMA 2014;311(5):507–520.

3. American Diabetes Association. Standards of medical care in diabetes—2016. Diabetes Care 2016;39(Suppl 1):S1–S112.

4. Rooke TW, Hirsch AT, Misra S, et al. 2011 ACCF/AHA focused update of the guidelines for the management of patients with peripheral artery disease (updating 2005 guidelines): a report of the American College of Cardiology Foundation/American Heart Association Task Force on Practice Guidelines. Circulation 2011;124:2020–2045.

5. 2013 ACC/AHA Guideline on the Treatment of Blood Cholesterol to reduce Atherosclerotic Cardiovascular Risk in Adults. A report of the American college of Cardiology/American Heart Association Task Force on Practice Guidelines. Circulation 2014;129(Suppl 2):S1–S45.

6. Smith SC, Benjamin EJ, Bonow RO, et al. AHA/ACCF secondary prevention and risk reduction therapy for patients with coronary and other atherosclerotic vascular disease: 2011 update: a guideline from the American Heart Association and American College of Cardiology Foundation. Circulation 2011;124:2458–2473.

7. Apovian CM, Aronne LJ, Bessesen DH, et al. Pharmacological management of obesity: an endocrine society clinical practice guideline. J Clin Endocrinol Metab 2015;100:342–362.

8. Hirsch AT, Haskal ZJ, Hertzer NR, et al. ACC/AHA guidelines for the management of patients with peripheral arterial disease (lower extremity, renal, mesenteric, and abdominal aortic): executive summary a collaborative report from the American Association for Vascular Surgery, Society for Cardiovascular Angiography and Interventions, Society of Interventional Radiology, Society for Vascular Medicine and Biology, and the ACC/AHA Task Force on Practice Guidelines. J Am Coll Cardiol 2006;47:1239–1312.

9. Alonso-Coello, P, Bellmunt S, McCorrian C, et al. Antithrombotic therapy in peripheral artery disease. Antithrombotic Therapy and Prevention of Thrombosis, 9th ed: American College of Chest Physicians Evidence-Based Clinical Guidelines. Chest 2012;141: e669S–e690S.

10. Bonaca MP, Scirica BM, Creager MA, et al. Vorapaxar in patients with peripheral artery disease: results from TRA2°P-TIMI 50. Circulation 2013;127:1522–1529.

28

HYPOVOLEMIC SHOCK

A Glass Half Full................................ Level II

Brian L. Erstad, PharmD, FCCP, FCCM, FASHP

Brian J. Kopp, PharmD, BCPS, FCCM

Yvonne C. Huckleberry, PharmD, BCPS

LEARNING OBJECTIVES

After completing this case study, the reader should be able to:

- Develop a plan for implementing fluid or medication therapies for treating a patient in the initial stages of shock.

- Outline the major parameters used to monitor hypovolemic shock and its treatment.

- List the major disadvantages of using only isolated hemodynamic recordings, such as blood pressure measurements, for monitoring the progression of shock.

- Compare and contrast fluids and medications used for treating hypovolemic shock.

PATIENT PRESENTATION

■ Chief Complaint

"I'm beat. I have vomited four times in the last 24 hours and had diarrhea last evening. Now is not a great time to get sick since I'm in college and have finals next week."

■ HPI

Four days PTA, Mr Hobbs, a 20-year-old college student, had abdominal pain that he attributed to a flare-up in his Crohn disease due to the stress of final examinations. He has an infliximab infusion scheduled for next week; he has them every 8 weeks and does not miss these infusions. However, he admits that he forgets to take his oral medications now that he lives away from his family. When he has Crohn pain, he does not feel like eating since eating causes more stomach pain. Furthermore, he has vomiting and diarrhea, which is aggravated by food intake. Per the recommendation of his community pharmacist, Mr Hobbs purchased a commercially available rehydration solution and attempted to drink the small but frequent volumes recommended by his pharmacist, but he could not keep up with fluid losses. His primary care physician referred him to the local hospital for rehydration and further evaluation.

■ PMH

Crohn disease, diagnosed 4 years ago
Ankylosing spondylitis, diagnosed 3 years ago
Pulmonary coccidioidomycosis (small ill-defined mass in lungs with positive cocci titers), diagnosed 1 year ago

■ FH

Noncontributory

■ SH

Does not smoke or use illicit drugs; admits to occasional ETOH use at parties

■ Meds

Infliximab 300 mg by IV infusion over 3 hours every 8 weeks
Azathioprine 100 mg PO daily
Fluconazole 400 mg PO daily
Fish oil (unknown strength) one capsule PO BID
Multivitamin one tablet PO daily
Whey shakes for protein supplementation, one shake PO daily

■ All

NKDA

■ ROS

The patient has had a recent increase in weight over the past month (6 kg), although this has decreased by 2 kg in the last few days. Hearing is intact with no vertigo. No dizziness or fainting episodes. Colorless sputum. No chest pain or dyspnea, but heart has been "racing." Has had one episode of diarrhea and four episodes of vomiting with abdominal pain in the past 24 hours. No musculoskeletal pain or cramping.

■ Physical Examination

Gen

Thin, somewhat anxious man in mild distress

VS

BP 84/58 (baseline 122/78), but possible orthostatic changes not determined, HR 132 (baseline 80), RR 16, T 38.2°C; admission Wt 60 kg, Ht 5'10"

Skin

Pale color (including nail beds) and dry, but not cyanotic; no lesions

HEENT

Normal scalp/skull; conjunctivae pale and dry with clear sclerae; PERRLA, dry oral mucosa; remainder of ophthalmologic exam not performed

Neck/Lymph Nodes

Supple, no lymphadenopathy or thyromegaly

Lungs/Thorax

Clear by palpation and auscultation

CV

RRR; S_1 and S_2 normal; apical pulse difficult to palpate; no MRG

Abd

Perigastric pain on light palpation, no hepatosplenomegaly or masses; bowel sounds present

Genit/Rect

Normal male genitalia; prostate smooth, not enlarged; no hemorrhoids noted; stool heme (–)

MS/Ext

No deformities with normal ROM of joints except for hips and knees (somewhat limited ROM); no edema, ulcers, or tenderness

Neuro

Mild muscular atrophy with weak grip strength; CN II–XII intact; 2+ reflexes throughout; Babinski downgoing

■ Labs

Na 149 mEq/L	Hgb 11.9 g/dL	Phos 2.9 mg/dL
K 3.3 mEq/L	Hct 34.3%	AST 35 IU/L
Cl 112 mEq/L	Plt 151 × 10³/mm³	ALT 23 IU/L
CO_2 30 mEq/L	WBC 13 × 10³/mm³	T. bili 1.1 mg/dL
BUN 32 mg/dL	PT 12.1 s	Alk phos 83 IU/L
SCr 1.4 mg/dL[a]	aPTT 33 s	CRP 16 mg/dL
Glu 105 mg/dL	Albumin 3.3 g/dL	ESR 48 mm/hour

[a]Baseline SCr 1.1 mg/dL.

■ Other Test Results

CXR negative. I/O 1200/75 (urinary catheter) for first 3 hours of hospitalization. Results pending for ABG with lactate level, blood and urine cultures, gastroenteric pathogens on stool culture, O & P, and *Clostridium difficile* titer.

■ Assessment

Volume depletion, possible acid–base disorder, possible infectious process, malnutrition, anemia.

QUESTIONS

Problem Identification

1.a. Create a list of the patient's drug-related problems.

1.b. What information (signs, symptoms, laboratory values) indicates the presence or severity of hypovolemic shock?

Desired Outcome

2. What are the goals of pharmacotherapy in this case?

Therapeutic Alternatives

3.a. What nondrug therapies might be useful for this patient?

3.b. What feasible pharmacotherapeutic alternatives are available for the treatment of shock and the associated laboratory alterations?

Optimal Plan

4. What drug, dosage form, dose, schedule, and duration of therapy are best for this patient?

Outcome Evaluation

5. What clinical and laboratory parameters are necessary to evaluate the therapy for the achievement of the desired therapeutic outcome and to detect or prevent adverse events?

Patient Education

6. What information should be provided to the patient to enhance adherence, ensure successful therapy, and minimize adverse effects?

■ CLINICAL COURSE

No evidence of infection was found, including a negative titer for *C. difficile*. All cultures were negative, and the elevated temperature abated within 12 hours of admission. However, the patient had a complicated clinical course since inadequate nonisotonic fluids were given early in his hospital course. After approximately 10 days, the patient had to be admitted to the ICU for renal failure precipitated by inadequate vascular expansion.

■ FOLLOW-UP QUESTION

1. Explain why hypotonic IV fluids such as 5% dextrose are not indicated in a patient with overt hypovolemia, who is going into shock.

■ SELF-STUDY ASSIGNMENTS

1. Search the literature and discuss the results of comparative trials involving crystalloids and colloids for plasma expansion.

2. Write a two-page report that compares the advantages and limitations of each type of fluid for the plasma expansion indication.

CLINICAL PEARL

Isotonic or near-isotonic IV crystalloid solutions are indicated in patients with extracellular fluid depletion, who cannot receive oral rehydration solutions due to the severity of presentation or inability to absorb adequate volumes. Isotonic solutions replenish the extracellular space and have minimal intracellular distribution.

REFERENCES

1. Dellinger RP, Levy MM, Rhodes A, et al. Surviving Sepsis Campaign: international guidelines for management of severe sepsis and septic shock: 2012. Crit Care Med 2013;41:580–631.

2. Yunos NM, Bellomo R, Hegarty C, et al. Association between chloride-liberal vs chloride-restrictive intravenous fluid administration strategy and kidney injury in critically ill adults. JAMA 2012;308:1566–1572.

3. Krajewski ML, Raghunathan K, Paluszkiewicz SM, et al. Meta-analysis of high- versus low-chloride content in perioperative and critical care fluid resuscitation. BJS 2015;102:24–36.

4. Finfer S, Bellomo R, Boyce N, et al. SAFE Study Investigators. A comparison of albumin and saline for fluid resuscitation in the intensive care unit. N Engl J Med 2004;350:2247–2256.

5. Brunkhorst FM, Engel C, Bloos F, et al. Intensive insulin therapy and pent starch resuscitation in severe sepsis. N Engl J Med 2008;358:125–139.

6. Myburgh JA, Finfer S, Bellomo R, et al. Hydroxyethyl starch or saline for fluid resuscitation in intensive care. N Engl J Med 2012;367:1901–1911.

7. Perner A, Haase N, Guttormsen AB, et al. Hydroxyethyl starch 130/0.42 versus Ringer's acetate in severe sepsis. N Engl J Med 2012;367:124–134.

SECTION 3
RESPIRATORY DISORDERS

29

ACUTE ASTHMA

A Little Influenza, a Big Asthma Attack .... Level I

Rebecca S. Pettit, PharmD, MBA, BCPS, BCPPS

LEARNING OBJECTIVES

After completing this case study, the reader should be able to:

- Recognize the signs and symptoms of an acute asthma exacerbation.

- Formulate therapeutic end points based on the initiation of a pharmacotherapy plan used to treat the acute asthma symptoms.

- Identify appropriate dosage form selection based on the patient's age, ability to take medication, or adherence to technique.

- Determine an appropriate home pharmacotherapy plan, including discharge counseling, as the patient nears discharge from a hospital setting.

PATIENT PRESENTATION

Chief Complaint

"My daughter has had a bad fever, and now she is having trouble breathing, and albuterol doesn't help."

HPI

Terri Collins is an 8-year-old African-American girl who presents to the ED with a 2-day history of fevers, malaise, and nonproductive cough. The mother gave acetaminophen and ibuprofen to help control the fever. Mother stated that "a lot of other kids in her class have been sick this fall, too." Terri started having trouble breathing the morning of admission, and the mother gave her albuterol, 2.5 mg via nebulization twice within an hour. Terri still sounded wheezy to the mother after the albuterol, and Terri stated it was "hard to breath." Terri was previously well controlled regarding asthma symptoms. Previous clinic notes reported symptoms during the day only with active play at school or at home and rare nighttime symptoms. She uses PRN albuterol to help with symptoms after playing. Her assessment in the emergency department revealed Terri to have labored breathing, such that she could only complete four- to five-word sentences. She had subcostal retractions, tracheal tugging with tachypnea at 54 breaths/min. Her other vital signs were a heart rate of 160 bpm, blood pressure of 115/59, temperature of 38.8°C, and a weight of 22.7 kg. The initial oxygen

saturation was 88%, and she was started on oxygen at 1 L/min via nasal cannula. Bilateral expiratory and inspiratory wheezes were noted on examination. A chest x-ray revealed a right lower lobe consolidation consistent with pneumonia and possible effusion. After receiving three albuterol/ipratropium nebulizations, her breath sounds and oxygenation did not improve; so she was started on albuterol via continuous nebulization at 10 mg/hour, and her oxygen was titrated to 3 L/min. She was also given a dose of 25 mg IV methylprednisolone and a dose of 600 mg IV magnesium sulfate. Terri was then transferred to the PICU for further treatment and monitoring.

PMH

Asthma; last hospitalization 4 years ago, and has had two courses of oral corticosteroids in the past year

FH

Asthma on father's side of the family

SH

Lives with mother, father, and two siblings, both of whom have asthma. There are two cats and a dog in the home. Father is a smoker, but states that he tries to smoke outside and not around the kids. She is in the second grade and is very active on the playground.

Meds

Albuterol 2.5 mg nebulized Q 4–6 H PRN wheezing
Fluticasone propionate 44 mcg MDI two puffs BID
Acetaminophen 160 mg/5 mL—10 mL Q 4 H PRN fever
Ibuprofen 100 mg/5 mL—10 mL Q 6 H PRN fever

All

NKA

ROS

(+) Fever, cough, increased work of breathing

Physical Examination

Gen

Alert and oriented but in mild distress with difficulty breathing

VS

BP 125/69, P 120, T 37.9°C, RR 40, O$_2$ sat 94% on 3 L/min nasal cannula

Skin

No rashes, no bruises

HEENT

NC/AT, PERRLA

Neck/LN

Soft, supple, no cervical lymphadenopathy

Chest

Wheezes throughout all lung fields, still with subcostal retractions

CV

RRR, no m/r/g

Abd

Soft, NT/ND

Ext

No clubbing or cyanosis

Neuro

A & O, no focal deficits

▣ Labs

Na 141 mEq/L	WBC $34.2 \times 10^3/mm^3$
K 3.1 mEq/L	Neut 91%
Cl 104 mEq/L	Lymph 5%
CO_2 29 mEq/L	Mono 4%
BUN 16 mg/dL	RBC $5.07 \times 10^6/mm^3$
SCr 0.52 mg/dL	Hgb 13 g/dL
Glu 154 mg/dL	Hct 41%
	Plt $310 \times 10^3/mm^3$

Respiratory viral panel nasal swab: positive for influenza A (probably H1N1 strain)

▣ Chest X-Ray

RLL consolidation

▣ Assessment

Asthma exacerbation with viral pneumonia

QUESTIONS

Problem Identification

1.a. Create a list of the patient's drug-related problems.

1.b. What information (signs, symptoms, laboratory values) indicates the severity of the acute asthma attack?

Desired Outcome

2. What are the acute goals of pharmacotherapy in this case?

Therapeutic Alternatives

3.a. What nondrug therapies might be useful for this patient?

3.b. What feasible pharmacotherapeutic alternatives are available for the treatment of acute asthma?

Optimal Plan

4.a. What drug, dosage form, dose, schedule, and duration of therapy are best for this patient's acute asthma exacerbation?

4.b. What other pharmacotherapy would you recommend in the acute treatment of this patient?

▣ CLINICAL COURSE

Within 48 hours of initiation of the treatment plan for management of the acute exacerbation, Terri was stable enough to transfer to the general pediatric floor. Her vital signs were BP 103/70, P 82, RR 35, T 37.2°C, and O_2 sat 99% on 1 L/min nasal cannula. Mother states that she is able to speak in full sentences now and no longer seems to have trouble breathing.

4.c. What drug, dosage form, dose, schedule, and duration of therapy are best for this patient's discharge plan?

Outcome Evaluation

5.a. Once the patient has transferred to the general medical floor and her vitals have improved (see the section "Clinical Course"), what clinical and laboratory parameters are necessary to evaluate the therapy for achievement of the desired therapeutic outcome and to detect or prevent adverse effects at that point in the patient's care?

5.b. What clinical parameters are necessary to evaluate the efficacy of the patient's asthma therapy after hospital discharge?

Patient Education

6.a. What should the family monitor for regarding the potential adverse effects from the drug therapy, and how should they be counseled on the use of the asthma medications, especially regarding the differences between quick-relief and controller medications?

6.b. Describe the information that should be provided to the family regarding medication delivery technique and possible asthma triggers.

▣ FOLLOW-UP QUESTIONS

1. Should any cough and cold products be used for asthma symptoms? Why or why not?

2. What information should be given to patients/families regarding influenza?

3. What information can be given to families who are concerned about giving their child "steroids" for asthma treatment (either in an acute asthma exacerbation or for controller therapy)?

▣ SELF-STUDY ASSIGNMENTS

1. Research the efficacy of systemic corticosteroids for treatment of acute asthma exacerbation when given intravenously versus orally (enterally).

2. Discuss the differences in acute asthma exacerbation symptoms in an adult patient versus a pediatric patient, and describe when you would refer a patient (or family) to the physician or emergency department based on an individualized asthma action plan.

3. Discuss the appropriate use of IV magnesium in an acute asthma exacerbation.

CLINICAL PEARL

For proper treatment of an acute asthma exacerbation, the patient (or family) needs to be aware of the first symptoms of an exacerbation and possible triggers. At this point, the patient (family) should initiate her asthma action plan to minimize the symptoms, duration of drug therapy, and severity of the exacerbation. This, in turn, should decrease the number of severe exacerbations and hospital admissions.

ACKNOWLEDGMENT

Special thanks to Jennifer Donaldson, PharmD, for her contribution in the initial development of this case.

REFERENCES

1. Basnet S, Mander G, Andoh J, et al. Safety, efficacy, and tolerability of early initiation of noninvasive positive pressure ventilation in pediatric patients admitted with status asthmaticus: a pilot study. Pediatr Crit Care Med 2012;13:393–398.

2. National Asthma Education and Prevention Program Expert Panel report 3: guidelines for the diagnosis and management of asthma. Bethesda, MD, National Institutes of Health, 2007. Available at: *http://www.nhlbi.nih.gov/guidelines/asthma/asthgdln.htm*. Accessed March 16, 2010.

3. Aldington S, Beasley R. Asthma exacerbations. 5: assessment and management of severe asthma in adults in hospital. Thorax 2007;62:447–458.

4. Andrew T, McGintee E, Mittal MK, et al. High-dose continuous nebulized levalbuterol for pediatric status asthmaticus: a randomized trial. J Pediatr 2009;155:205–210.

5. Vezina K, Chauhan BF, Ducharme FM. Inhaled anticholinergics and short-acting beta(2)-agonists versus short-acting beta2-agonists alone for children with acute asthma in hospital. Cochrane Database Syst Rev 2014;7:1–55.

6. Rowe BH, Camargo CA. The role of magnesium sulfate in the acute and chronic management of asthma. Curr Opin Pulm Med 2008;15:70–76.

7. Kokotajlo S, Degnan L, Meyers R, et al. Use of intravenous magnesium sulfate for the treatment of an acute asthma exacerbation in pediatric patients. J Pediatr Pharmacol Ther 2014;19(2):91–97.

8. Link HW. Pediatric asthma in a nutshell. Pediatr Rev 2014;35(7):287–298.

9. Rank MA, Li JT. Clinical pearls for preventing, diagnosing, and treating seasonal and 2009 H1N1 influenza infections in patients with asthma. J Allergy Clin Immunol 2009;124:1123–1126.

30

CHRONIC ASTHMA

Cat Got Your Tongue?........................... Level II

Julia M. Koehler, PharmD, FCCP

Meghan M. Bodenberg, PharmD, BCPS

Jennifer R. Guthrie, MPAS, PA-C

LEARNING OBJECTIVES

After completing this case study, the reader should be able to:

- Recognize signs and symptoms of uncontrolled asthma.

- Identify potential causes of uncontrolled asthma, and recommend preventive measures.

- Formulate a patient-specific therapeutic plan (including drugs, route of administration, and appropriate monitoring parameters) for management of a patient with chronic asthma.

- Develop a self-management action plan for improving control of asthma.

PATIENT PRESENTATION

Chief Complaint

"Please don't tell me we have to get rid of the cats!"

HPI

Shiloh Eddingfield is a 17-year-old female who presents to her primary care provider for follow-up and evaluation regarding her asthma. During her visit, she reports having had to use her albuterol MDI approximately 3–4 days per week over the past 2 months, but over the past week she admits to using albuterol once daily. She reports being awakened by a cough three nights during the last month. She states she especially becomes short of breath when she exercises, although she admits that her shortness of breath is not always brought on by exercise and sometimes occurs when she is not actively exercising. In addition to her albuterol MDI, which she uses PRN, she also has a fluticasone MDI, which she uses "most days of the week." She indicates that her morning peak flows have been running around 300 L/min (personal best = 400 L/min) over the past several weeks.

PMH

Asthma (previously documented as "mild persistent") diagnosed at age 7; no prior history of intubations; hospitalized twice in the last year for poorly controlled asthma; three visits to the ED in the last 6 months; treated with oral systemic corticosteroids during both hospitalizations and at each ED visit

Migraine headache disorder (without aura; diagnosed at age 15); currently taking prophylactic medication; has had only one migraine attack in the last year

FH

Mother 47 years old with HTN, migraine HA disorder; father 48 years old (smoker) with HTN and type 2 DM; brother, age 21 (smoker); twin sister, age 17 (nonsmoker).

SH

No alcohol or tobacco use. Single, sexually active. Lives at home with parents (father is a cabinet maker), twin sister, and two cats. Brother is currently away at college.

Meds

Flovent HFA 44 mcg, two puffs BID
Proventil HFA two puffs Q 4–6 H PRN shortness of breath
Yaz one PO daily
Propranolol 80 mg PO BID
Maxalt-MLT 5 mg PO PRN acute migraine

All

PCN (rash)

ROS

Denies fever, chills, headache, eye discharge or redness, rhinorrhea, sneezing, sputum production, chest pain, palpitations, dizziness or confusion

Physical Examination

Gen

Well-developed, well-nourished white female appearing stated age in NAD

VS

BP 110/68, HR 78, RR 16, T 37°C; Wt 58 kg, Ht 5′5″

HEENT

PERRLA; mild oral thrush present on tongue and buccal mucosa

Neck/Lymph Nodes

Supple; no lymphadenopathy or thyromegaly

Lungs/Thorax

Mild expiratory wheezes bilaterally

CV

RRR; no MRG

Abd

Soft, NTND; (+) BS

Genit/Rect

Deferred

Ext

Normal ROM; peripheral pulses 3+; no CCE

Neuro

A & O × 3

■ Labs

Na 136 mEq/L	Hgb 12 g/dL	WBC $6.0 \times 10^3/mm^3$
K 3.6 mEq/L	Hct 36%	PMNs 56%
Cl 99 mEq/L	RBC $5.0 \times 10^6/mm^3$	Bands 1%
CO_2 27 mEq/L	MCH 28 pg	Eosinophils 3%
BUN 18 mg/dL	MCHC 34 g/dL	Basophils 2%
SCr 0.6 mg/dL	MCV 90 μm³	Lymphocytes 33%
Glu 98 mg/dL	Plts $192 \times 10^3/mm^3$	Monocytes 5%
Ca 9.3 mg/dL		

■ Assessment

A 17-year-old girl with uncontrolled chronic asthma and mild oral thrush

QUESTIONS

Problem Identification

1.a. Create a list of the patient's drug therapy problems.

1.b. What information indicates the presence of uncontrolled chronic asthma?

1.c. What factors may have contributed to this patient's uncontrolled asthma?

1.d. How would you classify this patient's level of asthma control (well controlled, not well controlled, or very poorly controlled), according to NIH guidelines?

Desired Outcome

2. What are the goals of pharmacotherapy in this case?

Therapeutic Alternatives

3.a. What nonpharmacologic therapies might be useful for this patient?

3.b. What feasible pharmacotherapeutic alternatives are available for treatment of this patient's chronic asthma?

Optimal Plan

4.a. Outline an optimal plan of treatment for this patient's chronic asthma.

4.b. What alternatives would be appropriate if the initial therapy fails?

Outcome Evaluation

5. What clinical parameters are necessary to evaluate the therapy for achievement of the desired therapeutic effect and to detect or prevent adverse effects?

Patient Education

6. What information should be provided to the patient regarding the use of her asthma medications, and how can she use her peak flow readings to better manage her asthma?

■ SELF-STUDY ASSIGNMENTS

1. Review the NIH guidelines on the management of asthma during pregnancy, and develop a pharmacotherapeutic treatment plan for this patient's asthma if she were to become pregnant.

2. Review the literature on the impact of chronic inhaled corticosteroid use on the risk for development of osteoporosis, and write a two-page paper summarizing the available published literature on this topic.

CLINICAL PEARL

Patients with asthma who report that taking aspirin makes their asthma symptoms worse may respond well to leukotriene modifiers. Aspirin inhibits prostaglandin synthesis from arachidonic acid through inhibition of cyclooxygenase. The leukotriene pathway may play a role in the development of asthma symptoms in such patients, as inhibition of cyclooxygenase by aspirin may shunt the arachidonic acid pathway away from prostaglandin synthesis and toward leukotriene production. Although inhaled corticosteroids are still the preferred anti-inflammatory medications for patients with asthma and known aspirin sensitivity, leukotriene modifiers may also be useful in such patients based on this theoretical mechanism.

REFERENCES

1. National Asthma Education and Prevention Program. Executive Summary of the NAEPP Expert Panel Report 3: Guidelines for the Diagnosis and Management of Asthma. Bethesda, MD, U.S. Department of Health and Human Services, Public Health Service, National Institutes of Health, National Heart, Lung, and Blood Institute, 2007. Full report. Available at: http://www.nhlbi.nih.gov/guidelines/asthma/index.htm. Accessed April 15, 2016.

2. Global Initiative for Asthma (GINA). Global strategy for asthma management and prevention (updated 2016). Available at: http://www.ginasthma.com; 2016. Accessed April 1, 2016.

3. Lemanske RF, Mauger DT, Sorkness CA, et al. Step-up therapy for children with uncontrolled asthma while receiving inhaled corticosteroids. N Engl J Med 2010;362:975–985.

4. Busse W, Raphael GD, Galant S, et al. Fluticasone Propionate Clinical Research Study Group. Low-dose fluticasone propionate compared with montelukast for first-line treatment of persistent asthma: a randomized clinical trial. J Allergy Clin Immunol 2001;107:461–468.

5. Busse W, Nelson H, Wolfe J, Kalberg C, Yancey SW, Rickard KA. Comparison of inhaled salmeterol and oral zafirlukast in patients with asthma. J Allergy Clin Immunol 1999;103:1075–1080.

6. Humbert M, Beasley R, Ayres J, et al. Benefits of omalizumab as add-on therapy in patients with severe persistent asthma who are inadequately controlled despite best available therapy (GINA 2002 step 4 treatment): INNOVATE. Allergy 2005;60:309–316.

7. Food and Drug Administration (FDA) 2007. FDA alert: omalizumab (marketed as Xolair) information, February 2007 (updated April 2013). Available at: *http://www.fda.gov/NewsEvents/Newsroom/PressAnnouncements/2007/ucm108850.htm.* Accessed May 1, 2016.

8. Ortega HG, Liu MC, Pavord ID, et al. Mepolizumab treatment in patients with severe eosinophilic asthma. N Engl J Med 2014;371:1198–1207.

9. Peters SP, Kunselman SJ, Icitovic N, et al. Tiotropium bromide step-up therapy for adults with uncontrolled asthma. N Engl J Med 2010;363:1715–1726.

31

CHRONIC OBSTRUCTIVE PULMONARY DISEASE

Treading on Thin Air . . . . Level II

Joseph P. Vande Griend, PharmD, FCCP, BCPS

Joel C. Marrs, PharmD, FCCP, FASHP, FNLA, BCPS (AQ Cardiology), BCACP, CLS

LEARNING OBJECTIVES

After completing this case study, the reader should be able to:

- Recognize modifiable risk factors for the development of chronic obstructive pulmonary disease (COPD).

- Interpret spirometry readings and patient-specific factors to evaluate and appropriately provide a classification of COPD for an individual patient.

- Identify the importance of nonpharmacologic therapy in patients with COPD.

- Develop an appropriate medication regimen for a patient with COPD based on disease classification.

PATIENT PRESENTATION

Chief Complaint

"My wife says I need to get my lungs checked. Ever since we moved, I'm having a hard time breathing."

HPI

Dwayne Morrison is a 59-year-old man who is presenting to a new provider at the family medicine clinic today with complaints of increasing shortness of breath. He points out that he first noticed some difficulty catching his breath at his job 3 years ago. He had been able to carry heavy loads up and down a flight of stairs daily for the last 35 years without any problem. However, his shortness of breath began to make this very difficult. Coincidently at that time, he accepted a managerial position at his company that significantly reduced his activity level. After taking this position, he no longer noticed any problems, but admits that he avoids activities that cause him to physically exert himself. He noticed significant shortness of breath again after he moved to Colorado from a lower elevation 2 months ago to be closer to his grandchildren. His shortness of breath is worst when he is outside playing with his grandchildren. His previous physician had placed him on salmeterol/fluticasone (Advair Diskus) one inhalation twice daily 2 years ago. He thinks his physician initiated the medication for the shortness of breath, but he is not entirely sure. He is hoping to get a good medication that will help relieve his shortness of breath because the gardening season is right around the corner, and he enjoys this hobby.

PMH

CAD (MI 7 years ago, resulting in stent placement at that time; additional stent placed 2 years ago; normal echocardiogram and stress test 3 months ago)

Chronic bronchitis × 8 years (has had one exacerbation in the last 12 months; received oral antibiotic treatment but was not hospitalized)

Cervical radiculopathy

FH

Father with COPD (smoked a pipe for 40 years). Mother with coronary artery disease and cerebrovascular disease.

SH

He lives with his wife, who is a nurse. He has a 40 pack-year history of smoking. When he had an MI at age 52, he quit smoking temporarily. At present, he continues to smoke five to six cigarettes per day. He drinks two to three beers most nights of the workweek.

Meds

Aspirin 81 mg PO once daily
Bupropion SR 150 mg PO twice daily
Clopidogrel 75 mg PO once daily
Fluticasone/salmeterol 100/50, one inhalation BID
OTC ibuprofen 200 mg PO four to six times daily PRN neck pain
Rosuvastatin 20 mg PO once daily
Metoprolol succinate 50 mg PO once daily

All

NKDA

ROS

(+) Chronic cough with sputum production; (+) exercise intolerance

Physical Examination

Gen

WDWN man in NAD

VS

BP 110/68, P 60, RR 16, T 37°C; Wt 82 kg, Ht 5'9"; pulse ox 93% on RA

Skin

Warm, dry; no rashes

HEENT

Normocephalic; PERRLA, EOMI; normal sclerae; mucous membranes are moist; TMs intact; oropharynx clear

Neck/Lymph Nodes

Supple without lymphadenopathy

Lungs

Decreased breath sounds; no rales, rhonchi, or crackles

CV

RRR without murmur; normal S_1 and S_2

Abd

Soft, NT/ND; (+) bowel sounds; no organomegaly

Genit/Rect

No back or flank tenderness; normal male genitalia

MS/Ext

No CCE; pulses 2+ throughout

Neuro

A & O × 3; CN II–XII intact; DTRs 2+; normal mood and affect

■ Labs

Na 135 mEq/L	Hgb 13.5 g/dL	AST 40 IU/L	Ca 9.6 mg/L
K 4.2 mEq/L	Hct 41.2%	ALT 19 IU/L	Mg 3.6 mg/L
Cl 108 mEq/L	Plt 195 × 10³/mm³	T. bili 1.1 mg/dL	Phos 2.9 mg/dL
CO_2 26 mEq/L	WBC 5.4 × 10³/mm³	Alb 3.8 g/dL	
BUN 19 mg/dL			
SCr 1.1 mg/dL			
Glu 89 mg/dL			

■ Pulmonary Function Tests (During Clinic Visit Today)

Prebronchodilator FEV_1 = 2.98 L (predicted is 4.02 L)
FVC = 4.5 L
Postbronchodilator FEV_1 = 2.75 L

■ Assessment

This is a normal-appearing 59-year-old man presenting to the clinic with complaints of shortness of breath that is limiting his activity and affecting his quality of life. Given the results of spirometry and patient history, patient has COPD in addition to a history of CAD, daily pain from cervical radiculopathy, and chronic cough. Cardiac pathology as a cause of current symptoms is unlikely, given lack of chest pain and recent normal cardiovascular stress test. The patient states that he is adherent to his current medication regimen.

QUESTIONS

Problem Identification

1.a. Create a list of this patient's drug-related problems.

1.b. What objective information indicates the presence and severity of COPD?

1.c. What subjective information (eg, patient history) suggests the diagnosis of COPD in this patient?

1.d. How would you stage and classify this patient's COPD?

Desired Outcome

2. What are the desired goals of pharmacotherapy for the treatment of COPD in this patient?

Therapeutic Alternatives

3.a. What nonpharmacologic therapies would be useful to improve this patient's COPD symptoms?

3.b. What pharmacotherapeutic alternatives are available for the treatment of this patient's COPD based on the most recent GOLD guideline recommendations?

3.c. Should home oxygen therapy be considered for the patient at this time? Why or why not?

Optimal Plan

4. Evaluate the patient's current COPD regimen, and develop recommendations to continue or change the current COPD medications at his clinic visit today. Make sure to include specific doses, route, frequency, and duration of therapy.

Outcome Evaluation

5.a. What clinical parameters will you monitor to assess the COPD pharmacotherapy regimen in this patient?

5.b. What laboratory tests can be performed and how often should they be performed to assess the efficacy of the current COPD regimen as well as progression of the patient's lung disease?

Patient Education

6. What information should be provided to the patient to enhance adherence, ensure successful therapy, and minimize adverse effects?

■ SELF-STUDY ASSIGNMENTS

1. Describe and compare the expectations for deterioration in pulmonary function in patients with COPD who have quit smoking with those who continue smoking. In particular, emphasis should be placed on expected patterns of change in FEV_1, FVC, and general health over time in years.

2. Research and describe the appropriate use of inhaled corticosteroids for the management of stable COPD. Be able to compare and contrast the benefits and risks of this therapy.

CLINICAL PEARL

COPD can lead to exercise deconditioning, mood disorders such as depression, progressive muscle loss, and weight loss. A pulmonary rehabilitation program including mandatory exercise training of the muscles used in respiration is recommended for patients with COPD because of the established benefit related to improvements seen in dyspnea symptoms, health-related quality of life, reduced anxiety and depression, reduced number of hospital days secondary to exacerbations, and improved response to bronchodilators.[1]

REFERENCES

1. Global Initiative for Chronic Obstructive Lung Disease. Global strategy for the diagnosis, management, and prevention of chronic obstructive pulmonary disease. Updated 2015. Available at: *http://www.goldcopd.org*. Accessed September 2, 2015.

2. Qaseem A, Wilt TJ, Weinberger SE, et al. Diagnosis and management of stable chronic obstructive pulmonary disease: a clinical practice guideline update from the American College of Physicians, American College of Chest Physicians, American Thoracic Society, and European Respiratory Society. Ann Intern Med 2011;155:179–191.

3. Mahler DA, Wire P, Horstman D, et al. Effectiveness of fluticasone propionate and salmeterol combination delivered via the diskus device in the treatment of chronic obstructive pulmonary disease. Am J Respir Crit Care Med 2002;166:1084–1091.

4. Calverley PM, Anderson JA, Celli B, et al. Salmeterol and fluticasone propionate and survival in chronic obstructive pulmonary disease. N Engl J Med 2007;356:775–789.

5. Calverley P, Pauwels R, Vestbo J, et al. Combined salmeterol and fluticasone in the treatment of chronic obstructive pulmonary disease: a randomized controlled trial. Lancet 2003;361:449–456.

6. Szafranski W, Cukier A, Ramirez A, et al. Efficacy and safety of budesonide/formoterol in the management of chronic obstructive pulmonary disease. Eur Respir J 2003;21:74–81.

7. Jones PW, Willits LR, Burge PS, Calverley P. Disease severity and the effect of fluticasone propionate on chronic obstructive pulmonary disease exacerbations. Eur Respir J 2003;21:68–73.

8. Tashkin DP, Pearle J, Iezzoni D, Varghese ST. Formoterol and tiotropium compared with tiotropium alone for treatment of COPD. COPD 2009;6:17–25.

9. van Noord JA, Aumann JL, Janssens E, et al. Comparison of tiotropium once daily, formoterol twice daily, and both combined once daily in patients with COPD. Eur Respir J 2005;26:214–222.

10. Karner C, Cates CJ. Long-acting beta(2)-agonist in addition to tiotropium versus either tiotropium or long-acting beta(2)-agonist alone for chronic obstructive pulmonary disease. Cochrane Database Syst Rev 2012;4:CD008989.

32

PULMONARY ARTERIAL HYPERTENSION

Windy Cindy. . . . . Level II

Marta A. Miyares, PharmD, BCPS (AQ Cardiology), CACP

Brian C. Sedam, PharmD, BCPS, BCACP

LEARNING OBJECTIVES

After completing this case study, the reader should be able to:

- Determine risk factors for developing pulmonary arterial hypertension (PAH).

- Discuss common signs and symptoms associated with PAH.

- List the pharmacologic agents used to treat PAH.

- List the nonpharmacologic agents used to treat PAH.

- Recommend appropriate pharmacologic and nonpharmacologic education for a patient with PAH.

PATIENT PRESENTATION

■ Chief Complaint

"I felt really dizzy and short of breath, and I suddenly passed out on the bathroom floor."

■ HPI

Cindy Price is a 32-year-old woman who presents to the ED complaining of episodes of dyspnea and dizziness. While stepping out of the shower this morning, she became very weak and experienced a syncopal episode. She remembers falling to the floor and hitting her head but remembers nothing after that. She was brought to the ED this morning by her sister.

■ PMH

Hypertension × 4 years
Diabetes mellitus × 2 years
Asthma (intermittent)

■ FH

Father died of heart failure at the age of 62. Mother is 57 and was diagnosed with PAH 4 years ago. Cindy is single and lives with her sister (her only sibling).

■ SH

Denies tobacco or alcohol use. Admits to heavy cocaine use in her late 20s. Has tried various fad diets (including prescription amphetamines) since she was in college.

■ Meds

Hydrochlorothiazide 12.5 mg PO Q AM
Glyburide 5 mg PO daily with breakfast
Albuterol MDI one to two puffs Q 6 H PRN SOB

■ All

NKDA

■ ROS

Today, Cindy says she is comfortable at rest but complains of having experienced increased dyspnea, fatigue, and dizziness with her everyday activities for the past 6 months. She says that these symptoms only mildly limit her physical activity and denies experiencing these symptoms at rest. Over the past 2–3 months, she has developed palpitations and noticeable swelling in her ankles. She denies episodes of syncope before this acute incident. Approximately 9 months ago, Cindy was seen by her family physician for increasing shortness of breath. Her physician believed that her increasing dyspnea was attributed to asthma, so he prescribed an albuterol inhaler for her to use. The patient says that the albuterol inhaler did not improve her shortness of breath.

■ Physical Examination

Gen

Patient is lying in ED bed and appears to be in moderate distress

VS

BP 128/78, P 120, RR 26, T 37°C; Wt 128 kg, Ht 5'6", O_2 sat 88% on room air

Skin

Cool to touch; no diaphoresis

HEENT

PERRLA; EOMI; dry mucous membranes; TMs intact

Neck/Lymph Nodes

(+) JVD; no lymphadenopathy; no thyromegaly; no bruits

Lungs/Thorax

Clear without wheezes, rhonchi, or rales

Breasts

Deferred

CV

Split S_2, loud P_2, S_3 gallop

Abd

Soft; (+) HJR; liver slightly enlarged; normal bowel sounds; no guarding

Genit/Rect

Deferred

MS/Ext

Full range of motion; 2+ edema to both lower extremities; no clubbing or cyanosis; pulses palpable

Neuro

A & O × 3; normal DTRs bilaterally

■ **Labs**

Na 138 mEq/L	Hgb 14 g/dL	WBC $8.8 \times 10^3/mm^3$	Mg 2.1 mg/dL
K 3.8 mEq/L	Hct 40%	Neutros 62%	Ca 8.4 mg/dL
Cl 98 mEq/L	RBC $5.1 \times 10^6/mm^3$	Bands 2%	BNP 60 pg/mL
CO_2 28 mEq/L	Plt $311 \times 10^3/mm^3$	Eos 1%	
BUN 12 mg/dL	MCV 84 μm³	Lymphs 32%	
SCr 0.9 mg/dL	MCHC 34 g/dL	Monos 3%	
Glu 88 mg/dL			

■ **ECG**

Sinus tachycardia (rate 120 bpm); right-axis deviation; ST-segment depression in right precordial leads; tall P waves in leads 2, 3, and aVF

■ **Chest X-Ray**

Cardiomegaly; prominent main pulmonary artery; no apparent pulmonary edema

■ **Two-Dimensional Echocardiography**

Right ventricular and atrial hypertrophy; tricuspid regurgitation; estimated mean pulmonary arterial pressure (mPAP) 55 mm Hg

■ **Ventilation/Perfusion Scan**

Negative for pulmonary embolism

■ **Pulmonary Function Tests**

FEV_1 = 1.87 L (61% of predicted)
FVC = 2.10 L (57% of predicted)
FEV_1/FVC = 0.89

■ **Assessment**

A 32-year-old woman presents with signs/symptoms of PAH (likely familial)

QUESTIONS

Problem Identification

1.a. What potential risk factors does this patient have for developing PAH?
1.b. What subjective and objective clinical evidence is suggestive of PAH?

Desired Outcome

2. What are the initial and long-term goals of therapy in this case?

Therapeutic Alternatives

3.a. What pharmacologic alternatives are available for the treatment of PAH? Include each medication's role in disease state management/indication, mechanism of action, dose, potential adverse effects, contraindications, significant drug interactions, and monitoring parameters.
3.b. What nonpharmacologic alternatives are available for the treatment of PAH?

■ CLINICAL COURSE (PART 1)

After admission into the ED, the patient underwent a right heart catheterization for vasoreactivity testing. The results indicated that after receiving the short-acting vasodilator epoprostenol, the patient did not have significant reductions in mPAP and therefore was deemed a nonresponder. The patient's pulmonologist wants to start the patient on bosentan and asks for your recommendation.

Optimal Plan

4.a. Design a treatment plan for the initial management of this patient's PAH with bosentan. Include patient-specific information, including dosage form, dose, and schedule. Be sure to evaluate the patient's entire medication regimen.

■ CLINICAL COURSE (PART 2)

After 3 months of bosentan therapy the patient's liver function tests (LFTs) are elevated, so the patient's pulmonologist tells the patient to stop the bosentan for 1 month. It has now been 1 month and the patient returns with normal LFTs.

4.b. Recommend an appropriate alternative agent(s), including dosage form, dose, and schedule.

Outcome Evaluation

5. How should the recommended therapy be monitored for efficacy and adverse effects?

Patient Education

6. What information should be provided to the patient to enhance adherence, ensure successful therapy, and minimize adverse effects?

■ SELF-STUDY ASSIGNMENTS

1. Perform a literature search to determine which medications used for the treatment of PAH have been shown to be safe in pregnancy. Identify the risks associated with pregnancy in female patients with PAH.

2. Use primary and tertiary literature to identify the potential visual side effects associated with oral phosphodiesterase inhibitors. Identify the visual side effect that is a medical emergency.

3. Review primary and tertiary literature to compare the advantages and disadvantages of using the vasodilators epoprostenol, treprostinil, and iloprost for PAH.

4. Use two different drug information sources to develop a recommendation for transitioning a patient from intravenous epoprostenol to subcutaneous treprostinil.

CLINICAL PEARL

Calcium channel blockers should only be used in patients with PAH who respond favorably to short-acting vasodilators during right heart catheterization.

REFERENCES

1. Taichman DB, Ornelas J, Chung L, et al. Pharmacologic therapy for pulmonary arterial hypertension in adults: CHEST guideline and expert panel report. Chest 2014 Aug;146(2):449–475.

2. Galiè N, Humbert M, Vachiery JL, et al. 2015 ESC/ERS guidelines for the diagnosis and treatment of pulmonary hypertension: The Joint Task Force for the Diagnosis and Treatment of Pulmonary Hypertension of the European Society of Cardiology (ESC) and the European Respiratory Society (ERS): Endorsed by: Association for European Paediatric and Congenital Cardiology (AEPC), International Society for Heart and Lung Transplantation (ISHLT). Eur Respir J 2015 Oct;46(4):903–975.

3. McLaughlin VV, Archer SL, Badesch DB, et al. ACCF/AHA 2009 expert consensus document on pulmonary hypertension: a report of the American College of Cardiology Foundation Task Force on Expert Consensus Documents and the American Heart Association developed in collaboration with the American College of Chest Physicians; American Thoracic Society, Inc.; and the Pulmonary Hypertension Association. J Am Coll Cardiol 2009;53(17):1573–1619.

4. Raiesdana A, Loscalzo J. Pulmonary arterial hypertension. Ann Med 2006;38:95–110.

5. McGoon MD, Kane GC. Pulmonary hypertension: diagnosis and management. Mayo Clin Proc 2009;84(2):191–207.

6. Sitbon O, Humbert M, Jaïs X, et al. Long-term response to calcium channel blockers in idiopathic pulmonary arterial hypertension. Circulation 2005;111(23):3105–3111.

7. Bishop BM, Mauro VF, Khouri SJ. Practical considerations for the pharmacotherapy of pulmonary arterial hypertension. Pharmacotherapy 2012;32(9):838–855.

8. Archer SL, Michelakis ED. Phosphodiesterase type 5 inhibitors for pulmonary hypertension. N Engl J Med 2009;361:1864–1871.

9. McLaughlin VV, McGoon M. Pulmonary arterial hypertension. Circulation 2006;114:1417–1431.

33

CYSTIC FIBROSIS

Blood, Sweat, Lungs, and Gut . . . . Level II

Kimberly J. Novak, PharmD, BCPS, BCPPS

LEARNING OBJECTIVES

After completing this case study, the reader should be able to:

• Identify signs and symptoms of common problems in patients with cystic fibrosis (CF).

• Develop an antimicrobial therapy plan and appropriate monitoring strategy for treatment of an acute pulmonary exacerbation in CF.

• Devise treatment strategies for common complications of drug therapy in patients with CF.

• Provide education on aerosolized medications to patients with CF, including appropriate instructions for dornase alfa and inhaled tobramycin.

PATIENT PRESENTATION

■ Chief Complaint

As reported by patient's father: "My daughter's experiencing shortness of breath, fast breathing, increasing cough and sputum production, and decreased energy, and she has a poor appetite."

■ HPI

Jenna O'Mally is a 7-year-old girl with a lifetime history of CF; she was diagnosed with CF at birth after presenting with meconium ileus. She had been doing well until 4 weeks ago, when she developed cold-like symptoms, with a runny nose, dry cough, sore throat, and subjective fever. She was seen at her local pediatrician's office and prescribed a 5-day course of azithromycin suspension 200 mg/5 mL, 160 mg (10 mg/kg) PO on Day 1 and 80 mg (5 mg/kg) PO daily on Days 2–5 for possible pneumonia. After completing the antibiotic course, Jenna was not feeling any better. Father called the pulmonary clinic regarding her symptoms, and Jenna's pulmonologist called in a prescription to a local pharmacy for ciprofloxacin suspension 250 mg/5 mL, 325 mg PO BID (~40 mg/kg per day), and prednisolone syrup 15 mg/5 mL, one teaspoonful PO twice daily. Father was also instructed to perform three chest physiotherapy sessions (vest treatments) per day and increase her hypertonic saline schedule from once per day to twice daily with her vest treatments. The patient now presents to the pulmonary clinic for a follow-up to her outpatient treatment course. She describes worsening shortness of breath and chest pain, lung and sinus congestion, poor appetite, and severe fatigue. Father reports increasing cough productive of very dark green sputum but no fever. The patient has lost 2 lb since her last clinic visit and has missed 7 days of school. Her oxygen saturation is 88% in clinic on room air, and she was immediately placed on 1 L of O$_2$ by nasal cannula.

■ PMH

CF (Phe508del/G551D)

Significant for seven hospitalizations for acute pulmonary exacerbations of CF and two hospitalizations for distal intestinal obstruction syndrome (DIOS) since her initial NICU stay at birth; last hospitalization was 4 months ago

Sinus surgery × 2, last 1 year ago

Pancreatic insufficiency

Poor nutritional status

Recurrent constipation/DIOS

Pulmonary changes c/w long-standing CF with mild bronchiectasis

Seasonal allergies

Asthma

Broken clavicle previous summer after falling from a tree

ADHD

■ FH

Both parents are alive and generally well (father has hypercholesterolemia). Jenna has an older half-brother (age 15) without CF who had a recent bout of gastroenteritis and a younger sister (age 2) with CF who was recently diagnosed with RSV bronchiolitis. Two maternal uncles died at ages 13 and 17 from CF.

■ SH

Jenna is in first grade and is enrolled in the gifted program at her school. Family is considering home schooling due to frequent absences in the past school year. Lives with her mother, father, and younger sister approximately 100 miles from the nearest CF center. Her older half-brother visits every other weekend. They have well water and a small mixed-breed family dog; father smokes but only outside of the home. Family is experiencing financial difficulties due to a job layoff and recently lost health insurance. Family is in the process of applying for state Medicaid assistance.

■ Meds

Ciprofloxacin suspension 250 mg/5 mL, 325 mg PO BID

Prednisolone syrup 15 mg/5 mL, one teaspoonful PO BID

Aerosolized tobramycin 300 mg BID via nebulizer (every other month, currently "on")

Albuterol 0.083% 3 mL (one vial) BID via nebulizer with vest therapy (currently using TID)

Dornase alfa (Pulmozyme) 2.5 mg via nebulizer once daily with morning vest therapy

Sodium chloride 7% aerosol (Hyper-Sal) 4 mL via nebulizer once daily with evening vest therapy (currently using BID)

Fluticasone propionate (Flovent HFA) 44 mcg, one puff once daily

Budesonide (Rhinocort AQ) one spray each nostril once daily

Saline nasal rinse (neti pot) daily

Loratadine 5 mg PO once daily

Creon 12,000 two caps with meals (1500 units of lipase/kg/meal) and one cap with snacks and supplement shakes (750 units of lipase/kg/snack)

Omeprazole 20 mg PO once daily

Ferrous sulfate 324 mg PO BID

AquADEKs one chewable tablet PO once daily

Children's multivitamin with iron one chewable tablet PO once daily

Polyethylene glycol 17 g PO once daily

Atomoxetine 25 mg PO once daily

Ibuprofen 200 mg PO three to four times daily as needed for chest pain

Pediasure two cans per day

■ All

Codeine (itching), bacitracin cream (rash), strawberries (anaphylaxis)

■ ROS

Patient complains of chest pain when coughing and large amounts of expectorated green sputum. Reduced ability to perform usual daily activities and play because of SOB. No current hemoptysis, constipation, vomiting, or abdominal pain. Reports having three to four loose or partially formed stools each day. Patient usually has a large appetite but has not been able to finish a meal for the past week.

■ Physical Examination

Gen

A shy, thin, cooperative, 7-year-old girl who has shortness of breath with her oxygen cannula removed during the examination

VS

BP 100/65, P 144, RR 45, T 37.8°C; Wt 16 kg, Ht 3′10″; oxygen saturation 95% on 1 L of oxygen; 88% on room air

Skin

Normal tone and color, some eczematous lesions at the elbows

HEENT

EOMI, PERRLA; nares with dried mucus in both nostrils; sinuses tender to palpation; no oral lesions, but secretions noted in the posterior pharynx

Neck/Lymph Nodes

Supple; no lymphadenopathy or thyromegaly

Lungs

Crackles heard bilaterally in the upper lobes greater than in the lower lobes; mild scattered wheezes; chest pain not reproducible with palpation

Breasts

Tanner Stage I

CV

Tachycardic, regular rate without murmurs

Abd

Ticklish during examination; (+) bowel sounds; abdomen soft and supple; mild bloating noted, with palpable stool

Genit/Rect

Tanner Stage I, deferred internal exam

MS/Ext

Clubbing noted, with no cyanosis; capillary refill <2 seconds

Neuro

Jenna is alert and awake though reserved; CNs intact; somewhat uncooperative with the full neurologic examination

■ Labs

Na 149 mEq/L	Hgb 15.4 g/dL	WBC 16.5 × 10³/mm³	AST 30 IU/L
K 4.5 mEq/L	Hct 45.2%	Segs 72%	ALT 20 IU/L
Cl 108 mEq/L	MCV 78 μm³	Bands 10%	LDH 330 IU/L
CO₂ 34 mEq/L	MCH 31.1 pg	Lymphs 10%	GGT 75 IU/L
BUN 18 mg/dL	MCHC 34 g/dL	Monos 2%	T. Prot 7.3 g/dL
SCr 0.45 mg/dL	Ca, 4.6 mEq/Lᵃ	Eos 6%	Alb 3.1 g/dL
Glu 195 mg/dL	Phos 4.6 mEq/L	Mg 2.1 mg/dL	IgE 85 IU/mL

ᵃCaᵢ, ionized calcium.

■ Virology/Serology Results

Respiratory viral antigen panel: negative
Influenza A/B PCRs: negative
B. pertussis PCR: negative

■ Sputum Culture Results

Organism A: *Pseudomonas aeruginosa*
  Sensitive: piperacillin/tazobactam, cefepime, ceftazidime, meropenem, aztreonam, tobramycin, amikacin
  Intermediate: ciprofloxacin, levofloxacin
  Resistant: gentamicin

Organism B: *Stenotrophomonas maltophilia*
  Sensitive: trimethoprim–sulfamethoxazole, minocycline, moxifloxacin
  Resistant: ceftazidime, meropenem, levofloxacin, all aminoglycosides

Organism C: *P. aeruginosa*, mucoid strain
  Sensitive: piperacillin/tazobactam, cefepime, ceftazidime, meropenem, aztreonam, tobramycin
  Resistant: ciprofloxacin, levofloxacin, gentamicin, amikacin

Organism D: *Staphylococcus aureus*
  Sensitive: vancomycin, linezolid, trimethoprim–sulfamethoxazole, minocycline
  Resistant: nafcillin, cefazolin, clindamycin, erythromycin

Organism E: *Achromobacter xylosoxidans*
  Sensitive: piperacillin/tazobactam, ceftazidime, trimethoprim–sulfamethoxazole, minocycline
  Resistant: meropenem, cefepime, ciprofloxacin, all aminoglycosides

■ PFTs

FEV₁ 65% of predicted (baseline 90%); FVC 82% of predicted (baseline 95%)

■ Chest X-Ray

Bronchiectatic and interstitial fibrotic changes consistent with CF

■ High-Resolution Chest CT (HRCT)

Interval worsening of bronchiectasis in all lobes; increased mucus plugging in left lower lobe

■ Sinus CT

Panopacification of ethmoid and maxillary sinuses, possible polyp extending into right nasal passage

■ Assessment

A 7-year-old CF patient with failed outpatient management of acute pulmonary exacerbation and sinusitis, also with nutritional failure

QUESTIONS

Problem Identification

1.a. Identify this patient's drug-related problems. Include those relating to both her acute medical issue and her chronic CF management.

1.b. What information indicates the disease severity and the need to treat Jenna's acute pulmonary exacerbation pharmacologically?

1.c. Could any of her problems be caused by drug therapy?

Desired Outcome

2. What are the goals of pharmacotherapy in this case?

Therapeutic Alternatives

3.a. What nonpharmacologic therapies might be useful for this patient?

3.b. What pharmacotherapeutic alternatives are available for treatment of this patient's acute pulmonary exacerbation and chronic CF management?

3.c. What economic and psychosocial considerations are important in this patient's acute and chronic CF management?

Optimal Plan

4.a. What drugs, dosage forms, doses, schedules, and durations of therapy are best for this patient?

4.b. During the clinical course, serum tobramycin concentrations were drawn around the second dose of tobramycin, 160 mg (10 mg/kg/dose) IV Q 24 H. Levels are reported as follows:

• Random level: 7.4 mcg/mL collected 4 hours after the end of the 30-minute infusion

• Random level: 1.4 mcg/mL collected 10 hours after end of the 30-minute infusion

Based on this new information, evaluate her drug therapy. Calculate the maximum concentration at the end of infusion (C_{max}), true trough, AUC, elimination rate, half-life, volume of distribution, and clearance (standardized for BSA) of her tobramycin therapy. If necessary, suggest modifications. Assume that the previous doses were administered on time.

4.c. What pharmacologic therapies should be considered for Jenna's chronic CF management?

Outcome Evaluation

5. What clinical and laboratory parameters are necessary to evaluate the efficacy and safety of therapy for CF exacerbations?

Patient Education

6. What information should you provide the patient regarding the administration of aerosolized drug therapy? The patient will be going home on aerosolized dornase alfa, hypertonic saline, tobramycin, and albuterol.

7. Where can you obtain information about the patient assistance programs that are available for children, adolescents, and adults with CF on a national and state/local level?

■ SELF-STUDY ASSIGNMENTS

1. Investigate aztreonam lysine for inhalation (Cayston) and the unique drug delivery device required for administration (Altera Nebulizer System). How are these products prescribed and dispensed to patients?

2. Analyze the role of azithromycin in the chronic medical management of CF. What is/are the proposed mechanism(s) of action of azithromycin in CF management?

3. Review the recommendations for the administration of high-dose ibuprofen in patients with CF. When would you suggest that serum concentrations be drawn, and what levels are thought to be necessary to optimize therapy in a patient with CF?

4. Review the recommendations for use of fluoroquinolones in children. What data support these recommendations?

5. Investigate the new drug lumacaftor–ivacaftor (Orkambi) and its role in chronic CF management. What other research is being conducted in the new drug class of CFTR potentiators and modulators?

CLINICAL PEARL

Chronic gastric acid suppression (proton pump inhibitor or histamine-2 receptor antagonist) is often used in CF patients to improve efficacy of pancreatic enzyme replacement therapy regardless of the presence of gastroesophageal reflux symptoms. Due to defective bicarbonate transport in the small intestine and subnormal pH, enteric coating may not dissolve consistently in CF patients. Suppression of gastric acid can subsequently raise small intestine pH through mixing of gastrointestinal fluids.

REFERENCES

1. Solomon M, Bozic M, Mascarenhas M. Nutritional issues in cystic fibrosis. Clin Chest Med 2016;37:97–107.

2. Mogayzel PJ, Naureckas ET, Robinson KA, et al. Cystic fibrosis pulmonary guidelines. Chronic medications for maintenance of lung health. Am J Respir Crit Care Med 2013;187(7):680–689.

3. Patel K, Goldman JL. Safety concerns surrounding quinolone use in children. J Clin Pharmacol 2016 Feb 10 [Epublished ahead of print].

4. McCoy KS, Quittner AL, Oermann CM, Gibson RL, Retsch-Bogart GZ, Montgomery AB. Inhaled aztreonam lysine for chronic airway *Pseudomonas aeruginosa* in cystic fibrosis. Am J Respir Crit Care Med 2008:178(9):921–928.

5. Stevens DA, Moss RB, Kurup VP, et al. Allergic bronchopulmonary aspergillosis in cystic fibrosis—state of the art: cystic fibrosis foundation consensus conference. Clin Infect Dis 2003;37(Suppl 3): S225–S264.

34

GASTROESOPHAGEAL REFLUX DISEASE

A Burning Question . . . . Level II

Brian A. Hemstreet, PharmD, FCCP, BCPS

LEARNING OBJECTIVES

After completing this case study, the reader should be able to:

- Describe the clinical presentation of gastroesophageal reflux disease (GERD), including typical, atypical, and alarm symptoms.

- Discuss appropriate diagnostic approaches for GERD, including when patients should be referred for further diagnostic evaluation.

- Recommend appropriate nonpharmacologic and pharmacologic measures for treating GERD.

- Develop a treatment plan for a patient with GERD, including both nonpharmacologic and pharmacologic measures and monitoring for efficacy and toxicity of selected drug regimens.

- Outline a patient education plan for proper use of drug therapy for GERD.

PATIENT PRESENTATION

■ Chief Complaint

"I'm having a lot of heartburn. These pills I have been using have helped a little but it's still keeping me up at night."

■ HPI

Janet Swigel is a 68-year-old woman who presents to the GI clinic with complaints of heartburn four to five times a week over the past 5 months. She also reports some regurgitation after meals that is often accompanied by an acidic taste in her mouth. She states that her symptoms are worse at night, particularly when she goes to bed. She finds that her heartburn worsens and she coughs a lot at night, which keeps her awake. She has had difficulty sleeping over this time period and feels fatigued during the day. She reports no difficulty swallowing food or liquids. She has tried OTC Prevacid 24HR once daily for the past 3 weeks. This has reduced the frequency of her symptoms to 3–4 days per week, but they are still bothering her.

■ PMH

Atrial fibrillation × 12 years
Asthma × 10 years

Type 2 DM × 5 years
HTN × 10 years

■ SH

Patient is married with three children. She is a retired school bus driver. She drinks one to two glasses of wine 4–5 days per week. She does not use tobacco. She has commercial prescription drug insurance.

■ FH

Father died of pneumonia at age 75; mother died at age 68 of gastric cancer

■ MEDS

Diltiazem CD 120 mg PO once daily
Hydrochlorothiazide 25 mg PO once daily
Metformin 500 mg PO twice daily
Aspirin 81 mg PO daily
Fluticasone/salmeterol DPI 100 mcg/50 mcg one inhalation twice daily

■ All

Peanuts (hives)

■ ROS

Reports being tired all the time, (–) SOB or hoarseness; (+) cough at night, (+) frequent episodes of heartburn, sometimes after meals, but is worse at night; (–) N/V; (–) BRBPR or dark/tarry stools; (–) dysuria, nocturia, or frequency

■ Physical Examination

Gen

Well-developed African-American woman in NAD

VS

BP 142/85, P 90, RR 17, T 36°C; Wt 100 kg, Ht 5′7″

Skin

No lesions or rashes

HEENT

PERRLA; EOMI; moist mucous membranes; intact dentition; oropharynx clear

Neck/Lymph Nodes

Trachea midline; (–) thyromegaly; (–) lymphadenopathy; (–) JVD

Lungs/Thorax

Mostly CTA bilaterally, some intermittent wheezes

CV

Tachycardia with irregularly irregular rhythm; no MRG

Abd

Obese; NT/ND; (+) BS; (–) HSM

Genit/Rect

Gyn exam deferred; heme (–) brown stool

MS/Ext

No CVA tenderness

Neuro

A & O × 3, CN II–XII intact, 5/5 upper- and lower-extremity strength bilaterally

■ Labs

Na 138 mEq/L	Hgb 13 g/dL	WBC 8.7 × 10^3/mm³	AST 21 IU/L
K 3.8 mEq/L	Hct 39%		ALT 24 IU/L
Cl 108 mEq/L	RBC 4.6 × 10^6/mm³	Neutros 60%	Alk Phos 55 IU/L
CO_2 21 mEq/L	Plt 400 × 10^3/mm³	Bands 1%	*Fasting lipid panel:*
BUN 18 mg/dL		Eos 2%	TC 230 mg/dL
SCr 1.3 mg/dL		Lymphs 32%	LDL 130 mg/dL
Fasting Glu		Monos 5%	TG 170 mg/dL
220 mg/dL		A1C 9.0%	HDL 42 mg/dL
Ca 8.9 mg/dL			
Phos 4.1 mg/dL			

■ EGD

Grade B esophagitis; normal gastric and duodenal mucosa; small hiatal hernia. Biopsy results of esophagus and stomach are negative for atypical cells and *H. pylori*.

■ Assessment

A 68-year-old woman presenting with uncontrolled GERD symptoms despite self-treatment with OTC PPI therapy. EGD shows erosive esophagitis and a hiatal hernia.

QUESTIONS

Problem Identification

1.a. Develop a list of this patient's drug therapy problems.

1.b. Classify the GERD symptoms this patient is experiencing. Are they typical or atypical in nature? Are any alarm symptoms or features present?

1.c. What factors could be contributing to the development of GERD symptoms in this patient?

1.d. If you saw this patient in the community pharmacy setting, what factors would cause you to refer her for further diagnostic evaluation versus recommending empiric drug therapy?

1.e. What are other potential complications of long-standing untreated GERD?

Desired Outcome

2. Develop a list of pharmacotherapeutic goals for this patient.

Therapeutic Alternatives

3.a. What lifestyle modifications or nonpharmacologic therapies may improve this patient's GERD symptoms?

3.b. What drug therapies could be used to treat this patient's GERD symptoms?

Optimal Plan

4. Develop a complete treatment plan for managing this patient's GERD symptoms.

Outcome Evaluation

5. What parameters should be monitored to assess both the efficacy and toxicity of your selected drug regimen?

Patient Education

6. How will you educate the patient about her GERD therapy to enhance compliance, minimize adverse effects, and promote successful therapeutic outcomes?

■ CLINICAL COURSE

Four weeks later, Mrs Swigel returns to the clinic for follow-up. Her symptoms have greatly improved, but she is considering stopping therapy because she heard that "all sorts of bad side effects" can happen to her. She saw on television that she could get osteoporosis and that she should be taking calcium. Someone told her that she may also develop some "nasty infections." She does not think it is worth staying on the medication. She also states that she sometimes has brief episodes of heartburn after meals and wishes to know if she should take more of her medication to manage these symptoms.

■ FOLLOW-UP QUESTIONS

1. Should the patient be placed on calcium and vitamin D supplementation because of her acid-suppressive therapy?

2. How would you address her concerns regarding the potential for developing infections due to acid-suppressive therapy?

3. What recommendations could you give her regarding management of the breakthrough symptoms after meals?

■ SELF-STUDY ASSIGNMENTS

1. Surgical intervention is a well-accepted option for treating GERD in certain patients. Conduct a primary literature search and identify two articles that compare surgery with drug therapy for treatment of GERD. What conclusions can you draw from the results of these articles? When is surgery indicated in patients with GERD?

2. Pharmacy practice involves providing care to diverse patient populations. Identify and review tertiary drug references and internet websites that provide educational materials about GERD or its treatment in languages other than English.

CLINICAL PEARL

PPIs may cause false-negative results in patients undergoing urease-based *H. pylori* testing, such as with the urea breath test or rapid urease test, or stool antigen tests. Ideally, these drugs should be discontinued 2 weeks before performing these diagnostic tests.

REFERENCES

1. American Gastroenterological Association Institute. Guideline for the diagnosis and management and diagnosis of gastroesophageal reflux disease. Gastroenterology 2013;108:308–328.

2. American Gastroenterological Association Institute. Technical review on the management of gastroesophageal reflux disease. Gastroenterology 2008;135:1392–1413.

3. Haag S, Andrews JM, Katelaris PH, et al. Management of reflux symptoms with over-the-counter proton pump inhibitors: issues and proposed guidelines. Digestion 2009;80:226–234.

4. Chey WD, Wong BC. Practice Parameters Committee of the American College of Gastroenterology. American College of Gastroenterology guideline on the management of *Helicobacter pylori* infection. Am J Gastroenterol 2007;102:1808–1825.

5. Solomon M, Reynolds JC. Esophageal reflux disease and its complications. In: Pitchumoni CS, Dharmarajan TS, eds. Geriatric Gastroenterology. New York, NY: Springer Science; 2012:311–319.

6. Becher A, El-Serag HB. Mortality associated with gastroesophageal reflux disease and its non-malignant complications: a systematic review. Scand J Gastroenterol 2008;43:645–653.

7. Badillo R, Francis D. Diagnosis and treatment of gastroesophageal reflux disease. World J Gastrointest Pharmacol Ther 2014;5:105–112.

8. Brendenoord AJ, Pandolfino JE, Smout AJP. Gastroespohageal reflux disease. Lancet 2013;381:1933–1942.

9. Hershcovici T, Fass R. Pharmacological management of GERD: where does it stand now? Trends Pharmacol Sci 2011;32:258–264.

10. Chubineh S, Birk J. Proton pump inhibitors: the good, the bad, and the unwanted. South Med J 2012;105:613–618.

35

PEPTIC ULCER DISEASE

Feel the Burn . . . . Level II

Ashley H. Vincent, PharmD, BCACP, BCPS

LEARNING OBJECTIVES

After completing this case study, the reader should be able to:

- List the options for the evaluation and treatment of a patient with symptoms suggestive of peptic ulcer disease (PUD).
- Identify the desired therapeutic outcomes for patients with PUD.
- Identify the factors that guide selection of a *Helicobacter pylori* eradication regimen and improve adherence with the regimen.
- Compare the efficacy of three- and four-drug *H. pylori* treatment regimens and regimens lasting 7, 10 and 14 days or provided in sequential order.
- Create a treatment and monitoring plan for a patient diagnosed with PUD, given patient-specific information.

PATIENT PRESENTATION

Chief Complaint

"My stomach has been hurting really badly for the past month or so. It seems to get worse at night."

HPI

Justine Ward is a 67-year-old woman who presents to her primary care physician with complaints of episodic epigastric pain for the past 6 weeks. Her pain is nonradiating. It is sometimes worse with meals, but sometimes eating helps improve the pain. She has been experiencing occasional nausea, bloating, and heartburn. She denies

any change in color or frequency of bowel movements. She does not have a history of PUD or GI bleeding. She mentions that she has been having frequent headaches for the past month and has been taking naproxen sodium one to two times daily.

PMH

CAD with drug-eluting stent placement × 3 months
Hypothyroidism × 22 years
Hyperlipidemia × 10 years
Lactose intolerance × 47 years
Postmenopausal; LMP ~13 years ago

FH

Her mother died at the age of 75 from lymphoma. Her father is alive and has a history of glaucoma, prostate cancer, and AMI at age 70. She has five siblings who are alive. All siblings have a history of hypertension and hyperlipidemia.

SH

She is married and has raised three children; she is not employed outside the home. She has never smoked and drinks one to two glasses of wine most days of the week.

Meds

Plavix 75 mg PO daily
Lisinopril 5 mg PO daily
Metoprolol tartrate 25 mg PO twice daily
Aspirin 325 mg PO daily
Synthroid 125 mcg PO daily
Atorvastatin 80 mg PO daily
MVI tablet PO daily
Tums 500 mg PO PRN stomach pain
Naproxen sodium 220 mg PO PRN headache (one to two times daily for the past month)
Lactaid one tablet PO PRN dairy product consumption

All

NKDA

ROS

Unremarkable except for complaints noted above

Physical Examination

Gen

Slightly overweight woman in moderate distress

VS

BP 110/72 left arm (seated), P 99, RR 16 reg, T 37.2°C; Wt 68 kg, Ht 5′3″

Skin

Warm and dry

HEENT

Normocephalic; PERRLA; EOMI

Chest

CTA

CV

RRR; S_1 and S_2 normal; no MRG

Abd

Soft; mild epigastric tenderness; (+) BS; no splenomegaly or masses; liver size normal

Rect

Nontender; stool heme (+)

Ext

Normal ROM; no cyanosis, clubbing, or edema

Neuro

CN II–XII intact; A & O × 3

■ Labs

Na 142 mEq/L	Hgb 10.1 g/dL	Ca 9.5 mg/dL
K 4.7 mEq/L	Hct 30%	Mg 2.2 mEq/L
Cl 98 mEq/L	Plt 320 × 10³/mm³	Phos 3.8 mg/dL
CO_2 30 mEq/L	WBC 7.6 × 10³/mm³	Albumin 5.0 g/dL
BUN 8 mg/dL	MCV 72 μm³	TSH 2.4 μU/mL
SCr 0.7 mg/dL	Retic 0.4%	TC 142 mg/dL
FBG 92 mg/dL	Fe 48 mcg/dL	LDL 64 mg/dL
		HDL 53 mg/dL
		TG 127 mg/dL

■ Assessment

Suspected PUD

QUESTIONS

Problem Identification

1.a. Identify this patient's drug therapy problems.

1.b. What information (signs, symptoms, diagnostic tests, and laboratory values) indicates the presence of PUD?

■ CLINICAL COURSE (PART 1)

Justine's PCP referred her for a nonemergent EGD, which revealed a 5.5-mm superficial ulcer in the superior duodenum. The ulcer base was clear and without evidence of active bleeding (see Fig. 35-1).

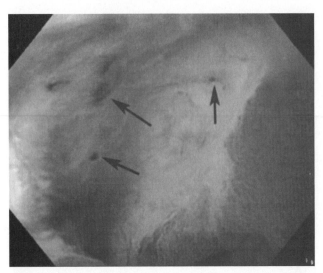

FIGURE 35-1: Endoscopy depicting duodenal ulcer with pigmented spots as noted by arrows. *(Reprinted with permission from Kasper DL, Fauci AS, Hauser SL, et al, eds. Harrison's Principles of Internal Medicine, 19th ed. New York, McGraw-Hill Education, 2015.)*

In addition, inflammation of the duodenum was detected and biopsied.

Desired Outcome

2. What are your treatment goals for treating this patient's PUD?

Therapeutic Alternatives

3.a. Considering the patient's presentation, what nonpharmacologic alternatives are available to treat her PUD?

3.b. In the absence of information about the presence of *H. pylori*, what pharmacologic alternatives are available to treat duodenal ulcers?

Optimal Plan

4. Based on the patient's presentation and the current medical assessment, design a pharmacotherapeutic regimen to treat her duodenal ulcer, anemia, and frequent headaches.

Outcome Evaluation

5. What clinical and laboratory parameters are necessary to evaluate therapy for achievement of the desired therapeutic outcomes and to detect or prevent adverse effects?

Patient Education

6. What information should be provided to the patient to ensure successful therapy, enhance compliance, and minimize adverse effects?

■ CLINICAL COURSE (PART 2)

At the time of the EGD, a biopsy of the duodenal mucosa was taken and indicated the presence of inflammation and abundant *H. pylori*–like organisms.

■ FOLLOW-UP QUESTIONS

1. What is the significance of finding *H. pylori* in the duodenal biopsy?

2. Based on this new information, how would you modify your goals for treating this patient's PUD?

3. What pharmacotherapeutic alternatives are available to achieve the new goals?

4. Design a pharmacotherapeutic regimen for this patient's ulcer that will accomplish the new treatment goals.

5. How should the PUD therapy you recommended be monitored for efficacy and adverse effects?

6. What information should be provided to the patient about her therapy?

7. How should her frequent headaches now be treated?

■ SELF-STUDY ASSIGNMENTS

1. Describe the advantages and limitations of both endoscopic and nonendoscopic diagnostic tests to detect *H. pylori*.

2. After performing a literature search on *H. pylori* eradication therapy, compare the efficacy of three- and four-drug regimens.

3. Based on the literature search on *H. pylori* eradication therapy, determine whether therapy should be continued for 7–14 days or provided in a sequential order.

4. Describe the role of pharmacists and nurse practitioners in treating patients with PUD.

REFERENCES

1. Gilard M, Arnaud B, Cornily JC, et al. Influence of omeprazole on the antiplatelet action of clopidogrel associated with aspirin: the randomized, double-blind OCLA (Omeprazole CLopidogrel Aspirin) study. J Am Coll Cardiol 2008;51:256–260.
2. Sibbing D, Morath T, Stegherr J, et al. Impact of proton pump inhibitors on the antiplatelet effects of clopidogrel. Thromb Haemost 2009;101:714–719.
3. Frelinger AL, Lee RD, Mulford DJ, et al. A randomized, 2-period, crossover design study to assess the effects of dexlansoprazole, lansoprazole, esomeprazole and omeprazole on the steady-state pharmacokinetics and pharmacodynamics of clopidogrel in healthy volunteers. J Am Coll Cardiol 2012;59:1304–1311.
4. Melloni C, Washam JB, Jones WS, et al. Conflicting results between randomized trials and observational studies on the impact of proton pump inhibitors on cardiovascular events when coadministered with dual antiplatelet therapy. Circ Cardiovasc Qual Outcomes 2015;8:47–55.
5. Bhatt DL, Cryer BL, Contant CF, et al. Clopidogrel with or without omeprazole in coronary artery disease. N Engl J Med 2010;363:1909–1917.
6. Drepper MD, Spahr L, Frossard JL. Clopidogrel and proton pump inhibitors—where do we stand in 2012? World J Gastroenterol 2012;18:2161–2171.
7. McColl KEL. *Helicobacter pylori* infection. N Engl J Med 2010;362:1597–1604.
8. Chey WD, Wong BCY; Practice Parameters Committee of the American College of Gastroenterology. American College of Gastroenterology guideline on the management of *Helicobacter pylori* infection. Am J Gastroenterol 2007;102:1808–1825.
9. Yang JC, Lu CW, Lin CJ. Treatment of *Helicobacter pylori* infection: current status and future concepts. World J Gastroenterol 2014;20:5283–5293.
10. Lanza FL, Chan FKL, Quigley EMM, et al. Guidelines for the prevention of NSAID-related ulcer complications. Am J Gastroenterol 2009;104:728–238.

36

NSAID-INDUCED ULCER DISEASE

To Protect and Serve. . . . . Level II

Carmen B. Smith, PharmD, BCPS

Jay L. Martello, PharmD, BCPS

LEARNING OBJECTIVES

After completing this case study, the reader should be able to:

- Determine whether patients with diabetes who have risk factors for NSAID-induced ulcer disease should remain on aspirin and at what dose.
- Identify the hallmark signs and symptoms of NSAID-induced PUD.
- Recommend appropriate therapy for the treatment of NSAID-induced PUD while taking into account *Helicobacter pylori* infection and its appropriate diagnosis and follow-up.
- Recommend alternative therapies besides traditional NSAIDs for treatment of pain and inflammation in patients with PUD.
- Educate patients effectively on treatment options for NSAID-induced PUD.

PATIENT PRESENTATION

Chief Complaint

"I have had some stomach pain in the last 2 weeks and am worried that my ulcers have come back."

HPI

Tom Jackson is a 55-year-old man who presents to his PCP with complaints of epigastric pain for 2 weeks. He stated that he started taking OTC Zantac for the pain with partial relief, but the symptoms persisted. They are consistent with those he experienced 3 months ago when he was diagnosed empirically with bleeding gastric ulcers. When questioned, he cannot recall what diagnostic tests were done, but he does recall having a prescription for several medications that he did not finish because he felt better after about a week and the medications gave him an odd taste in his mouth. He also says that acetaminophen has failed to provide much symptom relief from his osteoarthritis, so he currently uses a variety of OTC NSAID products. Additional review of his pharmacy records shows that he was prescribed a 14-day course of amoxicillin, clarithromycin, and omeprazole 3 months ago.

PMH

H/O PUD with *H. pylori*
GERD
OA primarily in right wrist and hand but also left hip
HTN
Type 2 DM
S/P appendectomy after appendicitis in the 1980s

FH

Father died of MI at age 45; mother died of cervical CA in her eighties

SH

Police officer; smokes one to two packs per week down from two packs per day 6 years ago; drinks one alcoholic drink per day but admits to occasionally having more; plays basketball one to two nights per week as he can tolerate with OA symptoms.

Meds

ASA 325 mg PO once daily
Lisinopril 20 mg PO once daily
Amlodipine 10 mg PO once daily
Metformin 1000 mg PO twice daily
Atorvastatin 40 mg PO nightly
OTC naproxen 200 mg, two tablets PO one to four times daily for OA pain
OTC ranitidine 75 mg, one tablet two to three times daily for stomach pain

All

Codeine (rash); tetracycline (rash/hives)

ROS

Denies headache or chest pain. Occasional SOB. No heartburn, weakness, polyphagia, polydipsia, or polyuria. Gait slow but steady. Complains of some chronic pain in left hip, which he has been told is from OA.

Physical Examination

Gen

The patient is a pleasant man in mild distress

VS

BP 130/60, P 80, RR 12, T 36.3°C; Wt 74.1 kg, Ht 5′8″

HEENT

PERRLA; funduscopic exam without hemorrhages, exudates, or papilledema; mild cataracts bilaterally

Neck/Lymph Nodes

Supple; no JVD or thyromegaly; no carotid bruits

Lungs

CTA

Cor

RRR, normal S_1, S_2.

Abd

Normal BS, moderate epigastric pain on palpation

Genit/Rect

Fecal occult blood test positive × 3

MS/Ext

No skin breakdown or ulcers; mild weakness of RUE; mild deformity of right first finger at MCP joint and swelling of DIP joints on first and second fingers

Neuro

A&O × 3; CN II–XII intact; negative Babinski. Normal sensation in hands bilaterally, decreased pain and vibratory sensation in right foot, normal in left

Labs

Na 141 mEq/L	Hgb 8.9 g/dL	*Fasting lipid profile:*
K 4.6 mEq/L	Hct 27%	T. Chol 171 mg/dL
Cl 107 mEq/L	Plt 390 × 10³/mm³	LDL-C 95 mg/dL
CO_2 27 mEq/L	WBC 7.0 × 10³/mm³	HDL-C 42 mg/dL
BUN 21 mEq/L	Retic 1.8%	TG 170 mg/dL
SCr 1.3 mg/dL	A1C 6.9%	TSH 2.93 μIU/mL
Glu 119 mg/dL		

H. pylori Testing

Rapid urease test of gastric biopsy negative but serology positive. Urea breath test not performed

EGD

Two small gastric ulcers approximately 6 mm in diameter, trace blood seen but no obvious active bleeding

QUESTIONS

Problem Identification

1.a. Create a list of the patient's drug therapy problems.

1.b. What signs, symptoms, and laboratory values indicate the presence of PUD in this patient?

1.c. What other diagnostic tests could be ordered to assess the patient's current *H. pylori* status?

1.d. What are the strengths and weaknesses of the different methods available for *H. pylori* diagnosis?

Desired Outcome

2. What are the goals of pharmacotherapy in this case?

Therapeutic Alternatives

3.a. What pharmacologic alternatives are available for treating the gastric ulcers in this patient?

3.b. What feasible pharmacotherapeutic options are available for preventing future gastric ulcers in this patient?

3.c. Should this patient remain on aspirin with his documented recurrent gastric ulcers?

Optimal Plan

4.a. What is the optimal pharmacotherapeutic regimen for treating this patient's gastric ulcers?

4.b. What pharmacotherapeutic regimen is best for treating this patient's osteoarthritis?

4.c. Is this patient a candidate for prophylaxis of future NSAID-induced ulcers? If so, what drug and regimen would you recommend?

Outcome Evaluation

5. What measures would you implement for monitoring the efficacy and toxicity of the treatment regimen for gastric ulcers in this patient?

Patient Education

6. What information should be shared with this patient about management of his gastric ulcers to enhance adherence, ensure successful therapy, and minimize adverse effects?

■ SELF-STUDY ASSIGNMENTS

1. Perform a literature search and assess current information on the efficacy of various agents for secondary prevention of NSAID-induced ulcers. Review expert opinion on the data specific to prevention of aspirin-induced PUD in the ACCF/ACG/AHA 2008 consensus document on antiplatelet therapy and PUD.

2. Review the Antithrombotic Trialists' (ATT) Collaboration study examining the cardiac benefits of low-dose aspirin and describe the risk of gastric bleeding in patients with and without coronary disease.

3. Perform a literature search and assess the cost-effectiveness of *H. pylori* screening in patients on chronic NSAID therapy.

CLINICAL PEARL

Documented or undocumented use of NSAIDs plays a role in 60% of peptic ulcers that occur in patients who are *H. pylori* negative.

Risk factors for developing NSAID-induced ulcer disease include: (1) prior history of PUD; (2) age >65 years; (3) high dose NSAID therapy; and (4) concomitant use of anticoagulants, antiplatelet agents, and/or corticosteroids.

REFERENCES

1. Chey WD, Wong BCY. Committee of the American College of Gastroenterology. American College of Gastroenterology guideline on the management of *Helicobacter pylori infection.* Am J Gastroenterol 2007;102:1808–1825.
2. Lanza FL, Chan FKL, Quigley EMM. Prevention of NSAID-related ulcer complications. Am J Gastroenterol 2009;104:728–738.
3. Laine L, Jensen DM. Management of patients with ulcer bleeding. Am J Gastroenterol 2012;107:345–360.
4. Singh G, Fort JG, Goldstein JL, et al. Celecoxib versus naproxen and diclofenac in osteoarthritis patients: SUCCESS-I Study. Am J Med 2006;119:255–66.
5. Antithrombotic Trialists' (ATT) Collaboration. Aspirin in the primary and secondary prevention of vascular disease: collaborative meta-analysis of individual participant data from randomized trials. Lancet 2009;373:1849–1860.
6. Bhatt DL, Scheiman J, Abraham N, et al. ACCF/ACG/AHA 2008 expert consensus document on reducing the gastrointestinal risks of antiplatelet therapy and NSAID use. Circulation 2008;118:1894–1909.
7. American Diabetes Association. Standards of medical care in diabetes—2016. Diabetes Care 2016;39:S1–S112.
8. Hochberg MC, Altman RD, April KT. American College of Rheumatology 2012 recommendations for the use of nonpharmacologic and pharmacologic therapies in osteoporosis of the hand, hip, and knee. Arthritis Care Res 2012;62:465–474.

37

STRESS ULCER PROPHYLAXIS/ UPPER GI HEMORRHAGE

A Bloody Good Time.............................Level I

Jay L. Martello, PharmD, BCPS

Lena M. Maynor, PharmD, BCPS

LEARNING OBJECTIVES

After completing this case study, the reader should be able to:

- Identify risk factors associated with stress gastritis/ulceration and determine which critically ill patients should receive pharmacologic prophylaxis.

- Recommend appropriate pharmacologic alternatives including agent, route of administration, and dose for the prevention of stress–induced gastritis/ulceration.

- Identify and implement monitoring parameters for the recommended stress gastritis/ulceration prophylactic regimens.

- Discuss the pharmacologic approaches to the management of stress ulcer–induced bleeding.

PATIENT PRESENTATION

◼ CHIEF COMPLAINT

No complaint—patient is unresponsive.

◼ HPI

Penny Robinson is a 26-year-old woman who presents to the ED with traumatic injuries following a motor vehicle accident. She was the restrained driver of a car who was hit on the driver's side by a tractor-trailer that ran a red light. When EMS arrived in the field, the patient was unresponsive with labored breathing. She was given fentanyl 50 mcg, succinylcholine 40 mg, midazolam 5 mg, and was intubated prior to transfer to the hospital. The EMS report indicates that the intubation was very difficult. The extraction time from the vehicle to the ED was 25 minutes.

◼ PMH (Provided by Patient's Mother)

PE × 1 about 2 months ago
IBS-C × 10 years
S/P cholecystectomy about 6 months ago

◼ FH

Both mother and father are still alive and in "good health."

◼ SH

Patient is a graduate student at a local university. She smoked cigarettes 1 ppd × 6 years until she was hospitalized for a PE and has since quit. She does not drink alcohol or use illicit drugs.

◼ ROS

Patient is unresponsive after an MVA

◼ Meds

Norethindrone 0.35 mg PO daily
Lubiprostone 24 mcg PO Q 12 H
Rivaroxaban 20 mg PO daily

◼ Allergies

Sulfamethoxazole/trimethoprim (shortness of breath)
Clindamycin (hives)
Cimetidine (shortness of breath and thrombocytopenia)

◼ Physical Examination

Gen

Young, unresponsive woman; no obvious bleeding on exam

VS

BP 108/68, P 106, RR 24, T 37.3°C; Wt 51 kg, Ht 5′11″

Skin

Warm, dry; small lacerations across forehead and chest; ecchymoses present on both legs and arms

Neck/Lymph Nodes

Supple, no palpable areas of deformity or masses

HEENT

No blood visible in the nose or ears; no obvious damage to the ears, eyes, or nose

Lungs

Patient is intubated

CV

S_1, S_2 normal; sinus tachycardia with no S_3, S_4

Abd

Firm; decreased bowel sounds

Genit/Rect

No obvious damage to the genital area

Neuro

Glasgow Coma Score = 7; negative Babinski; 2+ deep tendon reflexes

■ Labs

Na 135 mEq/L	Hgb 9.0 g/dL	PO_4 3.0 mg/dL
K 3.6 mEq/L	Hct 27.3%	Ca 10.2 mg/dL
Cl 101 mEq/L	WBC 8.0 × 10³/mm³	AST 29 IU/L
CO_2 22 mEq/L	Plt 122 × 10³/mm³	ALT 22 IU/L
BUN 20 mg/dL		Alk Phos 66 IU/L
SCr 0.8 mg/dL		T. bili 0.4 mg/dL
Glu 91 mg/dL		Alb 3.8 g/dL
		INR 1.1

■ ABG

pH 7.43, $PaCO_2$ 48 mm Hg, PaO_2 74 mm Hg, HCO_3^- 23 mEq/L, pulse ox 92%

■ AP Chest X-Ray

Multiple left and right rib fractures. There is evidence of a right hemopneumothorax with protrusion to the right lung.

■ Focused Assessment with Sonography in Trauma (FAST) Exam

No evidence of fluid in the perihepatic, hepatorenal, perisplenic, pericardial, or pelvic spaces

■ CT Abdomen/Pelvis with IV Contrast

There is no evidence for bowel obstruction. The common bile duct does not appear to be dilated. No free fluid present in the abdominal cavity.

■ CT Head with IV Contrast

No midline shift. No evidence for intracranial hemorrhage.

■ Urinalysis

Yellow color, specific gravity 1.026, pH 4.6, ketones negative, protein negative, nitrite negative, bilirubin negative, glucose negative, bacteria 0, WBC 0, RBC 3+, hCG negative

■ Clinical Course

The patient is given 1 L NS, increasing her BP to 122/76. She is also given 2500 units of 4-factor prothrombin complex concentrate (KCentra®) and 10 mg of IV phytonadione. She is transferred to the OR for repair of her rib fractures and hemopneumothorax. A central line is placed intraoperatively. She is given cefazolin 1 g Q 8 H for antimicrobial prophylaxis, which will continue for 24 hours after repair. Her fractures are repaired without significant incident and a chest tube is placed to drain fluid. During the surgery, the

patient was given 2 L of LR and 2 units of PRBC to correct for blood and fluid loss. The patient's vitals on exiting surgery and arriving in the surgical/trauma ICU are BP 106/62 and P 92. She is currently on assist/control mechanical ventilation. The patient's urine output has been 40 mL/hour for the past 2 hours. The Hgb is 9.6 g/dL, K 3.2 mEq/L, INR 2.0, and pulse ox 94%. She is started on NS at 100 mL/hour, enoxaparin 30 mg SQ Q 12 H, a fentanyl drip, and a midazolam drip. An NG tube is also placed.

QUESTIONS

Problem Identification

1.a. Prior to patient rounds, you review the medications the patient was taking prior to admission. Which of these chronic medications should be maintained during the hospitalization? Provide your rationale for continuing, discontinuing, or changing each drug regimen.

1.b. Identify all of the patient's drug therapy problems at this point in her hospital course (include both potential and actual drug therapy problems).

■ CLINICAL COURSE (PART 1)

Two days later, the patient is still in the surgical/trauma ICU. She is hemodynamically stable and is still mechanically ventilated. She has bowel sounds and is currently receiving tube feeds through her NG tube. Labs include: Na 138 mEq/L, K 3.5 mEq/L, Cl 103 mEq/L, CO_2 21 mEq/L, BUN 16 mg/dL, SCr 0.7 mg/dL, Hgb 8.6 g/dL, WBC 8.1 × 10³/mm³, platelets 102 × 10³/mm³, and INR 2.0. She has not had a bowel movement since admission and is given a glycerin suppository. The surgical resident realizes that no GI prophylaxis was provided initially but is not sure if it is needed at this point.

Follow-Up Questions

1.c. What are the risk factors for developing stress gastritis/ulceration in critically ill patients, and which risk factors does this patient have?

1.d. Do this patient's risk factors warrant prophylactic therapy to prevent stress ulceration? Provide the rationale for your answer.

Desired Outcome

2. What are the goals of pharmacotherapy for preventing stress gastritis and ulceration?

Therapeutic Alternatives

3. What pharmacologic options are available for prophylaxis of stress ulceration in this critically ill patient?

Optimal Plan

4. Create a pharmacotherapeutic plan for stress ulcer prophylaxis (SUP) in this patient.

Outcome Evaluation

5. What clinical and laboratory parameters should be monitored to assess the effectiveness and potential adverse effects of the regimen you selected?

■ CLINICAL COURSE (PART 2)

Early in the morning 2 days later (postoperative day 4), the patient is extubated and started on a clear liquid diet. Later that day, the patient has a large, dark red/black bowel movement that tests heme positive. The nurse checks the patient's vitals, which show BP 92/58 and P 100. A stat Hgb comes back 7.8 g/dL, with a repeat value of 7.9 g/dL. The patient is given 1 L of LR which increases the blood pressure to 112/68 and reduces her pulse to 88. Following her fluid bolus, the patient undergoes endoscopic evaluation. Multiple small gastric lesions oozing blood are visualized by EGD. The patient is diagnosed with an upper GI bleed.

■ FOLLOW-UP QUESTIONS

1. What are the differences in clinical presentation between an upper GI bleed and a lower GI bleed?
2. What are the pharmacotherapeutic goals for treating an upper GI bleed?
3. Discuss the pharmacologic options for treating an upper GI bleed.
4. Outline a pharmacotherapeutic plan for treating this patient's upper GI bleed.
5. What clinical and laboratory parameters should be monitored to assess the effectiveness and potential adverse effects of the regimen you recommended?

■ SELF-STUDY ASSIGNMENTS

1. Identify commercially available GI protective products that may be administered via nasogastric or orogastric tube.
2. Discuss how to mix, store, and administer IV pantoprazole, lansoprazole, and esomeprazole.
3. Identify potential drug interactions and adverse effects with antacids, sucralfate, H_2-receptor antagonists, and proton pump inhibitors.
4. Describe the impact of *Helicobacter pylori* infection on SUP and GI bleeding.
5. Identify methods of reversing direct-acting oral anticoagulants in the acute setting.

CLINICAL PEARL

When performing medication reconciliation, always be on the lookout for antiulcer agents on the patient's profile. They are often relics from a previous problem that has resolved and are no longer indicated. Patients on antiulcer agents without an indication incur increased health care costs and are at increased risk for drug interactions and side effects, including a greater risk of pneumonia and *Clostridium difficile* infection, as well as hypomagnesemia and hypocalcemia.

REFERENCES

1. American Society of Health-System Pharmacists. ASHP therapeutic guidelines on stress ulcer prophylaxis. Am J Health Syst Pharm 1999;56:347–379.
2. Guillamondegui OD, Gunter OL, Bonadies JA, et al. Practice Management Guidelines for Stress Ulcer Prophylaxis. Eastern Association for the Surgery of Trauma (EAST). 2008. Available at: https://www.east.org/education/practice-management-guidelines/stress-ulcer-prophylaxis. Accessed on January 18, 2016.
3. Ali T, Harty RF. Stress-induced ulcer bleeding in critically ill patients. Gastroenterol Clin North Am 2009;38:245–265.
4. Herzig SJ, Howell MD, Ngo LH, Marcantonio ER. Acid-suppressive medication use and the risk for hospital-acquired pneumonia. JAMA 2009;301:2120–2128.
5. Barkun AN, Bardou M, Pham CQ, Martel M. Proton pump inhibitors vs. histamine 2 receptor antagonists for stress-related mucosal bleeding prophylaxis in critically ill patients: a meta-analysis. Am J Gastroenterol 2012;107:507–520.
6. Marik PE, Vasu T, Hirani A, Pachinburavan M. Stress ulcer prophylaxis in the new millennium: a systematic review and meta-analysis. Crit Care Med 2010;38:2222–2228.
7. Compoginis JM, Gaspard D, Obaid A. Famotidine use and thrombocytopenia in the trauma patient. Am Surg 2011;77:1580–1583.
8. Kim YI, Park CK, Park DJ, Wi JO, Han ER, Koh YI. A case of famotidine-induced anaphylaxis. J Investig Allergol Clin Immunol 2010;20:166–169.
9. Gralnek IM, Barkun AN, Bardou M. Management of acute bleeding from a peptic ulcer. N Engl J Med 2008;359:928–937.
10. Barkun AN, Bardou M, Kuipers EJ, et al. International consensus recommendations on the management of patients with nonvariceal upper gastrointestinal bleeding. Ann Intern Med 2010;152:101–113.

38

CROHN DISEASE

A Sense of Urgency.............................. Level II

Brian A. Hemstreet, PharmD, FCCP, BCPS

LEARNING OBJECTIVES

After completing this case study, the reader should be able to:

• Describe the typical clinical presentation of active Crohn disease (CD), including signs, symptoms, and disease distribution and severity.
• Identify exacerbating factors and potential complications of CD.
• Recommend appropriate pharmacologic treatment for active CD.
• Review major toxicities of drugs commonly used for managing CD.
• Educate a patient on the proper use of medications used to treat CD.

PATIENT PRESENTATION

■ Chief Complaint

"I'm having occasional diarrhea, sometimes with blood. I occasionally have mild abdominal pain. I feel run down lately and have lost a few pounds."

■ HPI

John Jensen is a 32-year-old man who presents to the clinic with a 3-month history of intermittent episodes of diarrhea. He states that he has been having one to two loose bowel movements a day over this time. This is different from his typical bowel pattern. Over the past 4 weeks, he has also noticed blood in some of his stools. The episodes of diarrhea are infrequently accompanied by brief periods of mild abdominal pain. These symptoms have caused problems with his job, as he is a sales representative for a pharmaceutical company and spends a lot of time driving to appointments. He reports a 5-lb unintentional weight loss over this time period that he attributes to "not wanting to make his abdominal pain worse." He has tried OTC naproxen for the abdominal pain and Pepto-Bismol for the diarrhea, both of which have provided little relief. He does not recall any exposure to sick contacts. He reports no recent international travel. His PCP referred him to a gastroenterologist.

■ PMH

GERD
Sinusitis (last treated with antibiotics 8 months ago)
Seasonal allergic rhinitis
Exercise-induced bronchoconstriction
ACL repair of the right knee 2 years ago

■ FH

Father with DM, mother with HTN. Older sister with CD.

■ SH

Single. Works as a sales representative for a pharmaceutical company. Occasional alcohol use on the weekends. Smokes 0.5 ppd × 10 years.

■ Meds

Loratadine 10 mg PO once daily
Fluticasone two sprays each nostril PRN
Naproxen sodium 220 mg PO Q 8–12 H PRN pain
Albuterol HFA MDI PRN prior to exercise

■ All

Hydrocodone (GI upset)
Sulfa drugs (severe rash)

■ ROS

No sick contacts. Heartburn one to two times a week and rhinorrhea one to two times a week. No cough, SOB, HA, or mental status changes. No knee or joint pain. No jaundice or rashes. No mouth sores.

■ Physical Examination

Gen

Well-developed Caucasian male in no apparent distress

VS

Sitting: BP 139/89, P 82; standing: BP 136/70, P 85; RR 17, T 37.9°C; Wt 215 lb, Ht 5'9"

Skin

No lesions or rashes

HEENT

PERRLA, EOMI, pale conjunctivae, moist mucous membranes, intact dentition, oropharynx clear

Neck/Lymph Nodes

Trachea midline, (–) thyromegaly, (–) lymphadenopathy, (–) JVD

Lungs/Thorax

CTA bilaterally

CV

Regular rate and rhythm, no MRG

Abd

Nontender, nondistended, no rebound or guarding; (+) BS, (–) HSM

Genit/Rect

Prostate size WNL, (–) tenderness, heme (+) stool, no evidence of hemorrhoids

MS/Ext

No CVA tenderness

Neuro

A & O × 3, CN II–XII intact, 5/5 upper and lower extremity strength bilaterally

■ Labs

Na 139 mEq/L	Hgb 12 g/dL	AST 25 IU/L
K 3.0 mEq/L	Hct 37%	ALT 28 IU/L
Cl 100 mEq/L	RBC 2.86 × 10⁶/mm³	Alk phos 50 IU/L
CO₂ 26 mEq/L	Plt 400 × 10³/mm³	Total bili 1.2 mg/dL
BUN 15 mg/dL	MCV 80 μm³	Direct bili 0.6 mg/dL
SCr 1.1 mg/dL	WBC 12.7 × 10³/mm³	Albumin 4.1 g/dL
Glu 104 mg/dL	Neutros 67%	CRP 13 mg/dL
Ca 8.7 mg/dL	Bands 1%	Lipase 15 units/L
Phos 3.9 mg/dL	Eos 2%	ESR 105 mm/hour
	Lymphs 26%	Stool O & P (–)
	Monos 4%	Stool C. diff toxin (–)

■ Radiology

An abdominal x-ray reveals no evidence of obstruction, dilation, or free air.

■ Other

Colonoscopy: reveals a patchy "cobblestone" pattern of inflammation in the terminal ileum. The inflammatory process extends below the intestinal mucosa, and there is evidence of mucosal friability and recent bleeding. A biopsy of the intestinal mucosa revealed leukocyte infiltration and submucosal granulomas consistent with active CD.

■ Assessment

A 32-year-old man presenting with new-onset active CD involving the terminal ileum requiring treatment

QUESTIONS

Problem Identification

1.a. Create a list of this patient's drug therapy problems.

1.b. What signs, symptoms, and laboratory alterations in this patient are consistent with CD?

1.c. How would you classify the severity of this patient's CD? Provide the rationale for your answer.

1.d. What factors could lead to the development or exacerbation of CD in this patient?

1.e. What extraintestinal manifestations can develop in patients with CD?

Desired Outcome

2. Develop a list of pharmacotherapeutic goals for this patient.

Therapeutic Alternatives

3. What drug therapies could be used to treat this patient's CD?

Optimal Plan

4.a. Develop a complete treatment plan for managing this patient's CD.

4.b. How would your drug management differ if the disease involved the entire ileum and the colon?

Outcome Evaluation

5. What parameters should be monitored to assess both the efficacy and toxicity of your selected drug regimen?

Patient Education

6. How will you educate the patient about his CD therapy in order to enhance adherence, minimize adverse effects, and promote successful therapeutic outcomes?

■ CLINICAL COURSE

It is now 12 months after treatment was started. Mr Jensen achieved remission after 3 months of initial treatment. Following remission, he continued therapy for an additional 12-week period, after which he was withdrawn from drug treatment. He has had only a few intermittent episodes of diarrhea and abdominal pain over the next 6 months. However, over the past week he has had an increase in the frequency of bowel movements to three to four times per day with intermittent blood. He has developed significant abdominal pain, malaise, fever, and dehydration requiring hospitalization. He is admitted to the general medicine floor of the hospital with a recurrence of active moderate to severe CD.

■ FOLLOW-UP QUESTIONS

1. Given this new information, how would you modify the patient's drug therapy?

2. What baseline testing would be required if infliximab, adalimumab, or certolizumab were to be used in this instance?

■ SELF-STUDY ASSIGNMENTS

1. Search for Web sites containing information about local support groups in your area to which you may refer patients with CD for help and support.

2. Construct a table outlining the major differences between CD and ulcerative colitis.

3. Review the FDA recommendations for use of the major drug classes for treatment of both active CD and maintenance of remission in pregnant patients.

CLINICAL PEARL

Hospitalized patients with active CD are at high risk for blood clots due to their inflammatory state and should be placed on prophylactic therapy for deep vein thrombosis.

REFERENCES

1. Lichtenstein GR, Hanauer SB, Sandborn WJ; Practice Parameters Committee of the American College of Gastroenterology. Management of Crohn's disease in adults. Am J Gastroenterol 2009;104:465–483.

2. American Gastroenterological Association Institute Guidelines for the Identification, As-sessment and Initial Medical Treatment in Crohn's Disease Clinical Decision Support Tool. http://campaigns.gastro.org /algorithms/IBDCarePathway. Accessed November 16, 2015.

3. Cosnes J, Gower-Rousseau C, Seksik P, Cortot A. Epidemiology and natural history of inflammatory bowel diseases. Gastroenterology 2011;140:1785–1786.

4. Scharl M, Rogler G. Inflammatory bowel disease pathogenesis: what is new? Curr Opin Gastroenterol 2012;28:301–309.

5. Larsen S, Bendtzen K, Nielsen OH. Extraintestinal manifestations of inflammatory bowel disease: epidemiology, diagnosis, and management. Ann Med 2010;42:97–114.

6. Buchner AM, Blonski W, Lichtenstein GR. Update on the management of Crohn's disease. Curr Gastroenterol Rep 2011;3:465–474.

7. Cottone M, Renna S, Orlando A, Mocciaro F. Medical management of Crohn's disease. Expert Opin Pharmacother 2011;12:2505–2525.

8. Talley NJ, Abreu MT, Achkar JP, et al. An evidence-based systematic review on medical therapies for inflammatory bowel disease. Am J Gastroenterol 2011;106:S2–S25.

9. Ford AC, Bernstein CN, Khan KJ, et al. Glucocorticosteroid therapy in inflammatory bowel disease: systematic review and meta-analysis. Am J Gastroenterol 2011;106:590–599.

10. Prantera C, Scribano ML. Antibiotics and probiotics in inflammatory bowel disease: why, when, and how. Curr Opin Gastroenterol 2009;25:329–333.

39

ULCERATIVE COLITIS

Seriously? Four Times a Day?.....................Level I

Nancy S. Yunker, PharmD, BCPS

LEARNING OBJECTIVES

After completing this case study, the reader should be able to:

- Identify the common signs and symptoms of ulcerative colitis.

- Evaluate treatment options for an acute episode of ulcerative colitis and recommend a specific treatment plan that includes the medication, dosing regimen, potential side effects, and monitoring parameters.

- Develop a pharmacotherapeutic plan for an ulcerative colitis patient whose disease is in remission.

- Discuss recent advances in the pharmacotherapy of ulcerative colitis.

PATIENT PRESENTATION

■ Chief Complaint

"I can't take the pain and diarrhea anymore. I thought I could make it until I got home to see my doctor but today I realized I needed to see someone."

HPI

Bonnie Smith is a 32-year-old woman who presents to the ED with the chief complaint of a 1.5 week history of abdominal pain associated with cramping, bloody diarrhea, and mucus that she states is typical of her ulcerative colitis flares. She states that she has been having about four to five bloody bowel movements a day for most of the time that she has been in our city on vacation, but today she was dizzy when she stood up; she did not have any symptoms while sitting or lying down. She has been here on vacation for almost 2 weeks and is scheduled to return home in 3 days. She has not traveled outside the country, been hospitalized, or received antibiotics recently. She was diagnosed with UC approximately 3 years ago and has had approximately one exacerbation a year that her physician has treated with Pentasa capsules four times a day during each exacerbation. Each time her symptoms have resolved with 4–6 weeks of therapy. She has refused maintenance therapy because she does not want to take a medication four times a day; it is not conducive to her work and social life and she has refused rectal medications for the same reason. Her last exacerbation was approximately 10 months ago.

PMH

Ulcerative colitis, diagnosed 3 years ago
Type 1 DM

FH

Mother has a history of CAD and lung CA; father has a history of ulcerative colitis, S/P colectomy 18 years ago.

SH

Works as an office manager; lives with her fiancée; no children; denies tobacco use; drinks one to two glasses of wine every few weeks; acknowledges marijuana use from 2002 to 2005 but states none in the past 10 years

Meds

NPH insulin 22 units in the morning and evening; insulin aspart 6 units for blood glucose >300 mg/dL.
Vaccination history is unavailable.

All

NKDA

ROS

Negative for chest pain, SOB, dysuria, fever, chills, N/V, myalgias, arthralgias, polyuria, or recent allergic reaction. Positive for mild abdominal soreness, cramping, and bloody diarrhea.

Physical Examination

Gen

A & O, pleasant, healthy-appearing Caucasian woman in NAD

VS

At 8 AM:
BP (lying down) 100/58 mm Hg, P 60 bpm
BP (standing) 80/40 mm Hg, P 75 bpm
RR 18/min, T 37.0°C
Wt 66 kg (usual weight 68 kg), Ht 5'7", BMI 23.5 kg/m²

Skin

No lesions; warm, adequate turgor

HEENT

PERRLA; EOMI; mucous membranes without lesions or exudates; TMs intact

Lungs

CTA, no rales or rhonchi

CV

RRR, normal S_1 and S_2; no S_3, S_4

Abd

Normal active BS, soft, nondistended; tender to deep palpation but no palpable mass; no liver or spleen enlargement; no rebound tenderness or guarding

Rect

Somewhat tender; no hemorrhoids, fissures, or lesions by anoscopy; heme (+) stool

MS/Ext

No CCE; pulses 2+; normal ROM; strength 5/5 bilaterally

Neuro

A & O × 3; CN II–XII intact; DTRs 2+

Labs

At 10:00 AM:

Na 137 mEq/L	Hgb 13 g/dL	WBC 4.5 × 10³/mm³	AST 22 IU/L
K 3.4 mEq/L	Hct 38%	PMNs 52%	ALT 20 IU/L
Cl 105 mEq/L	Plt 242 × 10³/mm³	Bands 5%	Alk phos 36 IU/L
CO₂ 27 mEq/L	MCV 85.3 μm³	Lymphs 36%	T. Bili 0.5 mg/dL
BUN 26 mg/dL	MCH 29.1 pg	Basos 1%	PT 12.0 s
SCr 1.0 mg/dL	MCHC 34.1 g/dL	Monos 6%	INR 1.0
Glu 113 mg/dL			Ca 8.9 mg/dL
			Mg 1.9 mEq/L
			PO₄ 4.2 mg/dL
			Alb 3.9 g/dL
			A1C 6.2%

Urinalysis

Color yellow; transparency clear; negative for protein, leukocyte esterase, nitrite, blood, ketones, RBCs, WBCs, and bilirubin; pH 7.0; specific gravity 1.019

Clinical Course

The patient received 1 L of 0.9% saline with KCl 40 mEq over 4 hours starting at 11:00 AM. Vital signs at 3:00 PM were as follows: BP (lying down) 110/74 mm Hg, P 62 bpm; BP (standing) 112/74 mm Hg, P 64 bpm. Repeat laboratory tests were as follows:

Na 139 mEq/L	Hgb 12.5g/dL
K 3.9 mEq/L	Hct 36.3%
Cl 107 mEq/L	Plt 240 × 10³/mm³
CO₂ 27 mEq/L	MCV 85.2 μm³
BUN 14 mg/dL	MCH 25.8 pg
SCr 0.89 mg/dL	MCHC 31.4 g/dL
Glu 119 mg/dL	WBC 4.4 × 10³/mm³

◼ Assessment

Lower GI bleeding with a history of ulcerative colitis; patient is stable after volume repletion.

D/C with instructions to return to ED if symptoms worsen and to contact PCP on return home.

QUESTIONS

Problem Identification

1.a. List all of the patient's drug therapy problems, including those existing at her initial presentation to the ED.

1.b. List the signs, symptoms, and laboratory values that indicate the presence and severity of ulcerative colitis; also include pertinent negative findings.

1.c. Could the manifestations of the patient's ulcerative colitis have been precipitated by an event?

Desired Outcome

2. What are the short- and long-term pharmacotherapeutic goals for this patient?

Therapeutic Alternatives

3.a. What nondrug therapies might be useful for this patient?

3.b. What feasible pharmacotherapeutic alternatives should be considered for the treatment of ulcerative colitis?

3.c. What other general health maintenance issues and therapies should be considered in patients with ulcerative colitis?

Optimal Plan

4.a. What drug, dosage form, schedule, and duration of therapy are best for this patient based on your assessment of the patient's disease severity?

4.b. What alternatives should be considered if the patient fails to respond to initial therapy?

Outcome Evaluation

5. What clinical and laboratory parameters are necessary to evaluate the therapy for achievement of the desired therapeutic outcome and to detect or prevent adverse effects?

Patient Education

6. What information should be provided to the patient to enhance adherence, ensure successful therapy, and minimize adverse effects?

◼ CLINICAL COURSE

The patient presents to her local PCP for follow-up 1 month after her initial presentation to the ED. She states that her bowel movements are "completely normal" and she no longer has pain. She states that the symptoms started to resolve about 2 weeks after she started treatment. She has had no further complaints of weakness or dizziness. The repeat Hgb today is 12.9 g/dL.

◼ FOLLOW-UP QUESTIONS

1. Considering this new information, what therapeutic intervention(s) do you recommend at this time?

2. What additional information should be provided to the patient?

◼ SELF-STUDY ASSIGNMENTS

1. Review the literature comparing mesalamine, olsalazine, balsalazide, and sulfasalazine preparations regarding efficacy, adverse effects, and cost; include all currently available mesalamine dosage forms.

2. Perform a literature search to determine what new therapies are being evaluated for ulcerative colitis, including biologics and biosimilars.

3. Review the literature supporting use of cyclosporine, tacrolimus, anti-TNF-α agents in patients with severe, extensive disease poorly responsive to initial corticosteroid treatment.

4. Conduct a literature search to determine how pharmacogenomics is affecting therapy of ulcerative colitis patients.

CLINICAL PEARL

Infliximab, adalimumab, and golimumab are three TNF-α antagonists approved for the treatment of ulcerative colitis refractory to corticosteroids and other immunomodulators. While these agents have not been directly compared with one another, intravenous infliximab seems to be the most effective of the three based on analysis of current clinical trials. However, higher doses of adalimumab are being investigated, which may change this assessment.

REFERENCES

1. Dignass A, Lindsay JO, Sturm A, et al. For the European Crohn's and Colitis Organisation (ECCO). Second European evidence-based consensus on the management of ulcerative colitis Part 2: current management. J Crohn's Colitis 2012;6:991–1030.

2. Kornbluth A, Sachar DB. Practice Parameters Committee of the American College of Gastroenterology. Ulcerative colitis practice guidelines in adults: American College of Gastroenterology, Practice Parameters Committee. Am J Gastroenterol 2010;105:501–523.

3. Ye B, van Langenberg DR. Mesalazine preparations for the treatment of ulcerative colitis: are all created equal? World J Gastrointest Pharmacol Ther 2015;6:137–144.

4. Bressler B, Marshall JK, Bernstein CN, et al. On behalf of the Toronto Ulcerative Colitis Consensus Group. Clinical practice guidelines for the medical management of nonhospitalized ulcerative colitis: The Toronto Consensus. Gastroenterology 2015;148:1035–1058.

5. Hoy SM. Budesonide MMX®: a review of its use in patients with mild to moderate ulcerative colitis. Drugs 2015;75:879–886.

6. Dassopoulos T, Cohen RD, Scherl EJ, Schwartz RM, Kosinski L, Regueiro MD. Ulcerative colitis care pathway. Gastroenterology 2015;149:238–245.

7. Kopylov U, Ben-Horin S, Seidman E. Therapeutic drug monitoring in inflammatory bowel disease. Ann Gastroenterol 2014;27:304–312.

8. Blonski W, Buchner AM, Lichtenstein GR. Treatment of ulcerative colitis. Curr Opin Gastroenterol 2014;30:84–96.

9. Beery RM, Kane S. Current approaches to the management of new-onset ulcerative colitis. Clin Exp Gastroenterol 2014;7:111–132.

10. Hahn L, Beggs A, Wahaib K, Kodall L, Kirkwood V. Vedolizumab: an integrin-receptor antagonist for treatment of Crohn's disease and ulcerative colitis. Am J Health-Syst Pharm 2015;72:1271–1278.

40

NAUSEA AND VOMITING

In for a Tune-Up . . . . Level II

Kelly K. Nystrom, PharmD, BCOP

Amy M. Pick, PharmD, BCOP

LEARNING OBJECTIVES

After completing this case study, the reader should be able to:

- Develop a prophylactic antiemetic regimen based on the emetic risk associated with cancer chemotherapeutic agents to optimize the management of nausea and vomiting.

- Design an appropriate treatment regimen for anticipatory, breakthrough, acute, and delayed nausea and vomiting.

- Design a monitoring plan to assess the effectiveness of an antiemetic regimen.

- Discuss with patients and caregivers the reason for antiemetics, their appropriate use, and the management of side effects.

- Recommend appropriate alternative antiemetic strategies based on patient-specific conditions, such as previous response to chemotherapy and side effects.

PATIENT PRESENTATION

■ Chief Complaint

"I have stomach pain and back pain."

■ HPI

Mr Jones is a 57-year-old man who presents to the ED with complaints of lower back and abdominal pain, decreased appetite, and constipation since previous discharge from the hospital 3 days ago. He was recently hospitalized for prolonged abdominal pain, fatigue, a persistent cough, and a 14-lb weight loss over the previous 2 months. An ultrasound revealed marked cholelithiasis with changes of chronic cholecystitis for which he was started on amoxicillin/clavulanate. He was found to have a 1.4-cm pulmonary mass in the lower left lung associated with endobronchial obstruction, a 4-mm noncalcified left pulmonary nodule, slightly enlarged left hilar lymph nodes, and an enlarged liver with evidence of metastasis. A diagnosis of small-cell lung cancer was made with the plan to begin treatment in the outpatient setting. He currently reports that he does not have trouble swallowing but does have a productive cough. The sputum occasionally clears but is usually a brownish color.

■ PMH

BPH (untreated)
Cholelithiasis with chronic cholecystitis
Metastatic small-cell lung cancer
GERD

■ FH

Father died at age 82 of heart and renal failure; mother died at age 68 with emphysema, obesity, MI, hypertension; two sisters, one with diabetes; three adult children, alive and healthy.

■ SH

Single and works as a salesman at a car dealership. He has smoked 1–1.5 packs of cigarettes a day starting at the age of 14. He still smokes but has cut back because his employer has a campus-wide no smoking policy. History of alcohol and substance abuse, but he has not had alcohol for 14 years.

■ ROS

Complaints include hoarseness for 1 week and fatigue. Lower extremity weakness, productive cough with brownish sputum, abdominal pain and bloating, nausea, and constipation.

■ Home Meds

Ibuprofen 400 mg PO TID with food
Esomeprazole 40 mg PO daily
Oxycodone ER 10 mg PO Q 12 H
Oxycodone 5 mg PO Q 3 H PRN
Amoxicillin/clavulanate 875 mg PO BID × 6 more days

■ All

NKDA

■ Physical Examination

Gen

This is a pleasant thin Caucasian man who appears to be in acute distress due to back pain

VS

BP 160/82, P 91, RR 20, T 36.6°C; Wt 68 kg, Ht 6′0″

Skin

Warm and dry

HEENT

No discharge noted in the external ear canals. Oral mucosa is intact. Mouth is pink and dry

Neck/Lymph Nodes

Nontender, supple. No JVD, lymphadenopathy, or thyromegaly noted

Lungs/Thorax

Good air movement. No wheezes or rhonchi noted. No spinal abnormalities appreciated

CV

RRR. No rubs, murmurs, or gallops

Abd

Abdomen is firm and slightly distended; hypoactive bowel sounds; tender across his midsection with hepatomegaly

Genit/Rect

Deferred

MS/Ext

Normal range of motion and equal strength in upper and lower extremities. Positive for 2+ pitting edema in the feet and ankles

Neuro

Patient is awake, alert, and oriented. Cranial nerves intact. Gait was not assessed. Patient is very anxious about his diagnosis and chemotherapy

Labs

Na 141 mEq/L	Hgb 12.4 g/dL	T. bili 2.8 mg/dL
K 4.3 mEq/L	Hct 36.3%	Albumin 2.4 g/dL
Cl 106 mEq/L	Plt 148 × 10^3/mm^3	AST 154 IU/L
CO_2 21 mEq/L	WBC 18.4 × 10^3/mm^3	ALT 131 IU/L
BUN 21 mg/dL	Neutros 72%	Alk Phos 321 IU/L
SCr 0.7 mg/dL	Bands 8%	GGT 102 IU/L
Glu 97 mg/dL	Lymphs 11%	
	Monos 4%	
	Eos 1%	
	Basos 1%	
	Promyelo 1%	
	Meta 2%	

Clinical Course

Mr Jones is admitted to the hospital for severe abdominal and back pain. Although afebrile on admission, he is started on levofloxacin and metronidazole because of concerns of increased WBC count and possible abdominal infection. His oxycodone ER is increased to 20 mg PO Q 12 H for severe pain. He will receive his first chemotherapy cycle as an inpatient to try and improve his abdominal and back pain. He is very anxious about his diagnosis and the chemotherapy he is about to receive. Orders include:

Ondansetron 32 mg IV 30 minutes prior to chemotherapy × 3 days
Dexamethasone 20 mg IV 30 minutes prior to chemotherapy × 3 days
Fosaprepitant 150 mg IV 30 minutes prior to chemotherapy on day 1, and then aprepitant 80 mg PO daily on days 2 and 3
Cisplatin 75 mg/m2 IV on day 1
Etoposide 100 mg/m2 IV on days 1–3
Radiation therapy 250 cGy/fraction for a total dose of 3,500 cGy to the spine
Ondansetron 4–8 mg IV Q 8 H PRN nausea and vomiting

QUESTIONS

Problem Identification

1.a. Create a list of this patient's drug therapy problems.

1.b. What are this patient's risk factors for chemotherapy-induced nausea and vomiting?

1.c. What factors may be contributing to his nausea and vomiting?

Desired Outcome

2. What are the goals of therapy in this case?

Therapeutic Alternatives

3.a. Assess the patient's antiemetic regimen for prophylaxis of acute and delayed nausea and vomiting and for the treatment of breakthrough nausea and vomiting. Make any changes as necessary.

3.b. What nondrug therapies may be useful to prevent nausea and vomiting?

Patient Education

4. How would you educate this patient on his antiemetic regimen?

CLINICAL COURSE (PART 1)

You review Mr Jones' antiemetics, and the physician makes changes based on your recommendations. Mr Jones does well for the first 24 hours, but around hour 30, he develops nausea and vomiting. The nurse administers the patient a dose of ondansetron and is surprised when it does not work. Mr Jones is also given two other antiemetics ordered by the physician over the next 2 days with little relief.

FOLLOW-UP QUESTIONS

1. How might you educate the nurse about using ondansetron for breakthrough nausea and vomiting?

2. What pharmacologic alternatives may be helpful for the initial treatment of this patient?

CLINICAL COURSE (PART 2)

After implementation of your recommendations, Mr Jones' nausea and vomiting have resolved and he is ready to be discharged. He will return to the clinic in about 2 weeks to receive cycle 2 of his chemotherapy.

FOLLOW-UP QUESTIONS (Continued)

Optimal Plan

3. Design a plan for preventing delayed nausea and vomiting in this patient for subsequent chemotherapy cycles.

4. Design a plan to prevent anticipatory nausea and vomiting in this patient for subsequent chemotherapy cycles.

Outcome Evaluation

5.a. Describe how you will determine whether the antiemetic regimen he received was effective for preventing acute and delayed nausea and vomiting.

5.b. Describe the information you will need to assess the efficacy and adverse effects of the prophylactic antiemetic regimen prior to each future course of chemotherapy.

CLINICAL COURSE: ALTERNATIVE THERAPY

While discussing Mr Jones' antiemetic regimen, he says, "I remember that my sister used to take ginger to prevent sea sickness when she went on a cruise, and my cousin used ginger when he was having chemotherapy a few years ago. Would that be good for me to try?" See Section 19 in this Casebook for questions about the use of ginger for treatment of nausea and vomiting.

SELF-STUDY ASSIGNMENTS

1. Compare the indications, doses, and costs of the 5-HT$_3$ antagonists: dolasetron, ondansetron, granisetron, palonosetron, and the combination product netupitant/palonosetron.

2. Discern in which patients it would be appropriate to use palonosetron and/or one of the NK$_1$ receptor antagonists: aprepitant, fosaprepitant, rolapitant, or netupitant; discern the advantages and limitations of each drug.

3. Review various guidelines for antiemetic options for the treatment of refractory nausea and vomiting.

CLINICAL PEARL

Appropriate use of antiemetics is essential. The combination of a 5-HT$_3$ antagonist, dexamethasone and an NK$_1$ receptor antagonist is the regimen of choice for preventing acute nausea and vomiting with highly emetic and some moderately emetic chemotherapy regimens. The NK$_1$ receptor antagonists, dexamethasone and the palonosetron, or combination netupitant/palonestron are also useful for preventing delayed nausea and vomiting. Antiemetic therapy decisions should be based on efficacy, patient-specific factors, and cost.

REFERENCES

1. Ettinger DS, Berger MJ, Aston J, et al. NCCN Clinical Practice Guidelines in Oncology (NCCN Guidelines®) Guideline Antiemesis 2.2015. © 2015 National Comprehensive Cancer Network, Inc. Available at: NCCN.org. Accessed November 3, 2015.
2. Grunberg SM, Warr D, Grall RJ, et al. MASCC/ESMO guidelines: evaluation of new antiemetic agents and definition of antineoplastic agent emetogenicity—state of the art. Support Care Cancer 2011;19(Suppl 1):S43–S47.
3. Navari RM. Management of chemotherapy-induced nausea and vomiting: focus on newer agents and new uses for older agents. Drugs 2013;73:249–262.
4. Kris MG, Tonato M, Bria E, et al. MASCC/ESMO guidelines: consensus recommendations for the prevention of vomiting and nausea following high-emetic-risk chemotherapy. Support Care Cancer 2011;19(Suppl 1):S25–S32.
5. Jordan K, Jahn F, Aapro M. Recent developments in the prevention of chemotherapy-induced nausea and vomiting (CINV): a comprehensive review. Ann Oncol 2015;26:1081–1090.
6. Gold Standard, Inc. Rolapitant. Clinical Pharmacology [database online]. Available at: *http://www.clinicalpharmacology.com.cuhsl.creighton.edu*. Accessed November 3, 2015.
7. Navari RM. Treatment of breakthrough and refractory chemotherapy-induced nausea and vomiting. Biomed Res Int 2015; doi: 10.1155/2015/595894.

41

DIARRHEA

Diner's Diarrhea .... Level I

Marie A. Abate, BS, PharmD

Charles D. Ponte, BS, PharmD, BC-ADM, BCPS, CDE, CPE, DPNAP, FAPhA, FASHP, FCCP, FAADE

LEARNING OBJECTIVES

After completing this case study, the reader should be able to:

- Identify the common causes of acute diarrhea.

- Establish primary goals for the treatment of acute diarrhea.

- Recommend appropriate nonpharmacologic therapy for patients experiencing acute diarrhea.

- Explain the place of drug therapy in the treatment of acute diarrhea and recommend appropriate products.

PATIENT PRESENTATION

■ Chief Complaint

"I've had the runs for a couple of days, along with vomiting. I haven't been able keep anything down and I feel awful."

■ HPI

Mindy Colonada is a 25-year-old woman who comes to the Family Medicine Clinic with a complaint of nausea, vomiting, and diarrhea. She had been well until 1.5 days ago, when she began to experience severe nausea that occurred about 6 hours after eating out at a local sushi restaurant. She had eaten a plate of sushi along with two glasses of iced tea. She had a few sips of her boyfriend's beer, but did not have any milk or other dairy products. She woke up from sleep with severe nausea. She took two tablespoonfuls of Maalox Plus at that time. The nausea persisted, and she began to vomit "several times" with some relief. As the night progressed, she still felt "queasy" and took two extra Prilosec OTC tablets to settle her stomach. She began to feel dizzy, achy, and warm, and her temperature at the time was 38.2°C. These complaints continued to persist and she vomited a few more times. She has not tolerated any solid foods, but she has been able to keep down small amounts of fluid. Since yesterday, she has had four to six liquid stools along with crampy abdominal pain. She has not noticed any blood or mucus in the bowel movements. Her boyfriend brought her to the clinic because she was becoming weak and lightheaded when she tried to stand up. She denies antibiotic use, laxative use, or excessive caffeine intake. She usually drinks bottled water and has not been traveling outside the country. She often experiences stress-related constipation and occasionally (once every 2 months) has loose stools alternating with constipation. These are usually accompanied by abdominal discomfort that is relieved by a bowel movement. She states that this episode is different.

■ PMH

IBS × 2 years
Migraine headaches × 10 years
GERD × 5 years
Depression × 3 years
UTI—6 months ago (treated successfully with ciprofloxacin × 10 days)

■ FH

Noncontributory

■ SH

No current tobacco use, uses marijuana occasionally; drinks wine or a mixed drink socially, usually not more than one glass per week; has about two cups of caffeinated coffee daily. She works as an administrative associate for a local bank. Single, sexually active (one partner, monogamous relationship).

■ ROS

Dizzy on standing but no complaints of vertigo; denies headache, sore throat, ear pain, or nasal discharge. Denies coughing or congestion. Frequent bouts of nausea. Frequent loose stools associated with significant cramping. Decreased urination; no dysuria or frequency. Complains of generalized lassitude, mild aching, feels like her heart is skipping beats.

■ Meds

Valproic acid 500 mg PO BID × 6 years
Triphasil oral contraceptive 1 PO at bedtime × 3 years

Omeprazole 20–40 mg PO daily as needed
Women's Health Formula Multivitamin 1 PO daily
Metamucil one tablespoonful daily
St John's wort two 900 mg tablets daily

■ All

Penicillin → itching, rash on legs, 10 years ago; dust → nasal
congestion, watery eyes

■ Physical Examination

Gen

White female, appears ill, in moderate distress

VS

BP 125/82, P 80 (supine), BP 90/60, P 90 (standing), RR 16, T 38°C;
Wt 75 kg, Ht 5'4"

Skin

Slightly warm to touch, fair skin turgor (mild tenting noted)

HEENT

Dry mucous membranes, nonerythematous TMs, PERRLA, fundi
benign, slight erythema in throat

Neck/Lymph Nodes

Without masses, lymphadenopathy, or thyromegaly

Chest

Clear to A & P

CV

RRR without MRG

Abd

Diffuse tenderness, no guarding or rebound, without organomegaly, nondistended, hyperactive bowel sounds

Genit/Rect

Heme (–) stool in the rectal vault; no gross blood

MS/Ext

Normal muscle strength, no CCE

Neuro

A & O × 3; CN II–XII intact; normal reflexes, normal sensory and
motor function

■ Labs

Na 135 mEq/L	Hgb 12.0 g/dL	AST 35 IU/L
K 3.2 mEq/L	Hct 35%	ALT 30 IU/L
Cl 97 mEq/L	Plt 350 × 10³/mm³	T. bili 1.5 mg/dL
CO_2 25 mEq/L	WBC 12.0 × 10³/mm³	
BUN 25 mg/dL	PMNs 62%	
SCr 1.2 mg/dL	Lymphs 36%	
Glu 90 mg/dL	Monos 2%	

Serum pregnancy test—negative

■ UA

Clear, dark amber; SG 1.030; pH 6.0; protein (–); glucose (–);
acetone (–), bilirubin (–), blood (–); microscopic: 0–2 WBC/hpf,
0–2 RBC/hpf, several hyaline casts

■ Assessment

Probable acute gastroenteritis; R/O other causes
Depression
Migraine headaches
GERD
Irritable bowel syndrome

■ Plan

Admit to observation unit for acute therapy

QUESTIONS

Problem Identification

1.a. Create a list of the patient's drug therapy problems.

1.b. What signs and symptoms indicate the presence and severity of
the diarrhea?

1.c. What questions should you ask the patient or members of the
medical team to obtain the additional information needed for
a complete assessment of this patient?

1.d. Could any of this patient's problems have been caused by her
prescription drug therapy?

1.e. What are other possible causes of this patient's diarrhea?

Desired Outcome

2. What are the goals of therapy for this patient?

Therapeutic Alternatives

3.a. What nonpharmacologic therapies should be considered for
this patient?

3.b. What feasible pharmacotherapeutic alternatives are available
for treatment of diarrhea in this patient?

Optimal Plan

4. What nonpharmacologic interventions and specific pharmacotherapeutic regimens would you recommend for treating this
patient's diarrhea?

Outcome Evaluation

5. What clinical and laboratory parameters are necessary to evaluate the diarrhea therapy for achievement of the desired outcome
and to detect or prevent adverse effects?

Patient Education

6. What information should be provided to this patient to enhance
adherence, ensure successful therapy, minimize adverse effects,
and help prevent possible transmission to others?

■ FOLLOW-UP QUESTIONS

1. How should this patient's contraception be managed after she
is rehydrated and returns home?

2. Does the patient need any changes in her prophylactic migraine
headache therapy?

3. How should her IBS be managed?

4. Is there a relationship between the development of IBS and bacterial gastroenteritis?

■ CLINICAL COURSE

The treatment and monitoring plan you recommended was initiated on admission. The patient's diarrhea slowed by the evening of day 1. The patient had no further episodes of diarrhea or vomiting after midnight. On the morning of day 2, her orthostasis had resolved, her temperature was normal, the IV fluids were stopped, and she received clear liquids by mouth for breakfast and lunch. The patient was discharged during the late afternoon.

■ SELF-STUDY ASSIGNMENTS

1. Identify the infectious causes of diarrhea. Design an effective pharmacotherapy treatment regimen for each cause.

2. Provide recommendations for the prevention of traveler's diarrhea.

3. Describe whether or not antidiarrheal drug products can be safely recommended for use in very young children (<3 years old) or in patients with bloody diarrhea and, if so, the specific products that could be used.

4. Describe when oral rehydration products should be used, and recommend a specific product and dosage for young or older patients who present with mild to moderate diarrhea and minimal dehydration.

CLINICAL PEARL

Broad-spectrum antibiotics (especially clindamycin and the fluoroquinolones) are a common cause of *Clostridium difficile* colitis. Diarrhea is a common sign of the disease and may begin 3 days after initiating an antibiotic or up to 3 months after a course of antibiotics (the Rule of 3's).

REFERENCES

1. DuPont HL. Acute infectious diarrhea in immunocompetent adults. N Engl J Med 2014;370:1532–1540.

2. Barr W, Smith A. Acute diarrhea. Am Fam Physician 2014;89:180–189.

3. Pawlowski SW, Warren CA, Guerrant R. Diagnosis and treatment of acute or persistent diarrhea. Gastroenterology 2009;136:1874–1886.

4. Hatchette TF, Farina D. Infectious diarrhea: when to test and when to treat. CMAJ 2011;183:339–344.

5. Pulling M, Surawicz CM. Loperamide use for acute infectious diarrhea in children: safe and sound? Gastroenterology 2008;134:1260–1262.

6. Sarowska J, Choroszy-Król I, Regulska-Ilow B, Frej-Mądrzak M, Jama-Kmiecik A. The therapeutic effect of probiotic bacteria on gastrointestinal diseases. Adv Clin Exp Med 2013;22:759–766.

7. Sayuk GS, Gyawali CP. Irritable bowel syndrome: modern concepts and management options. Am J Med 2015;128:817–827.

8. Applegate JA, Walker CLF, Ambikapathi R, Black RE. Systematic review of probiotics for the treatment of community-acquired acute diarrhea in children. BMC Public Health 2013;13(Suppl 3):S16.

9. Ford AC, Talley NJ. Irritable bowel syndrome. BMJ 2012;345:e5836. doi:10.1136/bmj.e5836.

10. Beatty JK, Bhargava A, Buret AG. Post-infectious irritable bowel syndrome: mechanistic insights into chronic disturbances following enteric infection. World J Gastroenterol 2014;20:3976–3985.

42

IRRITABLE BOWEL SYNDROME

Life in the Slow Lane .... Level II

Nancy S. Yunker, PharmD, FCCP, BCPS

LEARNING OBJECTIVES

After completing this case study, the reader should be able to:

- Determine the signs and symptoms of irritable bowel syndrome associated with constipation (IBS-C).

- Devise patient management strategies for patients with IBS, including pharmacologic and nonpharmacologic options.

- Recommend parameters for monitoring the safety and efficacy of therapy used in patients with IBS-C.

- Discuss treatment options for IBS with diarrhea (IBS-D).

- Evaluate the efficacy of treatment options for patients with IBS.

PATIENT PRESENTATION

■ Chief Complaint

"My IBS is acting up again. I feel all bloated and I really have to strain to have a bowel movement. I have been really uncomfortable for the past 4 weeks. Most recently, I added Metamucil tablets to the docusate I was already taking because someone in the past told me that I would probably be able to tolerate the tablets better than Metamucil powder. I haven't seen much improvement in the 8 weeks that I have been using them, plus it is hard to remember to take them three times a day. I have tried to live with this but I really think I need to try something else. Is there anything you can give me?"

■ HPI

Jane Hoffman is a 28-year-old woman who presents to her PCP with the chief complaint of a 7-month history of hard pelletlike stools and difficulty passing stools. She was diagnosed with IBS her freshman year in college. She has been able to tolerate the minimal symptoms until about 8 months ago when she began to notice some bloating and a decrease in the number of bowel movements per week. She states that she now constantly feels bloated and has taken to wearing loose-fitting clothing because she cannot tolerate anything tight around her abdomen. She attributes the worsening symptoms to the stress associated with trying to complete classes for a graduate degree and serving as a TA for two courses. In addition to the 20 hours a week that she serves as a TA, she also works at least two weekends a month in a department store as a sales assistant. She also states the symptoms have gotten worse since she went back to school. In the last 2 years, they have been worse when she has midterms or finals or when she needs to complete a major college writing assignment. Other than stress, she cannot think of anything else that has changed in her life. She does not remember having any gastroenteritis symptoms in the last year, and she dislikes eating yogurt.

Prior to 8 months ago, she states that she averaged about six stools a week. She estimates that she has had one or two bowel movements a week for the past 6 weeks. She complains of straining to pass her stools and states that she is getting up 60 minutes early in the morning to allow for an attempt to pass a stool and uses the additional time exercising in order to "stimulate her bowels." She also tried eating more bran products, but felt like that made the pain and bloating worse, so she stopped. She states that the abdominal pain is not limited to when she passes a stool. She complains of abdominal pain and bloating almost continuously throughout the day for the past 2 months, although her symptoms are somewhat alleviated by passing a "good stool." She resumed taking docusate 8 months ago. She briefly took senna in addition to the docusate, but found that she sometimes had to go to the bathroom at inopportune times and felt that it caused additional cramping. She tried psyllium powder several years ago, but hated the taste. She thought about MiraLAX, but her mother took that prior to a GI procedure and said that it caused diarrhea, so the patient is hesitant to try it with all her responsibilities.

■ PMH

Seasonal allergies
Headaches
Anxiety
UTIs

■ PSH

Cholecystectomy 2 years ago

■ FH

Lives alone. She separated from her boyfriend 2 months ago due to school and other job commitments. She became solely responsible for the apartment rent when he left. He has been "hassling" her recently, and there is a question of verbal and physical abuse. Her mother is alive with HTN and recently had an MI, and her father is alive with hypercholesterolemia. No siblings.

■ SH

No alcohol use or smoking. No history of military service.

■ Meds

Diphenhydramine 25 mg orally Q 6 hours allergy symptoms
Ibuprofen 200 mg, two tablets orally Q 4–6 hours PRN headaches, menstrual cramps
Metamucil 0.52 g, 4 capsules orally three times a day
Docusate 100 mg orally twice daily
Ortho-Novum 1/35 (discontinued 2 months ago)

■ All

NKDA

■ ROS

Occasional headaches, usually associated with stress or allergy symptoms; occasional nausea, no vomiting; (−) blood in the stool or tarry stools; (+) flatulence and bloating. States that the abdominal symptoms may improve at night before bedtime especially if she uses a heating pad; she is not awakened at night with abdominal pain.

■ Physical Examination

Gen

A & O, WDWN pleasant Caucasian female appearing slightly anxious

VS

BP 116/78, P 68, RR 18, T 37.0°C; Wt 61 kg, Ht 5′6″

Skin

Dry skin on lower extremities, no rashes noted

HEENT

PERRLA, EOMI, moist mucus membranes, TMs intact

Neck/Lymph Nodes

No thyromegaly, lymphadenopathy, or JVD

Lungs

CTA; no rales or rhonchi

Breasts

Symmetric; no lumps or masses detected; nipples without discharge

CV

RRR, normal S_1 and S_2; no S_3 or S_4

Abd

(+) BS, slightly tender in LLQ, no HSM

Genit/Rect

Vulva normal; no palpable rectal masses; brown stool with no occult blood; no hemorrhoids

MS/Ext

No CCE, pulses 2+, normal ROM, normal strength bilaterally

■ Labs

Na 142 mEq/L	WBC 5.2×10^3/mm^3
K 4.0 mEq/L	Hgb 14.1 g/dL
Cl 106 mEq/L	Hct 42.4%
CO_2 27 mEq/L	
BUN 9 mg/dL	
SCr 0.8 mg/dL	
Glu 88 mg/dL	

Lactulose H_2 breath test: Negative
Serum pregnancy test: Negative

■ Other

FBDSI score: 66
IBS-SSS score: 300

■ Assessment

IBS associated with abdominal discomfort, bloating, and constipation

QUESTIONS

Problem Identification

1.a. Create a list of the patient's drug therapy problems.

1.b. What information (signs, symptoms, and laboratory values) indicates the presence and severity of IBS-C? What are the pertinent negative findings in this patient?

1.c. Could any of the patient's problems have been caused by drug therapy?

1.d. What additional information is needed to satisfactorily assess this patient?

Desired Outcome

2. Differentiate the patient's goals of therapy from those of her health care providers.

Therapeutic Alternatives

3.a. What nondrug therapies might be useful for this patient?

3.b. What feasible pharmacotherapeutic alternatives are available for the treatment of IBS-C?

3.c. What pharmacotherapeutic alternatives are available for the treatment of IBS-D?

Optimal Plan

4.a. What drug, dosage form, dose, schedule, and duration of therapy are best for this patient?

4.b. What alternatives would be appropriate if the initial therapy fails or cannot be used?

Outcome Evaluation

5. What clinical and laboratory parameters are necessary to evaluate the therapy for achievement of the desired therapeutic outcome and to detect or prevent adverse effects?

Patient Education

6. What information should be provided to the patient to enhance compliance, ensure successful therapy, and minimize adverse effects?

■ CLINICAL COURSE

The patient returns to the physician 6 weeks later and reports that her symptoms are much improved and that the abdominal pain has resolved. She is happy with her medication regimen, but her friends have suggested that herbal medications may be just as effective. She would like more information about the use of these products for IBS.

■ FOLLOW-UP QUESTIONS

1. What therapeutic regimen would you recommend for the patient at this time?

2. What information would you provide regarding the addition or substitution of alternative medications (eg, herbal medications) to this patient's regimen?

■ SELF-STUDY ASSIGNMENTS

1. Conduct a literature search to determine what types of alternative therapies, including probiotics, have been evaluated in IBS. Include a discussion of the scientific rigor of these studies.

2. Conduct an informal survey among friends, family members, coworkers, and fellow students about the incidence of IBS and what therapeutic options they would recommend to a person suffering from IBS.

3. Conduct a search of IBS drug treatment studies on www.clinicaltrials.gov and conduct a literature search to identify new and emerging therapies for IBS. Determine the commercial availability of these agents or potential research trial referral centers.

4. Discuss the hypothesized pathogenesis of irritable bowel syndrome including the disorder of the brain–gut axis, disturbed motility, impaired gut barrier function, visceral hypersensitivity, immunologic and infectious causation, genetic factors, psychosocial factors, and dietary alterations.

CLINICAL PEARL

Agents acting on serotonergic receptors have been used in IBS due to their ability to alter gastrointestinal transit. Ondansetron, a 5-HT$_3$ receptor antagonist approved for nausea and vomiting has been shown to improve stool consistency, urgency, and bloating in IBS patients with diarrhea but does not appear to result in pain relief.

REFERENCES

1. Ford AC, Moayyedi P, Lacy BE, Lembo AJ, for the Task Force on the Management of Functional Bowel Disorders. American College of Gastroenterology Monograph on the management of irritable bowel syndrome and chronic idiopathic constipation. Am J Gastroenterol 2014;109(Suppl 1):S2–S26.
2. Chey WD, Kurlander J, Eswaran S. Irritable bowel syndrome: a clinical review. JAMA 2015;313:949–958.
3. Thomas RH, Luthin DR. Current and emerging treatments for irritable bowel syndrome with constipation and chronic idiopathic constipation: focus on prosecretory agents. Pharmacotherapy 2015;35:613–630.
4. Chang L, Lembo A, Sultan S. American Gastroenterological Association Institute technical review on the pharmacological management of irritable bowel syndrome. Gastroenterology 2014;147:1149–1172.
5. Drossman DA, Chang L, Bellamy N, et al. Severity in irritable bowel syndrome: a Rome Foundation Working Team report. Am J Gastroenterol 2011;106:1749–1759.
6. Sayuk GS, Gyawali CP. Irritable bowel syndrome: modern concepts and management options. Am J Med 2015;128:817–827.
7. American College of Gastroenterology IBS Task Force. An evidence-based systematic review on the management of irritable bowel syndrome. Am J Gastroenterol 2009;104(Suppl 1):S8–S35.
8. Hookway C, Buckner S, Crosland P, Longson D. Irritable bowel syndrome in adults in primary care: summary of updated NICE guidance. BMJ 2015;350:h701.
9. Halland M, Saito YA. Irritable bowel syndrome: new and emerging treatments. BMJ 2015;350:h1622. doi:10.1136/bmj.h1622.
10. Moayyedi P, Quigley EMM, Lacy BE, et al. The effect of fiber supplementation on irritable bowel syndrome: a systematic review and meta-analysis. Am J Gastroenterol 2014;109:1367–1374.
11. Garnock-Jones KP. Eluxadoline: first global approval. Drugs 2015;75:1305–1310.

43

PEDIATRIC GASTROENTERITIS

One Thing You *Should* Try at Home .... Level II

William McGhee, PharmD

Laura M. Panko, MD, FAAP

LEARNING OBJECTIVES

After completing this case study, the reader should be able to:

- Recognize the signs and symptoms of diarrhea with dehydration and be able to assess the severity of the problem.

- Describe the two available rotavirus vaccines, compare their dosage and availability, compare their safety and efficacy with the previously available vaccine, and explain their potential impact on rotavirus-induced diarrhea.

- Recommend appropriate oral rehydration therapy (ORT) products and treatment regimens for varying degrees of dehydration severity.

- Properly assess the effectiveness of ORT using both clinical and laboratory parameters.

- Be able to educate parents about the limited usefulness of all antidiarrheal products and the role of ondansetron and probiotics in the treatment of acute diarrhea in children.

- Identify the signs and symptoms of severe dehydration that require referral to an ED for immediate IV volume replacement.

PATIENT PRESENTATION

■ Chief Complaint

Lydia Mason is a 9-month-old female who presented to the ED with a 3-day history of fever, vomiting, and diarrhea.

■ HPI

The child was in her baseline state of health, having just been seen by her pediatrician for her 9-month well-child check earlier in the week. Three days before presentation, she was noted to have a tactile fever, confirmed at 100.4°F (38.0°C) axillary, as well as diminished energy. Two days before presentation, she awoke from sleep, experiencing nonbilious, nonbloody emesis. Throughout that day, she had five similar episodes of vomiting, typically after attempts at oral intake. She continued to have low-grade fevers.

One day before presentation to the ED, she had only two episodes of emesis, but she developed diarrhea. The stools, totaling five that day, were initially described as slightly formed. As the day progressed, the stools became watery, voluminous, and contained small specks of blood. The patient's appetite continued to be poor, with very limited solid intake. On the pediatrician's recommendation, the family offered the patient liquids including formula, water, and Pedialyte, but she refused, preferring cola and diluted apple juice.

On the morning of presentation to the ED, the patient had another large, watery stool and was unusually fussy. Her diaper was dry, with no urine output the night prior. The family could

not accurately assess the number of wet diapers she had in the last 24 hours, given the difficulty distinguishing watery stool from urine. They also noted that her lips appeared dry and she had diminished tears.

■ PMH

Lydia was born at 38 weeks via spontaneous vaginal delivery without complications. She required 1 day of phototherapy for hyperbilirubinemia. She was discharged from the nursery within 3 days of birth. She has experienced approximately six upper respiratory tract infections and two episodes of otitis media, all after introduction into daycare at 7 weeks of age. These illnesses have not resulted in hospitalization or ED visitation.

No sick contacts were noted until the day she presented to the ED, when the patient's mother developed abdominal discomfort and loose stools. In addition, multiple infants at the daycare Lydia attends were experiencing similar symptoms.

Immunizations are up-to-date. Development is normal.

■ FH

Lydia's mother and father are 29 years old and in good health. There are two older siblings aged 3 and 6, who have been well.

■ SH

Lydia lives with her parents and siblings. There are two pet fish in the home but no reptile or other animal exposures. The patient attends daycare three times a week. The family uses city water and has not traveled out of state recently. Her diet consists of cow's milk-based infant formula and a myriad of solid foods. There has been no exposure to undercooked meats or fish.

■ Meds

Multivitamin. No prescriptions or over the counter medications.

■ All

NKDA, no food allergies

■ ROS

Negative except as noted in the HPI

■ Physical Examination

Gen

Patient is ill-appearing but nontoxic. She is very fussy during the examination but consoled by her mother with some effort.

VS

BP 92/50, P 145, RR 42, T 38.4°C (R); Wt 8.2 kg (50–75%) (Wt 5 days earlier at well-child check 9.0 kg)

Skin

Pink, mild tenting noted, capillary refill 2–3 seconds

HEENT

Anterior fontanelle sunken, eyes moderately sunken, scant tears, nose with clear rhinorrhea, lips and tongue dry, TMs gray and translucent

Neck/Lymph Nodes

Normal

Lungs/Thorax

Tachypneic; no focal findings, including wheezes, rales, or rhonchi; no retractions or grunting

Heart

Tachycardic, 1/6 flow murmur, normal pulses

Abd

Distended, hyperactive bowel sounds; no focal tenderness, masses, or hepatosplenomegaly

Genit/Rect

Normal female genitalia, mild diaper dermatitis

MS/Ext

Normal

Neuro

Sleepy but arousable; very fussy when awake; no focal defects

■ Labs

Na 137 mEq/L	Hgb 12.8 g/dL	WBC $14.0 \times 10^3/mm^3$
K 4.4 mEq/L	Hct 41%	Polys 52%
Cl 113 mEq/L	Plt $300 \times 10^3/mm^3$	Bands 5%
CO_2 14 mEq/L		Eos 0%
BUN 23 mg/dL		Basos 3%
SCr 0.4 mg/dL		Lymphs 24%
Glu 80 mg/dL		Monos 16%

■ UA

Specific gravity 1.029; ketones 2+; otherwise negative.

■ Assessment

1. Typical viral gastroenteritis, likely rotavirus infection
2. Dehydration with metabolic acidosis

QUESTIONS

Problem Identification

1.a. Create a list of the patient's drug therapy problems.

1.b. What information (signs, symptoms, laboratory values) indicates the presence or severity of gastroenteritis?

Desired Outcome

2. What are the goals of pharmacotherapy in this case?

Therapeutic Alternatives

3.a. What nondrug therapies might be useful for this patient?

3.b. What feasible pharmacotherapeutic alternatives are available for treating this patient's diarrhea?

Optimal Plan

4.a. What drug(s), dosage forms, schedule, and duration of therapy are best for this patient?

4.b. What is the efficacy and safety record of the available rotavirus vaccines, and what impact have they had on preventing rotavirus-induced diarrhea?

Outcome Evaluation

5. What clinical and laboratory parameters should be monitored to evaluate therapy for achievement of the desired therapeutic outcome?

Patient Education

6. What information should be provided to the child's parents to enhance compliance, ensure successful therapy, and minimize adverse effects?

■ SELF-STUDY ASSIGNMENTS

1. Explain the limitations of using probiotics for treating pediatric gastroenteritis including lack of FDA oversight, purity and standardization of products, lack of recognized treatment regimens, and safety concerns. Write a brief educational document explaining to parents when the use of probiotics should be considered in acute viral gastroenteritis.

2. What role does zinc supplementation have in the treatment of diarrhea in developing countries? Describe the rationale for its use and the most efficient way to administer it.

3. What barriers exist to the widespread implementation of ORT, including parents and physicians? How can these barriers be overcome? (*Hint*: Explore the advantages of ORT vs IV rehydration therapy, including ease of care at home vs hospitalization, insurance issues, and physician reluctance.)

4. Write a two-page essay describing the role of the community-based practitioner in the care of patients with pediatric gastroenteritis and dehydration. Emphasize how you would monitor patient safety and outcome and what you would tell the parents to optimize treatment at home.

CLINICAL PEARL

ORT is equivalent to IV therapy in rehydrating children with gastroenteritis and diarrhea with mild to moderate dehydration. It is the standard of care in the treatment of these patients and usually can be performed at home. Antidiarrheal, antiemetic, probiotic, and antimicrobial therapies are rarely necessary. IV rehydration is necessary only in patients with severe dehydration.

REFERENCES

1. Fischer TK, Viboud C, Parashur U, et al. Hospitalizations and deaths from diarrhea and rotavirus among children <5 years of age in the United States, 1993–2003. J Infect Dis 2007;195:1117–1125.

2. Tate JR, Burton AH, Boschi-Pinto C, et al. 2008 estimate of worldwide rotavirus-associated mortality in children younger than 5 years before the introduction of universal rotavirus vaccination programs: a systematic review and meta-analysis. Lancet Infect Dis 2012;12:136–141.

3. Centers for Disease Control and Prevention. Updated norovirus outbreak management and disease prevention guidelines. MMWR Morb Mortal Wkly Rep 2011;60(3):1–15.

4. Guarino A, Albano F, Ashkenazi S, et al. European Society for Paediatric Gastroenterology, Hepatology, and Nutrition/European Society for Paediatric Infectious Diseases evidence-based guidelines for the management of acute gastroenteritis in children in Europe. J Pediatr Gastroenterol Nutr 2008;46(Suppl 2):S81–S122.

5. Allen SJ, Martinez EG, Gregorio GV, Dans LF. Probiotics for treating acute infectious diarrhea. Cochrane Database Syst Rev 2010;(11):CD003048. doi:10.1002/14651858.CD003048.pub3.

6. Freedman SB, Steiner MJ, Chan KJ. Oral ondansetron administration in emergency departments to children with gastroenteritis: An economic analysis. PLoS Med 2010;7(10):e10000350. doi:10.1371/journal/pmed.1000350.

7. Carter B, Fedorowicz Z. Antiemetic treatment for acute gastroenteritis in children: an updated Cochrane systematic review with meta-analysis and mixed treatment comparison in a Bayesian framework. BMJ Open 2012;2:e000622. doi:10.1136/bmjopen-2011-000622.

8. Nunez J, Liu DR, Nager AL. Dehydration Treatment Practices Among Pediatrics-Trained and Non-Pediatrics Trained Emergency Physicians. Pediatric Emerg Care 2012;28:322–328.

9. Freedman SB, Uleryk E, Rumantir M, Finkelstein Y. Ondansetron and the risk of cardiac arrhythmias: a systematic review and postmarketing analysis. Ann Emerg Med 2014;64.19–25.

10. Boom JA, Tate JE, Sahni LC, et al. Effectiveness of pentavalent rotavirus vaccine in a large urban population in the United States. Pediatrics 2010;125:e199–e207. doi:10.1542/peds.2012-3804.

44

CONSTIPATION

All Bound Up . . . . Level II

Michelle Fravel, PharmD, BCPS

Beth Bryles Phillips, PharmD, FCCP, BCPS

LEARNING OBJECTIVES

After completing this case study, the reader should be able to:

- Identify medications that can exacerbate constipation.

- Describe the advantages and disadvantages of each class of laxatives and discuss the appropriate use of each class.

- Recommend an appropriate plan for the treatment of constipation, including lifestyle modifications and drug therapy.

- Educate patients regarding laxative therapy.

PATIENT PRESENTATION

Chief Complaint

"I feel just awful ever since starting these pain pills—I think I'd rather be in pain!"

HPI

Kerry Reynolds is a 64-year-old woman who presents to the ED complaining of increasing abdominal cramping and nausea for several days and now vomiting for the past several hours. She says this all started when she began Percocet therapy 2 weeks ago for postprocedural pain in association with right TKA. Her last bowel movement was 6 days ago. She began "not feeling well" 4 days ago, with bloating, decreased appetite, decreased thirst, and fatigue. She reports that yesterday, when her cramping was at its worst, she even used a couple doses of Metamucil, but it did not help. She says she was almost to the point where she thought about trying some powerful laxatives, but she has heard about the addiction they can cause and the last thing she wants is to be addicted to a laxative. She

has also tried to just quit taking the pain meds altogether, but she only makes it about halfway through the morning before the pain becomes unbearable. She reports that she has cut back on the pain pills and is only taking one pill four times a day now, compared with a week ago when she was taking two pills four times a day. On a scale of 1–10, with 1 being no pain and 10 being the worst pain ever experienced, she rates her pain at a 5 today. She does say the pain is improving every day. Her plan is to take one less pain pill every 3 days so that she can successfully taper the meds in about 2 weeks. She reports no fever, CP, or SOB. She states that she typically has daily bowel movements, with no straining, and spends less than 10 minutes, with little effort, having a bowel movement. Her last colonoscopy, performed 2 years ago, was unremarkable.

PMH

Hypothyroidism
Diabetes mellitus type 2
Hypertension
Dyslipidemia
Osteoarthritis

FH

Her mother is in her 80s and is healthy. Her father died in his 60s from heart disease. She has three brothers and three sisters; one brother has type 2 diabetes. She has two sons who are healthy.

SH

She is married and works as a social worker. She quit smoking >20 years ago. She does not drink alcohol and does not use illicit drugs.

ROS

(+) For constipation, lower abdominal fullness, N/V, right knee pain, (−) for SOB, CP, or fever/chills.

Meds

Diltiazem CR 240 mg PO daily
Chlorthalidone 25 mg PO daily
Levothyroxine 50 mcg PO daily
Metformin 1000 mg PO twice daily
Simvastatin 20 mg PO at bedtime
Multivitamin one tablet PO daily
Warfarin 5 mg daily × 5 weeks for VTE prophylaxis as directed by Anticoagulation Clinic
Oxycodone/acetaminophen 5 mg/325 mg one to two tablets Q 4–6 hours PRN

All
NKDA

Physical Examination

Gen

Pleasant woman in distress because of abdominal discomfort; is visibly uncomfortable and holding her stomach during the visit; appears tired

VS

BP 122/60, P 57, RR 16, T 36.2°C; Wt 112.4 kg, Ht 5′5″; waist circumference 37 in; pain rated 5 on scale of 1–10

Skin

Normal skin turgor and color

HEENT

PERRLA and EOM full without nystagmus; no scleral icterus; oral mucosa moist; no ulcerations noted

Neck/Lymph Nodes

Supple, no lymphadenopathy or JVD; no thyromegaly or bruits

CV

Regular, S_1 and S_2 without murmur

Lungs

Normal breath sounds; no crackles or wheezes

Abd

Soft, obese, tender; decreased bowel sounds; stool palpable on left side

Rectal

Stool present in rectal vault; no masses felt; tone fair; push strength fair; nontender

MS/Ext

S/P right TKA; surgical wound healing appropriately; no redness, swelling, exudation; range of motion within normal limits

Neuro

A & O × 3; CNs II–XII symmetric and intact; DTRs 2+

■ Labs

Na 138 mEq/L	Glu 133 mg/dL (fasting)	RBC 6.05 × 10⁶/mm³
K 3.7 mEq/L	A1C 6.4%	Hgb 15.5 g/dL
Cl 101 mEq/L	Ca 9.3 mg/dL	Hct 48%
CO_2 30 mEq/L	TSH 2.70 mIU/mL	MCV 79 μm³
BUN 14 mg/dL	INR 2.4	MCH 26 pg
SCr 0.8 mg/dL		MCHC 33%
ACR 227 mg/g		RDW 15.4%

■ Assessment

Constipation with fecal impaction; secondary symptoms of abdominal discomfort, nausea, and vomiting; etiology likely drug-induced.

■ Plan

Obtain abdominal x-ray and CT scan to rule out other potential causes of constipation; perform disimpaction.

■ Clinical Course

A plain x-ray of the abdomen showed gas-dilated loops in the colon. An abdominal CT scan was then performed and showed a large amount of stool in the colon and rectal vault. Disimpaction was successfully performed with no complications. A follow-up PEG-based bowel preparation was successful in clearing bowel and relieving the patient's abdominal pain. An appropriate medication regimen was recommended to maintain regular bowel function over the next 2 weeks while she continues her opioid therapy.

QUESTIONS

Identification

1.a. Develop a list of the potential therapy problems in this patient other than those related to her constipation.

1.b. What signs or symptoms are indicative of constipation in this patient?

1.c. What are some of the possible nonpharmacologic contributors to her constipation?

1.d. What are some of the possible pharmacologic contributors to constipation in this patient?

1.e. What information should be obtained from a patient who presents with a chief complaint of constipation?

Desired Outcome

2. What are the goals of pharmacotherapy in treating constipation?

Therapeutic Alternatives

3.a. What are some nonpharmacologic steps useful in treating constipation?

3.b. What are the pharmacologic options for the treatment of constipation?

3.c. Is this patient's current regimen for hypertension appropriate? If not, what recommendations can you make to optimize this regimen?

Optimal Plan

4. After nonpharmacologic measures have been attempted, what would be the most appropriate choice of drug therapy for her, including dose and schedule? Provide the rationale for your answer.

Outcome Evaluation

5.a. How would you monitor this patient to ensure that your pharmacotherapeutic goals have been achieved? How would you follow up with her to ensure resolution of the constipation?

■ CLINICAL COURSE

The recommendations you made were implemented, and Ms Reynolds returns to your clinic 1 month later. She reports that the drug therapy you recommended resulted in regular bowel function throughout the last 2 weeks of her opioid therapy. She does report, however, that her orthopedic physicians have now recommended TKA on the opposite leg. She says that after the last episode with constipation, she just does not think she wants to go through with it.

5.b. You reassure the patient that this problem can be prevented with her next surgery and that you will discuss options with her physicians. What regimen would you recommend for preventing opioid-induced constipation in this patient if she chooses to go through with the second TKA procedure?

Patient Education

6.a. What education would you provide to this patient who has concerns about recurrence of drug-induced constipation?

6.b. What education would you provide to this patient regarding her concerns about laxative addiction?

6.c. When instructing this patient on using a stimulant laxative, what information should you convey to ensure appropriate use of this product?

■ SELF-STUDY ASSIGNMENTS

1. Suggest pharmacotherapeutic options for the treatment of opioid-induced constipation in a pediatric patient. How does this approach compare with that used in treatment of adults?

2. Perform a literature search to find medications under investigation for the treatment of constipation. What different types of constipation will these new entities be used to treat? What place in therapy will these medications have?

CLINICAL PEARL

When a patient presents with constipation, obtain a detailed medication history, because medications commonly cause constipation. Management of medication-related constipation may include discontinuation of the offending agent with initiation of an appropriate alternative or initiation of a medication designed to address medication-related constipation. Failure to recognize medications as contributors to constipation may lead to inappropriate treatment and inadequate relief of constipation symptoms.

REFERENCES

1. American Diabetes Association. Standards of medical care in diabetes—2016. Diabetes Care 2016;39:S1–S112.

2. Panchal SJ, Muller-Schwefe P, Wurzelmann JI. Opioid-induced bowel dysfunction: prevalence, pathophysiology and burden. Int Clin Pract 2007;61:1181–1187.

3. Shah BJ, Rughwani N, Rose S. Constipation. Ann Intern Med 2015;162:ITC1. doi:10.7326/AITC201504070.

4. National Comprehensive Cancer Network. NCCN Clinical Practice Guidelines in Oncology: Palliative Care. V.1.2016 [Online]. Available at: *http://www.nccn.org/professionals/physician_gls/pdf/palliative.pdf.* Accessed September 3, 2016.

5. Thomas J, Darver S, Cooney GA, et al. Methylnaltrexone for opioid-induced constipation in advanced illness. N Engl J Med 2008;358:2332–2343.

6. Chey WD, Webster L, Sostek M, et al. Naloxegol for opioid-induced constipation in patients with noncancer pain. N Engl J Med 2014;370:2387–2396.

7. Davis M, Gamier P. New options in constipation management. Curr Oncol Rep 2015;17:55.

8. Tarumi Y, Wilson MP, Szafran O, et al. Randomized, double-blind, placebo-controlled trial of oral docusate in the management of constipation in hospice patients. J Pain Symptom Manage 2013;45:2–13.

45

ASCITES MANAGEMENT IN PORTAL HYPERTENSION AND CIRRHOSIS

Back to Drinking..............................Level II

Laurel A. Sampognaro, PharmD

Jeffery D. Evans, PharmD

LEARNING OBJECTIVES

After completing this case study, the reader should be able to:

- Identify signs and symptoms of cirrhosis and associated complications.

- Provide pharmacotherapeutic and lifestyle recommendations for managing ascites due to portal hypertension and cirrhosis.

- Develop a patient-specific regimen and monitoring parameters to meet the needs of a patient with ascites, esophageal varices, and hepatic encephalopathy.

- Interpret laboratory values associated with ascites.

- Provide appropriate patient education for the recommended pharmacologic and nonpharmacologic therapy to control complications of cirrhosis, as well as to prevent further complications.

PATIENT PRESENTATION

■ Chief Complaint

"I look like I'm pregnant and it's getting worse."

■ HPI

Robert Smith is a 38-year-old man with a history of alcoholic cirrhosis who has been admitted to the hospital due to an unexplained 8-kg weight gain over the past 6 days, abdominal swelling and pain, shortness of breath, and mild confusion.

■ PMH

Alcoholic cirrhosis diagnosed 2 years ago, Child–Pugh Grade A on diagnosis
EGD performed at time of cirrhosis diagnosis showed no esophageal varices
Allergic rhinitis
Hypertension

■ FH

Father is alive and well at the age of 70 without significant disease. Mother died at age 47 due to complications of type 1 DM.

■ SH

Recently separated from wife of 10 years and lives alone. Works as a plumber. History of extreme alcohol abuse but had quit drinking on cirrhosis diagnosis. Admits to heavy alcohol use over the past 2 months since separating from his wife and went on a drinking binge about 1 week ago.

■ Meds

Fluticasone furoate two sprays per nostril once daily
Levocetirizine 5 mg once daily
Lisinopril 10 mg once daily

■ All

NKDA

■ ROS

Abdominal discomfort described as occurring throughout the abdomen, shortness of breath, and mild confusion. Patient denies chills or fevers.

■ Physical Examination

Gen

Pleasant, chronically ill black man appearing to be in mild distress and fatigued

VS

BP 118/76, P 78, RR 27, T 37.2°C; Wt 94.2 kg, Ht 6′2″

Skin

(+) Palmar erythema, (+) spider angiomata, otherwise normal color

HEENT

PERRL, EOMI, clear sclerae, TMs normal, mucous membranes moist

Neck/Lymph Nodes

Supple, no thyroid nodules

Lung/Thorax

Mild bilateral crackles, decreased breath sounds in right lower lobe likely due to enlarged liver and ascites

Breasts

Nontender without masses

CV

RRR, S_1 and S_2 are normal, no MRG

Abd

Bulging, tender abdomen; hepatomegaly; (+) fluid wave; bowel sounds normal

Genit/Rect

Guaiac negative

MS/Ext

1+ pitting edema in both LE, palmar erythema; no clubbing or cyanosis

Neuro

Mildly confused, forgetful, A & O × 2 (oriented to person and time but does not know at which hospital he is)

■ Labs

Na 135 mEq/L	Hgb 16 g/dL	AST 88 IU/L	Ca 8.5 mg/dL
K 4.1 mEq/L	Hct 47%	ALT 116 IU/L	Mg 1.9 mEq/L
Cl 98 mEq/L	Plt 81 × 10³/mm³	LDH 167 IU/L	Phos 3.5 mg/dL
CO₂ 30 mEq/L	WBC 6.2 × 10³/mm³	T. bili 2.2 mg/dL	TSH 3.6 mIU/L
BUN 19 mg/dL	PT 14.3 s	D. bili 0.7 mg/dL	NH₃ 94 mcg/dL
SCr 0.7 mg/dL	PTT 47 s	T. prot 7.3 g/dL	HIV (−)
Glu 97 mg/dL	INR 1.33	Alb 2.8 g/dL	

■ Assessment

Worsening cirrhosis; now presenting with ascites and acute encephalopathy
Perform diagnostic and therapeutic paracentesis
R/O spontaneous bacterial peritonitis (SBP)

■ Clinical Course

After removal of 5 L of fluid by paracentesis, an analysis of the fluid was performed. The analysis reported a protein level of 1.4 g/dL, PMN 140 cells/mm³, and SAAG 1.4 g/dL.

The culture results were negative after 3 days.

The patient's mental status began to improve after paracentesis and the administration of lactulose 30 mL PO twice daily.

Once stabilized, an EGD was performed, which showed small esophageal varices.

QUESTIONS

Problem Identification

1.a. Create a list of the patient's drug therapy problems.

1.b. What information (signs, symptoms, lab values) indicates the presence of ascites in this patient?

1.c. What information (signs, symptoms, lab values) indicates the presence or absence of hepatic encephalopathy and SBP in this patient?

1.d. What classification system is used to evaluate the prognosis of chronic liver disease? Use this system to calculate the score and grade for this patient.

Desired Outcome

2. What are the goals of pharmacotherapy for managing ascites and related complications of cirrhosis?

Therapeutic Alternatives

3.a. What nonpharmacologic therapies might be considered for this patient?

3.b. What pharmacologic therapies should be considered for this patient?

Optimal Plan

4.a. Outline a suitable pharmaceutical care plan for the *acute* management of this patient. Include drug, dosage form, dose, dosing schedule, and duration of therapy.

4.b. Outline a suitable pharmacologic care plan for the *chronic* management of this patient. Include drug, dosage form, dose, dosing schedule, and duration of therapy.

4.c. If the initial therapy fails or is intolerable for the patient, what pharmacologic alternatives should be considered?

Outcome Evaluation

5. How should the recommended therapy be monitored for efficacy and adverse effects?

Patient Education

6. On discharge from the hospital, what information should be provided to the patient to enhance compliance, ensure successful treatment, and minimize or prevent adverse effects?

■ ADDITIONAL CASE QUESTIONS

1. What other diseases should the patient be tested for that could impact his liver function?

2. What vaccinations should he receive on discharge, assuming that he has not had any vaccinations for over 20 years?

■ SELF-STUDY ASSIGNMENTS

1. Identify which pain medications may be used safely in patients with cirrhosis and ascites.

2. Based on this patient's history, what 1-, 2-, and 5-year survival rates would be expected if the patient does not receive a liver transplant?

CLINICAL PEARL

Lactulose is considered by many and mentioned in the guidelines as a first-line agent in the prevention of recurrent hepatic encephalopathy secondary to cirrhosis. However, there is a limited amount of data justifying its use in these patients.

REFERENCES

1. Runyon B. Management of adult patients with ascites due to cirrhosis: update 2012. *American Association for the Study of Liver Diseases Practice Guidelines.* Available at: http://www.aasld.org/sites/default/files/guideline_documents/adultascitesenhanced.pdf. Accessed November 3, 2015.
2. Garcia-Tsao G, Sanyal A, Grace N, Carey W. Prevention and management of gastroesophageal varices and variceal hemorrhage in cirrhosis. Hepatology 2007;46:922–938.
3. Vilstrup H1, Amodio P, Bajaj J, et al. Hepatic encephalopathy in chronic liver disease: 2014 Practice Guideline by the American Association for the Study of Liver Diseases and the European Association for the Study of the Liver. Hepatology 2014;60:715–735.
4. Boyer T, Haskal Z. The role of transjugular intrahepatic portosystemic shunt (TIPS) in the management of portal hypertension. Hepatology 2010;51:1–16.
5. Garcia-Tsao G, Lim J. Members of Veteran Affairs Hepatitis C Resource Center Program. Management and treatment of patients with cirrhosis and portal hypertension: recommendations from the Department of Veterans Affairs Hepatitis C Resource Center Program and National Hepatitis C Program. Am J Gastroenterol 2009;104:1802–1829.
6. O'Shea RS, Dasarathy S, McCullough AJ, et al. Alcoholic liver disease. Hepatology 2010;51:307–328.
7. Gines P, Cardenas A, Arroyo V, et al. Management of cirrhosis and ascites. N Engl J Med 2004;350:1646–1654.
8. Han M, Hyzy R. Advances in critical care management of hepatic failure and insufficiency. Crit Care Med 2006;34(9 Suppl):S225–S231.
9. Moore KP, Aithal GP. Guidelines on the management of ascites in cirrhosis. Gut 2006;55(Suppl 6):vi1–vi12.
10. Ge P, Runyon B. The changing role of beta-blocker therapy in patients with cirrhosis. J Hepatol 2014;60:643–653.

46

ESOPHAGEAL VARICES

Banding the Bleeding . . . . Level I

Vanessa T. Kline, PharmD, BCPS

Jonathan M. Kline, PharmD, CACP, BCPS, CDE

LEARNING OBJECTIVES

After completing this case study, the reader should be able to:

- List nonpharmacologic options for managing patients with bleeding esophageal varices.

- Recommend appropriate pharmacologic therapy for controlling bleeding esophageal varices and adjunctive therapy in the setting of acute variceal bleeding.

- Provide appropriate education for patients receiving therapy for portal hypertension.

PATIENT PRESENTATION

■ Chief Complaint

"I've been throwing up blood, enough to fill my bathroom sink!"

■ HPI

Ethyl Johnson is a 55-year-old woman who presents to the ED with complaint of vomiting blood and bright red blood per rectum. She was in her usual state of health, until shortly after taking a dose of lactulose when she began to feel sick and subsequently vomited a large amount of blood into the bathroom sink. She also reports a 2-day history of BRBPR.

■ PMH

Cirrhosis secondary to hepatitis C (acquired from a blood transfusion in 1980s)
Hepatic encephalopathy
Hepatitis C
Peptic ulcer disease
Hypertension
Cellulitis (two admissions in the past 3 years)

■ FH

Father with CAD and CABG; no other history known.

■ SH

She lives alone and has been able to function independently. Quit smoking 10 years ago and does not drink alcohol. She works as an accountant.

■ ROS

Negative except for complaints noted in HPI.

■ Meds

Sucralfate 1 g PO BID
Omeprazole 20 mg PO BID
Bumetanide 1 mg PO BID
Spironolactone 50 mg PO once daily
Propranolol 40 mg PO BID (may not be taking)

■ All

NKDA

■ Physical Examination

Gen

Obese female looking older than stated age, looks somnolent but occasionally moves head

VS

BP 108/60, P 120, RR 14, T 37.8°C

Skin

Some spider angiomas on abdomen, thick skin, chronic venous stasis changes with lichenification

HEENT

PERRLA; icteric sclerae

Neck/Lymph Nodes

Neck supple; no masses

Lungs/Thorax

Clear to auscultation bilaterally

Breasts

No lumps or masses

CV

Tachycardia, RRR, no M/R/G

Abd

Obese, mildly distended, distant bowel sounds present, difficult to assess for hepatosplenomegaly

Rect

Frank blood

Ext

Bilateral 1+ pedal edema

Neuro

Sleepy, moves head occasionally; is arousable and oriented × 3; no asterixis

▇ Labs (on Admission)

Na 127 mEq/L	Hgb 7.8 g/dL	AST 104 IU/L
K 4.3 mEq/L	Hct 24.4%	ALT 49 IU/L
Cl 101 mEq/L	WBC 26.4 × 10³/mm³	Alk phos 114 IU/L
CO₂ 22 mEq/L	Neutros 59%	T. bili 4.3 mg/dL
BUN 57 mg/dL	Bands 17%	D. bili 3.3 mg/dL
SCr 1.9 mg/dL	Lymphs 23%	Protein 5.5 g/dL
Glu 155 mg/dL	Monos 1%	Alb 2.5 g/dL
	Plt 68 × 10³/mm³	Ca 8.4 mg/dL
	aPTT 42.1 s	Phos 4.4 mg/dL
	PT 16.5 s	
	INR 1.8	

▇ EGD

There is a large esophageal varix, with one large red spot and bulge that began spurting blood during the procedure. Two bands were applied to varices in that area but could not do more due to large amount of blood (Fig. 46-1).

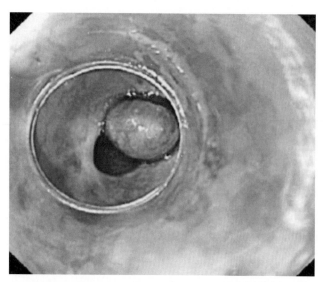

FIGURE 46-1. Endoscopic band ligation of esophageal varices. *(Reprinted with permission from Kasper DL, Fauci AS, Hauser SL, Longo DL, Jameson JL, Loscalzo J, eds. Harrison's Principles of Internal Medicine, 19th ed. New York, NY. McGraw Hill Education, 2015.)*

▇ Assessment

This is a 55-year-old woman with a history of chronic hepatitis C infection and cirrhosis who presents to the ED acutely ill after hematemesis secondary to bleeding esophageal varices. Labs show severe anemia, leukocytosis with left shift, hyponatremia, renal dysfunction, hypoalbuminemia, increased serum aminotransferases, and coagulopathy. The patient presents with Child–Pugh class C severity of disease. Will admit to an intensive care unit for further management.

QUESTIONS

Problem Identification

1.a. Create a list of the patient's drug therapy problems.

1.b. What information supports the diagnosis of bleeding esophageal varices, and what indicates the relative severity of disease?

Desired Outcome

2. What are the goals for managing this patient's clinical condition?

Therapeutic Alternatives

3.a. What nonpharmacologic interventions should be considered for this patient?

3.b. What pharmacologic interventions should be considered for this patient?

Optimal Plan

4. What pharmacotherapeutic plan should be implemented for managing the patient's current problems?

Outcome Evaluation

5. What clinical and laboratory parameters should be followed to evaluate the therapeutic interventions and to minimize the risk of adverse effects?

Patient Education

6. What information should be provided to the patient about her medication therapy?

▇ SELF-STUDY ASSIGNMENTS

1. Examine the relative effectiveness of nonpharmacologic therapies versus available pharmacologic treatments for the acute management of variceal bleeding.

2. Describe the effect of fluoroquinolone resistance on use of antibiotics in patients presenting with variceal hemorrhage.

3. Describe the dose-related side effects in patients receiving combination β-blocker and isosorbide mononitrate therapy.

CLINICAL PEARL

Although factor VII is often used in the setting of uncontrolled bleeding, randomized, controlled studies have not shown a significant benefit that outweighs the risk of thromboembolism in the management of variceal hemorrhage.

REFERENCES

1. Villanueva C, Colomo A, Bosch A, Concepción M, Hernandez-Gea V, Aracil C. Transfusion strategies for acute upper gastrointestinal bleeding. N Engl J Med 2013;368:11–21.

2. Garcia-Tsao G, Sanyal AJ, Grace ND, Carey W. Prevention and management of gastroesophageal varices and variceal hemorrhage in cirrhosis. Hepatology 2007;46:928–938.

3. Seo YS, Park SY, Kim MY, et al. Lack of difference among terlipressin, somatostatin, and octreotide in the control of acute gastroesophageal variceal hemorrhage. Hepatology 2014;60:954–963.

4. Satapathy SK, Sanyal AJ. Nonendoscopic management strategies for acute esophagogastric variceal bleeding. Gastroenterol Clin N Am 2014;43:819–833.

5. Bosch J, Thabut D, Albillos A, et al. Recombinant factor VIIa for variceal bleeding in patients with advanced cirrhosis: a randomized, controlled trial. Hepatology 2008;47:1604–1614.

6. Shah HA, Azam Z, Rauf J, et al. Carvedilol vs. esophageal band ligation in the primary prophylaxis of variceal hemorrhage: a multicenter randomized controlled trial. J Hepatol 2014;60:757–764.

7. Lo GH, Chen WC, Wang HM, Yu HC. Randomized controlled trial of carvedilol versus nadolol plus isosorbide mononitrate for the prevention of variceal rebleeding. J Gastroenterol Hepatol 2012;27:1681–1687.

8. Alaniz C, Mohammad RA, Welage LS. Continuous infusion of pantoprazole with octreotide does not improve management of variceal hemorrhage. Pharmacotherapy 2009;29:248–254.

9. Lo GH, Perng DS, Chang CY, Tai CM, Wang HM, Lin HC. A controlled trial of ligation plus vasoconstrictor versus proton pump inhibitor in the control of acute esophageal variceal bleeding. J Gastroenterol Hepatol 2013;28:684–689.

10. Deshpande A, Pasupuleti V, Thota P, et al. Acid-suppressive therapy is associated with spontaneous bacterial peritonitis in cirrhotic patients: a meta-analysis. J Gastroenterol Hepatol 2013;28:235–242.

47

HEPATIC ENCEPHALOPATHY

State of Confusion...........................Level I

Jeffrey T. Wieczorkiewicz, PharmD, BCPS

Carrie A. Sincak, PharmD, BCPS, FASHP

LEARNING OBJECTIVES

After completing this case study, the reader should be able to:

- Identify and correct the precipitating factors associated with the development of hepatic encephalopathy in a cirrhotic patient.

- Recommend appropriate nonpharmacologic and pharmacologic intervention for a cirrhotic patient who develops hepatic encephalopathy.

- Design a plan for monitoring the efficacy and adverse effects of recommended treatments for hepatic encephalopathy.

- Provide patient education for those receiving treatment for hepatic encephalopathy.

PATIENT PRESENTATION

■ Chief Complaint (from Son)

"My mother says she is dizzy and has felt a little off over the past 2 days."

■ HPI

Judy Sheddling is a 65-year-old woman who was brought to the ED by her son because of dizziness and confusion. The patient became increasingly confused over the past 2 days and on admission was alert to person only. The son states she is normally able to converse without difficulty but does require some assistance with ambulation. Over the past 2 days, she has had increasing difficulty with answering questions in conversations. He mentioned that his mother had forgotten to refill her prescription for rifaximin when she ran out a week ago. His mother had a scheduled endoscopy 2 days ago and did not take her lactulose the day prior to and the day of the test. She had also "retained a lot of water" and told her family that she was feeling bad.

■ PMH

ESLD secondary to NASH cirrhosis diagnosed 5 years ago; complicated by ascites
Grade 2 esophageal varices
Hypothyroidism
Colon cancer s/p resection (15 years ago)

■ FH

Not obtainable at this time

■ SH

Retired; lives with her husband; they have one son and two daughters

■ ROS

Constitutional: confused; weight gain
Eyes: no vision loss or pain
Ears, nose, mouth, throat: no hearing loss, nasal discharge, mouth or throat problems
Cardiovascular: no chest pains or palpitations
Respiratory: no shortness of breath, cough, or dyspnea on exertion
Gastrointestinal: (+) abdominal pain; no change in bowel habits, dysphagia, or odynophagia
Genitourinary: no dysuria or hematuria
Musculoskeletal: no joint pain or weakness
Neurologic: no weakness or headache
Psychiatric: no anxiety or depression
Endocrine: no diabetes; (+) thyroid disease
Hematologic: no enlarged lymph nodes

■ Meds

Folic acid 1 mg PO daily
Furosemide 40 mg PO daily
Lactulose 10 g/15 mL, one tablespoonful PO TID
Levothyroxine 100 mcg PO daily
Multivitamin one tablet PO daily
Pantoprazole 40 mg PO daily
Rifaximin 550 mg PO BID
Thiamine 100 mg PO daily

■ All

No known allergies

■ **Physical Examination**

Gen

Elderly woman in NAD who is disoriented to time and place

VS

BP 134/55, P 82, RR 20, T 36.7°C; Wt 79.4 kg, Ht 5′0″

Skin

Normal skin turgor

HEENT

PERRLA; dry mucous membranes; TMs intact; EOMI; fundi benign; anicteric sclerae; no sinus tenderness

Lungs

Chest symmetric; lungs CTA bilaterally; no wheezes or crackles

CV

S_1 and S_2 normal; RRR with no murmurs

Abd

Nontender; distended abdomen; no splenomegaly; liver edge not identifiable below the costal margin; hypoactive bowel sounds

Rect

Heme (−) stool; no masses

Ext

(+) LE edema; no clubbing or cyanosis

Neuro

Confused; oriented only to person; CNs II–XII intact; DTRs 2+; (+) asterixis

■ **Labs**

Na 135 mEq/L	Hgb 8.9 g/dL	WBC $5.2 \times 10^3/mm^3$	AST 63 IU/L
K 3.1 mEq/L	Hct 28%	PMNs 67%	ALT 23 IU/L
Cl 104 mEq/L	MCV 95 μm³	Bands 3%	Alk Phos 125 IU/L
CO_2 25 mEq/L	MCHC 34 g/dL	Eos 3%	T. bili 1.2 mg/dL
BUN 10 mg/dL	Retic 1.1%	Lymphs 25%	D. bili 0.4 mg/dL
SCr 1.4 mg/dL	Plt $112 \times 10^3/mm^3$	Monos 2%	Alb 3.1 g/dL
Glu 123 mg/dL			NH_3 70 mcg/dL
			Ca 9.4 mg/dL
			Mg 2.6 mg/dL
			Phos 3.5 mg/dL
			PT 15.2 s
			aPTT 39.8 s
			INR 1.5
			TSH 10.38 μIU/mL

■ **Assessment**

Hepatic encephalopathy (HE), type C, grade III, episodic, precipitated (by brief non-compliance with maintenance lactulose and rifaximin therapy).

QUESTIONS

Problem Identification

1.a. Create a list of the patient's drug therapy problems.

1.b. What information indicates the presence or severity of hepatic encephalopathy in this patient? (See Fig. 47-1.)

A Glasgow Coma Scale

Eye opening	Spontaneous	4
	To verbal command	3
	To pain	2
	None	1
Verbal responsiveness	Oriented	5
	Confused	4
	Inappropriate words	3
	Incomprehensible sounds	2
	None	1
Motor response	Obeys	6
	Localizes	5
	Withdraws (pain)	4
	Flexion (pain)	3
	Extension (pain)	2
	None	1
	Total: _____	

FIGURE 47-1. Glascow Coma Scale (GSC) is a clinical evaluation tool measuring the severity of hepatic encephalopathy. The scale includes an assessment of three separate areas of response: eyes, verbal and motor. The scores of the individual sections are then added together to reveal the overall severity score. The lowest score (3) indicates the highest level of severity and the highest score (15) indicates the lowest level of severity. *(Reprinted with permission from Stone CK, Humphries RL, eds. Current Diagnosis & Treatment: Emergency Medicine, 7th ed. New York, NY. Mc-Graw Hill Education, 2011.)*

1.c. What precipitating factors in this patient could potentially cause an episode of hepatic encephalopathy?

1.d. What additional information is needed to satisfactorily assess the hepatic encephalopathy of this patient?

Desired Outcome

2. What are the general principles for the management of hepatic encephalopathy and desired therapeutic outcomes?

Therapeutic Alternatives

3.a. What nondrug interventions are important before initiating pharmacotherapeutic agents for the treatment of hepatic encephalopathy?

3.b. What pharmacotherapeutic alternatives are available for the treatment of hepatic encephalopathy? Include the mechanism of action of each drug in your answer.

Optimal Plan

4. Outline a pharmacotherapeutic plan for this patient's drug therapy problems. Include the drugs, dosage forms, doses, schedules, and duration of treatment for each problem.

Outcome Evaluation

5. How would you monitor the efficacy and adverse effects of treatment that you recommended for this patient?

Patient Education

6. What medication-related information should be provided to the patient about her therapy on discharge?

■ CLINICAL COURSE

Two days after beginning treatment with the regimen you recommended, the patient is responding positively, and the dose has been titrated appropriately. The dizziness and confusion have subsided and she is now oriented to time, place, and person, and no asterixis is detected. The plan is to discharge the patient home tomorrow.

SELF-STUDY ASSIGNMENTS

1. Perform a literature search to assess the efficacy and role of rifaximin in the treatment of hepatic encephalopathy.

2. List the potential advantages and disadvantages of using antibiotics for the treatment of hepatic encephalopathy.

3. Perform a literature search to determine if protein restriction is appropriate in patients with liver disease, particularly patients with cirrhosis.

CLINICAL PEARL

Medication noncompliance, sedative–hypnotics, other CNS depressants, and narcotics may precipitate hepatic encephalopathy. A careful medication history is important in patients presenting with the disorder to identify and eliminate reversible causes.

REFERENCES

1. Cordoba J, Minguez B. Hepatic encephalopathy. Semin Liver Dis 2008;28:70–80.

2. Sundaram V, Shaikh OS. Hepatic encephalopathy: pathophysiology and emerging therapies. Med Clin North Am 2009;93:819–836.

3. Riggio O, Ridola L. Emerging drugs for hepatic encephalopathy. Expert Opin Emerg Drugs 2009;14:537–549.

4. Vilstrup H, Amodio P, Bajaj J, et al. Hepatic Encephalopathy in Chronic Liver Disease: 2014 Practice Guideline by American Association for the Science of Liver Diseases and European Association for the Study of the Liver. Hepatology 2014;60:715–735.

5. Mas A. Hepatic encephalopathy: from pathophysiology to treatment. Digestion 2006;73(Suppl 1):86–93.

6. Maclayton DO, Eaton-Maxwell A. Rifaximin for treatment of hepatic encephalopathy. Ann Pharmacother 2009;43:77–84.

7. Lawrence KR, Klee JA. Rifaximin for the treatment of hepatic encephalopathy. Pharmacotherapy 2008;28:1019–1032.

8. Bass NM, Mullen KD, Sanyal A, et al. Rifaximin treatment in hepatic encephalopathy. N Engl J Med 2010;362:1071–1081.

9. Eltawil KM, Laryea M, Peltekian K, Molinari M. Rifaximin vs conventional oral therapy for hepatic encephalopathy: a meta-analysis. World J Gastroenterol 2012;18:767–777.

10. Runyon B. Management of adult patients with ascites due to cirrhosis: Update 2012. American Association for the Study of Liver Diseases. Available at: https://www.aasld.org/sites/default/files/guideline_documents/adultascitesenhanced.pdf. Accessed on April 3, 2016.

48

ACUTE PANCREATITIS

A Sod Story. . . . . Level II

Scott W. Mueller, PharmD, BCCCP

Paul Reynolds, PharmD, BCPS

Robert MacLaren, BSc (Pharm), PharmD, MPH, FCCM, FCCP

LEARNING OBJECTIVES

After completing this case study, the reader should be able to:

• Evaluate precipitating factors associated with acute pancreatitis.

• Determine signs, symptoms, and laboratory abnormalities commonly associated with acute pancreatitis.

• Describe potential systemic complications associated with acute pancreatitis.

• Recommend appropriate pharmacologic and nonpharmacologic therapies for patients with acute pancreatitis.

• Develop monitoring parameters to assist in realizing desired therapeutic outcomes.

PATIENT PRESENTATION

■ Chief Complaint

"I've got a really bad pain in my stomach."

■ HPI

Bill Jones is a 42-year-old man who presents to the ED shortly after midnight on a Friday night because of intense midepigastric pain radiating to his back. He states that the pain started shortly after dinner the night before but has progressively worsened. The pain is unrelated to physical activity, and he began vomiting around midnight tonight.

■ PMH

Alcohol withdrawal seizures 5 months ago, which have not recurred. Hypertension, which is medically controlled.

■ FH

Father died at age of 56 from an MVA; mother is 72 years old and has type 2 DM and "cholesterol issues," for which she is taking an unknown medication. One sister, also with "cholesterol issues," taking an unknown medication. The sister has a remote history of pancreatitis as well.

■ SH

Divorced with three children. Employed as a groundskeeper at a golf course. Quit smoking 2 weeks ago, admits to a 40 pack-year history of smoking. He states that he used to consume 6–10 beers per day until 5 months ago when he had a withdrawal seizure but now drinks only on weekends a total of about 6 beers; he reports sharing a couple of pitchers with two friends last night with dinner. Drinks at least two cups of coffee each morning.

■ Meds

Phenytoin 200 mg twice daily since his seizure
Hydrochlorothiazide 25 mg once daily for blood pressure
Doxycycline 100 mg twice daily for 10 days for "cellulitis" (now cleared as today is day 10)
Ibuprofen 200 mg OTC several doses per day PRN sore back muscles

■ All

Amoxicillin/clavulanate makes his stomach upset

■ ROS

He states that he has been feeling well until last night. His back soreness from unloading pallets of heavy sod a week ago has resolved with occasional ibuprofen use. He just finished a course of antibiotics this morning for mild cellulitis that was limited to a 1 × 2-in area of the left lower tibia. He has vomited approximately six times since midnight. No complaints of diarrhea or blood in the stool or vomitus. No knowledge of any prior history of uncontrolled blood sugars or cholesterol.

■ Physical Examination

Gen

The patient is restless and in moderate distress but otherwise is a well-appearing, well-nourished male who looks his stated age

VS

BP 99/56, P 124, RR 30, T 38.9°C; Wt 89 kg, Ht 5′ 10″

HEENT

PERRLA; EOMI; oropharynx pink and clear; oral mucosa dry

Skin

Dry with poor skin turgor; location of previous cellulitis appears healed; nontender, (−) erythema, swelling, or warmth

Neck/Lymph Nodes

Supple; no bruits, lymphadenopathy, or thyromegaly

CV

Sinus tachycardia; no MRG

Lungs/Thorax

No external evidence of back injury; (−) spinal/CVA tenderness; normal range of motion; no abnormal breath sounds on auscultation

Abd

Moderately distended with active but diminished bowel sounds; (+) guarding; pain is elicited on light palpation of left upper and midepigastric region. No rebound tenderness, masses, or hepatosplenomegaly

MS/Ext

Extremities are warm and well perfused. Good pulses present in all extremities. No clubbing, palmar erythema, or spider angiomata.

Rect

Normal sphincter tone; no BRBPR or masses; stool is guaiac negative; prostate normal size

Neuro

A & O × 3; neuro exam benign; CN II–XII intact; strength is equal bilaterally in all extremities. Normal tone and reflexes. No asterixis.

■ Labs

Na 128 mEq/L	Hgb 17 g/dL	AST 342 IU/L	Ca 7.2 mg/dL
K 3.4 mEq/L	Hct 50%	ALT 166 IU/L	Mg 1.7 mEq/L
Cl 105 mEq/L	WBC 15.2 ×	Alk phos 285 IU/L	Phos 2.2 mg/dL
CO$_2$ 18 mEq/L	10^3/mm^3	LDH 255 IU/L	Trig 782 mg/dL
BUN 35 mg/dL	Neutros 72%	T. bili 0.6 mg/dL	Repeat Trig
SCr 1.5 mg/dL	Bands 4%	Alb 3.2 g/dL	1,010 mg/dL
Glu 375 mg/dL	Eos 1%	Prealb 25 mg/dL	PT 12.8 s
	Basos 1%	Amylase 1,555 IU/L	INR 1.1
	Lymphs 20%	Lipase 2,220 IU/L	aPTT 19.3 s
	Monos 2%		Phenytoin total
			13 mg/L
			BAC 4 mg/dL

■ Other Tests

Negative for serum ketones, ASA, acetaminophen, all other alcohols, viral hepatitis titers, and HIV

■ Arterial Blood Gases

pH 7.31, PaCO$_2$ 38 mm Hg, PaO$_2$ 88 mm Hg, HCO$_3^-$ 17 mEq/L, O$_2$ sat 98% in room air

■ UA

Color yellow; turbidity clear; SG 1.010; pH 7.2; glucose >1,000 mg/dL; bilirubin (−); ketones (−); Hgb (−); protein (−); nitrite (−); crystals (−); casts (−); mucous (−); bacteria (−); urobilinogen: 0.25 EU/dL; WBC 0–5/hpf; RBC 0/hpf; epithelial cells: 0–10/hpf.

■ Chest X-Ray

AP view of chest shows the heart to be normal in size. The lungs are clear without any infiltrates, masses, effusions, or atelectasis. No notable abnormalities.

■ Abdominal Ultrasound

Nonspecific gas pattern; no dilated bowel. Questionable opacity/abnormality of common bile duct. Cannot rule out gallstone/obstruction.

■ ECG

Sinus tachycardia; rate 140 bpm. No changes from his last ECG (5 months ago), no evidence of myocardial ischemia.

■ Assessment

Acute pancreatitis precipitating hyperglycemia, hypocalcemia, and nonanion gap metabolic acidosis
R/O choledocholithiasis

QUESTIONS

Problem Identification

1.a. What factors may have precipitated acute pancreatitis in this case?

1.b. What signs, symptoms, and laboratory tests are consistent with the diagnosis of acute pancreatitis? How can the severity of pancreatitis be classified?

1.c. Construct a drug therapy problem list for this patient.

Desired Outcome

2. What are the goals of therapy for this patient?

Therapeutic Alternatives

3. What therapies may be instituted to achieve the goals outlined above? Provide a rationale for each therapy.

Optimal Plan

4. Develop a pharmacotherapeutic care plan for this patient, including duration of therapy.

Outcome Evaluation

5.a. Outline the monitoring parameters for efficacy and adverse effects of therapy for pain management.

CLINICAL COURSE

IV morphine is initiated for pain control. Partial parenteral nutrition (without lipids) is considered but ultimately withheld as plans are made to initiate enteral nutrition during the daytime (ie, in about 12 hours). After several days of improvement in the hospital, the patient develops a WBC count of $23.4 \times 10^3/mm^3$ with neutrophils 77%, bands 15%, eosinophils 1%, basophils 0%, lymphocytes 3%, and monocytes 4%. He has a temperature of 39.8°C and is noted to be orthostatic (BP 128/76 sitting, 98/60 standing) with a glucose of 480 mg/dL. He has also experienced several episodes of diarrhea and steatorrhea.

Because of these setbacks in the patient's progress, a contrast-enhanced CT scan is obtained. The results demonstrate peripancreatic and retroperitoneal edema. The pancreas itself appears relatively normal with the exception of small nonenhancing areas around the neck of the pancreas, which are suggestive of necrosis.

5.b. What potential etiologies might explain this patient's fever and relapsing acute pancreatitis?

5.c. What are the new treatment goals for this patient?

5.d. Given this new information, what therapeutic interventions should be considered for this patient?

5.e. How should these new therapies be monitored for efficacy and adverse effects?

Patient Education

6. When this patient is stable, what information should be provided to him to reduce the likelihood of recurrent pancreatitis?

■ SELF-STUDY ASSIGNMENTS

1. Describe the pathophysiology of autodigestion during acute pancreatitis.

2. Describe the controversies of early enteral nutrition, probiotics, prophylactic antibiotics, and octreotide for management of acute pancreatitis.

3. Summarize published information regarding opioid effects on the sphincter of Oddi.

4. Compose a list of drugs believed to aggravate or cause pancreatitis and assess the level of association for each agent.

CLINICAL PEARL

Invasive placement of a nasojejunal tube is not uniformly required as nasojejunal feeding has not consistently shown benefit over nasogastric feeding. Therefore, gastric administration of nutrition is frequently preferred as this route is easily accessible.

REFERENCES

1. Lankisch PG, Apte M, Banks PA. Acute pancreatitis. Lancet 2015;386:85–96.

2. Johnson CD, Besselink MG, Carter R. Acute pancreatitis. BMJ 2014;349:g4859. doi:http://dx.doi.org/10.1136/bmj.g4859.

3. Working Group International Association of Pancreatology/American Pancreatic Association Acute Pancreatitis Guidelines. IAP/APA evidence-based guidelines for the management of acute pancreatitis. Pancreatology 2013;13:e1–15.

4. Tenner S, Baillie J, DeWitt J, Vege SW. American College of Gastroenterology Guideline: Management of acute pancreatitis. Am J Gastroenterol 2013;108:1400–1415.

5. Hung WY, Abreu Lanfranco O. Contemporary review of drug-induced pancreatitis: A different perspective. World J Gastrointest Pathophysiol 2014;5:405–415.

6. Olah A, Romics L Jr. Enteral nutrition in acute pancreatitis: a review of the current evidence. World J Gastroenterol 2014;20:16123–16131.

7. Poropat G, Giljaca V, Hauser G, Stimac D. Enteral nutrition formulation for acute pancreatitis. Cochrane Database Syst Rev 2015 Mar 23;3:CD010605. doi:10.1002/14651858.CD010605.pub2.

8. McClave SA, Martindale RG, Vanek VW, et al. Guidelines for the provision and assessment of nutrition support therapy in the adult critically ill patient: Society of Critical Care Medicine (SCCM) and American Society for Parenteral and Enteral Nutrition (A.S.P.E.N.). J Parenter Enteral Nutr 2009;33:277–316.

9. Bakker OJ, van Brunschot S, van Santvoort HC, et al. Early versus on-demand nasoenteric tube feeding in acute pancreatitis. N Engl J Med 2014;371:1983–1993.

10. Zerem E. Treatment of severe acute pancreatitis and its complication. World J Gastroenterol 2014;20:13879–13892.

49

CHRONIC PANCREATITIS

Like a Shot to the Gut .... Level II

Janine E. Then, PharmD, BCPS

Heather M. Teufel, PharmD, BCPS

LEARNING OBJECTIVES

After completing this case study, the reader should be able to:

- Identify subjective and objective findings consistent with chronic pancreatitis and acute exacerbations of chronic pancreatitis.

- Evaluate patient-specific data and develop a problem list for patients with acute exacerbations of chronic pancreatitis.

- Discuss therapeutic alternatives and outline a patient-specific plan for pain management during an acute exacerbation of chronic pancreatitis.

- Recommend appropriate pancreatic enzyme replacement therapy for management of steatorrhea in a patient with chronic pancreatitis.

PATIENT PRESENTATION

■ Chief Complaint

"I have had pain in my stomach for years, but now I just can't take it anymore. It feels like a shot to the gut."

■ HPI

Madeline Jane is a 35-year-old woman who presents to the ED complaining of pain in her abdomen and with radiation to her back. She also has noticed an increase in loose, foul-smelling stools and has observed a fatty content and consistency to her stool. Ms Jane has experienced pain in her abdomen for several years; she has also experienced chronic diarrhea with newly increased frequency in the last week. Concurrent with the pain are nausea and vomiting, which have also increased in intensity and frequency in the past week. Ms Jane presents to the ED today as she now has access to health insurance. She did not seek medical attention previously due to the financial implications of being uninsured.

■ PMH

There is no formal past medical history because the patient has not sought medical care since college due to being uninsured. Patient reports receiving the "usual" childhood vaccinations and medical care, but she has not seen a physician since college when she was dropped from her parent's medical coverage. Ms Jane states that she has had pain in her stomach and diarrhea for years but just dealt with it. Within the past week she noticed an increase in pain, increase in frequency of diarrhea, and change in the consistency and fatty content of her stool.

■ SH

Parents are alive and healthy. She is an only child. Patient does not drink alcohol, smoke cigarettes, or use illicit drugs per patient report. She is single and not sexually active. Ms Jane just started a new job as a medical claims processor at St. Anthony's hospital; she has completed a college-level education.

■ Meds

Multivitamin one tablet by mouth daily, has been taking for several years

Acetaminophen 500 mg by mouth Q 6 H PRN for abdominal pain; frequent daily use

Loperamide two tablets initially, and then one tablet by mouth PRN diarrhea; she usually takes two to four tablets per day

No prescription medications

■ All

Amoxicillin → rash when she received it as a child for an ear infection, no use since

■ ROS

Mild difficulty swallowing due to dry throat, (−) sore throat, or difficulty eating. No indigestion or bloating. Significant abdominal pain and diarrhea as described above. No constipation or fecal incontinence; normal flatus. No blood in the stool. No hemorrhoids. Urine is of normal color, volume, and odor.

■ Physical Examination

Gen

Thin, ill-appearing Caucasian woman, appearing anxious

VS

BP 106/70, P 104, RR 18, T 37.8°C; Wt 55 kg, Ht 5′5″

Skin

Normal skin turgor

HEENT

PERRLA, EOMI, oropharynx clear, mucous membranes dry, eyes chronically dry

Neck/Lymph Nodes

Supple; (−) JVD, thyromegaly, lymphadenopathy, or bruits

Lung/Thorax

Audible breath sounds in all lung fields; trachea at midline; normal rate, rhythm, and effort of breathing; (−) vertebral tenderness or deformity

CV

Regular rate and rhythm without gallops or murmur

Abd

Sparse bowel sounds, (+) rebound and guarding

Genit/Rect

No masses, guaiac (−)

MS/Ext

Pulses intact bilaterally; good capillary refill; no cyanosis, clubbing, or edema

Neuro

A & O × 3, CN II–XII intact

■ Labs

Na 140 mEq/L	Hgb 12 g/dL	WBC 8.2 × 10³/mm³	T. bili 1.5 mg/dL
K 4.2 mEq/L	Hct 37%	Neutros 65%	Alk Phos 140 IU/L
Cl 95 mEq/L	RBC 4.0 × 10⁶/mm³	Bands 5%	Alb 4.4 g/dL
CO₂ 31 mEq/L	Plt 400 × 10³/mm³	Eos 0%	Prealb 20 mg/dL
BUN 8 mg/dL	MCV 85.1 μm³	Lymphs 28%	Lipase 100 IU/L
SCr 0.6 mg/dL	MCHC 35 g/dL	Monos 2%	Amylase 110 IU/L
Glu 89 mg/dL	Antiplasminogen binding protein pending	Anti-SSA pending	IgG4 pending
ANA pending			

■ CT abdomen with IV contrast

Changes consistent with chronic pancreatitis: inflammation of the common bile duct (Fig. 49-1)

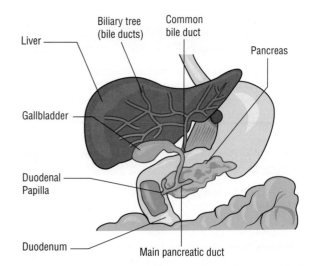

FIGURE 49-1. Anatomic structures depicting joining of common bile duct and the main pancreatic duct before emptying contents into the duodenum. (*Source: National Institute of Diabetes and Digestive and Kidney Diseases. Available at:* http://www.niddk.nih.gov/health-information/health-topics /diagnostic-tests/ercp/Pages/diagnostic-test.aspx)

■ Assessment

1. Chronic pancreatitis, idiopathic etiology—with acute exacerbation

2. Routine medical care needed

QUESTIONS

Problem Identification

1.a. Create a list of this patient's drug therapy problems.

1.b. What subjective and objective information is consistent with the diagnosis of chronic pancreatitis?

1.c. What signs, symptoms, and test results indicate that the patient is experiencing an acute exacerbation of chronic pancreatitis?

1.d. Which of the patient's problems are amenable to drug therapy?

1.e. What additional information is needed to satisfactorily assess the patient?

Desired Outcome

2. What are the goals of pharmacotherapy in this case?

Therapeutic Alternatives

3.a. What nondrug therapies could be useful in this patient?

3.b. What feasible pharmacotherapeutic alternatives are available for treating this acute exacerbation of chronic pancreatitis?

3.c. What additional care is required for a patient who has not seen a physician in about 15 years?

Optimal Plan

4. What drug, dosage form, and duration of therapy are best for this patient?

Outcome Evaluation

5. What clinical and laboratory parameters are necessary to evaluate the therapy for achievement of the desired therapeutic outcome and to detect or prevent adverse effects?

Patient Education

6. Ms Jane wants information on her inpatient medication regimen and the nurse refers her to you, the floor-based pharmacist. What information will you provide to enhance her understanding of the medications, maximize compliance with the new medication regimen, enhance the chance of success, and minimize adverse effects?

■ SELF-STUDY ASSIGNMENTS

1. Analyze the implication of an idiopathic diagnosis of disease. What other extrapancreatic diseases are associated with chronic pancreatitis?

2. What psychological factors will impact this patient's adherence to medical therapy or her willingness to seek further treatment given the patient's inattention to medical due diligence up to this point? How would this impact your ability to provide care for this patient?

CLINICAL PEARL

Chronic pancreatitis is of idiopathic etiology in up to 30% of cases.

REFERENCES

1. Tenner S, Baillie J, DeWitt J, Vege SS. American College of Gastroenterology Guideline: Management of Acute Pancreatitis. Am J Gastroenterol 2013;108:1400–1415.

2. DiMagno MJ, DiMagno EP. Chronic pancreatitis. Curr Opin Gastroenterol 2012;28:523–531.

3. Berry AJ. Pancreatic enzyme replacement therapy during pancreatic insufficiency. Nutr Clin Pract 2014;29:312–321.

4. Puylaert M, Kapural L, Van Zundert J, et al. Pain in chronic pancreatitis. Pain Pract 2011;11:492–505.

5. Trikudanathan G, Vavaneethan L, Vege SS. Modern treatment of patients with chronic pancreatitis. Gastroenterol Clin North Am 2012;41:63–76.

6. Giuliano CA, Dehoome-Smith ML, Kale-Pradhan PB. Pancreatic enzyme products: digesting the changes. Ann Pharmacother 2011;45:658–666.

50

VIRAL HEPATITIS A

Forbid Dual Infections . . . . Level II

Juliana Chan, PharmD, FCCP, BCACP

LEARNING OBJECTIVES

After completing this case study, the reader should be able to:

- Determine which patient populations are at greatest risk for contracting hepatitis A.

- Recommend hepatitis A immunization for appropriate individuals based on current guidelines of the Centers for Disease Control and Prevention (CDC).

- Assess the efficacy and adverse effects of hepatitis A vaccines.

- Counsel eligible patients on the benefits of hepatitis A vaccination and the possible adverse effects associated with its use.

PATIENT PRESENTATION

■ Chief Complaint

"My doctor sent me to follow up on my liver disease."

■ HPI

Hector is a 39-year-old Hispanic man, born and raised in Arizona, who will be visiting his family in Mexico in the next 2 weeks. He will be seeing his grandmother for her 90th birthday with his wife and daughter. He was diagnosed with NAFLD at the age of 32. He also has hepatitis C secondary to several blood transfusions in 1991 after having multiple surgeries following a motorcycle accident. Hector's PCP referred him to see the hepatologist again before traveling for vaccinations and follow-up as he has not seen the liver specialist in the last 5 years.

PMH

NAFLD diagnosed at age 32
Hepatitis C diagnosed at age 32
Hypercholesterolemia
HTN
Depression

Surgical History

Several surgeries after a motorcycle accident that required blood transfusions between 1991 and 1992

FH

Mother died at 57 secondary to breast cancer and father is alive with hepatitis B; one brother with gout, HTN, and DM

SH

Married for 13 years and lives with wife and daughter. He smokes tobacco; one ppd, and drinks two to three glasses of wine daily. He has several large tattoos that were done professionally. There is no history of IV drug use, cocaine use, or body piercings. He has worked as a chef since the age of 24.

ROS

Positive for fatigue, decrease in appetite. Denies weight loss/gain, fevers, chills, headaches, shortness of breath, and coughing. He does have some abdominal pain intermittently, also constipation off and on. No black stools or obvious blood in stools.

Meds

Multivitamin tablet PO once daily
Simvastatin 40 mg PO once daily
Lisinopril 40 mg PO once daily
Escitalopram 10 mg PO daily

All

PCN, sulfa

Physical Examination

Gen

The patient is a Hispanic-American man in no apparent distress

VS

BP 127/74, P 70, RR 22, T 36.9°C; Wt 121.8 kg, Ht 5′9″

Skin

Warm and dry. Spider angiomas are not present

HEENT

PERRLA, EOMI; fundi normal; TMs clear. Head is normocephalic and atraumatic; sclerae anicteric

Neck/Lymph Nodes

Supple; no masses or JVD

Chest

Clear without wheezes, rhonchi, or rales

CV

RRR, S_1, S_2 normal

Abd

(+) Bowel sounds, no masses, nontender, nondistended

Genit/Rect

Rectal exam deferred

MS/Ext

Normal range of motion throughout; no CCE

Neuro

A & O × 3; CN II–XII intact; no focal deficits, negative for asterixis

Labs (Nonfasting)

Na 144 mEq/L	Hgb 15.6 g/dL	AST 31 IU/L	T. chol 205 mg/dL
K 5.0 mEq/L	Hct 45.0%	ALT 63 IU/L	Anti-HBs (+)
Cl 107 mEq/L	WBC 6.9 ×	Alk phos 67 IU/L	HBsAg (−)
CO_2 30 mEq/L	$10^3/mm^3$	T. bili 1.0 mg/dL	Total anti-HAV (−)
BUN 16 mg/dL	Plt 305 ×	LDH 167 IU/L	
SCr 1.2 mg/dL	$10^3/mm^3$	PT 13.1 s	
Glu 119 mg/dL		Alb 4.5 g/dL	
HCV genotype 3a		HCV RNA PCR	
		400,000 IU/mL	

Abdominal Ultrasound

Findings

The liver has a course echotexture with smooth contour. No focal liver masses are seen. Hepatic steatosis is observed. There is no intrahepatic biliary dilatation. The common bile duct measures 3 mm. Multiple shadowing stones are seen within the gallbladder. There is no gallbladder wall thickening or pericholecystic fluid. The head and body of the pancreas are grossly unremarkable; views of the tail are obscured by overlying bowel gas. A limited survey of the kidneys was performed. The right kidney measures 10.0 cm in length. The left kidney measures 11.6 cm. No hydronephrosis is seen in either kidney. There is no splenomegaly. Visualized segments of the aorta and IVC are patent.

Impression

1. Coarse heterogeneous appearance of the liver is consistent with patient's history of hepatitis. No evidence for focal liver mass. Hepatic steatosis is present.

2. Cholelithiasis without evidence for cholecystitis.

Liver Biopsy

- Chronic hepatitis consistent with chronic HCV infection
- Minimal activity, grade 1 (0–4)
- No significant fibrosis, stage 1 (I–IV) by trichrome stain
- Moderate steatosis (2+ fat)
- Negative for dysplasia and negative for malignancy
- Hepatitis activity index (Batts and Ludwig criteria; 0–4):

   Portal inflammation: 1

   Piecemeal necrosis: 1

   Lobular inflammation: 1

   Fibrosis: 1

▪ Assessment

This is a 39-year-old Hispanic male with a history of chronic hepatitis C and NAFLD who is immune to hepatitis B and is here to be evaluated for the hepatitis A vaccine prior to his trip to Mexico.

QUESTIONS

Problem Identification

1.a. Does this patient need to be vaccinated against hepatitis A? Please review the patient's history and laboratory values to determine if the hepatitis A vaccine is needed.

1.b. What patient factors make this patient a candidate for the hepatitis A vaccination?

1.c. What other patient populations or environments present an increased risk for acquiring the hepatitis A infection?

Desired Outcome

2. What are the goals of hepatitis A vaccination?

Therapeutic Alternatives

3.a. What nonpharmacologic recommendations should be made to this patient and his family to minimize their risk of developing hepatitis A infection while in Mexico?

3.b. What commercial products are available for vaccination against hepatitis A, and how effective are they in providing protective efficacy?

Optimal Plan

4. Outline a vaccination regimen that includes dose, route of administration, and the number of doses required for the patient.

Outcome Evaluation

5.a. How should the regimen you recommended be monitored for efficacy?

5.b. What adverse effects may be experienced with the regimen you recommended, and how may these events be treated?

Patient Education

6. What information should be provided to the patient about the hepatitis A vaccine?

▪ CLINICAL COURSE

Hector's wife and daughter (who is 6 months pregnant) returned to Arizona from Mexico 8 days ago. His 39-year-old wife complains of nausea, weight loss, abdominal pain, and yellow eyes for 1 week. She was admitted to the hospital on day 9 since returning from vacation for medical evaluation. His daughter is symptom free, but it was recommended that she follow up with her obstetrician as soon as possible. The following labs were obtained during the first day of hospitalization for Hector's wife:

Na 137 mEq/L	Hgb 13.6 g/dL	AST 2,642 IU/L	Anti-HBs (+)
K 4.0 mEq/L	Hct 40.1%	ALT 2,166 IU/L	HBsAg (−)
Cl 100 mEq/L	WBC 7.7 × 10^3/mm^3	Alk phos 172 IU/L	Total anti-HAV (+)
CO_2 26 mEq/L		T. bili 20.5 mg/dL	Anti-HAV IgM (+)
BUN 12 mg/dL	Plt 141 × 10^3/mm^3	D. bili 12.9 mg/dL	Anti-HCV (−)
SCr 1.3 mg/dL		PT 12.9 s	Acetaminophen
Glu (nonfasting) 143 mg/dL		Alb 2.7 g/dL	< 10 mcg/mL

CT of the Abdomen With and Without IV Contrast

Clinical indication: 39 yo female with new hepatic failure

Impression:

1. Diffuse thickening of the transverse colon consistent with colitis, likely of infectious or inflammatory etiology

2. Diffuse low attenuation of the liver, perihepatic ascites, and edematous gallbladder wall consistent with underlying inflammatory process

▪ FOLLOW-UP QUESTIONS

1. Based on the information provided, what medical condition does Hector's wife have?

2. What is your treatment recommendation for Hector's wife?

3. Hector's daughter is not experiencing any symptoms since returning from Mexico. She visits her obstetrician the same day her mother was admitted to the hospital. She told her obstetrician that her mom is now hospitalized for acute hepatitis A. She will be 7 months pregnant in 1 week. What is your vaccination recommendation for Hector's daughter? When should the newborn be vaccinated?

▪ STUDY ASSIGNMENTS

1. Compare and contrast the mechanism of action, immunogenicity rate, and adverse effects of the two commercially available hepatitis A vaccines.

2. Determine which vaccines can be given simultaneously with the hepatitis A vaccine.

3. Compare the cost of administering the Havrix and Engerix-B vaccines separately versus the combination product Twinrix for an adult.

CLINICAL PEARL

The hepatitis A vaccine is highly effective in preventing hepatitis A infections when given immediately prior to departing to endemic areas.

According to the CDC, all children in the United States over 1 year of age should receive the hepatitis A vaccine.

REFERENCES

1. Advisory Committee on Immunization Practices (ACIP) Centers for Disease Control and Prevention (CDC). Update: prevention of hepatitis A after exposure to hepatitis A virus and in international travelers. Updated recommendations of the Advisory Committee on Immunization Practices (ACIP). MMWR Morb Mortal Wkly Rep 2007;56(41):1080–1084.

2. Advisory Committee on Immunization Practices (ACIP), Fiore AE, Wasley A, Bell BP. Prevention of hepatitis A through active or passive immunization. Recommendations of the Advisory Committee on Immunization Practices (ACIP). MMWR Morb Mortal Wkly Rep 2006;55(RR-7):1–23.

3. Centers for Disease Control and Prevention. Surveillance for Viral Hepatitis, 2013. Available at: http://www.cdc.gov/hepatitis/statistics/2013surveillance/commentary.htm#hepatitisA. Accessed November 7, 2015.

51

VIRAL HEPATITIS B

A Persistent Infection . . . . Level III

Juliana Chan, PharmD, FCCP, BCACP

LEARNING OBJECTIVES

After completing this case study, the reader should be able to:

- Outline a pharmacologic and nonpharmacologic regimen for patients with chronic hepatitis B.

- Determine clinical and laboratory end points for treatment of chronic hepatitis B.

- Assess the efficacy and adverse effects of chronic hepatitis B treatment with interferon, pegylated interferon, lamivudine, adefovir dipivoxil, entecavir, telbivudine, and tenofovir.

- Recommend hepatitis B immunization for appropriate individuals based on current guidelines of the Centers for Disease Control and Prevention (CDC).

- Provide patient education on interferon, pegylated interferon, lamivudine, adefovir dipivoxil, entecavir, telbivudine, and tenofovir treatment.

PATIENT PRESENTATION

■ Chief Complaint

"I'm here for my hepatitis B disease."

■ HPI

Trong Pan is a 21-year-old Chinese woman with no significant past medical history except for acquiring hepatitis B infection at birth from her mother. Over the summer, she was required to obtain a physical exam prior to entering her first year of nursing school. Laboratory test results indicated a positive HBsAg. She was referred to the liver clinic for further evaluation and possible treatment.

■ PMH

Seasonal allergies
Chronic hepatitis B

■ Surgical History

None

■ FH

Mother and father alive, both positive for HBsAg. Father has HCC. Has one younger sister, HBV status unknown.

■ SH

Single. She does not smoke or use IV drugs. She drinks socially on the weekends. She is in her first year of nursing school.

■ Meds

Phenylephrine 10 mg PO Q 4 H PRN for allergies
Dong quai three capsules PO daily for menstrual cramps
Calcium with vitamin D PO daily

■ All

None

■ ROS

Denies any symptoms. Her weight is stable with no loss of appetite. No nausea, vomiting, diarrhea, abdominal pain, or constipation. No melena or hematochezia. No changes in urine or stool color and no history of icteric sclerae.

■ Physical Examination

Gen

The patient is not in acute distress

VS

BP 128/82, P 76, RR 20, T 37.6°C; Wt 52.1 kg, Ht 5'5"

Skin

Warm and dry; no signs of jaundice. Good turgor

HEENT

Head is normocephalic, atraumatic. Sclerae are anicteric bilaterally. Neck is supple. No masses or palpable lymphadenopathy. PERRLA. Funduscopic exam normal

Cor

RRR, S_1, S_2 normal; no S_3 or S_4

Lungs

Clear to P & A

Abd

Good bowel sounds, soft, nontender; no evidence of ascites; no palpable hepatosplenomegaly

Rect

Guaiac negative

Ext

Normal range of motion throughout; no C/C/E, no gross lesions, ecchymosis, or peripheral edema

Neuro

CN II–XII intact; DTRs 2+ throughout; negative Babinski

■ Labs

Na 139 mEq/L	Hgb 12.4 g/dL	AST 64 IU/L	HBsAg (+)
K 4.0 mEq/L	Hct 37.3%	ALT 111 IU/L	Anti-HBs (−)
Cl 104 mEq/L	Plt 272 × 10³/mm³	Alk phos 71 IU/L	HBeAg (+)
CO_2 25 mEq/L	WBC 6.9 × 10³/mm³	T. bili 0.4 mg/dL	HBV DNA PCR Quant 6,368,844 IU/mL
BUN 12 mg/dL	TSH 1.96 μIU/mL	T. prot 7.2 g/dL	
SCr 0.9 mg/dL	T. chol 132 mg/dL	Alb 4.2 g/dL	Anti-HBc IgM (−)
Glu (nonfasting) 86 mg/dL	Trig 194 mg/dL	PT 10.8 s	Anti-HBc total (+)
			HCV RNA quant < 25 IU/mL
			Anti-HCV (−)
			Anti-HAV, total (+)
			Anti-HIV (−)

Other Tests

Complete Ultrasound of the Abdomen

Findings: There is no ascites. The liver is normal in contour and echogenicity. There is no intrahepatic biliary dilatation; the common bile duct is not dilated and measures 0.5 cm. The gallbladder is unremarkable and without calculi, wall thickening, or pericholecystic fluid. The head and body of the pancreas are grossly unremarkable; views of the tail are obscured by overlying bowel gas.

A limited survey of the kidneys was performed. The kidneys are normal in size and echogenicity. The right kidney measures 9.5 cm in length. The left kidney measures 9.6 cm. No hydronephrosis is seen in either kidney. The spleen is normal in echotexture and size, measuring 9.4 cm. The visualized portions of the abdominal aorta and IVC are unremarkable.

Impression: Unremarkable ultrasound of the abdomen, including limited survey of both kidneys.

Assessment

Truong Pan is a 21-year-old Chinese woman with elevated LFTs and chronic hepatitis B

QUESTIONS

Problem Identification

1.a. Create a list of this patient's drug therapy problems.

1.b. Which clinical findings, laboratory values, and items in the medical history suggest the presence of chronic hepatitis B virus (HBV) infection?

Desired Outcome

2. What are the goals of treatment for a chronic active HBV infection?

Therapeutic Alternatives

3.a. What nonpharmacologic measures should be considered for this patient?

3.b. What pharmacotherapeutic alternatives are available for treatment of this patient?

Optimal Plan

4. What drug, dose, dosage form, schedule, and duration of therapy should be recommended?

Outcome Evaluation

5.a. How should the therapy you recommended be monitored for efficacy and adverse effects?

5.b. Which baseline parameters are favorable predictors of response to HBV treatment for this patient (ie, sustained loss of HBeAg and undetectable HBV DNA)? Are there any predictors of an unfavorable response?

Patient Education

6. What information should be provided to this patient regarding the treatment?

■ CLINICAL COURSE (PART 1)

The patient tolerated the initial therapy very well with minimal adverse effects. After 52 weeks of therapy, her physician stopped the medication. However, 3 months posttreatment, her serum HBV DNA was detectable. She also states that since finishing her hepatitis B therapy, she is in a relationship and sexually active. Her lab results for the past few months of treatment were as follows:

Test	12 Weeks After Therapy Started	24 Weeks After Therapy Started	52 Weeks After Therapy Started	9 Months After Therapy Discontinued
AST (IU/L)	54	39	21	55
ALT (IU/L)	78	30	18	84
Alk phos (IU/L)	76	80	83	73
T. bili (mg/dL)	0.5	0.9	0.9	0.8
PT (s)	11.2	11.2	10.7	10.1
Alb (g/dL)	3.9	4.8	4.8	4.2
HBsAg	(+)	(+)	(+)	(+)
Anti-HBs	(−)	(−)	(−)	(−)
HBeAg	(+)	(+)	Nonreactive	(+)
HBeAb	(−)	(+)	(+)	(−)
HBV DNA (IU/mL)	904	<29[a]	<29[a]	1,122,971

[a]<29 IU/mL indicates undetectable HBV DNA level.

■ FOLLOW-UP QUESTIONS

1. Based on these results, what therapy would you recommend, if any? Include the drug name, dose, dosage form, schedule, and duration of therapy.

2. What adverse effects may occur with this new therapy, and how would you monitor for them?

3. What information should be provided to this patient about the new treatment?

4. What information or therapeutic intervention do you need to provide to the patient and for her new boyfriend?

5. What information does the patient need to know and give to patients she cares for as she practices nursing?

■ CLINICAL COURSE (PART 2)

Eighteen months after the completion of her initial course of therapy, Trong Pan is now married and is 23 years old. She is 3 months pregnant and continues on her hepatitis B therapy. Her HBsAg status is positive.

■ FOLLOW-UP QUESTIONS (Continued)

6. Would you recommend that the patient discontinue her hepatitis B medication because she is pregnant? Justify your answer.

7. Would you recommend hepatitis B vaccination for her newborn? If yes, include the doses and dosage schedule.

■ SELF-STUDY ASSIGNMENTS

1. Describe the ideal patient infected with hepatitis B to respond to antiretroviral HBV therapy and what you would monitor for therapeutic efficacy and adverse effects.

2. Compare and contrast the mechanism of action, immunogenicity rate, and adverse effects of the two available hepatitis B vaccines.

3. Survey several pharmacies to estimate the approximate retail cost of the antiretroviral HBV agents and pegylated interferon therapy for the treatment of hepatitis B.

4. Review the time course of serologic markers after an acute HBV infection and explain their significance to one of your peers (Fig. 51-1).

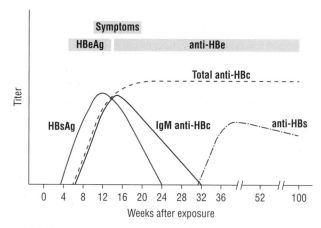

FIGURE 51-1. Typical serologic course of acute hepatitis B virus infection with recovery. *Note:* Serologic markers of infection vary depending on whether the infection is acute or chronic. *(Source: Centers for Disease Control and Prevention. Viral Hepatitis Resource Center.)*

CLINICAL PEARL

To eliminate HBV transmission that occurs during infancy and childhood, the Immunization Practices Advisory Committee of the Centers of Disease Control and Prevention recommends that all newborn infants be vaccinated regardless of the hepatitis B status of the mothers.

REFERENCES

1. World Health Organization (WHO). Guidelines for the prevention, care and treatment of persons with chronic hepatitis B infection. Geneva: WHO. Mar 2015. Available from: http://apps.who.int/iris/bitstream/10665/154590/1/9789241549059_eng.pdf?ua=1&ua=1. Last accessed November 8, 2015.
2. Martin P, Lau DT, Nguyen MH, et al. A Treatment Algorithm for the Management of Chronic Hepatitis B Virus Infection in the United States: 2015 Update. Clin Gastroenterol Hepatol 2015 Nov;13(12):2071–2087.e16.
3. Lok AS, McMahon BJ. Chronic hepatitis B: update 2009. Hepatology 2009;50:1–6.
4. Gish R, Jia JD, Locarnini S, Zoulim F. Selection of chronic hepatitis B therapy with high barrier to resistance. Lancet Infect Dis 2012;12:341–353.
5. Centers for Disease Control and Prevention. Hepatitis virus B: a comprehensive immunization strategy to eliminate transmission of hepatitis B virus infection in the United States: recommendations of the Advisory Committee on Immunization Practices (ACIP) part 1: immunization of infants, children, and adolescents. MMWR Morb Mortal Wkly Rep 2005;54(RR16):1–31.
6. Centers for Disease Control and Prevention. Hepatitis virus B: a comprehensive immunization strategy to eliminate transmission of hepatitis B virus infection in the United States: recommendations of the Advisory Committee on Immunization Practices (ACIP) part II: immunization of adults. MMWR Morb Mortal Wkly Rep 2006;55(RR16):1–33.
7. Centers for Disease Control and Prevention. Updated CDC recommendations for the management of hepatitis B virus-infected health-care providers and students. MMWR Morb Mortal Wkly Rep 2012;61(RR-3):1–12.
8. United States Department of Labor. Healthcare Wide Hazards (Lack of) Universal Precautions. Available at: *http://www.osha.gov/SLTC/etools/hospital/hazards/univprec/univ.html.* Accessed November 8, 2015.

52

VIRAL HEPATITIS C

Guidelines for Optimal Care De-LIVER-y . . . . Level II

Rima A. Mohammad, PharmD, BCPS

Randolph E. Regal, BS, PharmD

LEARNING OBJECTIVES

After completing this case study, the reader should be able to:

- Identify and evaluate the clinical manifestations and laboratory parameters relevant to the assessment and treatment of chronic hepatitis C virus (HCV) infection.

- Design a patient-specific pharmaceutical care plan for a patient with chronic HCV, including drugs, doses, and duration of therapy.

- Develop a plan for monitoring efficacy and adverse effects of the pharmacologic agents used in the management of chronic HCV.

- Identify and evaluate the drug interactions related to pharmacologic agents used in the treatment of chronic HCV, especially with direct-acting antivirals (DAAs).

- Provide patient education for patients with chronic HCV regarding their medications, nonpharmacologic interventions/behaviors, and vaccinations.

PATIENT PRESENTATION

Chief Complaint

"About two months ago, my internal medicine doctor informed me that my liver tests were abnormal. He referred me to your liver disease clinic for assessment and follow-up. I had my first liver clinic visit a month ago, and I'm here today to talk about treatment."

HPI

Jason Corey is a 38-year-old man who has been referred by his internal medicine physician to the liver clinic for assessment of his abnormal liver enzymes. After a conversation between the internal medicine physician and the hepatologist, Mr Corey had a battery of labs drawn and a liver biopsy done last week. He returns to the clinic today for a complete physical and further workup.

About 2 months ago, he went to his internal medicine physician for follow-up of his chronic left shoulder pain. The injury occurred 1.5 years ago from a body slam during a wrestling match with some friends. He was unable to treat the injury because he had no insurance at that time. He states that he has pain in his shoulder "all the time." He describes it as mild intensity, but it worsens during sleep, exercise, and physical therapy. He states that the pain is better with heat, and was improving with ibuprofen. However, his internal medicine physician discontinued ibuprofen in light of his potential liver disease. Since he was about 25 years old, he has worked out with weights about 3–4 days a week, and runs a few times a week. Although he continues to maintain his regimen despite working long hours, he has noticed a progressive decline in his stamina over the few months. He reports use of recreational drugs "on and off for the past 10 years," which included marijuana, alcohol, IV heroin, and intranasal cocaine. He states that he stopped use of these drugs around 6 months ago. He also has a history of alcohol abuse. His consumption of alcohol had gone from just an occasional social drink to drinking 8–12 drinks per day. He was treated for drug and alcohol abuse 6 months ago through an inpatient treatment program, and says he has been sober since that time. He does not recall ever having a blood transfusion. He denies any lower extremity edema, jaundice, or right upper quadrant pain. He also denies any hepatic encephalopathy or signs or stigmata of chronic liver disease at this time.

PMH

Major depressive disorder and anxiety: States he is currently on Seroquel and Zoloft and depression is well controlled.
GERD: Began several years ago, is often exacerbated by alcohol and spicy food. States he is currently on omeprazole.
Gastritis: Complaints of intermittent epigastric pain, increased in last 6 years (PUD never confirmed by EGD).
Chronic shoulder pain: Treated with applying heat and PRN ibuprofen (recently discontinued).

FH

No known family history of liver disease. Both parents are alive and living independently in their early 60s. He has two sisters (34 and 36 years old) and one brother (40 years old). His brother has some psychiatric issues, mainly anxiety, but otherwise his siblings are in good health.

SH

The patient earned his high school diploma. After being laid off as a customer service representative at a local bank where he had worked since his high school graduation, he recently found a job as a landscaper. He has been employed at that job for the past 6 months. He was divorced 1 year ago after 6 years of marriage, and has a 5-year-old daughter. He has since had one long-term relationship but never remarried. Currently, he is single and lives with his father and mother. He is a previous smoker who drank and used recreational drugs, including marijuana, alcohol, IV heroin, and intranasal cocaine for the past 10 years. About 6 months ago, he began counseling and treatment for his substance abuse, depression, and anxiety. His substance abuse and psychiatric problems worsened over the past year after his divorce. He states he has been clean for about 6 months. He smoked one and a half packs per day for the past 20 years, but recently quit smoking about 6 months ago.

Meds

MVI one tablet PO daily × 1 year
Omeprazole 40 mg PO BID × 5 years
Sertraline 150 mg PO at bedtime × 1 year
Quetiapine 400 mg PO BID × 6 months
Calcium carbonate 500 mg PO daily PRN × 5 years

Allergies and Intolerances

No known drug allergies.

ROS

General: He feels that overall his health is "pretty good" and it continues to improve in many respects as he exercises and makes healthier lifestyle choices. His GERD symptoms depend on the type of food he eats, and have been improved with weight loss, a better diet, and stopping drugs and alcohol. However, he reports a progressive decline in his exercise stamina over the past few months, occasional headache, and left shoulder pain with no apparent effect on ROM. The remainder of the review of systems was noncontributory, with no additional pertinent positives or negatives.

Physical Examination

Gen

General appearance of a well-nourished, well-built African-American man in NAD

VS

BP 138/92, P 88, RR 18, T 37.2°C; Wt 200 lb, Ht 5′10″

Skin

Intact without xanthomas, hematomas, or ecchymosis. No jaundice or palmar erythema

HEENT

PERRLA; EOMI; sclerae anicteric; funduscopic exam normal; TMs intact

Neck/Lymph Nodes

Neck supple; no lymphadenopathy or thyromegaly; no carotid bruits

Lungs/Thorax

Clear to auscultation with full and equal chest excursion. Normal breath sounds

CV

S_1, S_2 normal; no S_3 or S_4. No murmurs, rubs, or gallops

Abd

Soft, nontender. Normoactive bowel sounds. No organomegaly or bruits appreciated. No evidence of ascites

MS/Ext

No edema in LE bilaterally; peripheral pulses 2+ throughout; normal ROM. Some discomfort and pain with movement in left shoulder

Neuro

A & O × 3; CN II–XII intact; DTRs 2+

Labs Obtained 2 Months Ago from Patient's PCP

Na 138 mEq/L	Hgb 14 g/dL	AST 63 IU/L
K 4 mEq/L	Hct 39.8%	ALT 100 IU/L
Cl 103 mEq/L	Plt 237 × 10³/mm³	Alk phos 121 IU/L
CO_2 27 mEq/L	WBC 5.6 × 10³/mm³	T. bili 0.3 mg/dL
BUN 16 mg/dL	54% PMNS	Alb 4.4 g/dL
SCr 1.2 mg/dL	Bands 1%	GGT 42 IU/L
Glu 95 mg/dL	Lymphs 35%	HBsAg (−)
TSH 2.32 μIU/mL	Monos 10%	Anti-HAV (−)
PT 13.5 s	INR 1	Anti-HCV (+)

Labs Obtained at Preclinic Lab Draw About 1 Month Ago

Na 140 mEq/L	Hgb 14.0 g/dL	AST 58 IU/L	HBsAg (−)
K 4.1 mEq/L	Hct 39%	ALT 98 IU/L	Anti-HAV (−)
Cl 100 mEq/L	Plt 235 × 10³/mm³	Alk phos 112 IU/L	Anti-HCV (+)
CO_2 28 mEq/L		T. bili 0.4 mg/dL	HCV RNA (bDNA assay)
BUN 15 mg/dL	WBC 6 × 10³/mm³	Alb 4.1 g/dL	2.6 × 10⁶ copies/mL;
SCr 1.2 mg/dL		GGT 41 IU/L	1.3 × 10⁶ IU/mL
Glu 100 mg/dL	56% PMNs	Iron 95 mcg/dL	HCV genotype 1a
TSH 2.3 µIU/mL	Bands 1%	Ferritin 32 ng/mL	HIV (−)
T. chol 264 mg/dL	Lymphs 36%	TIBC 377 mcg/dL	IL28 gene homozygous
HDL 31 mg/dL	Monos 7%	T. sat. 25%	C/C
LDL 191 mg/dL	Uric acid 6 mg/dL		ANA (+)
TG 210 mg/dL	PT 12.0 sec		
	INR 1		

Liver Biopsy (Performed After Liver Clinic Visit 1 Month Ago)

Severe fibrosis (fibrosis 3/6) and severe chronic inflammation (a METAVIR score of A3) consistent with active severe chronic hepatitis with no indication of cirrhosis.

Assessment/Diagnosis

Newly diagnosed HCV, likely chronic

R/O cryoglobulinemia secondary to HCV (recently converted to positive ANA)

QUESTIONS

Problem Identification

1.a. Create a list of the patient's drug therapy problems. Prioritize the problems from most urgent to least urgent for addressing at this initial presentation. Other than the need for treating HCV, are any adjustments needed in his current medication regimen?

1.b. What physical findings and laboratory values indicate the presence of chronic HCV infection?

1.c. What risk factor(s) for HCV infection does the patient have?

1.d. What are the compelling reasons to treat this patient for chronic HCV?

Desired Outcome

2. What are the goals of treatment for chronic HCV infection?

Therapeutic Alternatives

3.a. What nonpharmacologic treatment measures should be implemented for this patient?

3.b. What pharmacotherapeutic alternatives are available for treatment of HCV infection in this patient?

3.c. Does this patient have any medical conditions that are considered at least relative contraindications to receiving the treatments discussed in the previous question?

Optimal Plan

4.a. Design a pharmacotherapeutic plan for this patient. Include the drug, dose, schedule, and duration of therapy.

4.b. Are there any potential drug interactions between his current medications and HCV medications? If any interactions are identified, what adjustments should be made to the patient's drug therapy based on these interactions?

4.c. What pharmacotherapeutic plan would you recommend to treat this patient's other active medical problems?

Outcome Evaluation

5.a. How should the therapy you recommended for HCV infection be monitored for efficacy and adverse effects?

5.b. Which baseline patient parameters may be predictors of poor response to the treatment you recommended?

5.c. What actions can be taken if the patient develops intolerable adverse effects to the treatment you recommended?

Patient Education

6. What information should be provided to this patient regarding his treatment?

■ CLINICAL COURSE: 4-WEEK VISIT

At his 4-week visit after initiation of HCV therapy, which included ribavirin, Mr Corey reports feeling more fatigue than at baseline; his AST and ALT are 37 and 40 IU/L, but his HCV RNA value is now 800 IU/mL (1600 copies/mL). He does report some SOB and DOE, but denies orthostatic symptoms. Other labs are similar to the initial presentation except for hemoglobin 11.3 g/dL, hematocrit 32.9%, WBC 9 × 10³/mm³, platelets 372 × 10³/mm³, and TSH 1.43 µIU/mL. He states that he has been adherent to therapy.

■ FOLLOW-UP QUESTIONS

1. Based on this information, should the therapy continue as planned? Why or why not?

2. What other laboratory tests would help you to monitor possible adverse effects of drug therapy?

■ CLINICAL COURSE: 8-WEEK VISIT

At his 8-week visit, Mr Corey reports feeling a little worse. Lab values include AST 32 IU/L, ALT 28 IU/L, and qualitative HCV RNA (−). Other labs are similar to the previous visit with the exception of hemoglobin 9 g/dL, hematocrit 29.1%, WBC 9.1 × 10³/mm³, and platelets 299 × 10³/mm³. He is experiencing more fatigue and SOB compared with the last visit. He is also experiencing severe seasonal allergies and his internal medicine physician prescribed Flonase one spray in each nostril once a day and albuterol inhaler two puffs every 6 hours as needed for SOB.

■ FOLLOW-UP QUESTIONS

3. Based on this information, should the therapy continue as planned? Why or why not?

4. What is the next option to treat anemia in this patient?

5. Are there any new drug therapy problems related to his new medications? If so, what are your recommendations to treat the current problems in this patient?

■ CLINICAL COURSE: 12-WEEK VISIT

At his 12-week visit, Mr Corey reports feeling better. Lab values include AST 41 IU/L, ALT 52 IU/L, and qualitative HCV RNA test (−). Other labs are similar to the previous visit with the exception of hemoglobin 11.0 g/dL, hematocrit 34.3%, WBC 3 × 10³/mm³, and platelets 142 × 10³/mm³. He appears well nourished and comfortable. He is more energetic and exercising more.

■ FOLLOW-UP QUESTIONS

6. Based on this information, should the therapy continue as planned? Why or why not?

7. What actions can be taken if the adverse effects are resolved in this patient?

8. Outline a plan for vaccinating the patient against other forms of viral hepatitis.

■ SELF-STUDY ASSIGNMENTS

1. Review the recent AASLD/IDSA guidelines for the treatment of chronic HCV genotype 1 infection and summarize the advantages and disadvantages of the various DAA regimens.

2. Perform a literature search to compare the differences in pharmacokinetic properties and tolerance between the DAAs.

3. Estimate the cost of a treatment course of DAA therapy in treatment-naïve HCV patients who achieve extended rapid virologic response (eRVR) during therapy.

4. Perform a literature search on new agents currently undergoing development and evaluation for the treatment of chronic HCV.

CLINICAL PEARL

DAA therapy is associated with many drug interactions due to DAAs being substrates, inducers and/or inhibitors of cytochrome P450 (CYP) 3A or 2C8, P-glycoprotein (P-gp), and organic anion transporting polypeptide (OATP) 1B1 and 2B1. Additional dosage adjustments and monitoring recommendations are reviewed in the prescribing information of each DAA medication; however, not all potential drug interactions have been studied and/or listed in the prescribing information. To supplement this information, pharmacokinetic properties of medications can be analyzed for the extent and pathway of metabolism. In the instances where there are no viable therapeutic alternatives, close monitoring of the interacting medication and dose titration could be recommended.

REFERENCES

1. Recommendations for testing, managing, and treating hepatitis C. American Association for the Study of Liver Diseases and Infectious Diseases Society of America. Available at: http://www.hcvguidelines.org/full-report-view. Accessed April 25, 2016.

2. Hepatitis C Information for Health Professionals. Division of Viral Hepatitis and National Center for HIV/AIDS, Viral Hepatitis, STD, and TB Prevention. Centers of Disease Control and Prevention Publication. March 14, 2011. Available at: http://www.cdc.gov/hepatitis/HCV/index.htm. Accessed April 25, 2016.

3. Burger D, Back D, Buggisch P, et al. Clinical management of drug–drug interactions in HCV therapy: challenges and solutions. J Hepatol 2013;58:792–800.

4. Deming P, Martin MT, Chan J, et al. Therapeutic advances in HCV genotype 1 infection: Insights from the Society of Infectious Diseases Pharmacists. Pharmacotherapy 2016;36:203–217.

5. Mohammad RA, Bulloch MN, Chan J, et al. Provision of clinical pharmacist services for individuals with chronic hepatitis C viral infection: Joint Opinion of the GI/Liver/Nutrition and Infectious Diseases Practice and Research Networks of the American College of Clinical Pharmacy. Pharmacotherapy 2014;34:1341–1354.

6. Zepatier package insert. Whitehouse Station, NJ; Merck&Co.; 2016.

7. Hep Drug Interactions. University of Liverpool. Available at: http://www.hep-druginteractions.org. Accessed April 25, 2016.

8. Franz CC, Egger S, Born C, Ratz Bravo AE, Krahenbuhl S. Potential drug–drug interactions and adverse drug reactions in patients with liver cirrhosis. Eur J Clin Pharmacol 2012;68:179–188.

9. Risser A, Donovan D, Heintzman J, Page T. NSAID prescribing precautions. Am Fam Physician 2009;80:1371–1378.

10. Benson GD, Koff RS, Tolman KG. Therapeutic use of acetaminophen in patients with liver disease. Am J Ther 2005;12:133–141.

53

DRUG-INDUCED ACUTE KIDNEY INJURY

Not a Cute Consequence .... Level II

Mary K. Stamatakis, PharmD

LEARNING OBJECTIVES

After completing this case study, the reader should be able to:

- Evaluate clinical and laboratory findings in a patient with AKI.

- Select pharmacotherapy for treatment of complications associated with AKI.

- Assess appropriateness of aminoglycoside serum concentrations in relation to efficacy and toxicity.

- Develop strategies to prevent drug-induced AKI, including the selection of pharmacologic alternatives that do not adversely affect kidney function.

- Adjust drug dosages based on a patient's estimated kidney function to maximize efficacy and minimize adverse events.

PATIENT PRESENTATION

▓ Chief Complaint

Not available

▓ HPI

Wilbur Elliott is a 79-year-old man who originally presented to the hospital 1 month ago with symptoms of heart failure that culminated in mitral valve replacement surgery. His surgery was complicated by a 1-hour hypotensive episode, with BP of 70/50 mm Hg during surgery. Three days postoperation, purulent drainage was noted from the surgical site, and he was subsequently diagnosed with mediastinitis. At that time, he was also found to have *Serratia* bacteremia (blood cultures × 4 positive for *Serratia marcescens*, sensitive to gentamicin, piperacillin, ceftazidime, ceftriaxone, and ciprofloxacin; resistance was noted to ampicillin). Therapy was initiated with gentamicin and ceftazidime. Thus far, he has completed day 21 of a 6-week course of antibiotics. A gradual increase in his BUN and serum creatinine concentrations from baseline has been noted (see Table 53-1) and signs of volume overload are present.

▓ PMH

Type 2 DM
CKD

Dyslipidemia
Osteoarthritis
HTN
Heart failure
Depression

▓ PSH

Mechanical mitral valve replacement surgery 28 days ago

▓ FH

Father had type 2 DM

▓ SH

Denies smoking or alcohol; retired coal miner (11 years ago)

▓ Meds

Gentamicin (see Table 53-1 for dosages and serum drug concentrations; gentamicin is currently on hold)

Ceftazidime 1 g IVPB Q 12 H
Warfarin 5 mg PO once daily
Enalapril 5 mg PO once daily
Colace 100 mg PO twice daily
Furosemide 40 mg PO Q 12 H × 2 days
Atorvastatin 20 mg PO daily
Escitalopram 10 mg PO daily
Glipizide 10 mg PO daily
Ibuprofen 400 mg PO Q 4–6 H PRN pain (started today for joint pain)

▓ All

NKDA

▓ ROS

Currently complains of trouble breathing, weakness, general malaise, and pain in right hand. No fever or chills

▓ Physical Examination

Gen

Confused-appearing man in mild distress

VS

BP 152/90 mm Hg, P 80 bpm, RR 26, T 37.7°C; current Wt 80 kg (admission Wt 75 kg), Ht 5′9″

Skin

Normal skin turgor, surgical incision site healing with no drainage

HEENT

PERRLA, EOMI, poor dentition

Neck/Lymph Nodes

(+) JVD

TABLE 53-1	Serum Creatinine, BUN, and Serum Gentamicin Concentrations During Hospitalization				
Postoperative Day	SCr (mg/dL)	BUN (mg/dL)	Gentamicin (mcg/mL)		Gentamicin Dosages
			Peak[a]	Trough[b]	
3	1.5	15			140 mg × 1, and then 120 mg Q 12 H
5	1.5	22	6.3	1.1	Continue current regimen
7	1.7	21			
10	2.1	22	6.9	1.8	Continue current regimen
14	2.7	21	8.3	2.5	Decrease to 120 mg Q 24 H
17	3.0	26			
21	3.2	27	9.4	2.7	Gentamicin on hold

BUN, blood urea nitrogen; SCr, serum creatinine.

[a]Serum drug concentrations drawn 30 minutes after a 30-minute infusion.

[b]Serum drug concentrations drawn immediately before a dose.

Chest

Basilar crackles, inspiratory wheezes

CV

S_1, S_2 normal, no S_3, irregular rhythm

Abd

Soft, nontender, (+) BS, (–) HSM

Genit/Rect

(–) Masses

MS/Ext

2+ ankle/sacral edema; some tenderness and limited motion in right hand

Neuro

A & O to person and place, but not to time

■ Labs (Current)

Na 139 mEq/L	Hgb 9.7 g/dL	Ca 8.6 mg/dL
K 3.7 mEq/L	Hct 29.5%	Mg 2.1 mg/dL
Cl 103 mEq/L	Plt 303 × 10³/mm³	Phos 4.4 mg/dL
CO_2 24 mEq/L	WBC 8.6 × 10³/mm³	INR 2.7
BUN 50 mg/dL	(BUN 19 mg/dL on admission)	
SCr 3.2 mg/dL	(SCr 1.5 mg/dL on admission)	
Glu 119 mg/dL		

■ UA

Color, yellow; character, hazy; glucose (–); ketones (–); SG 1.010; pH 5.0; protein 30 mg/dL; coarse granular casts 5–10/lpf; WBC 0–3/hpf; RBC 0–2/hpf; no bacteria; nitrite (–); osmolality 325 mOsm; urinary sodium 45 mEq/L; creatinine 33 mg/dL, FE_{NA} 3.1%.

■ Repeat Blood Cultures Today

Negative

■ Fluid Intake/Output and Daily Weights

Day	I/O	Weight (kg)
3 days ago	3200 mL/900 mL	N/A
2 days ago	2600 mL/1000 mL	76
Yesterday	2800 mL/1300 mL	N/A
Today	N/A	80

■ Assessment

AKI with extracellular fluid expansion

QUESTIONS

Problem Identification

1.a. Create a list of the patient's drug therapy problems.

1.b. What information (signs, symptoms, and laboratory values) indicates the presence or severity of the patient's problem(s)?

1.c. Based on his AKI, do any of his medications require dosage adjustment? If so, what adjustment would you recommend?

1.d. What additional laboratory information would assist in the assessment of this patient?

1.e. Could any of the patient's problems have been caused by drug therapy?

1.f. What risk factors did the patient have for gentamicin-induced AKI?

1.g. What therapeutic interventions could have been initiated to decrease the likelihood of developing drug-induced AKI?

1.h. Could extended-interval gentamicin dosing have minimized the likelihood of nephrotoxicity?

Desired Outcome

2. What are the goals of pharmacotherapy in this case?

Therapeutic Alternatives

3.a. What nondrug therapies might be useful for this patient?

3.b. What feasible pharmacotherapeutic alternatives are available for treating AKI in this patient?

Optimal Plan

4. What drugs, dosage forms, doses, schedules, and duration of therapy are best for this patient?

Outcome Evaluation

5. What clinical and laboratory parameters are necessary to evaluate therapy for achievement of the desired therapeutic outcomes and to detect or prevent adverse effects?

Patient Education

6. What information should be provided to the patient to enhance compliance, ensure successful therapy, and minimize adverse effects?

■ SELF-STUDY ASSIGNMENTS

1. Based on the patient's change in serum creatinine or urine output, classify the patient's AKI as Stage 1, Stage 2, or Stage 3.

2. Create a list of medication that may cause or worsen AKI and which should be avoided in this patient.

3. Assume that Mr Elliott's serum creatinine is 1.4 mg/dL at 1 month after discharge. At what point would you consider restarting the ACE inhibitor? Justify the use of ACE inhibitors in patients with chronic kidney disease.

4. What is the target INR in this patient? Do any of his medications interact with warfarin?

CLINICAL PEARL

Furosemide administration enhances sodium excretion, which results in an elevated FE_{NA} and limits the utility of the FE_{NA} calculation to assess AKI. To avoid misinterpretation of the FE_{NA} results, delay obtaining an FE_{NA} until the effect of the furosemide dose is complete (up to 10 hours in patients with kidney disease).

REFERENCES

1. Kidney Disease: Improving Global Outcomes (KDIGO) Acute Kidney Injury Work Group. KDIGO Clinical Practice Guideline for acute kidney injury. Kidney Inter Suppl 2012;2:1–138.

2. Mehta RL, Kellum JA, Shah SV, et al. Acute Kidney Injury Network: report of an initiative to improve outcomes in acute kidney injury. Crit Care 2007;11:R31.

3. Jelliffe R. Estimation of creatinine clearance in patients with unstable renal function, without a urine specimen. Am J Nephrol 2002;22:320–324.

4. Lopez-Novoa JM, Quiros Y, Vicente L, Morales AI, Lopez-Hernandez FJ. New insights into the mechanism of aminoglycoside nephrotoxicity: an integrative point of view. Kidney Int 2011;79:33–45.

5. Oliveira JF, Silva CA, Barbieri CD, Oliveira GM, Zanetta DMT, Burdmann EA. Prevalence and risk factors for aminoglycoside nephrotoxicity in intensive care units. Antimicrob Agents Chemother 2009;53:2887–2891.

6. Brater DC. Update in diuretic therapy: clinical pharmacology. Semin Nephrol 2011;31:483–494.

7. Wulf NR, Matuszewski KA. Sulfonamide cross-reactivity: Is there evidence to support broad cross-allergenicity? Am J Health-Syst Pharm 2013;7:1483–1494.

54

ACUTE KIDNEY INJURY

There's Nothing Cute About It . . . . Level II

Scott Bolesta, PharmD, BCPS, FCCM

LEARNING OBJECTIVES

After completing this case study, the reader should be able to:

- Assess a patient with AKI using clinical and laboratory data.

- Classify AKI in a patient.

- Distinguish between AKI resulting from prerenal and that from intrinsic injury.

- Recommend changes to the pharmacotherapeutic regimen of a patient with AKI.

- Justify appropriate therapeutic interventions for a patient with AKI.

PATIENT PRESENTATION

▪ Chief Complaint

"I feel really weak."

▪ HPI

Everit Mitchell is a 72-year-old man who presents to the ED with complaints of severe weakness that started this morning and recent stomach pain for the past week. He was feeling normal until he developed stomach pain 1 week ago that worsened with meals. Two days ago the pain worsened to the point where he avoided eating, and last evening he felt more tired than usual and went to bed early. He had difficulty sleeping due to the pain and since waking this morning he has been in too much pain and too weak to perform his normal ADLs. His wife brought him to the ED because his physician is away on vacation.

▪ PMH

HTN × 30 years
CAD × 20 years
MI × 2 with most recent 2 months ago s/p PCI with drug-eluting stent placement
s/p CABG 20 years ago
HF × 4 years
RA × 1 year

▪ FH

Father died of an acute MI at age 52; mother had diabetes mellitus and died of a stroke at the age of 65.

▪ SH

Retired and living at home with his wife. Before retirement, the patient was employed as an accountant. No alcohol, no tobacco use.

▪ Meds

Aspirin 81 mg PO daily
Amlodipine 10 mg PO once daily
Furosemide 40 mg PO once daily
Metoprolol succinate 50 mg PO once daily
Enalapril 20 mg PO once daily
Prasugrel 10 mg PO daily
Naproxen 500 mg PO BID

▪ All

NKA

▪ ROS

In addition to weakness and stomach pain, the patient complains of feeling cold but denies chills or fever. No changes in vision. Denies SOB, CP, and cough. Complains of feeling lightheaded. Has been having frequent loose black stools over the past 3 days and abdominal pain that has become severe in the last two days. Has noted a decrease in the frequency of his urination over the past 24 hours. Denies musculoskeletal pain or cramping.

Physical Examination

Gen

Pale, elderly Caucasian man who appears in moderate distress and generally weak and lethargic

VS

BP 89/43 mm Hg (77/32 mm Hg on standing), P 123 bpm, RR 25, T 36.1°C; Wt 78 kg, Ht 5′9″

Skin

Pale and cool with poor turgor

HEENT

PERRLA; EOMI; fundi normal; conjunctivae pale and dry; TMs intact; tongue and mouth dry

Neck/Lymph Nodes

No JVD or HJR; no lymphadenopathy or thyromegaly

Lungs

No crackles or rhonchi

CV

Tachycardic with regular rhythm; normal S_1, S_2; no S_3; faint S_4; no MRG

Abd

Rigid with guarding, epigastric tenderness, ND; no HSM; hyperactive BS

Genit/Rect

Stool heme (+); slightly enlarged prostate

MS/Ext

Weak pulses; no peripheral edema; mild swelling of MCP joints of both hands

Neuro

A & O × 3; CNs intact; DTRs 2+; Babinski (–)

Labs

Na 132 mEq/L	Ca 8.6 mg/dL
K 5.6 mEq/L	Mg 2.1 mg/dL
Cl 97 mEq/L	Phos 4.3 mg/dL
CO_2 22 mEq/L	WBC $8.6 \times 10^3/mm^3$
BUN 53 mg/dL	Hgb 7.6 g/dL
SCr 1.8 mg/dL	Hct 22.5%
Glu 123 mg/dL	Plt $96 \times 10^3/mm^3$

Assessment

A 72-year-old man with a suspected acute UGI bleed secondary to combined antiplatelet and NSAIDs use that has resulted in anemia and AKI from hypovolemia

QUESTIONS

Problem Identification

1.a. Create a list of the patient's drug therapy problems as they relate to his AKI.

1.b. What information (signs, symptoms, and laboratory values) indicates the presence or severity of hypovolemia and AKI in this patient?

Desired Outcome

2. What are the goals of pharmacotherapy in this case?

■ CLINICAL COURSE

On admission, the patient was resuscitated aggressively with IV normal saline and multiple transfusions (4 units of PRBCs). His home medications were held, and he underwent an emergent EGD. During endoscopy, a large ulcer in the gastric antrum was found with an exposed spurting artery. Endoscopic therapy was unsuccessful, and the patient was taken to the OR for surgical intervention. He was hypotensive in the OR (BP 70 mm Hg systolic on average) and was started on a norepinephrine infusion to maintain a stable BP. Postoperatively, he remained on mechanical ventilation, and his urine output was <100 mL total over the first 12 postoperative hours despite continued aggressive IV hydration and repeated transfusions in the OR. He also remained on norepinephrine for a continued low BP. On the morning of postoperative day 1, his labs were as follows:

Na 134 mEq/L	Ca 8.2 mg/dL
K 5.4 mEq/L	Mg 2.2 mg/dL
Cl 111 mEq/L	Phos 4.7 mg/dL
CO_2 19 mEq/L	WBC $14.6 \times 10^3/mm^3$
BUN 49 mg/dL	Hgb 10.3 g/dL
SCr 2.5 mg/dL	Hct 29.8%
Glu 145 mg/dL	Plt $112 \times 10^3/mm^3$

Urinalysis also showed muddy brown casts, urine sodium of 72 mEq/L, and specific gravity of 1.004. A diagnosis of ATN was made, and the patient was started on furosemide 80 mg IV Q 8 H. On postoperative day 2, the patient remained on mechanical ventilation and norepinephrine, his urine output had not improved, and his chest radiograph showed diffuse bilateral pulmonary edema with a decrease in O_2 saturation to 86%. An echocardiogram revealed hypokinesis of the anterior portion of the left ventricle and an EF of 25%. The patient was started on dobutamine, and an internal jugular vein catheter was inserted and CVVH-DF was begun. On postoperative day 5, his pulmonary edema had resolved, norepinephrine and dobutamine had been weaned off, the dialysis catheter was removed, and he was extubated. His subsequent hospital course was uneventful, and his kidney function gradually improved.

Therapeutic Alternatives

3.a. What nondrug therapies were used to manage this patient's AKI? Discuss the evidence that supports their use.

3.b. What pharmacotherapeutic alternatives have been studied for the treatment of AKI?

Optimal Plan

4. Design an optimal therapeutic plan for managing this patient's AKI postoperatively.

Outcome Evaluation

5. What clinical and laboratory parameters are necessary to evaluate the therapy for achievement of the desired therapeutic outcome and to detect or prevent adverse effects?

Patient Education

6. What information should be provided to the patient to help avoid future episodes of AKI?

■ SELF-STUDY ASSIGNMENTS

1. Compare and contrast the RIFLE criteria for defining and classifying AKI to that published by the Acute Kidney Injury Network, and describe how both of these definitions of AKI helped form the definition proposed by the KDIGO Guidelines.

2. Write a brief paper that discusses the pharmacotherapeutic interventions that have been studied for the prevention of AKI from causes other than IV contrast agents.

CLINICAL PEARL

Patients in the recovery (or "diuretic") phase of ATN produce large amounts of dilute urine due to resolution of tubular obstruction from sloughed tubular epithelial cells and inability of the recovering tubular cells to reabsorb sodium. This return of urine output does not signal complete recovery of kidney function, and medications eliminated to a large extent by active tubular secretion may still accumulate and require dosage adjustment.

REFERENCES

1. Kidney Disease: Improving Global Outcomes (KDIGO) Acute Kidney Injury Work Group. KDIGO Clinical Practice Guideline for acute kidney injury. Kidney Inter Suppl 2012;2:1–138.

2. Myburgh JA, Finfer S, Bellomo R, et al. Hydroxyethyl starch or saline for fluid resuscitation in intensive care. N Engl J Med 2012;367:1901–1911.

3. Prowle JR, Kirwan CJ, Bellomo R. Fluid management for the prevention and attenuation of acute kidney injury. Nat Rev Nephrol 2014;10:37–47.

4. Palevsky PM. Renal replacement therapy in acute kidney injury. Adv Chronic Kidney Dis 2013;20:76–84.

5. Ejaz AA, Mohandas R. Are diuretics harmful in the management of acute kidney injury? Curr Opin Nephrol Hypertens 2014;23:155–160.

6. Kellum JA, Lameire N. Diagnosis, evaluation, and management of acute kidney injury: a KDIGO summary (Part 1). Crit Care 2013;17:204.

7. Bellomo R, Wan L, May C. Vasoactive drugs and acute kidney injury. Crit Care Med 2008;36(Suppl):S179–S186.

55

PROGRESSIVE RENAL DISEASE

It Was Only a Matter of Time .... Level III

Michelle D. Furler, BSc Pharm, PhD

LEARNING OBJECTIVES

After completing this case study, the reader should be able to:

- Discuss various methods for estimating creatinine clearance and glomerular filtration rate.

- Differentiate AKI from CKD.

- Identify risk factors for progression of renal disease.

- Recommend nonpharmacologic and pharmacologic interventions to alter the rate of progression of renal disease.

- Recognize and treat potential comorbid or pathologic conditions that are frequently associated with chronic renal insufficiency.

- Educate patients about the common medications prescribed for chronic renal insufficiency.

- Provide recommendations for renal disease therapy during pregnancy.

PATIENT PRESENTATION

■ Chief Complaint

"I'm here to check the results of my labs."

■ HPI

Christine Karter-Davis is a 38-year-old woman with type 2 diabetes mellitus who returns to her PCP for a follow-up visit. At her routine physical examination 3 months ago, her annual kidney screening revealed 3+ protein and an ACR of 659 mg/g in spot urine collection. This is elevated from last year's screening which showed mildly increased albumin and SCr elevation of 1.2 mg/dL. A follow-up appointment was scheduled 6 weeks ago, and a second spot urine test showed persistent elevation of ACR 615 mg/g. Complete laboratory workup was ordered at that time along with a 24-hour urine collection (conducted 1 week ago). She has returned to the office today to review the results of this testing.

A pleasant woman with no current medical complaints, Ms Karter-Davis arrives in the office today with a printout of her home blood glucose monitor readings. Review of the report shows only six tests in the last month, all between 6:00 AM and 7:00 AM. From her past pregnancy she is known to have an aversion to needles, and on questioning reveals that she hates the lancing device, and the finger pricks really hurt so she does not test very often. She has started a new regimen of daily vitamin D and aspirin because she heard that it was good for her. She also shows you her new pill organizer (Dosette pack) that she picked up at the pharmacy on the way to the office. She says that with the new vitamins she has been forgetting to take some of her medications but feels that the pill organizer will help her remember.

■ PMH

Type 2 DM × 8 years (history of gestational diabetes with use of insulin required)
HTN × 6 years
Dyslipidemia × 5 years
Gastric ulcer treated several years ago with *H. pylori* regimen (antibiotics and PPI)
Appendectomy at age 16

■ FH

Father had DM and CHD and died at age 50 secondary to MI; mother (age 62) has HTN and dyslipidemia. Brother (age 31) has DM, and two sisters (age 27 and 29) have no known medical problems other than obesity.

■ SH

The patient is an administrative assistant, married for 6 months with one child (age 10) from a past relationship. Her job provides medical coverage and prescription drug benefits. She reports occasional alcohol consumption on weekends or when out with friends (one to two alcoholic beverages per month). She is a one ppd smoker; this is a decrease from her reported use of two ppd last year. No history of illicit drug use.

The patient admits to a somewhat sedentary lifestyle but says her husband and son have been trying to interest her in family outings with their new puppy. She drinks three to four cups of coffee per day. She tends to have fast food on her lunch hour but has begun making her lunches in an effort to save money for a belated honeymoon. Her husband is a weekend basketball player, and they have recently set up a home gym with a weight set that she has "played around with" but has not used in any serious way. She mentions that her husband enjoys protein shakes and bars that she has started taking occasionally in her lunches. She enjoys fried foods but indicates that her husband is now doing most of the cooking, barbequing several times per week. She has lost 4 kg since last year.

■ All

NKDA, seasonal allergies to grass and pollen

■ Meds

Metformin 1000 mg AM, 500 mg lunch and 1000 mg supper × 2 years; however, patient states she is taking 500 mg PO BID

Hydrochlorothiazide 50 mg PO daily × 1 year, increased last year from 25 mg daily

Atorvastatin 10 mg PO at bedtime × 1 year

Nasonex two sprays in each nostril BID (seasonal—not using currently)

Cetirizine 10 mg PO daily PRN allergies

Aleve PO PRN headaches

Omeprazole OTC 20 mg PO PRN "indigestion"

Multivitamin PO daily

Vitamin D₃ 1000 IU PO daily × 2 weeks

ASA 325 mg PO daily × 2 weeks

■ ROS

Occasional headaches, generally associated with menstruation; no c/o polyuria, polydipsia, polyphagia, sensory loss, or visual changes

No dysuria, flank pain, hematuria, pedal edema, chest pain, or SOB

■ Physical Examination

Gen

The patient is an obese African-American woman in NAD

VS

BP 162/94 mm Hg sitting and standing in both arms, HR 82, RR 18, T 37.5°C; Wt 87 kg, Ht 5′6″

Skin

Warm, dry, no rashes

HEENT

PERRLA, EOMI, fundi have microaneurysms consistent with diabetic retinopathy; no retinal edema or vitreous hemorrhage. TMs intact. Oral mucosa moist with no lesions.

Neck/Lymph Nodes

Supple without adenopathy or thyromegaly

Lungs/Thorax

Clear, breath sounds normal

CV

Heart sounds normal, no murmurs, no bruits

Abd

Soft NT/ND

Genit/Rect

Rectal exam deferred; recent Pap smear negative

MS/Ext

No CCE, normal ROM

Neuro

A & O × 3; CNs intact; normal DTRs

■ Labs (1 Week Ago, Fasting)

Na 140 mEq/L	Hgb 12.2 g/dL	*Fasting lipid profile:*
K 3.1 mEq/L	Hct 36.1%	T. chol 213 mg/dL
Cl 107 mEq/L	WBC 9.5 × 10³/mm³	Trig 149 mg/dL
CO₂ 26 mEq/L	Plt 148 × 10³/mm³	LDL 141 mg/dL
BUN 29 mg/dL	Ca 9.4 mg/dL	HDL 42 mg/dL
SCr 1.4 mg/dL	Phos 2.7 mg/dL	Alb 3.4 g/dL
Glu 196 mg/dL	Uric acid 6.2 mg/dL	
A1C 10.4%	eGFR_MDRD 40.6 mL/ min/1.73 m²	

■ UA (1 Week Ago)

pH 5.2, 1+ glucose, (–) ketones, 3+ protein, (–) leukocyte esterase and nitrite; (–) RBC; 3–4 WBC/hpf, ACR 673 mg/g

■ 24-Hour Urine Collection

Total urine volume 2.2 L, urine creatinine 64 mg/dL, urine albumin 873 mg/24 hour

■ Assessment

A 38-year-old woman recently diagnosed with diabetic nephropathy or diabetic kidney disease (DKD) and overt albuminuria complicated by inadequately controlled comorbid conditions.

QUESTIONS

Problem Identification

1.a. Create a list of the patient's drug therapy problems and include the evidence to support your assessment.

1.b. What signs, symptoms, or laboratory values indicate the presence, severity, and nature of renal disease in this patient?

1.c. What other risk factors for renal disease are present in this patient?

1.d. Are there alterative explanations for kidney disease in diabetic patients, and are additional laboratory evaluations indicated?

1.e. Discuss the value of the urine ACR. Calculate the ACR from the reported 24-hour urine and compare it to the spot urine results. Was collection of a 24-hour urine necessary in this patient?

1.f. What is the GFR in this patient both last year and last week, estimated using the 24-hour urine collection and the Cockcroft–Gault, MDRD, and CKD-EPI equations? Which of these estimates provides the best information for adjustment of drug dosing?

1.g. What degree of renal failure does this patient have?

1.h. Compare the definition, classification, and prognosis of CKD to AKI.

Desired Outcome

2. What are the goals of pharmacotherapy for the patient's medical conditions? Focus on renal insufficiency, diabetes, hypertension, and dyslipidemia.

Therapeutic Alternatives

3.a. What nonpharmacologic therapies might be useful to control this patient's medical conditions?

3.b. What are the pharmacotherapeutic alternatives for preventing renal disease progression and managing this patient's diabetes mellitus, hypertension, and dyslipidemia?

Optimal Plan

4. What drug regimens would provide optimal therapy for this patient's medical problems?

Outcome Evaluation

5. Outline the clinical and laboratory parameters necessary to evaluate the efficacy and safety of the recommended regimens for the patient's nephropathy, diabetes mellitus, hypertension, and dyslipidemia.

Patient Education

6. Based on the regimen you recommended, what information should be provided to the patient to ensure successful therapy and minimize adverse effects?

■ CLINICAL COURSE (PART 1)

The patient is started on the medications you recommended for renal protection, diabetes, hypertension, dyslipidemia, and cardiovascular protection. The patient returns to clinic 4 weeks later. She has a bit of a cough but reports tolerating her new medications well. She states that she is watching her diet and has been enjoying more outings with her family, exercising before work three times per week in the family weight room, and walking the dog for 20–30 minutes each evening after work with her husband and son. On evaluation, the following results are obtained: BP sitting and standing 150/87 mm Hg, HR 80, and ACR 420 mg/g. Fasting labs: BUN 29 mg/dL, SCr 1.6 mg/dL, Glu 146 mg/dL, K 4.3 mEq/L, Na 140 mEq/L, Alb 3.2 g/dL, Hct 36.1%, eGFR 42.2 mL/min/1.73 m², T. chol 203 mg/dL, TG 147 mg/dL, LDL 132 mg/dL, and HDL 42 mg/dL.

■ FOLLOW-UP QUESTIONS

1. Is the patient experiencing any adverse effects from her new medication regimen?

2. What additional information would be beneficial to you in evaluating her response to therapy?

3. For each of the major medical problems, describe any adjustments in pharmacotherapy that are required and outline a follow-up plan.

■ CLINICAL COURSE (PART 2)

After several months, the patient presents to the pharmacy for a refill of her medications. While speaking with the pharmacist, she asks for a recommendation regarding prenatal vitamins, indicating that she and her husband have recently discovered that she is pregnant.

■ FOLLOW-UP QUESTIONS

4. What impact, if any, will pregnancy have on the management and progression of nephropathy in this patient?

5. Are any changes required in her drug therapy at this time? If so, which ones and why? What nonpharmacological recommendations should be made?

■ SELF-STUDY ASSIGNMENTS

1. Discuss the role of diuretic therapy in patients with normal renal function compared to those with creatinine clearance values <20 mL/min.

2. Review and compare the effects of antihypertensive agents on renal blood flow and glomerular filtration rate in patients with hypertension and diabetic nephropathy.

CLINICAL PEARL

Both normotensive and hypertensive patients with type 2 diabetes and persistent albuminuria should be treated with either an ACE inhibitor or ARB to slow the progression of diabetic nephropathy and other microvascular and macrovascular diseases. A comprehensive treatment plan must include management of comorbid illnesses, with a particular focus on glycemic control and cardiovascular disease. Effective disease management must be tailored to patient needs and modified according to patient preferences and lifestyle.

REFERENCES

1. American Diabetes Association. Standards of medical care in diabetes—2016. Diabetes Care 2016:39(Suppl 1):S1–S112.

2. Canadian Diabetes Association Clinical Practice Guidelines Expert Committee. Canadian Diabetes Association 2013 clinical practice guidelines for the prevention and management of diabetes in Canada. Can J Diabetes 2013;37(Suppl 1):S1–S216. (2016 Interim Update to the Pharmacologic Management of Type 2 Diabetes chapter of these guidelines may be found at: http://guidelines.diabetes.ca/2016update.)

3. National Kidney Foundation. KDOQI clinical practice guidelines and clinical practice recommendations for diabetes and chronic kidney disease. Am J Kidney Dis 2007;49(Suppl 2):S1–S180.

4. National Kidney Foundation. KDOQI clinical practice guideline for diabetes and CKD: 2012 update. Am J Kidney Dis 2012;60:850–886.

5. Kidney Disease: Improving Global Outcomes (KDIGO) CKD Work Group. KDIGO 2012 Clinical practice guideline for the evaluation and management of chronic kidney disease. Kidney Intern Suppl 2013;3:1–150.

6. National Kidney Foundation. Frequently asked questions about GFR estimates. National Kidney Foundation, 2014. Available at: https://www.kidney.org/sites/default/files/docs/12-10-4004_abe_faqs_aboutgfrrev1b_singleb.pdf Accessed November 15, 2015.

7. Goff DC Jr, Lloyd-Jones DM, Bennett G, et al. 2013 ACC/AHA guideline on the assessment of cardiovascular risk: a report of the American College of Cardiology/American Heart Association Task Force on Practice Guidelines 2014;129:S49–S73.

8. Kidney Disease: Improving Global Outcomes (KDIGO) Lipid Work Group. KDIGO Clinical Practice Guideline for Lipid Management in Chronic Kidney Disease. Kidney inter., Suppl. 2013; 3: 259–305. http://www.kidney-international.org.

9. Kidney Disease: Improving Global Outcomes (KDIGO) Blood Pressure Work Group. KDIGO Clinical Practice Guideline for the Management of Blood Pressure in Chronic Kidney Disease. Kidney inter., Suppl. 2012; 2:337–414. Available at: http://www.kidney-international.org.

56

END-STAGE KIDNEY DISEASE

Urine Trouble .... Level II

Katie E. Cardone, PharmD, BCACP, FNKF, FASN

LEARNING OBJECTIVES

After completing this case study, the reader should be able to:

- Identify medication-related problems in a patient with end-stage kidney disease maintained on chronic hemodialysis.

- State the desired therapeutic outcomes of each problem.

- List therapeutic alternatives for managing each problem.

- Develop a plan for managing each problem that includes plans for monitoring patient response to interventions.

- Outline a plan for helping the patient understand and effectively implement medication-related interventions.

PATIENT PRESENTATION

■ Chief Complaint

"I feel tired, nauseated, and constipated."

■ HPI

Jane Lopez is a 42-year-old woman who presents to the outpatient dialysis center for her routine HD treatment. She has ESRD secondary to hypertension and has been on HD for 4 years. She has a failed AV fistula and graft and is currently dialyzed via central venous catheter. She has an upcoming appointment with the vascular surgeon to reevaluate her HD access. She also frequently leaves HD 30–60 minutes early against medical advice.

■ PMH

ESRD secondary to HTN
Anuria
HTN
Anemia
Secondary hyperparathyroidism
H/O gestational diabetes 12 years ago
GERD

■ PSH

Cesarean section 12 years ago
Tubal ligation 10 years ago
AV fistula creation 5 years ago (failed)
AV graft creation 3 years ago (failed)

■ FH

Father died of MI at age 60. Mother deceased due to breast cancer. No siblings. Has a 12-year-old son in good health.

■ SH

Married, lives with husband and a 12-year-old son. Occasional social alcohol use. Smokes 1/2 ppd (decreased from one ppd × 10 years). Denies caffeine consumption.

■ ROS

Complains of feeling tired and weak over the past several weeks. Reports some swelling in feet and lower legs. Also reports constipation, nausea, and heartburn.

■ Meds

Furosemide 80 mg PO daily
Metoprolol tartrate 50 mg PO BID
Lisinopril 20 mg PO daily
Calcium acetate 667 mg three caps PO TID with meals
Nephro-Vite PO daily
Omeprazole 20 mg PO daily
Ferrous sulfate 325 mg PO TID
Docusate 100 mg PO daily PRN
Calcium carbonate PO PRN heartburn
Epoetin alfa 10,000 units IV three times weekly with dialysis (dose stable for 3 months)
Iron sucrose 50 mg IV once weekly at dialysis
Paricalcitol 6 mcg IV three times weekly with dialysis

■ All

NKDA

■ Physical Examination

Gen

The patient is a WDWN Hispanic woman in NAD who appears her stated age

VS

BP 175/88 mm Hg (predialysis); 149/89 mm Hg (postdialysis)
Wt 88.6 kg (predialysis); 84.0 kg (postdialysis)
P 91 bpm, RR 16, T 36.5°C; Ht 5′4″

Skin

Dry, scaly arms and legs

Ext

Mild bilateral lower extremity edema
Remainder of the PE was WNL

■ Labs

Na 143 mEq/L	Hgb 9.3 g/dL	AST 21 IU/L	Alb 3.0 g/dL
K 4.3 mEq/L	Hct 27.5%	ALT 4 IU/L	Ca 9.4 mg/dL
Cl 95 mEq/L	RBC 2.84 ×	LDH 139 IU/L	Phos 6.7 mg/dL
CO₂ 26 mEq/L	10⁶/mm³	Alk phos 175 IU/L	iPTH 855 pg/mL
BUN 59 mg/dL	MCV 81.8 m³	T. bili 0.3 mg/dL	T. sat 12%
SCr 8.9 mg/dL	MCHC		Ferritin 99 ng/mL
Glu 88 mg/dL	32.4 g/dL		
	WBC 5.7 ×		
	10³/mm³		

Mrs Lopez's nephrologist provided the following dialysis prescription:

Dialyze 3.5 hours per session, three times per week (T, Th, Sat, morning shift)

Estimated dry weight: 83.5 kg

Dialyzer: F180 (high flux)

Blood flow rate: 400 mL/min

Dialysate flow rate: 800 mL/min

Dialysate: Bicarbonate

Na 145 mEq/L, K 2.0 mEq/L, Ca 2.5 mEq/L, HCO₃ 35 mEq/L

Heparin: 5000 unit IV bolus, and then 1000 units/hour until 1 hour before termination

QUESTIONS

Problem Identification

1.a. Create a list of the patient's drug therapy problems.

1.b. Could any of these problems have been caused or exacerbated by medications?

Desired Outcome

2. State the goal of pharmacotherapy for each problem identified.

Therapeutic Alternatives

3. What therapeutic options are available for each of this patient's drug therapy problems? Indicate the advantages and disadvantages of each option.

Optimal Plan

4. Which of the available therapeutic options identified in question 3 would you recommend for this patient? Provide a rationale for each recommendation. Include the name, dosage form, dose, schedule, and duration of therapy for any drugs recommended.

Outcome Evaluation

5. What clinical and laboratory parameters would you recommend to evaluate the desired and undesired consequences of each of your recommended interventions?

Patient Education

6. What information should be provided to the patient to enhance compliance, ensure successful therapy, and minimize adverse effects?

■ SELF-STUDY ASSIGNMENTS

1. Mrs Lopez develops a sinus infection for which she goes to an urgent care clinic. She is prescribed levofloxacin 500 mg PO daily × 14 days. Evaluate the appropriateness of this prescription for Mrs Lopez. What changes, if any, would you suggest regarding this prescription?

2. Mrs Lopez would like a kidney transplant but must first quit smoking to become eligible for transplant. Create a smoking cessation plan for her.

CLINICAL PEARL

The dose of ESAs should always be minimized. In the face of iron deficiency and low hemoglobin, iron should be replenished before increasing the ESA dose.

REFERENCES

1. Levin NW, Kotanko P, Eckardt KU, et al. Blood pressure in chronic kidney disease stage 5D—report from a Kidney Disease: Improving Global Outcomes controversies conference. Kidney Int 2010;77:273–384.
2. Kidney Disease: Improving Global Outcomes (KDIGO) Anemia Work Group. KDIGO clinical practice guideline for anemia of chronic kidney disease. Kidney Int Suppl 2012;2:1–335.
3. Epogen (epoetin alfa) package insert. Amgen Inc., Thousand Oaks, CA, 2014.
4. Kidney Disease: Improving Global Outcomes (KDIGO) CKD-MBD Work Group. KDIGO clinical practice guideline for the diagnosis, evaluation, prevention, and treatment of chronic kidney disease-mineral and bone disorder (CKD-MBD). Kidney Int 2009;76 (Suppl 113):S1–S130.
5. Triferic (ferric pyrophosphate citrate) package insert. Rockwell, Wixom, MI, 2015.
6. Pai AB, Jang SM, Wegrzyn N. Iron-based phosphate binders–a new element in management of hyperphosphatemia. Expert Opin Drug Metab Toxicol 2016;12:115–127.

57

SYNDROME OF INAPPROPRIATE ANTIDIURETIC HORMONE RELEASE

A Sudden Change of Mind . . . . Level I

Sarah A. Nisly, PharmD, BCPS

Jane M. Gervasio, PharmD, BCNSP, FCCP

LEARNING OBJECTIVES

After completing this case study, the reader should be able to:

- Identify the etiologies of hyponatremia and specifically the syndrome of inappropriate antidiuretic hormone (SIADH) release.
- Assess risk factors for developing hyponatremia and SIADH.
- Evaluate osmotic and fluid status in patients with hyponatremia.
- Recommend and monitor appropriate therapy and alternative treatments for SIADH.
- Discuss treatment options for SIADH, proper administration of selected treatments, and potential side effects.

PATIENT PRESENTATION

■ Chief Complaint

"There's nothing wrong with me, I don't know why she made me come here!"

■ HPI

Gerald O'Flannery is a 73-year-old man who presents to the ED after several episodes of "weird" behavior, according to his family and friends. He is accompanied by his wife who stated that Gerald had been the unrestrained driver in a car accident 3 days earlier. Gerald was driving himself home from the Caribou Lodge when he swerved off the road and hit a tree. His wife indicates that he hit his head on the steering wheel and lost consciousness for approximately 2 minutes but appeared otherwise unharmed except for a cut on his forehead. The paramedics cleaned and bandaged the patient's lesion and noted that he was combative and disoriented but refused to go to the hospital. The wife states that Gerald has not been "acting like himself" since the accident and she had observed him displaying worsening confused and disoriented behavior in the last 24 hours.

PMH

Exercise-induced asthma since childhood
Depression for 7 years

SH

Lives at home with wife; has two children, both living out of state. Employed part time as a cab driver. Social alcohol use. Denies smoking and use of illicit substances.

Meds

Albuterol inhaler 2 puffs by mouth Q 6 H PRN exercise; last used 1 week ago
Fluoxetine 20 mg by mouth daily for 6 years

All

Penicillin (reaction unknown)

ROS

Difficult to obtain because of decreased mental status. Wife states that he has no medical problems except asthma and depression.

Physical Examination

Gen

A & O × 3 but disoriented about recent events. Patient is agitated and confused.

VS

BP 131/87 mm Hg, P 90 bpm, RR 22, T 37°C; Wt 95 kg, Ht 5′9″

Skin

Diaphoretic centrally and very warm; small lesion above left eye

HEENT

NC/AT; EOMI; PERRL; TMs WNL bilaterally

Neck/Lymph Nodes

Supple without lymphadenopathy, masses, goiter, or bruits

Lung/Thorax

Clear to A & P bilaterally

CV

RRR; no MRG

Abd

Soft, NT/ND w/o masses or organomegaly; decreased bowel sounds in all four quadrants

Genit/Rect

Deferred

MS/Ext

Normal ROM; muscle strength 5/5 and equal bilaterally; pulses 2+ throughout; no CCE; capillary refill < 2 seconds

Neuro

CN II–XII intact; DTRs 2/4 and equal bilaterally; sensory intact; (−) Babinski

Labs

Na 112 mEq/L	Ca 9.2 mg/dL	T. chol 177 mg/dL
K 3.2 mEq/L	Phos 2.9 mg/dL	TSH 5.12 μIU/mL
Cl 90 mEq/L	Uric acid 3.2 mg/dL	Serum osmolality 238 mOsm/kg
CO_2 27 mEq/L	AST 87 IU/L	
BUN 16 mg/dL	ALT 59 IU/L	
SCr 0.9 mg/dL	T. bili 0.7 mg/dL	
Glu 115 mg/dL	LDH 256 IU/L	

UA

SG 1.008, pH 6.8, leukocyte esterase (−), nitrite (−), protein (−), ketones (−), urobilinogen nl, bilirubin (−), blood (−), glucose 80 mg/dL, spot urine sodium 125 mEq/L, osmolality 420 mOsm/kg

CT Head

Closed head injury (head trauma)

Assessment

1. Closed head injury
2. SIADH
3. Electrolyte disturbances

QUESTIONS

Problem Identification

1.a. Create a list of the patient's drug therapy problems.

1.b. What information (signs, symptoms, and laboratory values) indicates the presence or severity of SIADH as the cause of his hyponatremia?

1.c. Could any of the patient's problems have been caused by drug therapy?

Desired Outcome

2. What are the goals of pharmacotherapy in this case?

Therapeutic Alternatives

3.a. What nondrug therapies might be useful for this patient?

3.b. What pharmacotherapeutic alternatives are available for the treatment of hyponatremia?

Optimal Plan

4. What drug, dosage form, dose, schedule, and duration of therapy are most appropriate for initial treatment of this patient?

Outcome Evaluation

5. What clinical and laboratory parameters are necessary to evaluate the therapy for achievement of the desired therapeutic outcome and to detect or prevent adverse effects?

Patient Education

6. What information should be provided to the patient to enhance compliance, ensure successful therapy, and minimize adverse effects?

■ CLINICAL COURSE

After Mr O'Flannery's serum sodium returned to baseline, the team began to discuss his discharge regimen.

■ FOLLOW-UP QUESTION

1. Identify the appropriate discharge regimen for this patient. Should he continue his fluoxetine?

■ SELF-STUDY ASSIGNMENTS

1. Calculate this patient's serum osmolality and compare this to the measured serum osmolality.

2. What are the risk factors for hyponatremia caused by selective serotonin reuptake inhibitors (SSRIs)?

3. Perform a literature search to determine which SSRIs are most commonly associated with SIADH. Identify the general progression of SSRI-induced SIADH.

CLINICAL PEARL

Cerebral salt wasting (CSW) is another potential cause of hyponatremia, especially if the patient has had a head injury such as subarachnoid hemorrhage or stroke. It is often difficult to differentiate CSW from SIADH due to the overlap in their clinical features. Both CSW and SIADH present with inappropriately high urine osmolality and high urine sodium (usually >40 mEq/L). One difference is that CSW is associated with extracellular fluid depletion, whereas SIADH is associated with normal or slightly increased extracellular fluid volume. CSW can only be diagnosed in patients with clear evidence of volume depletion (hypotension, decreased skin turgor, and elevated hematocrit). SIADH is usually corrected through fluid restriction; however, establishing euvolemia through volume repletion with normal saline usually corrects CSW.

REFERENCES

1. Assadi F. Hyponatremia: a problem-solving approach to clinical cases. J Nephrol 2012;25:473–480.

2. Overgaard-Steensen C, Ring T. Clinical review: practical approach to hyponatraemia and hypernatraemia in critically ill patients. Crit Care 2013;17:206. doi:10.1186/cc11805.

3. Siragy HM. Hyponatremia, fluid–electrolyte disorders, and the syndrome of inappropriate antidiuretic hormone secretion: diagnosis and treatment options. Endocr Pract 2006;12:446–457.

4. Jacob S, Spinler SA. Hyponatremia associated with selective serotonin-reuptake inhibitors in older adults. Ann Pharmacother 2006;40:1618–1622.

5. Potts MB, DeGiacomo AF, Deragopian L, Blevins LS. Use of intravenous conivaptan in neurosurgical patients with hyponatremia from syndrome of inappropriate antidiuretic hormone secretion. Neurosurgery 2011;69:268–273.

6. Munger MA. New agents for managing hyponatremia in hospitalized patients. Am J Health Syst Pharm 2007;64:253–265.

7. Thompson CA. FDA approves oral vasopressin antagonist. Am J Health Syst Pharm 2009;66:1154.

8. Schrier RW, Gross P, Gheorghiade M, et al. Tolvaptan, a selective oral vasopressin V_2-receptor antagonist, for hyponatremia. N Engl J Med 2006;335:2099–2112.

58

ELECTROLYTE ABNORMALITIES IN CHRONIC KIDNEY DISEASE

Turn Down the 'Lytes . . . . Level II

Lena M. Maynor, PharmD, BCPS

Mary K. Stamatakis, PharmD

LEARNING OBJECTIVES

After completing this case study, the reader should be able to:

- Interpret clinical and biochemical findings in patients with CKD.

- Recommend a patient-specific therapeutic plan for treating electrolyte abnormalities and chronic kidney disease-mineral and bone disorder (CKD-MBD).

- Monitor the effectiveness of the pharmacotherapeutic plan for treating electrolyte abnormalities in CKD.

- Educate patients with CKD on nonprescription medications that can worsen electrolyte abnormalities in CKD.

PATIENT PRESENTATION

■ Chief Complaint

"I'm just don't feel like myself."

■ HPI

Robert Wolfe is a 67-year-old man with type 2 DM, HTN, and stage 5 CKD. He receives hemodialysis three times a week with a high-flux hemodialysis membrane. His wife brought him into the ED this morning after she noticed increased confusion and lethargy, worsening over the past 2–3 days. According to his wife, the patient missed his HD session 2 days ago. She reports no other new symptoms except for increased pain in his feet from his neuropathy for which his PCP increased his gabapentin dose last week.

■ PMH

Type 2 DM × 20 years

HTN × 30 years

Stage 5 CKD; he has been receiving HD for the past 5 years with a high-flux cellulose triacetate membrane; he has no residual renal function

Diabetic neuropathy

Anemia of CKD

Dyslipidemia

CKD-MBD

Uremic pruritus

■ FH

Father with CAD; mother with DM and HTN

■ SH

Retired from a glass factory; on disability; past history of smoking, quit 3 years ago; (–) ETOH for the past 7 years

■ Meds

Calcium acetate 667 mg, 2 PO TID

Gabapentin 300 mg PO BID (increased last week from 300 mg PO at bedtime)

Nephrocaps 1 PO daily

Sodium ferric gluconate 62.5 mg IV once weekly with HD

Metoprolol tartrate 25 mg PO BID

Amlodipine mg PO daily

Lipitor 10 mg PO daily

Glipizde XL 10 mg PO daily

Sitagliptin 25 mg PO daily

Epogen 6000 IU IV three times a week with HD

Calcijex 2 mcg IV three times a week with HD

Ensure® Original Vanilla nutritional supplement, one bottle (237 mL) PO TID

■ All

NKDA

■ ROS

Increased fatigue and confusion; reduced sensation in lower extremities

■ PE

Gen

Patient somnolent; does not appear to be in distress

VS

BP 168/82 mm Hg, P 82 bpm, RR 14, T 36.8°C; dry body Wt 68 kg, Ht 5′11″

Skin

Normal; intact, warm and dry

HEENT

NC/AT, PERRLA, EOMI, fundoscopy WNL, oropharyngeal mucosa clear

Neck/Lymph Nodes

Positive JVD; no lymphadenopathy, normal thyroid

Lungs

Crackles in bases bilaterally

CV

Normal S_1 and S_2; no S_3 or S_4

Abd

Soft, NT/ND, no HSM

Genit/Rect

Normal prostate, guaiac-negative stool

MS/Ext

1+ bilateral pedal edema, no clubbing or cyanosis

Neuro

A & O to person only, CN II–XII intact, normal DTRs bilaterally

■ Labs

Na 140 mEq/L	Hgb 11.2 g/dL	Ca 9.8 mg/dL
K 6.1 mEq/L	Hct 34.5%	Mg 2.4 mg/dL
Cl 99 mEq/L	Plt $182 \times 10^3/mm^3$	Phos 7.6 mg/dL
CO_2 18 mEq/L	WBC $7.8 \times 10^3/mm^3$	AST 12 IU/L
BUN 82 mg/dL		ALT 8 IU/L
SCr 8.2 mg/dL		T. bili 0.9 mg/dL
Glu 118 mg/dL		Alk phos 34 IU/L
		Alb 2.2 g/dL
		Intact PTH 140 pg/mL (last month 172 pg/mL)

■ ABG

pH 7.35, PaO_2 94, $PaCO_2$ 38, HCO_3 20 on room air

■ Chest X-Ray

No infiltrates or effusions

■ ECG

Sinus rhythm

■ Assessment

67-year-old man with type 2 DM, CKD on HD with altered mental status, hyperkalemia, hyperphosphatemia, and H/O CKD-MBD

■ Plan

Patient missed HD session yesterday. Will dialyze now to correct some of the electrolyte abnormalities.

Patient with altered mental status following missed HD session; likely worsened by increased dose of gabapentin. Will dialyze and change gabapentin dose to 300 mg PO at bedtime.

QUESTIONS

Problem Identification

1.a. Create a list of the patient's drug therapy problems.

Problem 1—Hyperkalemia

1.b. What information (signs, symptoms, and laboratory values) indicates the presence or severity of hyperkalemia?

1.c. Could any medications or nutritional supplements the patient is receiving be contributing to his hyperkalemia?

1.d. What is the pathophysiology of the patient's hyperkalemia?

1.e. What are the clinical consequences of hyperkalemia?

Desired Outcome

2. What are the goals for treating this patient's hyperkalemia?

Therapeutic Alternatives

3.a. What nondrug therapies are available for treating hyperkalemia?

3.b. What feasible pharmacotherapeutic alternatives are available for treating hyperkalemia?

Optimal Plan

4. What drug, dosage form, dose, schedule, and duration of therapy are best for treating hyperkalemia in this patient?

Outcome Evaluation

5. What clinical and laboratory parameters are necessary to evaluate the therapy for achievement of the desired therapeutic outcomes and to detect or prevent adverse effects?

Patient Education

6. What information should be provided to the patient regarding over-the-counter medications that may increase the risk of hyperkalemia?

Problem 2—Hyperphosphatemia, Hypercalcemia, and CKD-MBD

1.b. What information (signs, symptoms, and laboratory values) indicates the presence or severity of hyperphosphatemia and hypercalcemia?

1.c. Could any of the patient's medications be contributing to his hyperphosphatemia and hypercalcemia?

1.d. What is the pathophysiology of the patient's hyperphosphatemia and hypercalcemia?

1.e. What are the clinical consequences of hyperphosphatemia and hypercalcemia?

Desired Outcome

2. What are the goals of pharmacotherapy for treating this patient's hyperphosphatemia and hypercalcemia?

Therapeutic Alternatives

3.a. What nondrug therapies might be useful for treating this patient's hyperphosphatemia and hypercalcemia?

3.b. What pharmacotherapeutic alternatives are available for treating hyperphosphatemia?

3.c. What pharmacotherapeutic options are available for treating hypercalcemia?

Optimal Plan

4. What drugs, dosage forms, schedules, and duration of therapy are best for treating this patient's hyperphosphatemia and hypercalcemia?

Outcome Evaluation

5. What clinical and laboratory parameters are necessary to evaluate the therapy for achievement of the desired therapeutic outcome and to detect or prevent adverse effects?

Patient Education

6. What information should be provided to the patient regarding the administration of his phosphate binder to ensure an optimal outcome?

■ ADDITIONAL CASE QUESTIONS

1. What alternative regimens could be considered for this patient's painful diabetic neuropathy (include drug[s], dose, route of administration, and frequency)?

2. One month later, the following laboratory values and erythropoietin dosages were available from the outpatient hemodialysis unit. Formulate a treatment plan for the patient's anemia of CKD.

Time	Hgb (g/dL)	Ferritin (ng/mL)	Transferrin Saturation (%)	Erythropoietin Dosage
1 month ago	11.2	–	–	6000 IU IV three times per week
Current	9.2	210	25	6000 IU IV three times per week

■ SELF-STUDY ASSIGNMENT

Develop a protocol for switching patients from intravenous to subcutaneous erythropoietin administration in the hemodialysis setting.

CLINICAL PEARL

Uremic pruritus is a common and frustrating symptom in patients with CKD, with a poorly understood and complex pathophysiology. Patients who are inadequately dialyzed, have secondary hyperparathyroidism, anemia, elevated calcium × phosphorus product, or elevated serum magnesium and aluminum are more likely to suffer from pruritus. While the only definitive treatment for uremic pruritus is kidney transplantation, supportive treatment includes increasing dialysis efficiency, using biocompatible hemodialysis membranes, use of emollients with high water content, and treatment of known risk factors.

REFERENCES

1. Sanghavi S, Whiting S, Uribarri J. Potassium balance in dialysis patients. Semin Dial 2013;26:597–603.

2. KDIGO clinical practice guideline for the diagnosis, evaluation, prevention, and treatment of chronic kidney disease-mineral and bone disorder (CKD-MBD). Kidney Int Suppl 2009;76:S1–S130.

3. Tonelli M, Pannu N, Manns B. Oral phosphate binders in patients with kidney failure. N Engl J Med 2010;362:1312–1324.

4. Kasai S, Sato K, Murata Y, Kinoshita Y. Randomized crossover study of the efficacy and safety of sevelamer hydrochloride and lanthanum carbonate in Japanese patients undergoing hemodialysis. Ther Apher Dial 2012;16:341–349.

5. Floege J, Covic AC, Ketteler M, et al. Long-term effects of the iron-based phosphate binder, sucroferric oxyhydroxide, in dialysis patients. Nephrol Dial Transplant. 2015;30:1037–1046.

6. Kalantar-Zadeh K, Shah A, Duong U, Hechter RC, Dukkipati R, Kovesdy CP. Kidney bone disease and mortality in CKD: revisiting the role of vitamin D, calcimimetics, alkaline phosphatase, and minerals. Kidney Int Suppl 2010;78:S10–S21.

7. Pop-Busui R, Roberts L, Pennathur S, et al. The management of diabetic neuropathy in CKD. Am J Kidney Dis 2010;55:365–385.

8. Kidney Disease: Improving Global Outcomes (KDIGO) Anemia Work Group. KDIGO clinical practice guideline for anemia in chronic kidney disease. Kidney Int Suppl 2012;2:279–335.

9. Kfoury LW, Jurdi MA. Uremic pruritus. J Nephrol. 2012;25:644–652.

59

HYPERCALCEMIA OF MALIGNANCY

Up, Up, and Away .... Level I

Laura L. Jung, BS Pharm, PharmD

Lisa M. Holle, PharmD, BCOP, FHOPA

LEARNING OBJECTIVES

After completing this case study, the reader should be able to:

- Recognize the signs and symptoms of hypercalcemia.

- Evaluate laboratory data and clinical symptoms for assessment and monitoring of hypercalcemia, hypercalcemia treatment, and complications of hypercalcemia.

- Recommend a pharmacotherapeutic plan for the initial treatment of cancer-related hypercalcemia.

- Recognize and develop management strategies for toxicities associated with treatment options for hypercalcemia.

PATIENT PRESENTATION

■ Chief Complaint

"I can't stop throwing up."

■ HPI

Mary Krupp is a 62-year-old woman who presented to her family practitioner today with a 2-day history of nausea and vomiting. She states that her stomach has not felt normal for the past 3–4 days and is painful. Her daughter states that for the past several days she has complained of constipation, nausea, and extreme thirst, but because she has been vomiting, it has been hard to keep her mother drinking enough liquids. She also reports that her mother stopped taking the sustained-release morphine that was started last week because she thought these were side effects of the morphine. The daughter states that her mom's last bowel movement was 3 days ago despite administration of a stool softener daily. The daughter also reports her mother has gone "downhill" over the past month and spends 80% of her day in bed and the remainder in the recliner.

■ PMH

Stage IV non-small cell lung cancer diagnosed 1.5 years ago. At time of diagnosis, a CT scan revealed a 3-cm mass in the hilum of the right lung, extensive mediastinal lymphadenopathy, and a moderate right pleural effusion with pleural studding. A transbronchial biopsy identified the mass as adenocarcinoma, epidermal growth factor (EGFR) and anaplastic lymphoma kinase (ALK) negative. Cytology of the pleural effusion also revealed adenocarcinoma. She was treated with the following regimens: (1) carboplatin/paclitaxel × 4 cycles; (2) pemetrexed maintenance × 6 cycles; (3) nivolumab × 8 cycles; and (4) erlotinib monotherapy. Erlotinib was discontinued 2 days ago because of grade 4 skin rash. The last CT scan performed yesterday revealed a new tumor 3.5 × 4.2 mm in the left lower lobe and liver metastases.

COPD × 4 years

Dyslipidemia

■ FH

Mother died of NSCLC at age 80 years; father died of MI at 64 years; one sister died of breast cancer at 69 years; one sister and three brothers alive

■ SH

Tobacco: 2 ppd × 30 years; chronic alcohol use × 30 years EtOH (three to four drinks per day). Worked as an office assistant × 25 years. Lives at home with boyfriend of 16 years; has four grown daughters, ages 47, 44, 39, and 34 years. Had her first child at age 15.

■ Medications

Morphine sulfate sustained-release 30 mg PO Q 12 H (started 1 week ago)

Morphine sulfate oral solution 5 mg PO Q 2 H PRN pain (estimated use two times in the 24 hours before she stopped taking sustained-released)

Docusate sodium 200 mg PO at bedtime PRN

Simvastatin 20 mg PO daily

■ All

Cephalosporins, penicillin

■ ROS

No fever or chills. Daughter has noted that the patient is more tired than usual and is extremely thirsty, which she believes has affected her appetite over the past week. She denies polyuria, chest pain, unusual shortness of breath, dyspnea, or cough. Ms Krupp states her pain is 8/10 throughout the day.

■ Physical Examination

Gen

Thin Caucasian woman in obvious discomfort

VS

BP 95/70 mm Hg, P 105 bpm, RR 16, T 38°C; Wt 50 kg, Ht 5'1"

Skin

Slightly warm to touch, fair skin turgor (mild tenting noted)

HEENT

PERRLA, EOMI, fundi benign; nonerythematous TMs; oropharynx clear; mucous membranes dry

Neck/LN

Neck supple, slight axillary lymphadenopathy

Lungs

Decreased breath sounds; bilateral wheezes

Breasts

Breasts nontender. No palpable masses or nipple discharge

CV

RRR, S_1, S_2 normal; without MRG

Abd

Firm, distended, tender; decreased bowel sounds; stool palpable on left side

Genit/Rect

Normal female genitalia; stool heme (–)

MS/Ext

Bilateral lower extremity weakness graded at 4/5; otherwise normal

Neuro

A & O × 3; sensory and motor intact; strength 5/5 upper, 4/5 lower; CN II–XII intact; Babinksi (–)

■ Labs

Na 142 mEq/L	Glu 100 mg/dL	AST 63 IU/L	Ca 13.0 mg/dL
K 3.5 mEq/L	Hgb 12.7 g/dL	ALT 35 IU/L	Mg 1.5 mEq/L
Cl 109 mEq/L	Hct 40%	Alk phos 200 IU/L	Phos 3.5 mEq/L
CO_2 22 mEq/L	Plt 174 × 10³/mm³	LDH 160 IU/L	T. prot 5.1 g/dL
BUN 40 mg/dL	WBC 6.8 × 10³/mm³	T. bili 1.6 mg/dL	Alb 2.2 g/dL
SCr 0.9 mg/dL		D. bili 0.7 mg/dL	

■ Chest X-Ray

Osteolytic lesions on the right and left clavicles, masses in right and left lower lobes consistent with NSCLC

■ Assessment/Plan

62-year-old woman with metastatic NSCLC s/p three different treatment regimens. Poor performance status. Presenting with first episode of possible tumor-induced hypercalcemia with associated complications and uncontrolled pain.

Admit to inpatient oncology service for further management of hypercalcemia, related complications, and pain control.

QUESTIONS

Problem Identification

1.a. Create a list of the patient's drug therapy problems.

1.b. What information (signs, symptoms, and laboratory values) indicates the presence or severity of hypercalcemia?

1.c. What is the patient's corrected serum calcium level based on her serum albumin level?

1.d. Could any of the patient's problems have been exacerbated by her current drug therapy?

1.e. What are the possible etiologies of hypercalcemia in this patient?

1.f. What additional information is needed to satisfactorily assess this patient?

Desired Outcome

2. What are the goals of pharmacotherapy for this patient?

Therapeutic Alternatives

3.a. What nondrug therapies might be useful for this patient?

3.b. What feasible pharmacotherapeutic alternatives are available for treatment of hypercalcemia in this patient?

Optimal Plan

4.a. What drug, dosage form, dose, schedule, and duration of therapy are best for treating hypercalcemia in this patient?

4.b. What alternatives would be appropriate if the initial therapy fails or cannot be used?

Outcome Evaluation

5. What clinical and laboratory parameters are necessary to evaluate the therapy for achievement of the desired outcome and to detect or prevent adverse effects?

Patient Education

6. What information should be provided to the patient and her family to enhance compliance, ensure successful therapy, and minimize adverse effects?

■ CLINICAL COURSE

Ms Krupp's serum calcium level decreased to 8.8 mg/dL by day 3 with the treatment you recommended. She was discharged from the hospital on day 5 with improvement in her mental status. However, she returned to the hospital on day 10 with a serum calcium level of 15.2 mg/dL. She is very somnolent and lethargic.

■ FOLLOW-UP QUESTIONS

1. What pharmacologic and nonpharmacologic options might be considered at this time and why?

2. How would you monitor the therapy you recommended for efficacy and adverse effects?

■ SELF-STUDY ASSIGNMENTS

1. What nonmalignant disease states can induce hypercalcemia?

2. What treatment(s) can decrease the risk of developing hypercalcemia in patients receiving calcitriol for anticancer therapy?

CLINICAL PEARL

When evaluating a patient for hypercalcemia, a corrected calcium must be used to account for the patient's albumin level.

REFERENCES

1. Mirrakhimov AE. Hypercalcemia of malignancy: an update on pathogenesis and management. N Am J Med Sci 2015;7:483–493.

2. Santarpia L, Koch CA, Sarlis NJ. Hypercalcemia in cancer patients: pathobiology and management. Horm Metab Res 2010;42:153–164.

3. Tanvetyanon T, Stiff PJ. Management of the adverse effects associated with intravenous bisphosphonates. Ann Oncol 2006;17:897–907.

4. Ruggiero S, Gralow J, Marx RE, et al. Practical guidelines for the prevention, diagnosis, and treatment of osteonecrosis of the jaw in patients with cancer. J Oncol Pract 2006;2:7–14.

5. Major P, Lortholary A, Hon J, et al. Zoledronic acid is superior to pamidronate in the treatment of hypercalcemia of malignancy: a pooled analysis of two randomized, controlled clinical trials. J Clin Oncol 2001;19:558–567.

6. Zometa [package insert]. East Hanover, NJ, Novartis Pharmaceuticals Corporation, 2012.

7. Xgeva [package insert]. Thousand Oaks, CA, Amgen Inc, 2015.

8. Hu MI, Glezerman IG, Lebouleux S, et al. Denosumab for the treatment of hypercalcemia of malignancy. J Clin Endocrinol Metab 2014;99:3144–3152.

9. Non-Small Cell Lung Cancer NCCN Clinical Practice Guidelines in Oncology. V.2.2016. 2016 National Comprehensive Cancer Network, Inc. Available at: *NCCN.org*. Accessed November 5, 2015.

60

HYPOKALEMIA AND HYPOMAGNESEMIA

A Super Bowl Party . . . . Level III

Denise R. Sokos, PharmD, BCPS

LEARNING OBJECTIVES

After completing this case study, the reader should be able to:

- Analyze a patient case history and identify potential causes of electrolyte disorders.

- Select the appropriate route of administration and dose of electrolyte replacement therapy specific for a patient.

- Develop a monitoring plan for efficacy and toxicity in patients receiving electrolyte replacement therapy.

- Outline a patient education plan for a patient receiving electrolyte replacement supplements.

PATIENT PRESENTATION

Chief Complaint

"I'm short of breath."

HPI

Dorothy Snow is a 45-year-old woman with a history of nonischemic cardiomyopathy who presents to the ED with a 3-day history of shortness of breath with mild-to-moderate exertion. She reports three-pillow orthopnea × 2 days and cough during sleep. Denies chest pain; occasional palpitations. Reports a 10-lb weight gain in the last week and an increase in her lower extremity edema.

Two months ago, Mrs Snow was hospitalized briefly with atypical chest pain and had persistent hypokalemia for which her metolazone 5 mg daily was discontinued. Approximately one month ago, she subsequently developed significant fluid retention and her PCP restarted metolazone 5 mg PO MWF. About 2 weeks ago, she had an ED visit and her potassium was 7.2 mEq/L (hemolyzed sample). The potassium level was repeated with a result of 5.5 mEq/L. At that time, her potassium supplement dose was reduced from 80 mEq PO QID to 80 mEq PO BID.

PMH (Per Patient Report and Medical Records)

Nonischemic cardiomyopathy—echo LVEF 25% (11 months ago)
ICD placement (3 weeks ago)
Pulmonary hypertension—secondary to left heart disease

HTN
Asthma
Sleep apnea
Type 2 DM with peripheral neuropathy
Obesity
Chronic sinusitis
Anxiety disorder
Hypothyroidism

FH

Both parents are deceased

SH

Lives with husband. No alcohol use. Former smoker—quit 8 years ago. No illicit drugs.

Meds

Valsartan 160 mg PO BID
Omeprazole 20 mg PO daily
Carvedilol 25 mg PO BID
Digoxin 0.25 mg PO daily
Spironolactone 25 mg PO daily
Furosemide 80 mg PO BID
Citalopram 20 mg PO daily
Atorvastatin 20 mg PO daily
Insulin glargine 30 units SC Q 12 H
Insulin aspart 20 units SC TID with meals
Pregabalin 50 mg PO BID
Metolazone 5 mg PO MWF
Loratadine 10 mg PO daily
Tiotropium one puff daily
Fluticasone/salmeterol 500/50 one puff BID
Mometasone one spray each nostril daily
Meclizine 12.5 mg PO BID
Magnesium oxide 400 mg PO TID
Potassium chloride 80 mEq PO BID
Levothyroxine 75 mcg PO daily
Lorazepam 0.5 mg PO TID
Folic acid 1 mg PO daily

ALL

NKDA

ROS

Patient reports becoming short of breath for the past 3 days while walking up one flight of stairs or if she walks too quickly on a flat surface. Previously she could walk two flights of stairs before becoming short of breath. She uses three pillows at night to sleep but does not report PND symptoms. She reports increased swelling in her lower extremities, abdominal fullness, and early satiety. States that she has not changed her diet, but did attend an all-day Super Bowl party the previous weekend and ate foods that were not part of her normal diet (eg, chili, buffalo wings, veggies and dip, pizza). Denies ever having an ICD discharge.

Physical Examination

Gen

Appears older than her stated age; obese; mild dyspnea at rest

VS

P 106 bpm, RR 20, BP 115/70 mm Hg, T 35.8°C; Wt 192 lb (baseline weight 184 lb), Ht 5′5″, O_2 sat 88% room air

Skin

Skin warm, dry

HEENT

PERRLA; conjunctivae clear; moist mucous membranes; tongue midline

Neck/Lymph Nodes

Supple; JVP estimated at 14 cm; no carotid bruit; no lymphadenopathy; (+) thyroid nodules

Lungs

Bibasilar rales R > L; occasional wheezes

CV

Tachycardic; normal S_1, S_2; $+S_3$; $-S_4$; 2/6 holosystolic murmur best heard at second left intercostal space

Abd

Obese; good bowel sounds; no bruits; no hepatosplenomegaly, (+) hepatojugular reflux; no evidence of ascites

Genit/Rect

Deferred

Ext

No cyanosis; 3+ pitting edema to knees bilaterally; 2+ pulses bilaterally in upper and lower extremities

Back

No CVA tenderness

Neuro

Alert & oriented × 3; no focal deficits; mild sensory deficit in feet bilaterally; CN II–XII grossly intact

■ Labs

Na 130 mEq/L	Hgb 10.4 g/dL	Ca 8.3 mg/dL	Alb 3.0 g/dL
K 2.8 mEq/L	Hct 29.3%	Mg 1.3 mEq/L	PT 14 s
Cl 93 mEq/L	WBC 4.5 × 10^3/mm^3	Phos 3.1 mEq/L	INR 1.2
CO_2 30 mEq/L		AST 100 IU/L	aPTT 21 s
BUN 17 mg/dL	Plt 165× 10^3/mm^3	ALT 110 IU/L	CK 30 IU/L
SCr 1.0 mg/dL	BNP 1533 pg/mL	Troponin I < 0.01 ng/mL	
Glu 143 mg/dL			

■ Chest X-Ray

Bilateral pulmonary edema; moderate R pleural effusion; small L pleural effusion; (+) cardiomegaly

■ 12-Lead ECG

Sinus tachycardia; LBBB; no evidence of acute ischemia

■ Assessment

Admit to inpatient monitored bed.

1. Acute exacerbation of chronic heart failure
2. NYHA class III symptoms, ACC stage C
3. Volume overload
4. Electrolyte abnormalities
5. Hyperglycemia

QUESTIONS

Problem Identification

1.a. Create a list of the patient's drug therapy problems.

1.b. What information (signs, symptoms, and laboratory values) indicates the presence and severity of the electrolyte abnormalities?

1.c. What are the potential causes of the electrolyte disorders in this patient?

1.d. What additional information is needed to satisfactorily assess this patient's electrolyte disorders?

Desired Outcome

2. What are the goals of pharmacotherapy in this patient?

Therapeutic Alternatives

3. What feasible pharmacotherapeutic alternatives are available for treatment of hypervolemia, hypokalemia, and hypomagnesemia in this patient?

Optimal Plan

4.a. Given the therapeutic alternatives outlined above, what is the most appropriate therapy for treatment of hypervolemia, hypokalemia, and hypomagnesemia in this patient?

4.b. What therapy changes should be made for the patient's heart failure and hyperglycemia?

Outcome Evaluation

5. What clinical and laboratory parameters are necessary to evaluate the therapy for the desired therapeutic outcome and prevention of adverse effects?

Patient Education

6. What information should be provided to the patient to enhance adherence, ensure successful therapy, and minimize adverse effects?

■ CLINICAL COURSE

The medical team implemented the pharmacotherapy plan you recommended. Today is day 4 of hospitalization, and her clinical status is improved. She states she can walk farther without becoming short of breath and only needs one pillow to sleep. Additionally, she describes less swelling in her legs. On physical exam, her HR is 73 BP is 108/57 mm Hg, and O_2 saturation is 96% on room air. Her lungs are clear and she has 1+ edema in her legs. Pertinent laboratory results indicate serum potassium 3.8 mEq/L, SCr 1.2 mg/dL, Mg 1.8 mg/dL, CO_2 26 mEq/L, and Glu 129 mg/dL. Her JVP is 8 cm and she has no hepatojugular reflex. She is scheduled for discharge today.

■ FOLLOW-UP QUESTIONS

1. What changes should be made to the patient's medication regimen at hospital discharge to prevent future electrolyte imbalances?

2. Develop a plan to monitor this patient's electrolytes after hospital discharge.

3. What vaccinations should this patient receive?

SELF-STUDY ASSIGNMENTS

1. Outline a therapeutic plan for the treatment of pulmonary hypertension in this patient.

2. Describe how a patient's acid–base status can affect serum electrolyte concentrations.

CLINICAL PEARL

Hypokalemia and hypomagnesemia often coexist. In patients refractory to potassium replacement, magnesium concentrations should be evaluated, and any magnesium deficit must be corrected before potassium can be appropriately replaced.

REFERENCES

1. Cohn JN, Kowey PR, Whelton PK, Prisant M. New guidelines for potassium replacement in clinical practice. A contemporary review by the National Council on Potassium in Clinical Practice. Arch Intern Med 2000;160:2429–2436.

2. Huang CL, Kuo E. Mechanism of hypokalemia in magnesium deficiency. J Am Soc Nephrol 2007;18:2649–2652.

3. Ayuk J, Gittoes NJL. How should hypomagnesaemia be investigated and treated? Clin Endo 2011;75:743–746.

4. Yancy CW, Jessup M, Bozkurt B, et al. 2013 ACCF/AHA guideline for the management of heart failure: a report of the American College of Cardiology Foundation/American Heart Association Task Force on Practice Guidelines. Circulation 2013;128:e240–e327.

5. Kraft MD, Btaiche IF, Sacks GS, Kudsk KA. Treatment of electrolyte disorders in adult patients in the intensive care unit. Am J Health-Syst Pharm 2005;62:1663–1682.

61

METABOLIC ACIDOSIS

Oh, My Aching Acidosis . . . . Level II

Brian M. Hodges, PharmD, BCPS, BCNSP

LEARNING OBJECTIVES

After completing this case study, the reader should be able to:

- Recognize the clinical and laboratory manifestations of metabolic acidosis.

- Differentiate among different causes of metabolic acidosis.

- Develop a patient-specific pharmacotherapeutic plan for treating chronic metabolic acidosis.

- Provide medication education for patients with chronic metabolic acidosis.

PATIENT PRESENTATION

Chief Complaint

"I just feel so weak all the time."

HPI

Sue Rider is a 67-year-old woman with progressively declining renal function, due to hypertension, who is being seen in the nephrology clinic for management of fatigue, dyspnea, somnolence, and lethargy. She further reports that over the past few months she has experienced a decrease in appetite and occasionally feels nauseated without vomiting. She reports frequent nonadherence to her antihypertensive regimen "when I feel good." She also reports no history of diarrhea.

PMH

HTN
Declining renal function due to HTN
Seasonal allergic rhinitis

SH

She is a retired schoolteacher who lives with her husband of 38 years and has three grown children. She denies alcohol use. There is no history of tobacco habituation or recreational drug use.

FH

History of CAD in her mother's family

ROS

As per HPI

Meds

Amlodipine 5 mg PO daily
Metoprolol succinate 25 mg PO daily
Metolazone 2.5 mg PO daily, taken intermittently for lower extremity edema (reports that she has not taken any for the past few months)

ALL

NKDA

Physical Examination

Gen

Pleasant African-American woman in NAD

VS

BP 145/85 mm Hg, P 78 bpm, RR 22, T 37.2°C; Wt 75 kg, Ht 5′4″

HEENT

No hemorrhages or exudates on funduscopic examination

Neck/Lymph Nodes

JVP was 5 cm; carotid pulses were 2+ bilaterally; no thyromegaly or lymphadenopathy

Lungs

CTA and P

CV

Unable to palpate PMI; regular rate and rhythm; normal S_1 and S_2; no murmurs

Abd

Obese, soft, nontender; normoactive bowel sounds; no organomegaly

MS/Ext

Minimal sternal and quadriceps tenderness

Neuro

No focal cranial nerve deficits; strength 5/5 in all extremities. DTRs are 1+ brachioradialis, 2+ biceps, 2+ quadriceps, 1+ ankle jerks, toes downgoing bilaterally.

■ Labs

Na 131 mEq/L	Hgb 12.2 g/dL	AST 13 IU/L
K 4.4 mEq/L	Hct 37%	ALT 7 IU/L
Cl 101 mEq/L	Plt 225 × 10³/mm³	Alk phos 113 IU/L
CO_2 19 mEq/L	WBC 7.6 × 10³/mm³	GGT 14 IU/L
BUN 37 mg/dL	Ca 7.4 mg/dL	T. bili 0.4 mg/dL
SCr 2.9 mg/dL	Mg 2.2 mg/dL	Alb 3.6 g/dL
Glu 89 mg/dL	Phos 4.3 mg/dL	

■ ABG on RA

pH 7.32; $PaCO_2$ 38 mm Hg; PaO_2 106 mm Hg; bicarbonate 19 mEq/L

■ UA

SG 1.025; pH 5.8; protein reagent strip +

■ KUB

No nephrocalcinosis

■ Assessment

1. Acidosis
2. CKD
3. Hypertension
4. Hyponatremia
5. Hypocalcemia

QUESTIONS

Problem Identification

1.a. Identify the type of acidosis (metabolic vs respiratory) this patient exhibits, calculate the anion gap, and identify the potential causes.

1.b. What medical conditions present in this patient are either untreated or inadequately treated?

1.c. What information obtained from the patient's symptoms, physical examination, and laboratory analysis indicates the presence of a chronic metabolic acidosis due to CKD?

1.d. What are the proposed mechanisms of metabolic acidosis in patients with CKD?

1.e. What are the complications associated with prolonged acidosis in patients with CKD?

Desired Outcome

2. What are the pharmacotherapeutic goals for this patient?

Therapeutic Alternatives

3. What treatment alternatives are available to achieve the desired therapeutic outcomes?

Optimal Plan

4. Design a pharmacotherapeutic plan for the management of metabolic acidosis and its complications in this patient.

Outcome Evaluation

5. Outline a clinical and laboratory monitoring plan to assess the patient's response to the pharmacotherapeutic regimen you recommended.

Patient Education

6. How should the patient be counseled about the drug therapy to treat chronic metabolic acidosis?

■ CLINICAL COURSE

At the patient's 3-month clinic visit, 2+ pedal edema is noted. During the patient interview, she states that her adherence to her medications has improved. Labs are as follows:

Na 135 mEq/L	Ca 8.6 mg/dL
K 3.9 mEq/L	Mg 1.9 mg/dL
Cl 101 mEq/L	Phos 5.0 mg/dL
CO_2 22 mEq/L	Alb 3.0 g/dL
BUN 36 mg/dL	
SCr 3.0 mg/dL	
Glu 99 mg/dL	

■ FOLLOW-UP CASE QUESTIONS

1. How might the patient's buffer therapy requirement change if she is started on sevelamer carbonate to limit dietary phosphorus absorption?

2. What clinical and laboratory parameters should be monitored to assess the adequacy of the patient's ACE inhibitor dosing to slow the progression of her CKD?

■ SELF-STUDY ASSIGNMENTS

1. Differentiate between the bone disease of metabolic acidosis versus that associated with chronic renal failure and osteoporosis.

2. Discuss the types of metabolic acidoses that may be present in patients with CKD and how they may be differentiated.

CLINICAL PEARL

While the chronic metabolic acidosis associated with CKD is usually not progressive, there is increasing evidence that correction of the acidosis is related to decreased progression of CKD. Appropriate sodium bicarbonate therapy may result in improved nutritional status, renal function, and quality of life for patients with CKD.

REFERENCES

1. Kraut JA, Madias NE. Metabolic acidosis of CKD: An Update. Am J Kidney Dis 2016;67:307–317.
2. Kidney Disease: Improving Global Outcomes (KDIGO) CKD Work Group. KDIGO 2012 Clinical Practice Guideline for the Evaluation and Management of Chronic Kidney Disease. Kidney inter., Suppl. 2013;3:1–150.
3. KDIGO Blood Pressure Work Group. KDIGO clinical practice guideline for the management of blood pressure in chronic kidney disease. Kidney Int 2012;2(Suppl):337–414.

4. Raphael KL. Approach to the treatment of chronic metabolic acidosis in CKD. Am J Kidney Dis 2016;67:696–702.

5. Mahajan A, Simoni J, Sheather SJ, et al. Daily oral sodium bicarbonate preserved glomerular filtration rate by slowing its decline in early hypertensive nephropathy. Kidney Int 2010;78:303–309.

6. Goraya N, Simoni J, Jo C, Wesson DE. A comparison of treating metabolic acidosis in CKD stage 4 hypertensive kidney disease with fruits and vegetables or sodium bicarbonate. Clin J Am Soc Nephrol 2013;8:371–381.

7. Foque D, Pelletier S, Mafra D, Chauveau P. Nutrition and chronic kidney disease. Kid Int 2011;80:348–357.

8. Kidney Disease: Improving Global Outcomes (KDIGO) CKD–MBD Work Group. KDIGO clinical practice guideline for the diagnosis, evaluation, prevention, and treatment of chronic kidney disease–mineral and bone disorder (CKD–MBD). Kid Int 2009;76(Suppl 113):S1–S130.

Note: All KDIGO clinical practice guidelines are available online at *http://kdigo.org/home/guidelines/*.

62

METABOLIC ALKALOSIS

Keep Me in the Loop . . . . Level I

Jennifer Confer, PharmD, BCPS, BCCCP

LEARNING OBJECTIVES

After completing this case study, the reader should be able to:

- Recognize the signs and symptoms of metabolic alkalosis.

- Interpret laboratory findings that are consistent with metabolic alkalosis.

- Describe patient-specific factors that contribute to the development of metabolic disorders.

- Recommend appropriate first-line treatment regimens and alternatives for metabolic alkalosis.

- Formulate a patient-specific pharmacotherapeutic plan for the treatment and monitoring of metabolic alkalosis.

PATIENT PRESENTATION

■ Chief Complaint

"I feel very weak and tired."

■ HPI

Lois Strickland is a 60-year-old woman who presents to the ED with complaints of generalized weakness, fatigue, myalgias, and polyuria over the past 2 days. She states that recently she has felt bloated and has been taking an extra dose of her "water pill" every day for the past week and a half. She also mentioned that she may have eaten something bad because she has thrown up three times since dinner last night.

■ PMH

Hypertension (diagnosed 15 years ago)
HF (diagnosed 2 years ago)
Diabetes, type 2—diet controlled
Dyslipidemia (diagnosed 2 years ago)

■ FH

Mother is alive with a history of HTN and dyslipidemia. Father is alive with HTN. Younger sister is alive with dyslipidemia.

■ SH

Patient reports she does not consume alcohol except a glass of wine "at special occasions." She denies tobacco or illicit drug use. Lives at home with her husband of 35 years and their two dogs.

■ Meds

Lisinopril 10 mg PO once daily
Carvedilol 25 mg PO BID
Furosemide 40 mg PO once daily
Atorvastatin 40 mg PO at bedtime
Last dose of all medications was this morning 3 hours before arriving at the ED (except atorvastatin, which was taken yesterday evening)

■ All

Codeine—patient reports "I get short of breath"

■ ROS

Denies unusual weight gain or loss. She denies fever, chills, or night sweats, but reports dizziness that has occurred off and on over the past week in addition to generalized fatigue and weakness. No reported chest pain, palpitations, shortness of breath, or cough. She denies diarrhea, constipation, or change in bowel habits. She reports a recent increase in thirst and urination, but no change in urine color. She reports myalgias and perioral numbness that began recently with the fatigue and weakness.

■ Physical Examination

Gen

The patient is ill-appearing and feels warm to the touch

VS

BP 93/62 mm Hg, HR 101, RR 20, T 37.9°C; Wt 80 kg, Ht 5′7″; O$_2$ sat 96% on RA

Skin

Soft, intact, warm, dry

HEENT

EOMI; PERRLA; no sinus tenderness; dry mucous membranes; no oral lesions; no nasal congestion present

Neck/Lymph Nodes

No JVD or bruits; no lymphadenopathy or thyromegaly

Chest

CTA bilaterally

Breasts

Deferred

CV

RRR; normal S_1, S_2; no S_3 or S_4; no murmurs, rubs, gallops

Abd

Soft, NTND; (+) bowel sounds

GU/Rect

WNL

Ext

No CCE; feet are dry and wrinkled

Neuro

A & O × 3. CN II–XII intact.

▓ Labs

Na 132 mEq/L	Hgb 12.4 g/dL	Alb 3.8 g/dL
K 2.9 mEq/L	Hct 36.7%	AST 19 IU/L
Cl 85 mEq/L	Plt 324 × 10³/mm³	ALT 16 IU/L
CO_2 39 mEq/L	WBC 12.1 × 10³/mm³	Alk phos 62 IU/L
BUN 24 mg/dL	Mg 1.7 mEq/L	T. bili 0.4 mg/dL
SCr 1.1 mg/dL	Phos 3.6 mg/dL	PT 11.3 s
Glu 118 mg/dL	Ca 7.6 mg/dL	INR 0.96

▓ ABG

pH 7.54, $PaCO_2$ 46 mm Hg, PaO_2 86 mm Hg, HCO_3 38.3 mEq/L on RA

▓ UA

Urine sodium 18 mEq/L; potassium 33 mEq/L; chloride 9 mEq/L, urine pH 6.1

▓ Chest X-Ray

Mild pulmonary congestion, otherwise unremarkable

▓ ECG

Sinus tachycardia, rate 101, no acute ST-segment or T-wave changes

▓ Assessment

Admit patient for hypotension, flulike symptoms, electrolyte and acid-base abnormalities

QUESTIONS

Problem Identification

1.a. Identify the type of acid–base disturbance present in this patient. Interpret the patient's arterial blood gas results and identify potential causes to support your response.

1.b. Create a list of this patient's drug therapy problems.

1.c. Describe the physical exam and laboratory findings that are consistent with metabolic alkalosis and those that are inconsistent with this acid–base disorder.

1.d. What is the pathophysiology underlying this patient's metabolic alkalosis?

1.e. What medications, dietary supplements, and medical procedures could contribute to metabolic alkalosis? Include those that may not apply to this patient.

Desired Outcome

2. What are the desired therapeutic outcomes for this patient?

Therapeutic Alternatives

3. What pharmacologic and nonpharmacologic alternatives should be considered for the treatment of metabolic alkalosis in this patient?

Optimal Plan

4.a. What drug, dosage form, dose, schedule, and duration of therapy are best for this patient?

4.b. What other modifications in the patient's current drug regimen are warranted? Include your rationale.

Outcome Evaluation

5.a. What clinical and laboratory parameters are necessary to evaluate the therapy for achievement of the desired outcome and to detect or prevent adverse effects?

▓ CLINICAL COURSE

The patient was started on IV fluids, and 24 hours later the patient is observed to have 1+ pitting edema in her lower extremities. Laboratory values are as follows:

Na 140 mEq/L	BUN 14 mg/dL	*ABG*
K 3.8 mEq/L	SCr 0.8 mg/dL	pH 7.46
Cl 103 mEq/L	Mg 2.1 mEq/L	$PaCO_2$ 39 mm Hg
CO_2 30 mEq/L		PaO_2 92 mm Hg
		HCO_3 31 mEq/L

5.b. What is your assessment of the patient's response to the IV fluids? What modifications in therapy are warranted, if any?

Patient Education

6. What information should be provided to the patient to help enhance adherence, ensure successful outcomes, and prevent future complications?

▓ SELF-STUDY ASSIGNMENTS

1. Prepare a paper on the three phases (initiation, maintenance, and compensation) of the pathogenesis of metabolic alkalosis. Describe the mechanisms behind each phase and the treatments, if appropriate.

2. Describe how assessment of urine electrolytes is useful in the diagnosis and treatment of metabolic alkalosis.

CLINICAL PEARL

Although most cases of metabolic alkalosis are asymptomatic, the disorder can lead to serious complications from electrolyte abnormalities (eg, tetany, arrhythmias, mental status changes).

In addition to assessing arterial blood gas and laboratory tests, it is important to obtain a thorough patient history to identify underlying cause of metabolic alkalosis and treat it appropriately.

REFERENCES

1. Shah N, Shaw C, Forni LG. Metabolic alkalosis in the intensive care unit. Neth J Crit Care 2008;12(3):113–119.

2. Gennari FJ, Weise WJ. Acid–base disturbances in gastrointestinal disease. Clin J Am Soc Nephrol 2008;3:1861–1868.

3. Soifer JT, Kim HT. Approach to metabolic alkalosis. Emerg Med Clin N Am 2014;32:453–463.

4. Seifter JL. Integration of acid-base and electrolyte disorders. N Engl J Med 2014;371(19):1821–1831.

5. Dellinger RP, Levy MM, Rhodes A, et al. Surviving sepsis campaign: International guidelines for management of severe sepsis and septic shock: 2012. Crit Care Med 2013;41:580–637.

6. Moviat M, Pickkers P, van der Hoeven PHJ, et al. Acetazolamide-mediated decrease in strong ion difference accounts for the correction of metabolic alkalosis in critically ill patients. Crit Care 2006;10:R14. doi:10.1186/cc3970.

7. Oh YK. Acid–base disorders in ICU patients. Electrolyte Blood Press 2010;8:66–71.

63

ALZHEIMER DISEASE

Not Going Gently Into That Good Night . . . . Level II

Carol A. Ott, PharmD, BCPP

LEARNING OBJECTIVES

After completing this case study, the reader should be able to:

- Assess cognitive deficits and noncognitive/behavioral symptoms of Alzheimer disease (AD).

- Evaluate the drug therapy regimens for medications that could interfere with the AD process and future drug therapy recommendations.

- Recommend appropriate pharmacotherapy to manage the cognitive and behavioral symptoms of AD.

- Determine appropriate education and counseling to provide to patients and caregivers about AD, the possible benefits and adverse effects of pharmacotherapy for the disorder, and the importance of adherence to therapy.

- Propose at least three theories of AD etiologies and agents under investigation based on those theories.

PATIENT PRESENTATION

▪ Chief Complaint

"Mom has become apathetic and tearful in the last month. She complains that someone is stealing from her and she is not always cooperative. She lives on her own, but I am considering moving her to a nursing home."

▪ HPI

Norma Dale is a 74-year-old woman who presents to the geriatric care clinic for a routine visit accompanied by her daughter Ann. Norma was diagnosed with AD 6 years ago. Her initial symptoms included forgetting times and dates easily, misplacing and losing items, repeating questions and current events, inability to answer questions, and increasing difficulty with managing finances. She was initially treated with rivastigmine which was eventually discontinued due to intolerable side effects although it worked well to slow her decline. Treatment with donepezil 10 mg at bedtime has been well tolerated for the past 4 years, and Norma has been participating more actively in family and social functions. Behavioral problems have been infrequent since diagnosis and have not been treated in the past. Since her last clinic visit, Norma began using Depend undergarments as extra protection for urinary incontinence.

Norma lives on her own; her daughter and son share the duties of visiting her twice a day. They have been able to maintain a regular routine with her mother's daily activities, nutrition, and financial responsibilities, using lists and notes to help Norma orient herself. Ann sets up a medication box weekly for Norma. Ann is moving in 1 month to live closer to her own daughter to help with grandchildren and has asked her youngest unmarried brother, Sam, to help take care of their mother. Sam has agreed to be his mother's caregiver. He lives and works across town and is not sure if he wants to move his mother into his home. There has been discussion about placing Norma in a long-term care facility. Norma displays lack of interest, apathy, and tearfulness lately, especially when Ann and Sam are talking about her care. Ann asks about Norma's current Alzheimer's medication and her recent lack of cooperation and mood.

▪ PMH

Osteoarthritis in hands and hip × 6 years
Hypertension × 15 years
Dyslipidemia × 6 years
AD diagnosed 6 years ago
Urinary incontinence × 6 months

▪ FH

Noncontributory, both parents deceased. Five children, four who live nearby

▪ SH

Lives at home; has been widowed for 10 years (husband died of cancer); negative for tobacco use; occasional alcohol use socially, none for ~5 years

▪ Meds

Donepezil 10 mg PO at bedtime
Vitamin E 400 IU PO once daily
Lisinopril 10 mg PO once daily
Simvastatin 20 mg PO every evening
Aspirin 81 mg PO once daily
Oxybutynin 5 mg PO twice daily (× 2 months)
Ensure drinks PRN
Acetaminophen PRN

▪ All

NKDA

▪ ROS

Reports occasional bladder incontinence and knee pain; no c/o heartburn, chest pain, or shortness of breath

▪ Physical Examination

Gen

Well-developed woman who appears her stated age

VS

BP 144/82 mm Hg, P 76 bpm, RR 18, T 37°C; Wt 165 kg, Ht 5'6"

Skin

Normal texture and color

HEENT

WNL, TMs intact

Neck/Lymph Nodes

Neck supple without thyromegaly or lymphadenopathy

Lungs/Thorax

Clear, normal breath sounds

Breasts

No masses or tenderness

CV

RRR, no murmurs or bruits

Abd

Soft, NT/ND

Genit/Rect

Normal external female genitalia

MS/Ext

No CCE, Heberden's nodes on both hands, decreased ROM (L) hip

Neuro

Motor, sensory, CNs, cerebellar, and gait normal. Folstein MMSE score 16/30, compared to a score of 19/30 and 24/30, last year and at the initial diagnosis, respectively. Disoriented to season, month, date, and day of week. Disoriented to country. Good registration but impaired attention and very poor short-term memory. Unable to remember any of three items after 3 minutes. Able to follow commands. Displayed apathy, tearfulness, and frustration during MMSE.

■ Labs (Fasting)

Na 139 mEq/L	Hgb 13.5 g/dL	T. bili 0.9 mg/dL	*Fasting lipid panel*
K 3.7 mEq/L	Hct 39.0%	D. bili 0.3 mg/dL	T. chol 212 mg/dL
Cl 108 mEq/L	AST 25 IU/L	T. prot 7.5 g/dL	LDL 130 mg/dL
CO_2 25.5 mEq/L	ALT 24 IU/L	Alb 4.5 g/dL	HDL 45 mg/dL
BUN 16 mg/dL	Alk phos 81 IU/L	Ca 9.7 mg/dL	TG 180 mg/dL
SCr 1.4 mg/dL	GGT 22 IU/L	Phos 4.5 mg/dL	
Glu 102 mg/dL	LDH 85 IU/L	Vit B_{12} 430 pg/mL	Free T4 0.9 ng/dL
		TSH 2.5 mIU/L	UA 6.8 mg/dL

■ Urinalysis

Specific gravity 1.010, color dark yellow, appearance clear, glucose (+), bilirubin (−), ketones (−), pH 7.4, protein (−), blood (−), nitrite (+), WBC/hpf 25–50, RBC/hpf 0, leukocyte esterase 2+, bacteria 1+

■ CT Scan (Head, 4 Years Ago)

Mild-to-moderate generalized cerebral atrophy

■ Assessment

1. AD, stage 5 on the Global Deterioration Scale (moderate AD—early dementia)

2. Behavioral problems reported by caregiver as lack of interest, apathy, uncooperative behavior, and tearfulness

3. Occasional urinary incontinence

4. Occasional hip and hand pain secondary to osteoarthritis; generally well controlled with acetaminophen PRN

5. Dyslipidemia not optimally controlled with current drug therapy

6. Possible urinary tract infection

QUESTIONS

Problem Identification

1.a. Create a list of the patient's drug therapy problems.

1.b. What information (signs, symptoms, and laboratory values) indicates the presence or severity of the cognitive and noncognitive problems of this patient with AD?

1.c. Rank the drug therapy problems according to the urgency of need to address.

Desired Outcome

2.a. What are the goals of pharmacotherapy in this case?

2.b. What drugs or disease states may interfere with achieving these goals?

Therapeutic Alternatives

3.a. What nondrug therapies might be useful for this patient?

3.b. What feasible pharmacotherapeutic alternatives are available for treatment of the cognitive deficits of AD?

3.c. What pharmacologic treatments may be useful to treat the noncognitive symptoms and behaviors of this patient?

3.d. What economic and psychosocial considerations are applicable to this patient?

Optimal Plan

4.a. What drug, dosage form, dose, schedule, and duration of therapy are best for the cognitive and noncognitive symptoms of this patient?

4.b. What alternatives would be appropriate if the initial therapy fails or cannot be used?

Outcome Evaluation

5. What clinical and laboratory parameters are necessary to evaluate the therapy for achievement of the desired therapeutic outcome and to detect or prevent adverse effects?

Patient Education

6. What information should be provided to the patient to enhance compliance, ensure successful therapy, and minimize adverse effects?

■ CLINICAL COURSE

Norma's uncooperative behavior and apathy improve with your recommended drug therapy changes. She remains tearful at times and is now not sleeping well at night. She continues to be fearful of someone coming into her house and insists that some of her things are missing.

■ FOLLOW-UP QUESTIONS

1. What further evaluation should be done to address the patient's continued tearfulness and sleep problems?

2. Discuss the use of antipsychotic medications for the treatment of psychiatric and behavioral problems in AD. Include a discussion of the pros and cons of treatment.

3. What is the impact of vitamin B_{12} and thyroid function on the presentation and progression of dementia symptoms?

4. What options are available for the treatment of urinary incontinence in this patient after discontinuation of oxybutynin?

5. Determine the clinical utility of combination therapy with a cholinesterase inhibitor and memantine. What improvements in clinical condition may be expected? Is the potential benefit worth the risk?

6. Discuss the treatment of medical conditions, including hypertension and dyslipidemia, in the patient with progressing dementia. What are the pros and cons of treatment relative to the patient's quality of life; cost, side effects, and complexity of the drug regimen; and ethical treatment?

■ SELF-STUDY ASSIGNMENTS

1. Describe neurofibrillary tangles and neuritic plaques and their roles in AD development.

2. List at least three theories of the etiology of AD. What therapies are under investigation to support these theories?

3. Characterize the stages of cognitive decline as described by the Global Deterioration Scale and define the stage where AD may be identified.

4. Differentiate cognitive deficits from noncognitive/psychiatric symptoms and behaviors of AD.

5. Evaluate potential therapies under investigation for Alzheimer dementia.

6. Discuss the utility of clinical amyloid imaging in the diagnosis of Alzheimer dementia, focusing on the FDA-approved amyloid imaging agent florbetapir.

7. Debate the link between type 2 diabetes mellitus and the risk of developing Alzheimer dementia.

8. Evaluate the diagnostic criteria for Neurocognitive Disorder, Alzheimer's type in the Diagnostic and Statistical Manual, 5th edition (DSM-5).

CLINICAL PEARL

The elderly, especially those with dementia, can develop delirium very easily, and it may appear acutely as a behavioral problem. Causes may include medications (eg, anticholinergic agents) and medical conditions (eg, UTI); therefore, a thorough assessment should be performed.

REFERENCES

1. Rabins PV, Blacker D, Rovner BW, et al. American Psychiatric Association practice guideline for the treatment of patients with Alzheimer's disease and other dementias. 2nd edition. Am J Psychiatry 2007;164(Suppl 12):5–56.

2. Herholz K, Ebmeier K. Clinical amyloid imaging in Alzheimer's disease. Lancet Neurol 2011;10:667–670.

3. Sadowsky CH, Galvin JE. Guidelines for the management of cognitive and behavioral problems in dementia. J Am Board Fam Med 2012;25:350–366.

4. Vogel T, Dali-Youcef N, Kaltenbach G, Andrés E. Homocysteine, vitamin B_{12}, folate and cognitive functions: a systematic and critical review of the literature. Int J Clin Pract 2009;63:1061–1067.

5. Jaturapatporn D, Isaac MG, McCleery J, Tabet N. Aspirin, steroidal and non-steroidal anti-inflammatory drugs for the treatment of Alzheimer's disease (Review). Cochrane Database Syst Rev 2012. doi:10.1002/14651858.CD006378.pub2.

6. Chang-Quan H, Hui W, Chao-min W, et al. The association of antihypertensive medication use with risk of cognitive decline and dementia: a meta-analysis of longitudinal studies. Int J Clin Pract 2011;65:1295–1305.

7. Jeste DV, Blazer D, Casey D, et al. ACNP white paper: update on use of antipsychotic drugs in elderly persons with dementia. Neuropsychopharmacology 2008;33:957–970.

8. Romeo R, Knapp M, Hellier J, et al. Cost-effectiveness analyses for mirtazapine and sertraline in dementia: randomised controlled trial. Br J Psychiatry 2013;202:121–128.

9. Ehret MJ, Chamberlin KW. Current practices in the treatment of Alzheimer disease: where is the evidence after the phase III trials? Clin Ther 2015;37:1604–1616.

10. Campbell N, Boustani M, Limbil T, et al. The cognitive impact of anticholinergics: a clinical review. Clin Interv Aging 2009;4:225–233.

64

MULTIPLE SCLEROSIS

White Dots and Black Holes. . . . . Level I

Jacquelyn L. Bainbridge, BS Pharm, PharmD, FCCP

Augusto Miravalle, MD

Felecia Hart, PharmD

LEARNING OBJECTIVES

After completing this case study, the reader should be able to:

• Describe the signs and symptoms of multiple sclerosis (MS) that often mimic those of other neurologic diseases.

• Design a pharmacotherapeutic regimen for treating an acute exacerbation of MS.

• Identify patients for whom disease-modifying therapy (DMT) would be appropriate and recommend the most appropriate alternative for an individual patient.

- Implement a pharmacotherapeutic plan for a patient with worsening MS.
- Educate patients and health care practitioners on the proper dosing, self-administration (if appropriate), adverse effects, and storage of various medications used in MS.

PATIENT PRESENTATION

■ Chief Complaint

"My legs are numb and weak, and I'm having trouble walking and urinating."

■ HPI

Loretta Mansfield is a 26-year-old woman who was in excellent health until 4 days ago, when she developed numbness and tingling in her left foot. Over the course of the next 4 days, the numbness extended higher up her leg to her lower abdomen, stopping at the umbilicus, and then going down the right leg. She also developed weakness in both of her legs, is having trouble walking, and is bothered by urinary urgency.

■ PMH

Frequent migraine headaches since adolescence, that have been difficult to control despite therapy with acetaminophen, aspirin, and caffeine (Excedrin) and oral sumatriptan.
Mild recurrent bouts of depression that have not been treated pharmacologically.
Obesity most of her life.

■ FH

English descent. She was born in Arizona and moved at the age of 12 to Ohio. She has no siblings, and both parents are alive and well. There is no family history of neurologic disease.

■ SH

Married; employed as an accountant; smoked one pack per day for 8 years; use of alcohol is limited to an occasional glass of wine or beer on weekends.

■ Meds

Acetaminophen, aspirin, and caffeine (Excedrin) two tablets PO PRN headache
Sumatriptan 50 mg PO PRN migraine, at the onset of pain

■ Allergies

NKDA

■ ROS

Unremarkable except that she reports feeling run down and tired most of the day. No previous history of visual disturbance (eg, pain, blurred, or double vision), sensory, motor, bowel, bladder, or gait disturbance.

■ Physical Examination

Gen

The patient is a Caucasian woman who appears to be slightly anxious but is otherwise in NAD

VS

BP 120/72 mm Hg, P 88 bpm and regular, RR 20, T 36.6°C; Wt 86.4 kg, Ht 5′2″, BMI 34.7

Skin

Normal turgor; no obvious lesions, tumors, or moles

HEENT

NC/AT, TMs clear

Neck/Lymph Nodes

Supple, without lymphadenopathy or thyromegaly

CV

RRR; S_1, S_2 normal; no MRG

Lungs

Clear to A & P

Abd

NTND

Genit/Rect

Deferred

MS/Ext

Normal ROM; pulses 2+ throughout

Neuro

CNs II–XII are intact with the exception of abnormal saccadic movements on horizontal gaze; no signs of optic neuropathy.
Motor: Tone, bulk, and strength are 5/5 in both arms, with good fine motor movements. In the legs, she has 4/5 strength in an upper motor neuron pattern, with normal tone and bulk.
Sensory: Moderately diminished light touch, pain, and temperature in both legs with a cord level at the umbilicus, and decreased vibratory sensation in both great toes. (+) Romberg sign.
Coordination: Finger-to-nose and alternating movements with the hands are normal, as is heel to shin bilaterally.
Gait: Mildly unsteady on tandem walking. Timed 25-foot walk was 5.2 seconds.
Reflexes: 2/2 in UE, 3/3 in LE; (+) Babinski bilaterally.
The patient is alert, oriented, and cooperative. No Lhermitte's sign is noted.

■ Labs

Na 142 mEq/L	Anion Gap 16 mEq/L	AST 12 IU/L
K 4.1 mEq/L	Ca 9.4 mg/dL	ALT 40 IU/L
Cl 99 mEq/L	Bilirubin 0.8 mg/dL	GGT 33 IU/L
CO_2 23 mEq/L	Protein total 8.1 g/dL	ESR 20 mm/hour
BUN 11 mg/dL	Albumin 4.9 g/dL	TSH 1.0 μIU/mL
SCr 0.9 mg/dL	B_{12} 510 ng/L	ANA negative
Glu 109 mg/dL	Anti-JC virus	CRP 1.0 mg/dL
25(OH) vitamin D 17 ng/mL	antibody negative	Lyme serology negative

■ Lumbar Puncture

CSF analysis shows opening pressure 140 mm H_2O, 10 WBC/μL, 97% lymphocytes; protein 30 mg/dL, glucose 65 mg/dL; IgG index 1.7; 12 oligoclonal bands unique to CSF.

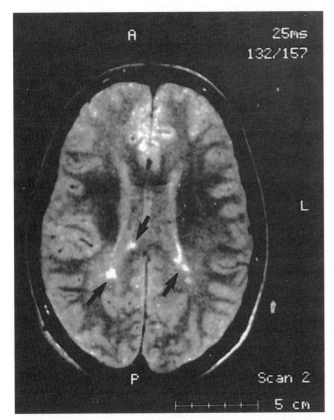

FIGURE 64-1. Brain MRI scan. *Arrows* highlight typical periventricular white matter lesions seen in multiple sclerosis.

MRI Scan

Thoracic spine MRI with and without injection of contrast material reveals a one-segment long enhancing lesion in the posterior thoracic spine at level T10.

Brain MRI shows multiple areas of T2 and FLAIR hyperintense lesions; four were periventricular, one was in the left cerebellum, two were juxtacortical; none of the areas enhance after injection of contrast material. A total of 12 T2 and FLAIR lesions were seen in the brain; see Fig. 64-1.

Assessment/Plan

1. Medical history, physical exam findings, and other diagnostic tests are consistent with MS. Because this is her first episode of MS-like symptoms, diagnosis is clinically isolated syndrome (CIS). Diagnostic tests suggest high risk of recurrent disease activity over 5–20 years.

2. Plan to initiate therapy to treat acute signs/symptoms. We will consider long-term therapy with a disease-modifying agent and symptomatic therapies.

3. Patient counseling on lifestyle and dietary modifications will be provided to assist in improving quality of life and slowing or preventing disease progression.

QUESTIONS

Problem Identification

1.a. What clinical information (patient demographics, signs, symptoms, and lab values) suggests the diagnosis of MS in this patient?

1.b. What additional information (laboratory tests, diagnostic procedures) may be useful in assessing this patient?

Desired Outcome

2. What are the goals of therapy for this patient?

Therapeutic Alternatives

3.a. What pharmacotherapeutic options are available to treat this patient's acute neurologic signs and symptoms?

3.b. What pharmacotherapeutic options are available to reduce the risk of recurrent disease activity in this patient?

3.c. What symptomatic treatments may be indicated for this patient?

3.d. What behavioral or dietary changes may be beneficial?

Optimal Plan

4. Design a comprehensive pharmacotherapeutic plan for this patient on her initial presentation.

Outcome Evaluation

5. What clinical and laboratory parameters are necessary for assessment of both efficacy and toxicity?

Patient Education

6. What information would you provide to this patient about her initial therapy?

■ CLINICAL COURSE

The patient was treated with the regimen you recommended, with gradual resolution of her symptoms. Six months after the initial presentation, she returns to clinic with complaints of painful loss of vision in her left eye, which evolved over 3 days. On exam, she has a visual acuity of 20/200 in the left eye and 20/20 in the right eye. Visual fields are normal, but she has loss of color sensitivity in the left eye. There is a left relative afferent pupillary defect (Marcus Gunn pupil). There is no disc swelling or atrophy in either eye on funduscopic examination. The remainder of the physical exam is notable only for a mild Romberg sign and increased reflexes in the lower extremities. Her affect is sad, and she is tearful during the examination. She is concerned that she has now progressed to a diagnosis of clinically definite MS.

■ OPTICAL COHERENCE TOMOGRAPHY (OCT)

OCT was completed because of her complaint of left eye pain and visual loss. OCT was performed on the right and left optic nerves for evaluation of vision loss and eye pain. The signal strength was 9 in the right eye and 6 in the left eye.

Right eye: The average peripapillary retinal nerve fiber layer thickness was 104 μm. There was no retinal nerve fiber layer loss in any quadrant or sector.

Left eye: The average peripapillary retinal nerve fiber layer thickness was 80 μm. There were significant changes in the superior and inferior quadrants consistent with optic neuritis.

■ FOLLOW-UP QUESTION

1. Would you consider the new information gathered at the follow-up visit to be evidence of significant disease progression that would prompt you to change your treatment strategy? If so, what therapies would be appropriate for the patient?

■ SELF-STUDY ASSIGNMENTS

1. Obtain relevant information and formulate an opinion on the role of plasmapheresis in the treatment of MS.

2. Review the clinical studies evaluating comparative trials of DMTs for MS. How does glatiramer acetate compare with interferon β-1b and interferon β-1a in terms of both efficacy and toxicity?

3. Outline a plan for providing patient education on the dosing, administration, monitoring, and storage of interferon β-1b, interferon β-1a, and glatiramer acetate.

4. Identify recent clinical trials assessing the efficacy and toxicity of natalizumab, rituximab, alemtuzumab, fingolimod, teriflunomide, and dimethyl fumarate for MS. Considering the data available, define the potential role(s) of these agents for patients with MS.

CLINICAL PEARL

Many patients do not feel better with interferon therapy and may experience unpleasant adverse effects. It is important to reinforce that the first-generation or self-injected DMTs (Avonex, Betaseron, Copaxone, Rebif) medications do not reduce disease symptoms but will reduce attacks and progression of disability over time. Adequate counseling about the potential benefits and expected side effects is essential to ensuring adherence to the therapy.

REFERENCES

1. Tullman MJ. A review of current and emerging therapeutic strategies in multiple sclerosis. Am J Manag Care 2013;19(2 Suppl):S21–S27.

2. Kaufman DI, Trobe JD, Eggenberger ER, Whitaker JN. Practice parameter: the role of corticosteroids in the management of acute monosymptomatic optic neuritis. Report of the Quality Standards Subcommittee of the American Academy of Neurology. Neurology 2000;54:2039–2044.

3. Martinelli V, Rocca MA, Annovazzi P, et al. A short-term randomized MRI study of high-dose oral vs intravenous methylprednisolone in MS. Neurology 2009;73(22):1842–1848.

4. Goodin DS, Frohman EM, Garmany GP, et al. Disease modifying therapies in multiple sclerosis. Report of the Therapeutics and Technology Assessment Subcommittee of the American Academy of Neurology and the MS Council for Clinical Practice Guidelines. Neurology 2002;58:169–178.

5. Corboy JR, Goodin DS, Frohman EM. Disease-modifying therapies for multiple sclerosis. Curr Treat Options Neurol 2003;5:35–54.

6. Ali R, Nicholas RS, Muraro PA. Drugs in development for relapsing multiple sclerosis. Drugs 2013;73(7):625–650.

7. O'Conner P, Wolinsky JS, Confavreux C, et al. Randomized trial of oral teriflunomide for relapsing multiple sclerosis. N Engl J Med 2011;365:1293–1303.

8. Gold R, Kappos L, Arnold DL, et al. Placebo-controlled phase 3 study of oral BG-12 for relapsing multiple sclerosis. N Engl J Med 2012;367:1098–1107.

9. Schapiro RT. Managing symptoms of multiple sclerosis. Neurol Clin 2005;23(1):177–187, vii.

10. Egeberg MD, Oh CY, Bainbridge JL. Clinical overview of dalfampridine: an agent with a novel mechanism of action to help with gait disturbances. Clin Ther 2012;34:2185–2194.

11. Mikol DD, Barkhof F, Chang P, et al. Comparison of subcutaneous interferon beta-1a with glatiramer acetate in patients with relapsing multiple sclerosis (the REbif vs. Glatiramer Acetate in Relapsing MS Disease [REGARD] study): a multicentre, randomised, parallel, open-label trial. Lancet Neurol 2008;7:903–914.

65

COMPLEX PARTIAL SEIZURES

An Overdue Visit to a Neurology Clinic . . . . Level I

James W. McAuley, RPh, PhD, FAPhA

LEARNING OBJECTIVES

After completing this case study, the reader should be able to:

- Identify necessary data to collect for patients with complex partial seizures.

- Define potential drug-related problems for antiepileptic drugs.

- List desired therapeutic outcomes for patients with complex partial seizures.

- Based on patient characteristics, choose appropriate pharmacotherapy for treatment of partial seizures and develop a suitable care plan.

- Identify key issues for a woman of childbearing potential taking antiepileptic drugs.

PATIENT PRESENTATION

■ Chief Complaint

"My family doctor told me I should see a neurologist about my seizures."

■ HPI

Peggy Livingston is a 36-year-old woman referred to the neurology clinic by her PCP for evaluation of her seizures and anticonvulsant therapy. She is enduring quite a heavy seizure burden. Her last seizure was 10 days ago, which resulted in her falling down her basement stairs. Her seizures started at a very early age, and she said no one has been able to identify why she started having seizures. She remembers having them in grade school and being confused a lot throughout her schooling. She was briefly tried on phenobarbital initially but has been on phenytoin most of her life. She has poor seizure control with no extended seizure-free periods. She has not seen a neurologist for years, if ever. She has not had any neuroimaging studies and provides no previous EEG results.

On speaking with the patient and her husband of 2.5 years, most of her events involve "blackouts" and losing track of time. Occasionally, she has "grand mal" seizures. She is more likely to have a seizure if she gets overly tired or stressed. She has no history of severe head injury with loss of consciousness, or other significant risk factors for seizures. She states that at some time in her past, she "felt really bad, almost drunk" on higher doses of phenytoin. She states that she is very adherent, although she has run out of medication more than once. Because she is having seizures, she does not drive and therefore must rely on others for transportation. This lack of independence is a major concern for Peggy.

Data gathered from reviewing her seizure calendar over the past 2 months (Fig. 65-1) suggest that she is experiencing approximately eight "small" seizures per month (complex partial seizures with no secondary generalization) and one "big" seizure per month (a secondarily generalized tonic–clonic seizure). Her interview

Patient Instructions: Please record the number and type of seizures you have each day.

S = Small, B = Big, ? = Possible seizure   **Patient: P. Livingston**

March

Sunday	Monday	Tuesday	Wednesday	Thursday	Friday	Saturday
		1	2	3	4	5 S
6	7	8	9	10	11 S	12 S
13	14 S→B	15	16	17	18	19
20	21	22 S, S	23 S	24	25	26
27	28	29	30 S	31		

April

Sunday	Monday	Tuesday	Wednesday	Thursday	Friday	Saturday
					1	2
3	4 S	5	6 S	7 S	8	9
10	11	12	13	14	15 S	16 S, S→B
17	18	19 S	20	21	22	23
24	25 ? S	26	27	28	29 S	30

FIGURE 65-1. Seizure calendar (S, small; B, big; ?, possible seizure).

details and her overall score on her responses to the QOLIE-31 questions show a significant impact of the seizures on her quality of life. Her scores on the energy/fatigue, seizure worry, and social function domains are especially low in comparison with a cohort of other patients with epilepsy. The score on her NDDI-E was 11, indicating that she had some mood issues, but she was not depressed. On asking if there is anything else the patient would like to discuss, Peggy and her husband state that they desire to start a family in the near future.

■ PMH

Noncontributory, except as described previously

■ FH

Both parents deceased; one younger brother in good health; no seizure disorder, cancer, or CV disease

■ SH

Married; works in a local restaurant; denies tobacco and alcohol use; finished high school with a "C" average; no children

■ ROS

Tired a lot, but no problems with balance or double vision

■ Meds

Phenytoin (Dilantin) 300 mg PO at bedtime

■ All

NKDA

■ Physical Examination

Gen

Pleasant woman showing some anxiety during this initial visit

VS

BP 132/87 mm Hg, P 72 bpm, RR 18, T 36.2°C; Wt 66.8 kg, Ht 5'1"

Skin

Normal color, hydration, and temperature

HEENT

Mild hirsutism; (+) gingival hyperplasia

Neck/Lymph Nodes

(–) JVD; (–) lymphadenopathy

Lungs/Thorax

CTA

Breasts

Deferred

CV

Normal S_1 and S_2, RRR, NSR, normal peripheral pulses

Abd

NT/ND, (+) BS, no HSM

Genit/Rect

Deferred

MS/Ext

Significant burn on palm of right hand. This happened within the last week when she had a seizure while frying eggs on the stovetop. Her husband stated that he witnessed her put hand directly in the frying pan during her seizure.

Neuro

CNs II–XII intact; slight lateral gaze nystagmus noted. Motor: 4/5 muscle strength on left side, 5/5 on right side. DTRs: 2+ RUE, 1+ LUE, 0 RLE, 0 LLE. Sensory: normal light touch and pinprick. Station: normal.

■ Labs

Na 137 mEq/L	Hgb 14.5 g/dL	AST 31 IU/L
K 4.1 mEq/L	Hct 41.7%	ALT 22 IU/L
Cl 100 mEq/L	RBC 4.71×10^6/mm³	Alk phos 187 IU/L
CO_2 29 mEq/L	MCV 88.6 μm³	GGT 45 IU/L
BUN 9 mg/dL	MCHC 34.7 g/dL	Ca 7.3 mg/dL
SCr 0.6 mg/dL	Plt 212×10^3/mm³	Alb 3.9 g/dL
Glu 107 mg/dL	WBC 5.4×10^3/mm³	

■ EEG

Abnormal for bitemporal slowing, which is more significant in the left temporal region, as characterized by polymorphic and epileptiform discharges consistent with a history of seizure disorder

■ Assessment

Uncontrolled complex partial seizures, with occasional secondary generalization

QUESTIONS

Problem Identification

1.a. Create a list of the patient's drug therapy problems.

1.b. Which information (signs, symptoms, and laboratory values) indicates the presence or severity of complex partial seizures?

Desired Outcome

2. What are the goals of pharmacotherapy in this case?

Therapeutic Alternatives

3.a. What nonpharmacologic therapies might be useful for this patient?

3.b. What feasible pharmacotherapeutic alternatives are available for treatment of complex partial seizures in this patient?

3.c. What economic and psychosocial considerations are applicable to this patient?

Optimal Plan

4. What drug, dosage form, dose, schedule, and duration of therapy are best for this patient?

Outcome Evaluation

5. Which clinical and laboratory parameters are necessary to evaluate the therapy for achievement of the desired therapeutic outcome and to detect or prevent adverse effects?

Patient Education

6. What information should be provided to the patient to enhance adherence, ensure successful therapy, and minimize adverse effects?

■ CLINICAL COURSE

A collective decision was made among the health care practitioners, the patient, and her husband to add another antiepileptic drug to her current drug regimen and to see her back in 6 weeks. She was given written and verbal information on this new drug and instructed to call or use the patient portal with any questions, problems, or concerns. She and her husband verbalized an understanding. At her next visit, the patient reported that there had been an initial response to the addition of the new antiepileptic drug (ie, fewer seizures), but she still has some "small" seizures and one "big" seizure per month. There are no recent laboratory data. Her neurologic examination is unchanged. She and her husband would like to further discuss their desire to start a family.

■ FOLLOW-UP QUESTION

1. What is known about long-term effects on cognition and behavior in children exposed to antiepileptic drugs in utero?

■ SELF-STUDY ASSIGNMENTS

1. Outline a plan for assessing this patient's adherence with her medication regimen.

2. What risk factors does this patient have for osteoporosis? What interventions should be made?

3. Would switching this patient from brand Dilantin to generic phenytoin be an appropriate alternative? What are the ramifications of making this change?

4. What role can community pharmacists play in the care of patients with epilepsy?

CLINICAL PEARL

Although epilepsy affects men and women equally, there are many women's health issues, including menstrual cycle influences on seizure activity, drug interactions between contraceptives and antiepileptic drugs, and teratogenicity of antiepileptic drugs.

REFERENCES

1. Taylor RS, Sander JW, Taylor RJ, Baker GA. Predictors of health-related quality of life and costs in adults with epilepsy: a systematic review. Epilepsia 2011;52:2168–2180.
2. Gilliam FG, Barry JJ, Hermann BP, Meador KJ, Vahle V, Kanner AM. Rapid detection of major depression in epilepsy: a multicentre study. Lancet Neurol 2006;5:399–405.
3. Fraser LA, Burneo JG, Fraser JA. Enzyme-inducing antiepileptic drugs and fractures in people with epilepsy: A systematic review. Epilepsy Res 2015;116:59–66.
4. Pennell PB. Hormonal aspects of epilepsy. Neurol Clin 2009;27:941–965.
5. Holmes LB, Baldwin EJ, Smith CR, et al. Increased frequency of isolated cleft palate in infants exposed to lamotrigine during pregnancy. Neurology 2008;70:2152–2158.
6. Meador KJ, Baker GA, Browning N, et al., for the NEAD Study Group. Fetal antiepileptic drug exposure and cognitive outcomes at age 6 years (NEAD study): a prospective observational study. Lancet Neurol 2013;12:244–252.
7. McAuley JW, Chen AY, Elliott JO, Shneker BF. An assessment of patient and pharmacist knowledge of and attitudes toward reporting adverse drug events due to formulation switching in patients with epilepsy. Epilepsy Behav 2009;14:113–117.
8. McCagh J, Fisk JE, Baker GA. Epilepsy, psychosocial and cognitive functioning. Epilepsy Res 2009;86:1–14.
9. England MJ, Liverman CT, Schultz AM, Strawbridge LM. Epilepsy across the spectrum: promoting health and understanding. A summary of the Institute of Medicine report. Epilepsy Behav 2012;25:266–276.
10. Mula M, Kanner AM, Schmitz B, Schachter S. Antiepileptic drugs and suicidality: An expert consensus statement from the Task Force on Therapeutic Strategies of the ILAE Commission on Neuropsychobiology. Epilepsia 2013;54:199–203.

66

GENERALIZED TONIC–CLONIC SEIZURES

Senior Seizures .... Level II

Jennifer A. Donaldson, PharmD

LEARNING OBJECTIVES

After completing this case study, the reader should be able to:

- Define epilepsy.
- Differentiate seizure types based on clinical presentation and description.
- Recommend drugs of choice and alternative therapies for different types of seizures.
- Identify appropriate dosing, the most common adverse effects, and monitoring parameters for anticonvulsants.
- Develop an appropriate pharmaceutical care plan for a patient with epilepsy.

PATIENT PRESENTATION

■ Chief Complaint

"I had a seizure a few weeks ago and banged up my head."

■ HPI

Carter McNeely is a 68-year-old man whose seizures are well controlled with carbamazepine monotherapy. The seizure from 2.5 weeks ago was the first seizure in 20 months. During the seizure, he fell to the floor and sustained a laceration to his occipital region that required staples for closure. The description of his seizures is vague because there have been only six seizures documented since he developed epilepsy 3 years ago. Because Mr McNeely lives alone in an assisted living facility, only half of the documented seizures have been witnessed by another individual who could provide a description. Two seizures were witnessed by other residents who described him as "falling to the ground and starting to shake." One seizure occurred in the day room when a facility nurse was in the room, and he documented that Mr McNeely fell to the ground, developed rhythmic extensions to both his legs, became incontinent of urine, and was sleepy and disoriented for 2 hours after the episode.

He has only been treated with carbamazepine. This was started by his family practice physician after his second seizure. An EEG was obtained at that time and was unremarkable. Because the seizures are so infrequent, the dose of carbamazepine has never been adjusted.

■ PMH

Tonic–clonic seizures diagnosed 3 years ago
HTN adequately controlled with lisinopril monotherapy
Dyslipidemia controlled with atorvastatin and low-cholesterol diet
BPH, currently symptom-free on dutasteride

■ FH

Mother died at age 74 of "natural causes"; had HTN for many years. Father died at age 70 of "natural causes"; did not have any known medical illnesses. All of his children and grandchildren are alive and well. One son and one daughter have HTN.

■ SH

Retired factory worker; resides in an assisted living facility. He is widowed and has six children and nine grandchildren, whom he sees frequently. He denies past or present tobacco and illicit drug use. He reports a history of regular alcohol use but now only drinks one beer that his grandson brings to him every Saturday evening.

■ Meds

Aspirin 81 mg PO once daily
Atorvastatin 40 mg PO once daily
Carbamazepine XR 200 mg PO twice daily
Dutasteride 0.5 mg PO once daily
Lisinopril 20 mg PO once daily
Multivitamin with minerals one tablet PO once daily

■ All

NKDA
Adverse drug effect history—none

■ Physical Examination

Gen

Exam reveals an elderly Caucasian man who appears his stated age in NAD

VS

BP 126/78 mm Hg, HR 72, RR 16, temperature not measured; Ht 5′10″, Wt 72.5 kg

HEENT

Normocephalic; scalp: healing 3-cm lesion in the occipital region with corresponding mild tenderness and bruising; PERRL

Neck/LN

No thyromegaly, lymphadenopathy, or carotid bruits

Chest/Lungs

Lungs CTA

CV

RRR, no m/r/g

Abd

Soft, nontender; no HSM; (+) BS

MS/Ext

Normal tone; 5/5 strength in all extremities

Neuro

Awake; A & O × 3; CN II–XII intact, reflexes 2+ and symmetric throughout

■ Labs

		Fasting Lipid Profile
Na 127 mEq/L	Hgb 13.5 g/dL	
K 4.7 mEq/L	Hct 41%	T. Chol 155 mg/dL
Cl 90 mEq/L	RBC 3.9 × 10⁶/mm³	TG 123 mg/dL
CO_2 25 mEq/L	WBC 5.1 × 10³/mm³	HDL-C 39 mg/dL
BUN 10 mg/dL	Diff WNL	LDL-C 91 mg/dL
SCr 0.6 mg/dL	MCV 97 μm³	
Glu 100 mg/dL	Carbamazepine 6 mcg/mL	

■ EEG

Sleep-deprived EEG unremarkable. Photic stimulation failed to produce any other changes

■ Assessment

Sixty-eight-year-old man with fairly well-controlled seizures on carbamazepine monotherapy

QUESTIONS

Problem Identification

1.a. What are this patient's drug therapy problems?

1.b. What additional information is needed to fully assess the patient's problems related to epilepsy or his drug therapy?

1.c. What are the age-specific management issues for this patient?

Desired Outcome

2. What are the goals of pharmacotherapy in this case?

Therapeutic Alternatives

3.a. What nonpharmacologic interventions may be helpful for this patient?

3.b. What pharmacotherapeutic options are available to treat his epilepsy?

Optimal Plan

4. What is the best pharmacotherapeutic plan for this patient?

Outcome Evaluation

5. Which clinical and laboratory parameters are needed to evaluate the therapy to ensure the best possible outcome?

Patient Education

6. What information should the patient receive to ensure successful therapy and to minimize adverse effects?

■ SELF-STUDY ASSIGNMENTS

1. Smoking can affect serum concentrations of drugs. Perform a literature search to determine why this occurs and what effect it might have on anticonvulsants.

2. Perform a literature search to identify articles that have concluded that seizure medications can be withdrawn after a certain seizure-free interval.

3. Write a concise paper outlining the current recommendations for assisting a person who is having a seizure.

4. Assume that a patient taking valproic acid has poorly controlled seizures and a decision is made to add lamotrigine. What precautions, if any, should be taken? How should you initiate lamotrigine therapy?

CLINICAL PEARL

Many important historical figures had epileptic seizures, including Buddha, Socrates, Alexander the Great, Julius Caesar, St. Paul the Apostle, Mohammed, Peter the Great, Handel, Napoleon, Paganini, Kierkegaard, Alfred Nobel, and Dostoyevsky. It may be useful to share some of these names with patients to break the stigma of mental illness associated with epilepsy.

REFERENCES

1. Johnston A, Smith PEM. Epilepsy and the elderly. Expert Review of Neurotherapeutics 2010;10(12):1899–1910.
2. Tanaka A, Akamatsu N, Shouszki T, et al. Clinical characteristics and treatment responses in new-onset epilepsy in the elderly. Seizure 2013;22:772–775.
3. Leppik IE, Walczak TS, Birnbaum AK. Challenges of epilepsy in elderly people. Lancet 2012;380:1128–1130.
4. Baker GA, Jacoby A, Buck D, et al. The quality of life of older people with epilepsy: findings from a UK community study. Seizure 2001;10:92–99.
5. Stefan H. Epilepsy in the elderly: facts and challenges. Acta Neurol Scand 2011;124:223–237.
6. Glauser T, Ben-Menachem E, Bourgois B, et al. Updated ILAE evidence review of antiepileptic drug efficacy and effectiveness as initial monotherapy for epileptic seizures and syndromes. Epilepsia 2013;54:551–563.

67

STATUS EPILEPTICUS

Tempest in a Tom Collins . . . . Level I

Jennifer A. Donaldson, PharmD

LEARNING OBJECTIVES

After completing this case study, the reader should be able to:

- Define status epilepticus and its precipitating causes.

- Identify measures that should be taken in the ED for a patient in status epilepticus.

- Recommend appropriate drug treatment for status epilepticus.

- Recommend an optimal care plan for a patient with status epilepticus.

PATIENT PRESENTATION

Chief Complaint

As given by a friend of the patient: "I walked back into the room after getting breakfast and Josh was having a seizure. He kept shaking for a couple of minutes so I went to get the RA and he said we needed to get him to the ED."

HPI

Joshua Banch is a 20-year-old man brought to the university ED by his college roommate and dormitory resident assistant (RA). The roommate reported that he and Joshua went out partying the night before because all the fraternities were throwing rush parties. The roommate left Joshua partying at the Delta Tau Chi fraternity house at about 2:00 AM. He heard Joshua return to the room at approximately 4:30 AM and he was clearly intoxicated.

PMH

Medical records revealed that the patient developed generalized tonic–clonic seizures in childhood. Phenobarbital was initiated and controlled the seizures for many years. Withdrawal of phenobarbital was attempted 10 years ago after several years of being seizure-free. The drug was restarted when seizures occurred during the attempted taper. Phenobarbital was replaced with carbamazepine because of sedation and lethargy. Phenytoin was added 8 years ago because of frequent and prolonged breakthrough seizures. He has had occasional breakthrough seizures since his admission to the university 2 years ago. Breakthrough seizures are typically associated with Joshua's non-adherence with medications or sleep deprivation due to prolonged study sessions. He is routinely followed in the university neurology clinic.

FH

Negative for epilepsy; the patient has two siblings, all alive and well. No other information on family history was obtained.

SH

Single with no children; no tobacco use; reports drinking up to six beers per week

Meds

Carbamazepine 500 mg PO TID
Phenytoin 100 mg PO BID

All

NKDA

ROS

Unobtainable

Physical Examination

Gen

WDWN Caucasian man who is unarousable; clothes are wet from urinary incontinence

VS

BP 150/90 mm Hg, P 150 bpm, RR 25, T 37.5°C; Ht 5′7″, Wt 68.3 kg

Skin

Warm, dry, and pale; nail beds are pale

HEENT

Mucous membranes are dry

Neck/Lymph Nodes

Supple; no thyromegaly or lymphadenopathy

Lungs/Chest

Symmetric, lungs CTA

CV

RRR, no m/r/g

Abd

Soft, no HSM, BS normal in all four quadrants

MS/Ext

Muscle mass normal, full ROM

Neuro

Unarousable; reflexes 3+ bilaterally

■ Labs

Na 136 mEq/L	Hgb 12.8 g/dL	Drug screen: pending
K 4.5 mEq/L	Hct 41%	Carbamazepine: pending
Cl 97 mEq/L	Plt 320 × 10³/mm³	Phenytoin: pending
CO₂ 28 mEq/L	WBC 9.0 × 10³/mm³	
BUN 16 mg/dL	Diff WNL	
SCr 1.0 mg/dL		
Glu 60 mg/dL		

■ EEG

Baseline from medical record: Diffuse background slowing; no focal changes or epileptiform activity present; photic stimulation failed to produce other changes

■ Assessment

Twenty-year-old man with a history of tonic–clonic seizures now in status epilepticus

QUESTIONS

Problem Identification

1.a. What are this patient's drug therapy problems?

1.b. What steps should be taken when the patient is first seen in the ED?

Desired Outcome

2. What are the goals of pharmacotherapy in this case?

Therapeutic Alternatives

3. What pharmacotherapeutic options are available to treat status epilepticus?

Optimal Plan

4. What is the best pharmacotherapeutic plan for this patient?

Outcome Evaluation

5. What clinical and laboratory parameters are needed to evaluate the therapy to ensure the best possible outcome?

Patient Education

6. What information should the patient receive to ensure successful therapy and to minimize adverse effects?

■ SELF-STUDY ASSIGNMENTS

1. There are several drug interactions with phenytoin and carbamazepine. Describe the effects that these drugs have on each other. What, if anything, should be done to compensate for these drug interactions?

2. There are several sports in which patients with epilepsy should not participate. What are some of these sports, and why should these individuals not participate in them?

3. Finger-stick assays are available for phenytoin, carbamazepine, and phenobarbital. What role might they play in the emergent therapy of status epilepticus? Characterize the accuracy of these tests.

4. Prepare a two-page paper summarizing the hematologic adverse effects of all of the anticonvulsants.

CLINICAL PEARL

EEG studies have demonstrated that benign self-limited tonic-clonic seizures in adults last about 1 minute on average and rarely last more than 2 minutes.

REFERENCES

1. Betjemann JP, Lowenstein DH. Status Epilepticus in adults. Lancet Neurol 2015;14:615–624.
2. Brophy GM, Bell R, Claassen J, et al. Guidelines for the evaluation and management of status epilepticus. Neurocrit Care 2012;17(1):3–23.
3. Sharvon S. The treatment of status epilepticus. Curr Opin Neurol 2011;24:165–170.
4. Trinka E. What is the relative value of the standard anticonvulsants: phenytoin and fosphenytoin, phenobarbital, valproate, and levetiracetam? Epilepsia 2009;50(Suppl 12):40–43.
5. Prasad M, Krishnan PR, Sequeira R, Al-Roomi K. Anticonvulsant therapy for status epilepticus. Cochrane Database Syst Rev 2014;10(9):CD003723. doi:10.1002/14651858.CD003723.pub3.
6. Silbergleit R, Durkalski V, Lowenstein D, et al. Intramuscular versus intravenous therapy for prehospital status epilepticus. N Engl J Med 2012;366:591–600.
7. Glauser T, Ben-Menachem E, Bourgois B, et al. Updated ILAE evidence review of antiepileptic drug efficacy and effectiveness as initial monotherapy for epileptic seizures and syndromes. Epilepsia 2013;54:551–563.

68

ACUTE MANAGEMENT OF THE BRAIN INJURY PATIENT

The Agony of Defeat............................Level III

Denise H. Rhoney, PharmD, FCCP, FCCM

Dennis Parker, Jr., PharmD

LEARNING OBJECTIVES

After completing this case study, the reader should be able to:

• Discuss the goals of cerebral resuscitation.

• Interpret parameters beneficial in assessing the severity of the brain injury.

- Describe the impact of prior antithrombotic therapy on traumatic brain injury and devise an appropriate treatment plan for patients with traumatic brain injury while on antithrombotic therapy.

- Discuss the therapeutic management of traumatic brain injury and increased intracranial pressure associated with acute brain injury.

- Recommend appropriate therapy to prevent medical complications after brain injury.

PATIENT PRESENTATION

▣ Chief Complaint

Not available—the patient was brought to the ED by EMS as a trauma code.

▣ HPI

Oliver Johnson is a 55-year-old man who was brought to the ED after suffering a ski accident while on vacation with his wife. His wife reports that he was unarousable at the scene of the accident.

▣ PMH (As Per Patient's Wife)

Dyslipidemia
NSTEMI (1 year ago)

▣ FH

Unknown

▣ SH

Unknown

▣ ROS

Unobtainable

▣ Meds

Aspirin 325 mg PO daily
Clopidogrel 75 mg PO daily
Simvastatin 40 mg PO daily

▣ All

NKDA

▣ Physical Examination

Gen

WDWN man who does not speak, open his eyes, or move on verbal stimuli. On painful stimuli, he does not speak or open his eyes but does exhibit flexor posturing.

VS

BP 87/60 mm Hg, P 126 bpm, RR 30, T 38.3°C; Wt 85 kg, Ht 6′0″

Skin

Multiple bruises on the face and extremities bilaterally

HEENT

The patient has multiple soft tissue injuries to the face. The left pupil is 5 mm and nonreactive to direct light, and the right pupil is 2 mm and slowly reactive to light. EOMs are not reactive and not moving. External inspection of ears and nose reveals no acute abnormalities.

There is some dried blood in the mouth. The head has a large open scalp laceration on the forehead with surrounding ecchymoses. Neck is in a cervical collar; therefore, movement was not attempted. There are no gross masses in the neck.

Lungs

Rhonchi and crackles present bilaterally with thick secretions

Heart

Sinus tachycardia with S_1 and S_2 present

Abd

Soft with no masses or tenderness but decreased bowel sounds. There is no gross hepatosplenomegaly.

Ext

No nontraumatic edema is noted

Neuro

There is no response other than flexor posturing to pain. The Glasgow Coma Scale score is 5.

▣ Labs

Na 140 mEq/L	Hgb 13.8 g/dL	Ca 8.4 mg/dL	*ABG*
K 3.7 mEq/L	Hct 40.9%	Mg 1.8 mg/dL	pH 7.49
Cl 106 mEq/L	Plt 166 × 10³/mm³	Phos 2.4 mEq/L	HCO_3 22 mEq/L
CO_2 20 mEq/L	WBC 26.0 × 10³/mm³	Alb 3.4 g/dL	$PaCO_2$ 33 mm Hg
BUN 15 mg/dL	Diff N/A		PaO_2 66 mm Hg
SCr 1.1 mg/dL			O_2 sat 86% on RA
Glu 285 mg/dL			Urine drug screen (−)
			Blood alcohol <20 mg/dL

▣ Portable Chest X-Ray

Right upper lobe atelectasis. No rib fractures. The ET tube is above the carina.

▣ Head CT

There is a left parietal open depressed skull fracture. There is an area of hemorrhagic contusion in the left frontal region. There are multiple left temporal and parietal epidural hematomas with midline shift.

▣ Assessment

1. S/P head trauma secondary to ski accident

2. Skull fracture and temporal and parietal epidural hematomas with midline shift

3. Coma

4. Respiratory distress

5. Hyperglycemia

■ CLINICAL COURSE

On arrival in the ED, IV access was initiated, and the patient was intubated orally using a rapid sequence intubation technique (fentanyl 200 mcg IV followed by lidocaine 100 mg IV, midazolam 2 mg IV, and rocuronium 5 mg IV). The patient was started on 3% sodium/acetate solution at 75 mL/hour and midazolam infusion at 12 mg/hour. Other medications include levetiracetam 2 g IV load followed by 1g IV Q 12 H, fentanyl 25 mcg IV Q 1 H PRN, and insulin aspart correction dose protocol as needed hourly.

A ventriculostomy was placed for monitoring of ICP with an initial ICP reading of 18 mm Hg. The patient was then transferred to the neurointensive care unit for monitoring.

Over the next 48 hours, pertinent laboratory measurements included serum sodium 158 mEq/L, serum osmolality 290 mOsm/L, urine osmolality 250 mOsm/L, and urine specific gravity 1.010 g/cm³. See ICU Flowsheet for other important parameters for the first 24 hours (Fig. 68-1) and second 24 hours (Fig. 68-2) in the ICU.

QUESTIONS

Problem Identification

1.a. Could any of the patient's prehospital medications have contributed to the extent of the brain injury?

1.b. What information (signs, symptoms, and laboratory values) indicates the severity of this patient's brain injury?

1.c. What patient factors may complicate assessment of the neurologic examination?

1.d. What poor prognostic indicators do this patient exhibit?

Desired Outcome

2.a. What are the immediate goals of therapy for this patient?

2.b. What are the goals of fluid resuscitation and hemodynamic monitoring for this patient?

2.c. What are the goals of therapy for patients with traumatic brain injury and prehospital use of antiplatelet medications?

Therapeutic Alternatives

3.a. What therapeutic alternatives are available for reversal of the antiplatelet effects of clopidogrel and aspirin?

3.b. What therapeutic alternatives are available for fluid resuscitation, and which would be the most appropriate for this patient?

3.c. What nondrug therapies may be useful for preventing or treating increased ICP?

3.d. What pharmacotherapeutic alternatives are available for treating increased ICP?

Optimal Plan

4.a. Develop an optimal pharmacotherapeutic plan to treat the patient's increased ICP.

Time	Temp (°C)	HR (bpm)	BP (mm Hg)	ICP (mm Hg)	CPP (mm Hg)	BG (mg/dL)	Fluid A (mL)	Fluid B (mL)	Fluid C (mL)	Nutrition	UOP (mL)	Meds given
0600	37.6	85	120/86	18	79	306	80		12	NPO	60	Insulin aspart 8 units
0700		88	128/88	22	77		80		12		105	
0800		89	119/67	15	69		80		12	NPO	100	
0900		85	125/89	16	70		80	100	12		60	Levetiracetam 1000mg IV
1000	38.2	86	110/65	20	60	288	80		12	NPO	55	Insulin aspart 6 units APAP 325 mg
1100		92	115/79	22	71		80		12		60	Fentanyl 25 mcg × 2
1200		94	129/55	18	62		80		12	NPO	67	
1300		100	100/68	19	60		80		12		100	
1400	38.1	92	113/70	17	67	270	80		12	NPO	55	Insulin aspart 6 units APAP 325 mg
1500		98	130/85	21	79		80		12		70	
1600		89	129/75	18	75		80		12	NPO	60	
1700		94	119/88	20	76		80		12		60	
1800	37.5	85	115/66	22	75	240	80		12	NPO	60	Aspart 2 units
1900		86	124/50	22	53		80		12		80	
2000		83	144/54	16	68		80		12	NPO	60	
2100		89	140/87	24	81		80	100	12		70	Levetiracetam 1000mg IV
2200	38.6	86	139/84	24	78	220	80		12	NPO	75	Aspart 2 units APAP 325 mg
2300		90	120/86	20	77		80		12		60	
2400		70	132/75	12	82		80		12	NPO	50	
0100		78	140/70	20	73		80		12		110	
0200	37.5	72	135/68	20	70	190	80		12	NPO	120	
0300		79	149/75	19	81		80		12		80	
0400		75	137/68	28	63		80		12	NPO	110	
0500		77	130/68	27	62		80		12		60	

Fluid A = 3% sodium chloride/acetate; Fluid B = levetiracetam IVPB; Fluid C = midazolam infusion (concentration = 1 mg/mL).

HR, heart rate; BP, blood pressure; ICP, intracranial pressure; CPP, cerebral perfusion pressure; BG, blood glucose; UOP, urine output; IVPB, intravenous piggy bag.

FIGURE 68-1. Neurointensive care unit flowsheet. Day 1 (0–24 hours postadmission).

Time	Temp (°C)	HR (bpm)	BP (mm Hg)	ICP (mm Hg)	CPP (mm Hg)	BG (mg/dL)	Fluid A (mL)	Fluid B (mL)	Fluid C (mL)	Nutrition	UOP (mL)	Meds given
0600	37.4	85	121/76	19	72	226	80		12	NPO	70	Insulin aspart 4 units IV
0700		78	125/80	20	75		80		12		150	
0800		80	129/66	25	62		80		12	NPO	100	
0900		82	135/87	26	77		80	100	12		200	Levetiracetam 1000 mg IV
1000	38.2	86	120/60	20	60	188	80		12	NPO	350	Insulin aspart 2 units IV APAP 325 mg
1100		95	110/70	28	55		125		12		300	Fentanyl 25 mcg × 2
1200		98	119/65	28	55		125		12	NPO	150	
1300		97	110/78	29	60		125		12		350	
1400	38.3	90	118/77	35	55	286	125		12	NPO	300	Insulin aspart 8 units IV APAP 325 mg
1500		88	135/80	31	67		125		12		500	
1600		89	129/85	28	72		125		12	NPO	350	
1700		77	120/87	20	78		125		12		200	
1800	38.1	80	135/68	23	67	240	125		12	NPO	250	Aspart 2 units IV APAP 325 mg
1900		76	128/60	24	59		125		12		200	
2000		80	141/70	26	68		125		12	NPO	150	
2100		78	140/86	14	90		125	100	12		250	Levetiracetam 1000 mg IV
2200	37.8	80	129/89	24	78	220	125		12	NPO	300	Aspart 4 units IV
2300		80	130/76	18	84		125		12		300	
2400		76	137/70	25	80		125		12	NPO	250	
0100		78	140/80	17	83		125		12		250	
0200	37.9	78	145/78	22	78	190	125		12	NPO	100	Aspart 2 units IV
0300		88	145/70	28	77		125		12		250	
0400		80	127/78	25	76		125		12	NPO	300	
0500		75	138/69	27	75		125		12		250	

Fluid A = 3% sodium chloride/acetate; Fluid B = levetiracetam IVPB; Fluid C = midazolam infusion (concentration = 1 mg/mL).

HR, heart rate; BP, blood pressure; ICP, intracranial pressure; CPP, cerebral perfusion pressure; BG, blood glucose; UOP, urine output; IVPB, intravenous piggy bag.

FIGURE 68-2. Neurointensive care unit flowsheet. Day 2 (24–48 hours postadmission).

4.b. Outline a pharmacotherapeutic plan for prevention of medical complications that may occur in this patient.

Outcome Evaluation

5. What monitoring parameters should be instituted to ensure efficacy and prevent toxicity for the therapy recommended for increased ICP and other medical issues?

Patient Education

6. What medication education should this patient receive if he is discharged on clopidogrel and aspirin?

■ SELF-STUDY ASSIGNMENTS

1. Review the different types of neurologic monitoring devices that are available and how drug therapy might influence these monitoring parameters.

2. Review paroxysmal autonomic instability or "sympathetic storming" and its treatment options and monitoring parameters.

3. Evaluate the role of serum biomarkers in predicting outcome after traumatic brain injury.

4. Review the guidelines for managing the neurobehavioral sequelae of traumatic brain injury.

CLINICAL PEARL

There are only three standards of care for severe brain injury patients: (1) use of corticosteroids is not recommended for improving outcome or reducing ICP; (2) in the absence of increased ICP, chronic prolonged hyperventilation ($PaCO_2$ < 25 mm Hg) should be avoided; and (3) prophylactic use of antiepileptic drugs is not recommended for preventing late posttraumatic seizures (>7 days).

REFERENCES

1. McMillian WD, Rogers FB. Management of prehospital antiplatelet and anticoagulant therapy in traumatic head injury: a review. J Trauma 2009;66:942–950.

2. Le Roux P, Menon DK, Citerio G, et al. Consensus Statement of the International Multidisciplinary Consensus Conference on Multimodaltity Monitroing in Neurocritical Care. Neurocrit Care 2014;21(Suppl 2):S297–S361.

3. Batchelor JS, Grayson A. A meta-analysis to determine the effect of preinjury antiplatelet agents on mortality in patients with blunt head trauma. Br J Neurosurg 2013;27:12–18.

4. Beynon C, Hertle DN, Unterberg AW, Sakowitz OW. Clinical Review: Traumatic brain injury in patients receiving antiplatelet medication. Crit Care 2012;16:228. doi: 10.1186/cc11292.

5. Forsyth LL, Liu-DeRyke X, Parker D Jr, Rhoney DH. Role of hypertonic saline for the management of intracranial hypertension after stroke and traumatic brain injury. Pharmacotherapy 2008;28:469–484.

6. Brain Trauma Foundation, American Association of Neurological Surgeons, Congress of Neurological Surgeons, Joint Section on Neurotrauma and Critical Care, AANS/CNS. Guidelines for the management of severe traumatic brain injury. J Neurotrauma 2007;24(Suppl 1):S1–S106.

7. Barr J, Fraser GL, Puntillo K, et al. Clinical practice guidelines for the management of pain, agitation, and delirium in adult patients in the intensive care unit. Crit Care Med 2013;41:263–306.

8. Wakai A, McCabe A, Roberts I, Schierhout G. Mannitol for acute traumatic brain injury. Cochrane Database Syst Rev 2013;8:CD001049.

9. Rowe AS, Goodwin H, Brophy GM, et al. Seizure prophylaxis in neurocritical care: a review of evidence-based support. Pharmacotherapy 2014;34:396–409.

10. McClave SA, Martindale RG, Vanek VW, et al. Guidelines for the Provision and Assessment of Nutrition Support Therapy in the Adult Critically Ill Patient: Society of Critical Care Medicine (SCCM) and American Society for Parenteral and Enteral Nutrition (A.S.P.E.N.). J Parenter Enteral Nutr 2009;33:277–316.

69

PARKINSON DISEASE

Slow and Shaky. . . . . Level III

Mary L. Wagner, PharmD, MS

Margery H. Mark, MD

LEARNING OBJECTIVES

After completing this case study, the reader should be able to:

- Recognize motor and nonmotor symptoms of Parkinson disease (PD).

- Develop an optimal pharmacotherapeutic plan for a patient with PD as he or she progresses through different stages of the disease.

- Recommend alterations in therapy for a patient experiencing adverse drug effects, drug–drug interactions, and drug–food interactions.

- Educate patients with PD about the disease, its drug therapy, and nonpharmacologic treatments.

PATIENT PRESENTATION

Chief Complaint

"My work performance has declined because my tremor makes it difficult to type on the computer, and I am slower with most tasks."

HPI

Lisa Farmer is a 53-year-old, right-handed woman who presents to the neurology clinic because of a mild tremor in her right hand that has worsened over the past 6 months. It takes her longer to do things because it takes a little more effort to get movement started, and her muscles feel a little stiff. She also admits to waking up several times during the night. The stiffness, slowness, tremor, and sleep problems have affected her job performance as a graphic designer, resulting in her contemplating early retirement. She also complains of constipation, loss of sense of smell for about 2 years, decreased libido for 6–8 months, night sweats that cause nighttime awakenings, and very irregular menstrual periods for the past year.

PMH

HTN × 1 year
Broken left wrist after fall 2 years ago

FH

Mother died at age 89 of complications associated with a hip fracture, osteoporosis, and Alzheimer disease (clinical diagnosis without postmortem confirmation); father died from an ischemic stroke; two daughters are in good health

SH

(–) Alcohol, (–) tobacco, married for 23 years

ROS

No complaints other than those noted in the HPI. She denies any other symptoms of autonomic dysfunction such as problems with swallowing, urination, drooling, or dizziness. She also denies any psychological problems such as depression, panic attacks, vivid dreams, acting out dreams, hallucinations, or paranoia.

Meds

Verapamil SR 180 mg PO every morning for 1 year
Calcium carbonate 600 mg PO every morning and night

All

None

Physical Examination

Gen

The patient is a Caucasian woman who appears to be her stated age but with minimal hypomimia

VS

BP 118/74 mm Hg sitting, 116/70 mm Hg standing, P 70 bpm, RR 13; T 36.8°C; Wt 53 kg, Ht 5′2″

Skin

Small amount of dry yellow scales in her eyebrows

HEENT

Decreased facial expression, decreased eye blinking; PERRLA; EOMI

Neck/Lymph Nodes

Supple, no masses, normal thyroid, no bruits

Lungs/Thorax

Clear, normal breath sounds, CTA

CV

RRR, no murmurs, no bruits

Abd

Soft, nontender, no palpable masses

Genit/Rect

No nodules palpated; no rectal polyps

MS/Ext

Normal peripheral pulses and postural stability. No CCE

Neuro

General neurologic exam intact, MoCA 30/30, HAM-D Scale 3/66 (sleep and libido problems)
UPDRS: Total 19
Part 1: Mentation, behavior, and mood score 0/16.
Part 2: ADL score 5/52 (mild trouble with handwriting, cutting food, tremor, and dressing [putting on nylon stockings and buttoning small buttons]). She has no problems with gait. She has some reduced arm swing on the right when she walks. She has no problems with speech, salivation, swallowing, hygiene, turning in bed, falling, freezing, walking, or sensory effects.
Part 3: Motor exam 7/108 (mild problems with facial expression and overall bradykinesia). She has right-sided rigidity and rest tremor, appearing like classic pill-rolling tremor. She has problems with fine motor coordination on her right side noted by the rapid alternating movements, finger taps, hand movements, and foot tap tests. She has no problems arising from a chair or problems with posture or postural stability.
Handwriting sample: Somewhat slow and progressively smaller in size indicating signs of micrographia

■ Labs

Na 136 mEq/L	Hgb 13.5 g/dL	AST 20 IU/L
K 4.3 mEq/L	Hct 40.5%	ALT 24 IU/L
Cl 101 mEq/L	RBC 4.42 × 10⁶	Alk phos 80 IU/L
CO₂ 23 mEq/L	WBC 5.0 × 10³/mm³	GGT 18 IU/L
BUN 12 mg/dL	Plt 395 × 10³/mm³	Ferritin 100 ng/mL
SCr 0.73 mg/dL	Homocysteine 6 μmol/L	TSH 2.0 mIU/L
Glu 83 mg/dL	Vitamin D, 25-hydroxy 25 ng/mL	T4 total 7.5 mcg/dL

■ Assessment

Based on the HPI and UPDRS, the patient's symptoms are consistent with early, mild PD

■ Clinical Course

The patient is told that she has PD, and the various treatment options are presented to her. She asks about treatment options that may delay disease progression.

QUESTIONS

Problem Identification

1.a. List and assess each one of the patient's complaints. Determine if there are multiple potential etiologies that could account for the symptoms.
1.b. Assess the abnormalities in the physical examination and laboratory findings.
1.c. List the cardinal motor and nonmotor symptoms of PD, and describe which signs and symptoms of PD are present in this patient.
1.d. According to the Hoehn–Yahr Scale, what stage is the patient's disease?

Desired Outcome

2. What are the goals of therapy for patients with PD?

Therapeutic Alternatives

3.a. What nonpharmacologic alternatives may be beneficial for the treatment of PD in this patient both now and in the future?
3.b. Based on the patient's signs and symptoms, what pharmacotherapeutic alternatives are viable options for her at this time?

Optimal Plan

4. What drug, dosage form, dose, schedule, and duration of therapy are best for this patient's current problems?

Outcome Evaluation

5. Which monitoring parameters should be used to evaluate the patient's response to medications and to detect adverse effects?

Patient Education

6. What information should be provided to the patient to ensure successful therapy, enhance compliance, and minimize adverse effects?

■ CLINICAL COURSE—1 YEAR LATER

Six months later, Ms Farmer returns to the clinic. After taking rasagiline for 3 months, her PD symptoms did not improve as much as she expected, so she started pramipexole, which was gradually increased to 1 mg three times a day. Her slowness, stiffness, and tremor have improved since then. She is better able to perform her job, enjoys the work, and is no longer planning her retirement. Her constipation has improved only marginally with the increased fluids and addition of the Metamucil that she takes one tablespoonful twice daily. Her libido and night sweats improved after starting conjugated equine estrogens 0.45 mg per day and medroxyprogesterone acetate 1.5 mg per day. She no longer complains of itchy eyebrows and scalp. She continues to take verapamil SR, multivitamin, calcium carbonate 600 mg, and vitamin D and rasagiline 1 mg daily. The patient reports no side effects from the medicine. However, her husband complains that her personality has changed because she shops excessively, often buying duplicates of things, which is straining their budget.

Vitals: BP 116/70 mm Hg sitting; P 70 bpm
UPDRS (patient states she is "on"): Mental 0, ADLS = 3 and motor = 6, total 9

Medications:

Verapamil SR 180 mg PO every morning
Multivitamin one PO daily
Calcium carbonate 600 mg PO every morning and night
Vitamin D 1000 IU PO daily
Conjugated equine estrogens 0.45 mg PO daily
Medroxyprogesterone acetate 1.5 mg PO daily
Metamucil one tablespoonful PO twice daily
Pramipexole 1 mg PO three times daily
Rasagiline 1 mg PO daily

■ FOLLOW-UP QUESTIONS

1. What is your assessment of the effectiveness of the PD therapy the patient is now receiving?

2. What potential side effects from therapy is the patient now experiencing?

3. What adjustments in drug therapy do you recommend for each of the patient's problems?

4. What information should the patient receive about her medical problems and therapy at this visit?

5. What additional tests could be ordered to assess comorbid conditions?

■ CLINICAL COURSE—7 YEARS LATER

Ms Farmer returns to the neurology clinic for a routine follow-up visit. She is now 60 years old and still working with reduced hours. She no longer has trouble with compulsive behaviors. Her constipation initially improved with a bowel regimen but now has worsened since starting supplements that she purchased over the internet. Her symptoms are now bilateral and include tremor, rigidity, stiffness, and gait problems. She also reports that she is slower and clumsier in almost all activities but especially when driving, handling utensils, dressing, turning in bed, and getting out of a chair. She still has good postural stability without falls. There are no difficulties with mood, autonomic symptoms, or hallucinations. She started an exercise program, converted to organic food, reads extensively about her symptoms on the internet, and purchases various treatments that she hears about from her friends in the local PD support group. About a month prior to the visit, she purchased coenzyme Q10 and cowage (an herbal supplement that contains natural levodopa), thinking they would be a natural way to help her PD. She read about RLS and, thinking that her nighttime restlessness, trouble falling asleep, and daytime fatigue were related to RLS, she started iron supplements and kava several months ago and was planning to tell her doctor about her findings at the next visit.

She claims that the restlessness occurs only at night after dinner when she is sitting. She notes that she has a bubbling feeling in her veins that leads to restlessness, which is relieved by walking or movement. Her husband says that she kicks him at night and the bed covers are quite tousled in the morning; she also often shouts in her sleep.

BP 120/74 mm Hg and weight 50 kg

She has a positive glabellar reflex (Myerson's sign)

Hamilton Psychiatric Rating Scale for Depression 3/66

MoCA 29/30

UPDRS scores while "on" are: mood 3, ADL 12, and motor 43

Laboratory values are normal and similar to previous labs: Ferritin 150 ng/mL

DXA scan (6 years ago) T-score: spine –1.0 and left hip –1.4

Patient diary (day prior to visit)—Table 69-1

TABLE 69-1

Time	Meds	Symptoms	Comments
7 AM	Carbidopa/levodopa 25/100	Mild stiffness and slowness	Med onset 30 min
8 AM	Verapamil SR 180	Good control of symptoms	Breakfast
	Cowage (*Mucuna pruriens*) 30 g		
	Calcium 600 mg		
	Benefiber one tablespoon		
	Rasagiline 1 mg		
	Coenzyme Q10 100 mg		
8:30–10 AM		Dancelike movements in extremities (chorea)	Noted this since I started supplements
11:30 AM	Carbidopa/levodopa 25/100	"Off"	Onset 30 min but does not take full effect. It feels like half a dose since supplements started
	Ferrous sulfate 300 mg		
	Benefiber one tablespoon		
	MVI		
	Colace 100 mg		
Noon		"On" without chorea	Lunch
4:30 PM		"Off" with tremor, stiffness, and slowness	11:30 dose wearing off earlier since supplements started
5:30 PM	Carbidopa/levodopa 25/100	"Off" with tremor, stiffness, and slowness	Dinnerz
	Coenzyme Q10 100 mg		Delayed onset 60 min
10 PM	Carbidopa/levodopa 25/100	"On" without chorea	I fall asleep between 10:30 and 11:30 PM depending on restlessness and funny sensations in my legs
	calcium 600 mg		
	Vitamin D 1,000 IU		
	Kava 100 mg		
	Coenzyme Q10 100 mg		
10 PM–7 AM			My husband says that I have restless sleep and kick him during the night. I wake up between 1 AM and 2 AM to go to the bathroom and have a hard time going back to sleep because of feeling stiff all over and restlessness in my legs

FOLLOW-UP QUESTIONS

1. List the patient's problems at this visit.

2. List and explain any drugs or foods that could be causing any drug–drug or drug–food interactions.

3. For each of the problems identified, what adjustments in drug therapy do you recommend?

4. What information should be provided to the patient to ensure successful therapy, enhance compliance, and minimize adverse effects with medications that have been added since the last visit?

CLINICAL COURSE: ALTERNATIVE THERAPY

Ms Farmer has been taking coenzyme Q10 for about a month before coming in for reevaluation. Unlike the kava and cowage, which could be actively worsening her symptoms or posing other safety problems, coenzyme Q10 might actually have some benefit for PD. Should Ms Farmer continue taking the supplement? See Section 19 in this Casebook for questions about the use of coenzyme Q10 for treatment of PD.

SELF-STUDY ASSIGNMENTS

1. Review the pharmacology and efficacy reports of investigational drugs for PD.

2. Investigate the treatment of other nonmotor symptoms of PD such as autonomic dysfunction, depression, anxiety, and psychosis.

3. Investigate the use of deep brain stimulation for the treatment of advanced PD.

CLINICAL PEARL

As PD progresses, the timing of medication needs to coincide with symptoms. Evaluate the onset and duration of each dose and make modifications accordingly. Symptoms may worsen when patients are forced to receive medications at predetermined dosing times such as those used in hospitals and nursing homes. Thus, let the patient's symptoms guide the dosing times.

REFERENCES

1. Kalia LV, Lang AE. Parkinson's disease. Lancet 2015;386:896–912.

2. Pedrosa DJ, Timmermann L. Review: management of Parkinson's disease. Neuropsychiatr Dis Treat 2013;9:321–340.

3. Connolly BS, Lang AE. Pharmacologic Treatment of Parkinson Disease: a review. JAMA 2014;311:1670–1683.

4. Zesiewicz TA, Sullivan KL, Arnulf I, et al. Practice parameter: treatment of nonmotor symptoms of Parkinson disease: report of the Quality Standards Subcommittee of the American Academy of Neurology. Neurology 2010;74:924–931.

5. Seppi K, Weintraub D, Coelho M, et al. The Movement Disorder Society Evidence-Based Medicine Review Update: treatment for the non-motor symptoms of Parkinson's Disease. Mov Disord 2011;26(S3):S42–S80.

6. Zigmond MJ, Cameron JL, Hoffer BJ, Smeyne RJ. Neurorestoration by physical exercise: moving forward. Parkinsonism Relat Disord 2012;18(Suppl 1):S147–S150.

7. Fox SH, Katzenschlager R, Lim SY, et al. The Movement Disorder Society Evidence-Based Medicine Review Update: treatment for the motor symptoms of Parkinson's disease. Mov Disord 2011;26(Suppl 3):S2–S41.

8. Zesiewicz TA, Evatt ML. Potential influences of complementary therapy on motor and non-motor complications in Parkinson's disease. CNS Drugs 2009;23(10):817–835.

9. Groenendaal H, Tarrants ML, Armand C. Treatment of advanced Parkinson's disease in the United States: a cost-utility model. Clin Drug Investig 2010;30:789–798.

10. Goetz CG, Fahn S, Martinez-Martin P, et al. Movement Disorder Society-sponsored revision of the Unified Parkinson's Disease Rating Scale (MDS-UPDRS): Process, format, and clinimetric testing plan. Mov Disord 2007;22:41–47.

70

CHRONIC PAIN MANAGMENT

Using Opioid Medication in a Troubled Time. . . . Level II

Ernest J Dole, PharmD, PhC, FASHP, BCPS

LEARNING OBJECTIVES

After completing this case study, the reader should be able to:

- Define the goals for pain management in a patient with chronic nonmalignant pain.

- Apply the principles and tools discussed when prescribing, assessing, monitoring, and dispensing chronic opioid therapy (COT) in chronic non-cancer pain (CNCP).

- Assess patients to identify possible presence of risk factors for aberrant behavior surrounding COT for CNCP.

- Describe strategies to identify and manage medication related aberrant behavior and risks associated with COT, including use of current guidelines for prescribing COT, Prescription Drug Monitoring Programs (PMP), urine drug monitoring (UDM), patient and prescriber agreements (PPAs), and treatment modification.

PATIENT PRESENTATION

Chief Complaint

"Everything hurts. My pain is 10/10, it is always at a 10/10! I have tried the medications that everyone has prescribed me, but they never seem to work and I'm still in pain. I've tried PT and it makes my pain worse! I'm told to wear my CPAP mask, that it will help my sleep and help my pain. But every time I wear it, I get claustrophobic and my anxiety increases, so I don't wear it anymore. I have been in pain for 30 years, and every time I ask for a medication that works, like oxycodone, which I know works, I am told to try another medication I have never tried, and to see PT and the psychologist. Well, I'm sick of trying medications that don't work, and I'm sick of being told the pain is in my head! The pain isn't in my head, it's all over my body! I just want a shot or a pill that will take all my pain away!"

HPI

Danica Mole is a 56-year-old female with pain from temporomandibular-joint disorder, fibromyalgia, and ruptured L4-L5. She states that her pain began when she was assaulted by one of her high school students 25 years ago. There was never a report filed of an assault, and she has been on disability since the time of the assault. She has been a patient in this pain clinic for five years during which she has failed multiple medications; every time a new nonopioid medication began to work, she developed adverse reactions to it. Thus, she has been prescribed and using opioid medications to control her pain. While she has never overtly misused her opioid medications, she has been calling and asking for early refills of her opioid medications due to overuse, and lost or stolen prescriptions. She bristles at any suggestion that she may be "chemically coping." She states proudly that she used to have an alcohol problem, but "took care of herself" and did not need any "12 Step program or rehab hospital." She has never embraced PT, and states that her pain is made worse by PT. She is antagonistic to behavioral therapy and has been fired as a patient by two of the clinic's psychiatrists in five years. The clinic's interventionists have declined to offer her epidural or facet injections because they fear further complaints from her regarding complications from the procedure. She has tried trigger-point injections (TPI) only once, stating that they made her pain worse.

PMH

Fibromyalgia × 25 years
Degenerative disk disease × 25 years
TMJ disorder × 30 years
Obesity × 20 years
OSA × 20 years
PTSD × 25 years
HTN × 10 years
Hyperlipidemia × 10 years
Remote history of substance use disorder, alcohol, "clean" for 6 years

FH

Noncontributory

SH

Patient is a retired high school teacher. She retired after she was assaulted by one of her students and placed on medical disability over 30 years ago. She has been married for 30 years. She spends her days caring for their 22-year-old daughter who cannot work due to severe migraine headaches and fibromyalgia. She and her husband are pursuing medical disability for their daughter. She often sleeps until one in the afternoon and then stays up most of the night talking to her daughter. She has one younger sister and one younger brother. She makes multiple plans to volunteer and to take care of her elderly in-laws, but never is able to complete these plans.

Medications

Oxycodone IR 15 mg PO Q 6 H PRN for pain
Morphine ER 30 mg PO TID for pain
Atorvastatin 10 mg PO HS
Hydrochlorothiazide 25 mg PO Q AM
Diazepam 5 mg PO TID PRN

All

APAP: increased pain, stomach upset
Amitriptyline: rash
Duloxetine: stomach upset, "mania"
NSAIDs (all): ulcer
Gabapentin: "could not think"
Pregabalin: weight gain
Venlafaxine: stomach upset, increased depression

ROS

Positive for total body pain. She states all her muscles hurt, that she has electrical, shooting stinging pain from her back, legs, and feet bilaterally. Her mood is agitated.

Physical Examination

Gen

Patient is a 56-year-old obese woman with wide spread allodynia

VS

BP 150/96 mm Hg, P 96 bpm, RR 15, T 37.5°C; Wt 137.6 kg, Ht 158 cm, BMI 55 kg/m²

HEENT

PERRLA, EOMI, TMs intact

Neck

Supple, no JVD, no bruits

Resp

CTA and P; no crackles or wheezes

CV

NSR without MRG

Breasts

Negative

Abd

Soft, NT, liver and spleen not palpable, (+) BS

Genit/Rect

Heme (–) stool, pelvic exam deferred

MS/Ext

Widespread, extreme allodynia with any touch; axial spine had good alignment of the spine. Spine demonstrated excellent range of motion; however, there was widespread allodynia on her spinous muscles. Thoracic spine was normal except for allodynia. Cervical spine demonstrated good range of motion; positive allodynia. She had spasm and tenderness in the trapezius muscles bilaterally (left greater than right), in the rhomboid muscles (right side principally), and in the scalene muscles (the right side of her neck greater than the left side although both sides were affected).

Neuro

CN II–XII intact, A & O × 3
Normal motor strength in the upper extremities with reflexes 1+ and symmetric and normal sensation extremities, no CCE

Labs

Chem 7: WNL
LFTs: WNL
CBC: WNL except for elevated Hgb and Hct
MRI: Slight degenerative disk disease, that is appropriate for age

Assessment

1. Fibromyalgia

2. Depression

3. Anxiety

4. Obesity

5. Possible medication related aberrant behavior

6. HTN

7. Hyperlipidemia

QUESTIONS

Problem Identification

1.a. Create a list of the patient's drug therapy problems.

1.b. What information indicates the presence or severity of chronic nonmalignant pain?

1.c. Could any of the patient's problems have been caused by drug therapy?

1.d. What additional information is needed to satisfactorily assess this patient's pain?

1.e. Address the patient's concerns and expectation regarding her pain and medication therapy.

1.f. Determine if the patient is at risk for medication-related aberrant behavior.

1.g. Assess the patient's risk for additional morbidity from her medications.

Desired Outcome

2.a. What are the patient's goals of pharmacotherapy in this case?

2.b. What are the clinician's goals of pharmacotherapy in this case?

Therapeutic Alternatives

3.a. What nonpharmacologic therapies might be useful for this patient?

3.b. What behavioral therapies might be useful for this patient?

3.c. Compare the opioid medication pharmacotherapeutic alternatives available for treatment of this patient's pain.

Optimal Plan

4.a. What is the best approach to safe prescribing of opioid medications for DM?

4.b. What drug, dosage, form, schedule, and duration of therapy are best for treating this patient's pain, based on DM's total daily opioid dose in morphine-equivalent dose (MED)?

4.c. What are the advantages and disadvantages of using an extended release (ER) opioid medication compared with an immediate release (IR) opioid medication?

Outcome Evaluation

5.a. What outcome parameters can be utilized to gauge DM's progress?

5.b. What tools can be employed to monitor for medication-related aberrant behavior?

5.c. What steps can be taken if DM begins to exhibit medication-related aberrant behavior, yet has a valid reason to continue opioid medications?

5.d. If DM continues to exhibit medication-related aberrant behavior, what strategies can be used to wean her opioid medications?

5.e. Compare and contrast the terms: physical dependence, tolerance, pseudo-addiction, addiction, and withdrawal.

Patient Education

6. What information should be provided to the patient to enhance compliance, ensure successful therapy, and minimize adverse effects?

■ CLINICAL COURSE

The physician in the clinic decides that DM is at a very high risk for accidental opioid overdose because she refuses to wear a CPAP mask and because of her high total daily opioid dose. The physician also states that DM's recent UDS came back positive for opiates and oxycodone and asks for a consult.

■ FOLLOW-UP QUESTIONS

1. How would you consult the physician regarding the use of buprenorphine for pain?

■ SELF-STUDY ASSIGNMENTS

1. Prepare a list of opioids and their corresponding equianalgesic dosing.

2. The use of opioid medication is a controversial topic; often it is driven more by passion than by scientific data. In 3–4 sentences per viewpoint, discuss this issue from the perspective of (1) a provider, and (2) the patient.

CLINICAL PEARL

Opioids are not first-line therapy for any CNCP conditions. No therapeutic guidelines for fibromyalgia advocate for the use of opioids.

REFERENCES

1. Centers for Disease Control and Prevention. Prescription painkiller overdoses in the U.S. http://www.cdc.gov/vitalsigns/PainkillerOverdoses/index.html. Accessed May 9, 2016.

2. Cobaugh DJ, Gainor C, Gaston C, et al. The opioid abuse and misuse epidemic: implications for pharmacists in hospitals and health systems. Am J Health-Syst Pharm 2014;71:1539–1554.

3. U.S. Food and Drug Administration. Introduction to FDA blueprint for prescriber education for extended-release and long-acting opioid analgesics. http://www.fda.gov/downloads/ForIndustry/UserFees/PrescriptionDrugUserFee/UCM361069.htm. Accessed May 9, 2016.

4. Federation of State Medical Boards. Model policy on the use of opioid analgesics in the treatment of chronic pain, 2013. http://www.fsmb.org/Media/Default/PDF/FSMB/Advocacy/pain_policy_july2013.pdf. Accessed May 10, 2016.

5. Center for Disease Control and Prevention. Draft CDC guideline for prescribing opioids for chronic pain—United States, 2016. https://www.regulations.gov/#!documentDetail;D=CDC-2015-0112-0002. Accessed May 10, 2016.

6. Chou R, Turner JA, Devine EB, et al. The Effectiveness and risks of long-term opioid therapy for chronic pain: a systematic review for a National Institutes of Health Pathways to Prevention workshop. Ann Intern Med 2015;162:276–286.

7. American Academy of Pain Management. Co-prescribing of naloxone in conjunction with opioid therapy: a statement from the American Academy of Pain Management. http://blog.aapainmange.org/co-prescribing-of-naloxone-in-conjunction-with-opioid-therapy/ Accessed May 10, 2016.

8. Center for Substance Abuse Treatment. Managing chronic pain in adults with or in recovery from substance use disorders. Rockville (MD): Substance Abuse and Mental Health Services Administration (US); 2012. (Treatment Improvement Protocol (TIP) Series, No. 54.)

http://store.samhsa.gov/shin/content/SMA12-4671/TIP54.pdf. Accessed May 10, 2016.

9. Christo PJ, Manchikanti L, Ruan X, et al. Urine drug testing in chronic pain. Pain Physician 2011;14:123–143.

10. Center for Substance Abuse Treatment. Clinical drug testing in primary care. Rockville (MD): Substance Abuse and Mental Health Services Administration (US) https://store.samhsa.gov/shin/content/SMA12-4668/SMA12-4668.pdf. Accessed May 10, 2016.

71

ACUTE PAIN MANAGEMENT

No Pain, Much Gain. . . . . Level I

Gina M. Carbonara Baugh, PharmD

Charles D. Ponte, BS, PharmD, BC-ADM, BCPS, CDE, CPE, FAADE, FAPhA, FASHP, FCCP, FNAP

LEARNING OBJECTIVES

After completing this case study, the reader should be able to:

- Differentiate acute pain from chronic pain.

- Describe the typical clinical findings associated with acute pain.

- Describe the subjective and objective assessment of pain.

- Identify appropriate nonopioid and opioid analgesics for selected patients with acute pain.

- Choose suitable drug and nondrug therapy for the management of common opioid analgesic side effects.

- Develop an appropriate therapeutic plan (including monitoring parameters) for a patient with acute pain.

PATIENT PRESENTATION

■ Chief Complaint

"My belly hurts, and I can't stand the sight of food."

■ HPI

Charles Porter is a 58-year-old man who presents to the Family Practice Center with a 2-day history of nausea, vomiting, and epigastric and RUQ abdominal pain. The patient states that the pain began several hours after eating a large platter of cheese ravioli with sausage and meatballs at a local restaurant. The pain intensified and was associated with escalating nausea followed by several episodes of vomiting. The vomiting finally ceased but the abdominal pain has persisted and is made worse after meals. The pain is now dull, constant, and "bores" to his back. Lying up in bed or sitting in a chair seems to relieve some of the pain. Since the initial episode, his appetite has decreased and he has been avoiding fried or fatty foods. He denies any change in stool color or consistency.

■ PMH

HTN × 18 years; poorly controlled
Type 2 DM × 23 years; under fair control
History of gout; last attack 15 years ago
Dyslipidemia × 23 years
Alcoholic hepatitis without cirrhosis × 5 years

■ FH

Father deceased (esophageal varices), age 76; mother deceased (MI), age 83; brother alive and well, age 65; sister with breast cancer and gallbladder disease, age 48

■ SH

Is a retired bar owner. He lives with his wife (married for 25 years) on a 10-acre farm a few miles from town. He has two dogs and a cat. He has a 50 pack-year history of smoking and a history of chronic alcohol abuse.

■ ROS

As per HPI; otherwise negative

■ Meds

Atorvastatin 20 mg PO once daily
Hydrochlorothiazide 25 mg PO once daily
Losartan 100 mg PO once daily
Exenatide 10 mcg subQ twice daily
Metformin 500 mg PO BID
Aspirin 81 mg PO once daily
Insulin glargine 10 units subcutaneously at bedtime
Pepcid AC 20 mg PO PRN heartburn
MVI one PO once daily

■ All

Erythromycin—abdominal pain
Morphine—hives and mild wheezing

■ Physical Examination

Gen

A pleasant, middle-aged white man in mild-to-moderate acute distress; appears his stated age

VS

BP 160/95 mm Hg (sitting), P 84 bpm, RR 20, T 37.8°C; pain 6/10; Wt 90 kg, Ht 5′10″

HEENT

PERRLA, fundi with mild AV nicking; TMs intact; mucous membranes moist

Chest

Clear to A & P

Heart

Normal S_1 and S_2; without murmur, rub, or gallop

Abd

Normal bowel sounds, without organomegaly, moderate diffuse epigastric pain with deep palpation with mild guarding

Genit/Rect

Slightly enlarged prostate; guaiac (–) stool

Ext

Good strength throughout, reflexes intact, mild decreased pinprick sensation to both lower extremities; no CCE

■ Labs

Na 138 mEq/L	Hgb 12.6 g/dL	AST 98 units/L
K 3.3 mEq/L	Hct 36%	ALT 77 units/L
Cl 97 mEq/L	Platelets 340 × 10³/mm³	Alk phos 200 units/L
CO₂ 23 mEq/L	WBC 14.0 × 10³/mm³	T. bili 3.4 mg/dL
BUN 15 mg/dL	Neutros 76%	D. bili 2.6 mg/dL
SCr 1.3 mg/dL	Bands 4%	Amylase 435 units/L
Glu 210 mg/dL	Eos 2%	Lipase 367 units/L
	Lymphs 18%	*Fasting lipid profile*
		T. chol 210 mg/dL
		HDL 30 mg/dL
		LDL 120 mg/dL
		TG 300 mg/dL

■ Assessment

Acute epigastric abdominal pain; R/O cholelithiasis, acute cholecystitis, ascending cholangitis, acute pancreatitis, hepatitis

QUESTIONS

Problem Identification

1.a. Create a list of the patient's drug therapy problems.

1.b. What clinical information indicates the presence of an acute pain syndrome?

1.c. What is the pathophysiologic basis for the development of acute pain?

1.d. Could the patient's problem have been caused by drug therapy?

Desired Outcome

2. What are the goals of pharmacotherapy in this case?

Therapeutic Alternatives

3.a. What feasible pharmacotherapeutic alternatives are available for the treatment of acute pain?

3.b. What economic, psychosocial, and ethical considerations are applicable to this patient?

Optimal Plan

4.a. What drug, dosage form, dose, schedule, and duration of therapy are best for this patient?

4.b. What alternatives would be appropriate if the initial therapy fails or cannot be used?

Outcome Evaluation

5. What clinical and laboratory parameters are necessary to evaluate the therapy for achievement of the desired therapeutic outcome and to detect or prevent adverse effects?

Patient Education

6. What information should be provided to the patient to enhance adherence, ensure successful therapy, and minimize adverse effects?

■ CLINICAL COURSE

The patient was admitted to the inpatient service for presumed cholecystitis/acute pancreatitis/hepatitis and pain control. An abdominal ultrasound and abdominal CT were ordered. Blood cultures were obtained. Gastroenterology and general surgery services were consulted. The patient was made NPO except for his home medications. A sliding scale insulin regimen was also ordered.

The drug therapy regimen that you recommended for the patient was initiated. At the end of the first hospital day, the patient states that the medication "eases the pain some" but the pain is inadequately controlled. The pain is rated as an 8/10 using a single-dimensional visual analog pain scale. The patient also complains of some nausea and urinary hesitancy.

■ FOLLOW-UP QUESTIONS

1. What is the most likely cause of this patient's inadequate pain control?

2. What are the revised management goals for this patient?

3. What therapeutic alternatives would be appropriate for this patient?

4. What clinical and laboratory parameters are necessary to evaluate the therapy for achievement of the desired therapeutic outcome and to detect or prevent adverse effects?

5. What is the role of the pharmacist in the management of patients with acute pain?

■ SELF-STUDY ASSIGNMENTS

1. Describe the role of NMDA antagonists in the management of pain.

2. Describe the pathophysiology and management of opioid-induced respiratory depression.

3. What types of pain do *not* typically respond to opioid analgesics?

4. Explain the pathophysiology behind the development of opioid tolerance.

5. Explain the concepts of equianalgesic doses and relative analgesic potency.

6. Explain the WHO analgesic ladder and list representative analgesic classes (or individual agents) associated with each step of the ladder.

7. Describe the advantages and disadvantages of single- and multi-dimensional pain assessment instruments.

CLINICAL PEARL

Analgesic tolerance can be overcome by switching from one opioid to another. Because cross-tolerance is not complete among opioids, use only 50–75% of the equianalgesic dose of an opioid when changing from one drug to another and titrate accordingly.

REFERENCES

1. Steeds CE. The anatomy and physiology of pain. Surgery 2013;31:49–53.
2. Fink WA. The pathophysiology of acute pain. Emerg Med Clin North Am 2005;23:277–284.
3. Trivedi CD, Pitchumoni CS. Drug-induced pancreatitis: an update. J Clin Gastroenterol 2005;39:709–716.
4. Li L, Shen J, Bala MM, et al. Incretin treatment and risk of pancreatitis in patients with type 2 diabetes mellitus: systematic review and meta-analysis of randomised and non-randomised studies. BMJ 2014;348:g2366.
5. Etienne D, Reda Y. Statins and their role in acute pancreatitis: Case report and literature review. World J Gastrointest Pharmacol Ther 2014;5:191–195.
6. American Diabetes Association. Standards of Medical Care in Diabetes–2016. Diabetes Care 2016;39(S1):S1–S112.
7. American Pain Society. Principles of Analgesic Use in the Treatment of Acute Pain and Cancer Pain, 6th ed. Glenview, IL, American Pain Society, 2008.
8. Ghelardini C, Di Cesare Mannelli L, Bianchi E. The pharmacological basis of opioids. Clin Cases Miner Bone Metab 2015;12:219–221.
9. Prommer EE. Pharmacological Management of Cancer-Related Pain. Cancer Control 2015;22:412–425.
10. Thompson DR. Narcotic analgesic effects on the sphincter of Oddi: a review of the data and therapeutic implications in treating pancreatitis. Am J Gastroenterol 2001;96:1266–1272.
11. Spiegel B. Meperidine or morphine in acute pancreatitis? Am Fam Physician 2001;64:219–220.

72

MIGRAINE HEADACHE

Oh, My Aching Head! . . . . Level II

Susan R. Winkler, PharmD, BCPS, FCCP

Brittany N. Hoffmann-Eubanks, PharmD, MBA

LEARNING OBJECTIVES

After completing this case study, the reader should be able to:

- Develop pharmacotherapeutic goals for preventing and treating migraine headaches.

- Provide appropriate pharmacotherapeutic recommendations for an individual patient based on the patient's headache type and severity, medical history, previous drug therapy, concomitant problems, and pertinent laboratory data.

- Educate patients on the use of abortive and prophylactic agents for migraine headaches and menstrual migraines.

- Describe the appropriate use of a headache diary and how it may be used to refine headache treatment.

PATIENT PRESENTATION

Chief Complaint

"This new medication is not working for my migraines. My headaches are worse around my period and I have gained 10 pounds!"

HPI

Sarah Miller is a 34-year-old woman who presents to the Neurology Clinic for a follow-up of migraine headaches. She states that she used to get about two migraines every month; however, she recently went back to work full-time and has two young children, ages 3 and 5, to care for. Since then, the frequency of her migraines has increased to about four to five per month. She states her migraines usually occur in the morning and are more frequent around her menses. Her typical headache evolves quickly (within 1 hour) and involves severe throbbing pain which is unilateral and temporal in distribution. Her headaches are preceded by an aura which consists of nausea and pastel lights flashing throughout her visual field. Photophobia occurs frequently, and vomiting may occur with an extreme headache. She reports experiencing severe migraine attacks that cause her to miss 1 day of work each month. She is unable to complete household chores and has a difficult time caring for her children on the days she has severe migraine attacks. She also complains of having mild migraine attacks lasting 3 days per month during which her productivity at work and at home is reduced by half. She typically has to retreat to a dark room and avoid any noise, or the severity of the migraine increases. She rates her migraines as 7–8 on a headache scale of 1–10, with 10 being the worst. At her previous visit to the Neurology Clinic 3 months ago, she was prescribed naratriptan 2.5 mg orally to be taken at the onset of headache. However, naratriptan has not been effective for half of the migraines she has had in the last 3 months. During two of the attacks, she experienced partial pain relief, with the pain returning later in the day. She mentions that she was prescribed naratriptan when the Cafergot she was taking stopped working. She states she has taken her medications exactly as advised. She prefers to use medications that can be taken orally. She was started on valproic acid at her last clinic visit for headache prophylaxis and has noticed a 10-lb weight gain. She inquires about switching from valproic acid to another medication.

PMH

Migraine with aura since age 29; previous medical workup, including an EEG and a head MRI, demonstrated no PVD, CVA, brain tumor, infection, cerebral aneurysm, or epileptic component. Drug therapies have included the following:

Abortive therapies:

1. Simple analgesics, NSAIDs, and Cafergot (good efficacy until 3 months ago)
2. Narcotics (good efficacy, but puts her "out of commission for days")
3. Midrin (no efficacy)
4. Naratriptan (minimal efficacy)

Prophylactic therapies:

1. Valproic acid 500 mg daily (weight gain)
2. Propranolol 20 mg BID (increased episodes of dizziness and lightheadedness; patient self-discontinued medication)

Mild depression for 8 months, treated with:

1. Bupropion SR 150 mg PO TID (minimal efficacy, self-discontinued 3 months ago)
2. Sertraline 50 mg PO at bedtime (recently started 1 month ago)

FH

Positive for migraines (both parents); hypertension and type 2 diabetes (mother)

SH

Secretary; recently changed jobs to a full-time position. Mother of two boys, ages 3 and 5. Denies alcohol use; started smoking cigarettes again 3 months ago due to stress, 1 ppd. Occasional caffeine intake.

ROS

Complains of increased frequency of migraine headaches starting about 6 months ago; increased frequency around menses. Limited efficacy with naratriptan; no nausea, vomiting, diarrhea, or flashing lights at present.

Meds

Naratriptan 2.5-mg tablets, one tablet PO at onset of migraine, repeat dose of 2.5 mg PO in 4 hours if partial response or if headache returns. Maximum dose 5 mg per 24 hours.
Metoclopramide 10 mg PO at onset of migraine.
Valproic acid 500 mg PO at bedtime.
Sertraline 50 mg PO at bedtime.

All

NKDA

Physical Examination

Gen

WDWN woman in mild distress

VS

BP 142/86 mm Hg, HR 76, RR 18, T 37.2°C; Wt 75 kg, Ht 5′3″

Skin

Normal skin turgor; no diaphoresis

HEENT

PERRLA; EOMI; no funduscopic exam performed

Neck

Supple; no masses, thyroid enlargement, adenopathy, bruits, or JVD

Chest

Good breath sounds bilaterally; clear to A & P

CV

RRR; S_1, S_2 normal; no murmurs, rubs, or gallops

Abd

Soft, NT/ND, no hepatosplenomegaly; (+) BS

Genit/Rect

Deferred

MS/Ext

UE/LE strength 5/5 with normal tone; radial and femoral pulses 3+ bilaterally; no edema; no evidence of thrombophlebitis; full ROM

Neuro

A & O × 3; no dysarthria or aphasia; memory intact; no nystagmus; no fasciculations, tremor, or ataxia; (−) Romberg; CN II–XII intact; sensory intact; DTRs: 2+ throughout; Babinski (−) bilaterally

Labs

Na 142 mEq/L	Hgb 13 g/dL	AST 23 IU/L
K 4.2 mEq/L	Hct 40%	ALT 25 IU/L
Cl 101 mEq/L	Plt 302 × 10³/mm³	Alk phos 35 IU/L
CO_2 23 mEq/L	WBC 8 × 10³/mm³	Urine pregnancy test (−)
BUN 12 mg/dL	Differential WNL	
SCr 0.8 mg/dL		
Glu 95 mg/dL		

Assessment

1. Increase in frequency of migraines related to menses and increased stress.
2. Minimal efficacy of naratriptan 2.5 mg PO as an abortive treatment.
3. Previous prophylactic treatments have been unsuccessful and have caused unwanted adverse effects.
4. Tobacco use restarted due to stress; currently smoking 1 ppd.

QUESTIONS

Problem Identification

1.a. Create a list of the patient's drug therapy problems at this clinic visit.

1.b. Calculate the patient's MIDAS score and describe the severity of her migraine headaches. (See Fig. 72-1 for MIDAS questionnaire.)

1.c. What clinical information is consistent with a diagnosis of migraines in this patient?

1.d. Could any of the patient's problems have been caused or exacerbated by her drug therapy?

Desired Outcomes

2. What are the goals of therapy for this patient?

Therapeutic Alternatives

3.a. What pharmacotherapeutic alternatives are available for treatment of the patient's nausea, and how will they impact potential acute therapies?

3.b. What pharmacotherapeutic alternatives are available for the acute treatment of this patient's migraine attacks?

3.c. What pharmacotherapeutic alternatives are available for prevention of this patient's migraine attacks?

Optimal Plan

4.a. Considering this patient's past successes and failures in treating her migraine attacks, design an optimal pharmacotherapeutic plan for the acute treatment of her migraine headaches.

4.b. Design an optimal pharmacotherapeutic plan for prevention of her migraine headaches.

INSTRUCTIONS: Please answer the following questions about ALL the headaches you have had over the last 3 months. Write your answer in the box next to each question. Write zero if you did not do the activity in the last 3 months.

Days

1. How many days in the last 3 months did you miss work or school because of your headaches?

2. How many days in the last 3 months was your productivity at work or school reduced by half or more because of headaches? *(Do not include days you counted in question 1 where you missed work or school.)*

3. How many days in the last 3 months did you NOT do household work because of your headaches?

4. How many days in the last 3 months was your productivity in household work reduced by half or more because of your headaches? *(Do not include days you counted in question 3 where you did not do household work.)*

5. On how many days in the last 3 months did you miss family, social, or leisure activities because of your headaches?

MIDAS Score: Add the total number of days from questions 1–5.   **Total**

NOTE: Scores from A and B below are not included in the MIDAS score, but are used to assess frequency and intensity of pain.

A. How many days in the last 3 months did you have a headache? *(If a headache lasted more than 1 day, count each day.)*

B. On a scale of 0–10, on average how painful were these headaches? *(0 = no pain, and 10 = pain as bad as it can be.)*

Interpretation

The MIDAS questionnaire is scored in units of lost days. Depending on the MIDAS score, patients are assigned to 1 of 4 grades:

MIDAS Grade	Definition	Score
I	Minimal or infrequent disability	0–5
II	Mild or infrequent disability	6–10
III	Moderate disability	11–20
IV	Severe disability	≥ 21

FIGURE 72-1. MIDAS questionnaire. *(Reprinted with permission from Bigal ME, Lipton RB, Krymchantowski AV. The medical management of migraine. Am J Ther 2004;11:130–140. Lippincott Williams & Wilkins, www.lww.com.)*

Outcome Evaluation

5. What clinical and/or laboratory parameters should be assessed regularly to evaluate the therapy for achievement of the desired therapeutic outcome and to detect or prevent adverse effects?

Patient Education

6.a. What information should be provided to the patient regarding migraine triggers?

6.b. What information should be provided to the patient regarding her new acute and preventive therapies?

■ CLINICAL COURSE: ALTERNATIVE THERAPY

While discussing possible alternatives to her valproic acid therapy, Ms Miller says that a friend who also has migraines had read about some herbal remedies used for migraine prevention. She asks whether any products like that could be used instead of or along with her prescription medications. Ms Miller is very interested in a more "natural" therapy, but only if it would reduce the number of migraines she experiences. For questions related to the use of butterbur and feverfew for the prevention of migraine headaches, please see Section 19 (Complementary and Alternative Therapies) of this Casebook.

■ FOLLOW-UP QUESTION

1. Describe how a headache diary could help the treatment of this patient's migraine headaches. (See Fig. 72-2 for headache diary.)

■ SELF-STUDY ASSIGNMENTS

1. Evaluate the literature regarding the efficacy of IV agents (eg, dihydroergotamine, valproate sodium) for acute migraines.

2. Evaluate the literature on intranasal ketorolac and intranasal oxytocin for acute migraine.

Name: _____ Month: _____ Year: _____

Date of Headache														
Headache Intensity														
Excruciating pain	10	10	10	10	10	10	10	10	10	10	10	10	10	10
	9	9	9	9	9	9	9	9	9	9	9	9	9	9
Severe pain	8	8	8	8	8	8	8	8	8	8	8	8	8	8
	7	7	7	7	7	7	7	7	7	7	7	7	7	7
Severe pain	6	6	6	6	6	6	6	6	6	6	6	6	6	6
	5	5	5	5	5	5	5	5	5	5	5	5	5	5
Moderate pain	4	4	4	4	4	4	4	4	4	4	4	4	4	4
	3	3	3	3	3	3	3	3	3	3	3	3	3	3
Mild pain	2	2	2	2	2	2	2	2	2	2	2	2	2	2
Aura only	1	1	1	1	1	1	1	1	1	1	1	1	1	1
Headache Duration (hours)														
Level of Disability														
Hospitalized														
Treatment by health care professional														
Bedrest required														
Decrease in activity by 50%														
Decrease in activity by 25%														
Normal activity														
Other (comment below)														
Associated Symptoms														
Nausea														
Vomiting														
Visual disturbances														
Menstrual period														
Neurological														
Other (comment below)														
Medications Taken														
1.														
2.														
3.														
4.														
5.														
Treatment Results														
Complete relief														
75% relief														
50% relief														
25% relief														
No relief														
Other (comment below)														
General Comments														

Note: A normal diary includes space to record a full month of headache activity. This form has been truncated for space purposes.

FIGURE 72-2. A headache diary.

3. Review the literature on the efficacy of the calcitonin gene-related peptide receptor antagonists, telcagepant and olcegepant, for acute treatment of migraines.

4. Explain the role of onabotulinum toxin type A (Botox) for prevention of chronic migraine.

CLINICAL PEARL

Migraines are three times more prevalent in women and are associated with estrogen levels. Sixty percent of women migraineurs report menstrually associated migraines, and 7–14% have migraines exclusively with menses.

REFERENCES

1. Bigal ME, Lipton RB, Krymchantowski AV. The medical management of migraine. Am J Ther 2004;11:130–140.

2. Yang M, Rendas-Baum R, Varon SF, Kosinski M. Validation of the Headache Impact Test (HIT-6) across episodic and chronic migraine. Cephalalgia 2010;31:357–367.

3. Lipton RB. Risk factors for and management of medication-overuse headache. Continuum (Minneap Minn) 2015;21(4):1118–1131.

4. Banzi R, Cusi C, Randazzo C, Sterzi R, Tedesco D, Moja L. Selective serotonin reuptake inhibitors (SSRIs) and serotonin-norepinephrine reuptake inhibitors (SNRIs) for the prevention of migraine in adults. Cochrane Database Syst Rev 2015. doi:10.1002/14651858.CD011681.

5. Evans RW, Tepper SJ, Shapiro RE, Sun-Edelstein C, Tietjen GE. The FDA alert on serotonin syndrome with use of triptans combined

with selective serotonin reuptake inhibitors or selective serotonin-norepinephrine reuptake inhibitors: American Headache Society position paper. Headache 2010;50:1089–1099.

6. Silberstein SD. Preventive migraine treatment. Continuum (Minneap Minn) 2015;21(4):973–989.

7. Lipton RB, Silberstein SD. Episodic and chronic migraine headache: breaking down barriers to optimal treatment and prevention. Headache 2015;55(S2):103–122.

8. Silberstein SD, Holland S, Freitag F, et al. Evidence-based guideline update: pharmacologic treatment for episodic migraine prevention in adults. Report of the Quality Standards Subcommittee of the American Academy of Neurology and the American Headache Society. Neurology 2012;78:1337–1345.

9. Linde M, Mulleners WM, Chronicle EP, McCrory DC. Gabapentin or pregabalin for the prophylaxis of episodic migraine in adults. Cochrane Database Syst Rev 2013. doi:10.1002/14651858.CD010609.

10. Nierenburg HDC, Ailani J, Malloy M, Siavoshi S, Hu NN, Yusuf N. Systematic review of preventive and acute treatment of menstrual migraine. Headache 2015;55:1052–1071.

73

ATTENTION-DEFICIT HYPERACTIVITY DISORDER

He Is So Energized, He Keeps
Going and Going and . . . . Level I

Darin C. Ramsey, PharmD, BCPS, BCACP

Laura F. Ruekert, PharmD, BCPP, CGP

LEARNING OBJECTIVES

After completing this case study, the reader should be able to:

- Describe the signs and symptoms of attention-deficit hyperactivity disorder (ADHD) as defined by the *Diagnostic and Statistical Manual of Mental Disorders (DSM)*-5.

- Differentiate treatment options for ADHD with regard to effectiveness, tolerability, safety, monitoring parameters, and potential for drug interactions.

- Compare the advantages and disadvantages of once-daily stimulant preparations with immediate-release stimulants.

- Develop useful dosing schedule strategies that may be employed in the management of patients with ADHD to enhance medication adherence.

- Perform patient assessment to determine efficacy with selected therapy and appropriate monitoring for any adverse effects.

PATIENT PRESENTATION

Chief Complaint

"My son has trouble focusing and sitting still while completing his afternoon homework."

HPI

David Handlon is a 10-year-old boy who returns for a routine visit to his psychiatrist with his mother. He was diagnosed 2 years ago with ADHD and is currently being treated with Adderall XR 20 mg every morning. His mother states that during the last parent–teacher meeting, his teacher indicated that David's behavior is well controlled during the day. Despite David's good behavior during the day, his mother reports difficulty getting David to complete any afternoon tasks or assignments after school. David's rules include no playtime activities until he has completed his afternoon homework assignments. Instead of focusing on homework, David insists on playing Guitar Hero® in his room, and he sometimes carelessly

throws his guitar. David has also exhibited impulsive and reckless behavior when interacting with his younger 8-year-old brother. Initially David's mother thought the medication was working. However, within the past year, David's afternoon antics have progressively gotten worse. Mrs Handlon is afraid that uncontrolled afternoon antics will have serious repercussions on David's daytime behavior and grades. She questions, "What are my options?"

PMH

Asthma × 3 years
ADHD × 2 years
Tonsillectomy (1 year ago)
Broken wrist at age 8 (fell from tree)
Vaccinations up to date

FH

Both father and uncle have a history of hyperactivity and are currently receiving treatment as adults

SH

Lives with both parents and younger brother in the suburbs

Meds

Adderall XR 20 mg daily (given every morning at 7:00 AM)
Albuterol inhaler two puffs Q 4–6 H PRN shortness of breath
Singulair 5 mg PO daily

All

NKDA

ROS

Physical assessment was difficult to assess in David as he could not sit still for more than 30 seconds and was jumping off of the exam table. Asthma symptoms appear controlled with PRN inhaler use at bedtime only and daily Singulair.

Physical Examination

Gen

Well-nourished, healthy-appearing male child, normal physical development

VS

BP 110/72 mm Hg, P 82 bpm, RR 25, T 37.5°C; Wt 50 kg, Ht 5′2″

Skin

No signs of rash, skin irritation, or bruising noted. Scar noticed on left wrist from where he fell from tree. Minor cuts on knees from frequent falls on school playground.

HEENT

Unable to assess

Neck/Lymph Nodes

Unable to assess

Lungs/Thorax

No rales, rhonchi, or wheezing

CV

RRR

Abd

Deferred

Genit/Rect

Deferred

MS/Ext

Unable to assess

Neuro

A & O × 3; no underlying tics noted

■ Labs

Na 138 mEq/L	Hgb 14 g/dL	WBC 9 × 10³/mm³	Mag 1.8 mg/dL
K 3.8 mEq/L	Hct 44.5%	Neutros 66%	Serum iron
Cl 106 mEq/L	RBC 4.6 × 10⁶/mm³	Bands 2%	95 mcg/dL
CO₂ 23 mEq/L	Plt 278 × 10³/mm³	Eos 3%	TSH 3.6 mIU/L
BUN 18 mg/dL	MCV 85 μm³	Lymphs 24%	
SCr 0.8 mg/dL	MCHC 33 g/dL	Monos 5%	
Glu 110 mg/dL			

■ ECG

NSR; changes not clinically significant

■ Assessment

1. ADHD

2. Mild-persistent asthma, well controlled with PRN albuterol and daily Singulair

QUESTIONS

Problem Identification

1.a. Create a list of the patient's drug therapy problems.

1.b. What information (signs, symptoms, and laboratory values) indicates the presence or severity of ADHD?

Desired Outcome

2. What are the goals of treatment (pharmacotherapy and non-pharmacotherapy) for a patient diagnosed with ADHD?

Therapeutic Alternatives

3.a. What nondrug therapies might be beneficial for patients diagnosed with ADHD?

3.b. What pharmacotherapeutic stimulant and nonstimulant dosage formulations are available for the treatment of ADHD?

Optimal Plan

4.a. What drug, dosage form, dose, schedule, and duration of therapy are best for this patient?

4.b. What therapeutic alternatives would be appropriate if the patient fails to respond to stimulant therapy?

Outcome Evaluation

5. What clinical and laboratory parameters are necessary to evaluate the therapy for achievement of the desired therapeutic outcome and to detect or prevent adverse effects?

Patient Education

6. What information, specific to this case, should be provided to the patient and his family to enhance adherence, ensure successful therapy, and minimize adverse effects?

■ SELF-STUDY ASSIGNMENTS

1. Many parents are apprehensive about starting stimulants in children with the fear of the potential for stimulant abuse when they become older. After performing a literature search, prepare an educational brochure addressing the question, "Does stimulant treatment of ADHD increase the risk for drug abuse?"

2. Provide a summary that addresses the long-term effect stimulants have on growth and appetite.

3. Review the boxed warning that the Drug Safety and Risk Management Advisory Committee of the FDA recommended to be added to the product labeling of stimulants used to treat ADHD. What patient population does this boxed warning affect, and what events prompted this recommendation by the FDA?

4. Develop an appropriate recommendation for product conversion in a patient who is switching from oral methylphenidate (Concerta®) 36 mg PO daily to methylphenidate (Daytrana®) transdermal patch. Also, convert doses of mixed amphetamine salts (Adderall IR/Adderall XR®) to lisdexamfetamine (Vyvanse®).

5. Perform a literature search and defend or refute the role of modafinil, selective serotonin reuptake inhibitors, tricyclic antidepressants, and atypical antipsychotics in the treatment of ADHD.

CLINICAL PEARL

Stimulant medications are considered first-line therapy in children with ADHD. The American Academy of Pediatrics reports at least an 80% response rate when these agents are used appropriately in the management of ADHD. If a patient does not respond adequately to initial stimulant therapy, a second or even third stimulant should be tried before initiating a nonstimulant medication. Most patients will be successfully treated by an alternative stimulant.

REFERENCES

1. American Psychiatric Association. Diagnostic and Statistical Manual of Mental Disorders, 5th ed. Washington, DC, American Psychiatric Association, 2013.

2. Pliszka S, Bernet W, Bukstein O, et al., for the American Academy of Child and Adolescent Psychiatry Work Group on Quality Issues. Practice parameter for the assessment and treatment of children and adolescents with attention-deficit-hyperactivity disorder. J Am Acad Child Adolesc Psychiatry 2007;46:894–921.

3. Dopheide JA, Pliszka SR. Attention-deficit-hyperactivity disorder: an update. Pharmacotherapy 2009;29:656–679.

4. Wolraich M, Brown L, Brown RT, et al. ADHD: clinical practice guideline for the diagnosis, evaluation, and treatment of attention-deficit/hyperactivity disorder in children and adolescents. Pediatrics 2011;128:1007–1022.

5. Dobie C, Donald WB, Hanson M, et al. Institute for Clinical Systems Improvement. Diagnosis and Management of Attention Deficit

Hyperactivity Disorder in Primary Care for School-Age Children and Adolescents, 9th ed. March 2012. Available at: *https://www.icsi.org /_asset/60nzr5/ADHD-Interactive0312.pdf.* Accessed March 30, 2016.

6. Sonuga-Barke EJS, Brandeis D, Cortese S, et al. Nonpharmacological interventions for ADHD: systematic review and meta-analyses of randomized controlled trials of dietary and psychological treatments. Am J Psychiatry 2013;170:275–289.

7. The Medical Letter. Drugs for ADHD. Med Lett Drugs Ther 2015;15;57(1464):37–40.

8. Stuhec M, Munda B, Svab V, et al. Comparative efficacy and acceptability of atomoxetine, lisdexamfetamine, bupropion and methylphenidate in treatment of attention deficit hyperactivity disorder in children and adolescents: a meta-analysis with focus on bupropion. J Affect Disord 2015;178:149–159.

9. Daughton J, Corr L, Liu H, West M. Clonidine extended-release tablets for the treatment of ADHD. Neuropsychiatry 2012;2(2):117–123.

10. Bernknoph A. Guanfacine (Intuniv) for attention-deficit/hyperactivity disorder. Am Fam Physician 2011;83:474–475.

74

BULIMIA NERVOSA

Self-Conscious Socialite.........................Level I

Laura F. Ruekert, PharmD, BCPP, CGP

Cheen T. Lum, BSc, PharmD, BCPP

LEARNING OBJECTIVES

After completing this case study, the reader should be able to:

- Define bulimia nervosa (BN) according to the *Diagnostic and Statistical Manual of Mental Disorders (DSM)-5* criteria.

- Assess signs and symptoms commonly associated with the presentation of BN.

- Name effective pharmacologic and nonpharmacologic treatment options for the management of BN.

- Compare and contrast short-term and long-term complications of BN and discuss the associated therapeutic options for prevention and management.

- Design a treatment plan including monitoring parameters and counseling points for a patient with BN.

PATIENT PRESENTATION

Chief Complaint

"I'm so unpopular, I just want to die!"

HPI

Cady Greenwald is a 21-year-old female presenting to a behavioral acute care hospital referred by her outpatient psychiatrist for suicidal ideations and symptoms of an eating disorder. She reported worsening depressive symptoms after she was cut from the college dance team 6 months ago. She expressed anxious feelings of inadequacy and obsessions with her image after that incident, and she is now binge eating and purging up to 8 episodes a week. She explains she tries to withhold food for as long as possible and then loses control and impulsively binges on large amounts of food usually in private. She becomes overwhelmed with guilt and anxiety and subsequently purges. In addition, she uses laxatives about three to four times a week and engages in self-injurious behavior by cutting her forearm. She has now dropped out of school and expresses suicidal ideations with a plan, stating "no one would miss me." She admitted daily use of alcohol and marijuana to help her depressive thoughts, calm her anxieties, and to regulate her appetite. Compounding the eating disorder is that Cady has a diagnosis of bipolar disorder, type II, treated with escitalopram, bupropion, and ziprasidone, and she has been experiencing a depressive episode.

PMH

Bipolar disorder, type II
Cluster B personality disorder traits

FH

Parents married for 25 years. Father has a history of depression. Maternal aunt diagnosed with bipolar disorder. Maternal uncle and paternal aunt have with a history of depression and substance use.

SH

Completed 2 years of college as a dance major but dropped out 2 weeks ago due to increasing stress. She lives alone in her apartment. She admits to smoking marijuana daily, because she claims "everything is OK after I smoke." She also drinks until she passes out about two nights a week and just occasionally drinks otherwise. She uses tobacco 1 PPD × 2 years

Meds

Ziprasidone 40 mg PO BID (3 years)
Bupropion SR 200 mg PO BID (1 year)
Escitalopram 20 mg PO once daily (3 years)

All

NKDA

ROS

Cady expresses feelings of hopelessness and frustration with her life in general. She states she has never experienced relief from depressive symptoms and uses marijuana and alcohol daily to cope. She endorses suicidal ideations with a plan of cutting her wrists, but denies any previous attempts. She reports high anxieties and obsessions with her image. She reports fatigue, weakness, dizziness, and low energy increasing the past couple weeks. Her LMP was 2 months ago, and her periods have been irregular.

Physical Examination

Gen

Tearful, thin, anxious-appearing Caucasian female

Skin

Abrasion on dorsum of right hand (Russell's sign), numerous superficial scars and cuts on the left forearm. No findings of lanugo on arms/upper body area.

VS

BP 98/72 mm Hg, P 52 bpm, RR 20, T 36.4°C; Wt 54 kg, Ht 5′4″

HEENT

Normocephalic; brittle/coarse hair; PERRLA, EOMI; mild parotid gland enlargement

Neck/Lymph Nodes

No JVD

Lungs/Thorax

Lungs CTA; no rales, rhonchi, wheezes

CV

Hypotensive; bradycardic

Abd

Slightly distended, (−) BS

Genit/Rect

Unremarkable

MS/Ext

No cyanosis, clubbing, edema

Neuro

A & O × 3

■ Labs

Na 135 mEq/L	Hgb 14 g/dL	WBC 7.3 × 10^3/mm³	AST 20 IU/L
K 3.3 mEq/L	Hct 39%		ALT 15 IU/L
Cl 100 mEq/L	RBC 5 × 10⁶/mm³	Neutros 60%	Ca 8.6 mg/dL
HCO_3 22 mEq/L	Plt 247 × 10³/mm³	Bands 3%	Mg 1.3 mg/dL
BUN 25 mg/dL	MCV 83 fL	Eos 2%	Serum iron 96 mcg/dL
SCr 1.0 mg/dL	MCHC 34 g/dL	Lymphs 31%	Folic acid 9.3 ng/mL
Glu 74 mg/dL	Albumin 3.4 g/dL	Monos 4%	Ferritin 110 ng/mL

Other:

UDS: +THC	BAL <0.2	Hcg (−)
HAM-D score 20		EKG shows QTc interval of 506 sec

■ Assessment

New diagnosis of bulimia nervosa (BN), severe, complicated by self-mutilating behaviors, a depressive episode associated with bipolar disorder type 2, and current misuse of multiple substances

QUESTIONS

Problem Identification

1.a. Create a list of the patient's drug therapy problems.

1.b. What signs, symptoms, and laboratory values indicate the severity of the BN, secondary complications, and depression?

Desired Outcome

2. What are the goals of therapy for this patient?

Therapeutic Alternatives

3.a. What nondrug treatment strategies would be beneficial for this patient?

3.b. What drug treatment strategies are available for the treatment of eating disorders?

Optimal Plan

4.a. What drug, dosage form, route, schedule, and duration of therapy is appropriate in this patient?

4.b. What pharmacologic alternatives would be appropriate if initial treatment interventions fail or are insufficient to achieve desired outcomes?

Outcome Evaluation

5. What clinical and laboratory parameters are necessary to evaluate the therapy for achievement of the desired therapeutic outcome and to detect or prevent adverse effects?

Patient Education

6. What information should be provided to the patient to enhance adherence, ensure successful therapy, and minimize adverse effects associated with BN treatment?

■ SELF-STUDY ASSIGNMENTS

1. Compare and contrast the differences in the etiologies and presentations of the various eating disorders.

2. Review the literature and discuss the incidence, types, and implications of psychiatric comorbidities associated with eating disorders and how these impact treatment.

3. Prepare a table highlighting the different laboratory parameters seen in a patient presenting with acidosis secondary to laxative abuse versus a patient presenting with alkalosis secondary to excessive purging.

4. Review the literature and prepare a one-page paper describing the complications of eating disorders and the overall implications of eating disorders on long-term health.

CLINICAL PEARL

Therapeutic management of eating disorders involves both comprehensive and intensive therapy with a multidisciplinary team using a combination of methods to address the complex nature of the disorder. Nonpharmacologic and pharmacologic approaches are intended to address the symptoms of eating disorders and any comorbid psychiatric disease states (substance abuse, depression, anxiety are highly concomitant) as well as to prevent or treat potential complications.

REFERENCES

1. American Psychiatric Association. Diagnostic and statistical manual of mental disorders, 5th ed. Washington, DC, American Psychiatric Association, 2013.

2. Finzi-Dottan R, Zubery E. The role of depression and anxiety in impulsive and obsessive–compulsive behaviors among anorexic and bulimic patients. Eat Disord 2009;17:162–182.

3. American Psychiatric Association (APA). Practice Guidelines for the Treatment of Patients with Eating Disorders, 3rd ed. Washington, DC, American Psychiatric Association (APA), June 2006.

4. Aigner M, Treasure J, Kaye W, Kasper S, and the WFSBP Task Force on Eating Disorders. World Federation of Societies of Biological Psychiatry (WFSBP) guidelines for the pharmacological treatment of eating disorders. World J Biol Psychiatry 2011;12:400–443.

5. Tortorella A, Fabrazzo M, Monteleone AM, Steardo L, Monteleone P. The role of drug therapies in the treatment of anorexia and bulimia nervosa: a review of the literature. J Psychopathol 2014;20:50–65.

6. Yager J, Devlin MJ, Halmi KA, et al. Guideline watch (August 2012): practice guideline for the treatment of patients with eating disorders, 3rd ed. American Psychiatric Association, 2012.

7. Setnick, J. Micronutrient deficiencies and supplementation in anorexia and bulimia nervosa: a review of the literature. Nutr Clin Pract 2010;25:137–142.

75

ALCOHOL WITHDRAWAL

Cold Turkey Can Land You in Hot Water . . . . Level I

Kevin M. Tuohy, PharmD, BCPS

LEARNING OBJECTIVES

After completing this case study, the reader should be able to:

- Describe the signs and symptoms of acute alcohol withdrawal syndrome.
- Explain the common laboratory abnormalities seen in alcohol-dependent patients.
- Develop a treatment plan for acute alcohol withdrawal and alcohol-related seizures.
- Recommend an appropriate pharmacotherapeutic regimen for electrolyte replacement in an alcohol-dependent patient.

PATIENT PRESENTATION

Chief Complaint

"My husband has been acting strange, sweating, and shaking all day. I think he had a seizure an hour ago."

HPI

Brian Johnson is a 54-year-old man who is brought to the ED by his wife. She states that her husband has abused alcohol since she met him while in college. She states that his typical daily consumption for the past 25 years has averaged about 14–18 alcoholic beverages. She reports that he has not been able to afford to drink recently due to a recent layoff from his job. In an effort to save money, he has decided to quit drinking "cold turkey." He has not had any alcohol to drink in the previous 48 hours.

PMH

Alcohol abuse and dependence
Alcohol withdrawal with seizure 4 years prior
Hypertension × 10 years
GERD × 4 years

SH

The patient is an unemployed construction worker. He has not worked for the past 6 months. He has been married for 22 years. He has been a heavy drinker for past 25 years. Drinks an average of 16 drinks (usually beer- or whiskey-containing drinks) per day. (+) Tobacco history—quit 5 years ago.
Denies any illicit drug use.

Meds

Hydrochlorothiazide 25 mg PO daily
Amlodipine 5 mg PO daily
OTC omeprazole 20 mg PO as needed for heartburn symptoms

All

NKDA

ROS

The patient exhibits overall confusion and is not responsive to questions. Wife states his mental status was normal until this afternoon when his confusion, sweating, and shakiness started.

Physical Examination

Gen

Tall, thin, undernourished-appearing male, in mild distress who is acutely confused and tremulous

VS

BP 162/85 mm Hg, P 107 bpm, RR 20, T 38.3°C; Wt 76 kg, Ht 6′6″

Skin

Moist, diaphoretic

HEENT

Head—atraumatic, icteric sclera, PERRLA, EOMI, mild AV nicking on funduscopic exam

Neck/Lymph Nodes

Supple, no thyromegaly or lymphadenopathy

Lungs/Thorax

Symmetric, lungs CTA

CV

RRR, no MRG

Abd

Soft, nontender; (+) bowel sounds; (+) hepatomegaly

Genit/Rect

(–) Occult blood in stool

MS/Ext

Confused, tremor in both hands

Neuro

A & O only to person, DTRs exaggerated

Labs

Na 139 mEq/L	Phos 2.8 mg/dL	PT 14.5 seconds
K 3.2 mEq/L	Ca 9.5 mg/dL	INR 1.30
Cl 88 mEq/L	GGT 310 IU/L	ETOH (–)
CO_2 26 mEq/L	AST 250 IU/L	
BUN 14 mg/dL	ALT 120 IU/L	
SCr 1.1 mg/dL	T. bili 1.7 mg/dL	
Glu 99 mg/dL	D. bili 1.1 mg/dL	
Mg 1.6 mg/dL	Alb 2.1 g/dL	

■ **Assessment**

Acute alcohol withdrawal with possible witnessed seizure

QUESTIONS

Problem Identification

1.a. Create a list of patient's drug therapy problems.

1.b. What information (signs, symptoms, and laboratory values) indicates that this patient is experiencing alcohol withdrawal?

1.c. What signs, symptoms, and history are consistent with alcohol dependence in this patient?

1.d. What laboratory abnormalities may be expected in a patient with a history of alcohol abuse?

Desired Outcome

2. What are the goals of pharmacotherapy in this case?

Therapeutic Alternatives

3.a. What pharmacotherapeutic alternatives are available for the treatment of alcohol withdrawal?

3.b. How should alcohol withdrawal seizures be managed pharmacologically?

3.c. What electrolyte imbalances need to be corrected in this patient, and what vitamin deficiencies should be corrected?

3.d. What pharmacotherapeutic agent can be recommended to treat this patient's acutely elevated blood pressure and heart rate?

Optimal Plan

4. Design an appropriate pharmacotherapy regimen for the treatment of alcohol withdrawal in this patient. Include recommendations for electrolyte replacement and correction of vitamin deficiencies, as well as for the management of the patient's other medical problems.

Outcome Evaluation

5. What clinical and laboratory parameters are necessary to evaluate your therapy for the achievement of desired therapeutic outcome and to detect or prevent adverse effects?

Patient Education

6. What information should be provided to the patient to enhance adherence, ensure successful therapy, and minimize adverse effects?

■ SELF-STUDY ASSIGNMENTS

1. Research alcohol-related treatment Web sites that can be recommended to patients with alcohol dependence.

2. Discuss the pharmacologic options that are currently marketed in the United States (FDA-approved drugs) for the treatment of alcohol dependence.

CLINICAL PEARLS

1. All benzodiazepines appear similarly efficacious in reducing signs and symptoms of alcohol withdrawal. The choice of the agent should be determined based on patient-specific factors and the pharmacokinetic profile of the drug.

2. Very high doses of benzodiazepines are often needed to control the symptoms of alcohol withdrawal. This is due to cross tolerance between alcohol and benzodiazepines.

REFERENCES

1. Mayo-Smith MF. Pharmacological management of alcohol withdrawal: a meta-analysis and evidence-based practice guideline. American Society of Addiction Medicine Working Group on Pharmacological Management of Alcohol Withdrawal. JAMA 1997;278:144–151.

2. Muzyk AJ, Leung JG, Nelson S, Embury ER, Jones SR. The role of diazepam loading for the treatment of alcohol withdrawal syndrome in hospitalized patients. Am J Addict 2013;22:113–118.

3. Martinotti G, diNicola M, Frustaci A, et al. Pregabalin, tiapride, and lorazepam in alcohol withdrawal syndrome: a multi-centre, randomized, single-blind comparison trial. Addiction 2010;105:288–299.

4. Lyon JE, Khan RA, Gessert CE, Larson PM, Renier CM. Treating alcohol withdrawal with oral baclofen: a randomized, double-blind, placebo-controlled trial. J Hosp Med 2011;6:469–474.

5. Muzyk AJ, Fowler JA, Norwood DK, Chilipko A. Role of a2-agonists in the treatment of acute alcohol withdrawal. Ann Pharmacother 2011;45:649–657.

6. Mueller SW, Preslaski CR, Kiser TH, et al. A randomized, double-blind, placebo-controlled dose range study of dexmedetomidine as adjunctive therapy for alcohol withdrawal. Crit Care Med 2014;42:1131–1139.

7. Rathlev NK, Ulrich AS, Delanty N, D'Onofrio G. Alcohol-related seizures. J Emerg Med 2006;31:157–163.

8. Hillbom M, Pieninkeroinen I, Leone M. Seizures in alcohol-dependent patients. Epidemiology, pathophysiology and management. CNS Drugs 2003;17:1013–1030.

9. Sullivan JT, Sykora K, Schniederman J, Naranjo CA, Sellers EM. Assessment of alcohol withdrawal: the revised clinical institute withdrawal assessment for alcohol scale (CIWA-Ar). Br J Addict 1989;84:1353–1357.

76

NICOTINE DEPENDENCE

What Is That Smell? .... Level II

Gabriella A. Douglass, PharmD, BCACP

Julie C. Kissack, PharmD, BCPP, FCCP

LEARNING OBJECTIVES

After completing this case study, the reader should be able to:

• Explain the adverse effects of secondhand smoke exposure.

• Interpret the stage of change exhibited by a specific patient, and prepare an action plan to promote smoking cessation and nicotine abstinence based on the 5A plan.

• Design patient-specific recommendations for initiating lifestyle modifications and pharmacologic treatment to encourage reduction or elimination of cigarette smoke exposure.

• Recommend alternative treatments for nicotine dependence if an initial plan fails.

• Develop patient counseling on the use of pharmacotherapeutic agents used to treat nicotine dependence for a specific patient.

PATIENT PRESENTATION

▇ Chief Complaint

"I don't know why I'm feeling so bad, but giving up these coffin sticks might be a good thing to do. The one time I tried to quit using nicotine gum for two days, it made me sick to my stomach, my jaw really hurt and I really craved a cigarette."

▇ HPI

Phil Morris is a 32-year-old man who presents to the primary care clinic complaining of extreme thirst, excessive urination, and generally feeling unwell for the past 2 weeks. "I have missed 2–3 days of work each week in the last month so there is less money to stretch for our expenses. My insurance premiums are high and I struggle to pay for the coverage. My wife and three kids are hungry and I can only afford to buy one cigarette at a time. And one more thing, it is so hard for me to remember to take that medication that was prescribed to control my sugar. Can you help me get right so I can get back to work?"

▇ PMH

Type 2 diabetes mellitus (diagnosed at age 29)

▇ FH

Mother (age 52) has history of type 2 diabetes and ovarian cancer. Father (age 57) has history of hypertension, myocardial infarction, and obesity. Patient is the oldest child of six siblings. All siblings have smoked cigarettes, but in the last 5 years, two of the siblings have quit smoking. Wife is a nonsmoker and son has asthma; one daughter has ADHD, and one daughter has no identified health problems.

▇ SH

Works at a local convenience store. Smokes a pack of cigarettes daily, when he can afford to buy them, and has smoked for the past 18 years. Drinks 10 cans of Mountain Dew a day when he is working. States that he only drinks a six pack of beer on Friday nights after he gets paid. Lives with his wife of 14 years and their three children who are 12, 9, and 3 years old. Wife is a stay-at-home mother. The family has insurance coverage through a state program which they signed up for through the Health Insurance Marketplace Web site.

▇ Meds

Metformin 500 mg PO BID with meals (started at time of diagnosis)

▇ All

NKDA

▇ ROS

General feeling of being unwell. Denies history of goiter; has no intolerance to heat or cold. Has had polyuria for the past week.

▇ Physical Examination

Gen

Heavy-set African-American man who has dark circles under his eyes, looks sad, and appears his stated age. Strong odor of cigarette smoke. Yellowed skin on fingers. Yellow teeth.

VS

BP 128/85 mm Hg, P 89 bpm, RR 20, T 98.7°F; Wt 125 kg, Ht 5'8"

▇ Labs

FBG 150 mg/dL; A1C 7.5%; Total cholesterol 140 mg/dL, Triglycerides 175 mg/dL, HDL 25 mg/dL, VLDL calculated 35 mg/dL, LDL calculated 80 mg/dL. All labs were documented in the clinic chart 1 month prior to this visit.

▇ Assessment

1. Nicotine dependence—patient may be ready to quit smoking

2. Type 2 diabetes—not adequately controlled

3. Evaluate risk for ASCVD

4. Obesity—he is struggling to buy food for his family and not making healthy beverage choices

5. Poor adherence to medication regimen—limited financial resources and regimen complexity may adversely impact ability to comply with pharmacotherapy

6. Compromised quality of life secondary to work absences

QUESTIONS

Problem Identification

1.a. Create a list of this patient's drug therapy problems.

1.b. What information in the patient's history can be identified as disease or symptoms directly related to the patient's smoking history (Fig. 76-1)?

1.c. Identify the stage of change that the patient is currently in at this time of his life, and describe your intervention plan using one of the A's from the 5A intervention plan for smokers (Table 76-1). State monitoring parameters that indicate uncontrolled disease states in addition to the nicotine dependence.

1.d. Describe aspects of the case that reveal the severity of nicotine dependence.

1.e. Identify the most likely reason that the patient's previous quit attempt was unsuccessful with nicotine gum.

A Cigarette and Select Smoke Components

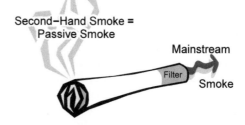

Cigarette Smoke

Gaseous Component	Particulate Component
Carbon monoxide	Nicotine
Hydrogen cyanide	Tobacco alkaloids
Toluene	Tar
Methanol	Polynuclear Aromatic
Acetone	Hydrocarbons (PAH)

FIGURE 76-1. A cigarette and select smoke components.

TABLE 76-1 Stages of Change and Smoking Cessation Counseling

Stage of Change	Patient's Mindset	Response
Precontemplation	Not interested in quitting, fails to recognize smoking as a problem	Provide concise and relevant statement about why the smoker should think about quitting smoking
Contemplation	Smoking is a problem and might consider quitting	State that there is good evidence that cigarette smoke and secondhand smoke are dangerous. Encourage smoker to quit
Preparation	Cigarette smoking is problematic and now ready to think about quitting	Discuss options for treatment—both pharmacotherapeutic and nonpharmacotherapeutic
Action	Motivated to quit, instituting a plan with an identified quit date and developing a plan to cope with stressors	Encourage quit attempt, offer to be a resource during the quit attempt, and praise former smokers' abstinent status
Maintenance	Former smokers who have not smoked for a period of time	Great job staying quit. Continued cessation is a positive move in becoming healthier

Desired Outcome

2. What are the goals of smoking cessation pharmacotherapy and disease state management for this patient?

Therapeutic Alternatives

3.a. Describe nondrug therapies that may help this patient reach his smoking cessation pharmacotherapy treatment goals and improve work attendance.

3.b. What pharmacotherapeutic options are available for the treatment of this patient's nicotine dependence and other disease states, and which would be an acceptable recommendation to make for this patient?

3.c. What economic, psychosocial, racial, and ethical issues need to be considered in this patient's treatment?

Optimal Plan

4. What drugs, dosage forms, doses, schedules, and duration of therapy are best to control this patient's disease states?

Outcome Evaluation

5. What clinical and laboratory parameters are necessary to evaluate the therapy for achievement of the desired therapeutic outcome and to detect or prevent adverse effects?

Patient Education

6. What information should be provided to the patient about the medications you recommended to enhance adherence, ensure successful outcomes, and minimize adverse effects?

■ SELF-STUDY ASSIGNMENTS

1. Evaluate current literature concerning the use of quitlines to enhance quit-smoking attempts. What is the status of quitlines in your state? In a one-page paper, explain how you could educate your community about quitlines.

2. Visit the *smokefree.gov* Web site and select two studies—one nonpharmacological and one pharmacological—that are currently enrolling smokers (eg, veterans, pregnant women) to help them quit smoking. Compare and contrast the two studies. Create a flyer that could be used to recruit patients to one of the two studies.

3. Review the Surgeon General's report about secondhand smoke found at http://www.surgeongeneral.gov/library/reports /50-years-of-progress/exec-summary.pdf.

4. Develop a 10-item list stating how secondhand smoke acts as a toxin to cause disease. Write a two-page paper delineating how

you could use this information to encourage parents and other caregivers to quit smoking.

5. Describe the legal status (both federal and state) and explain the role of commercially used e-cigarettes.

CLINICAL PEARL

Blood glucose levels may be increased while using the nicotine patch because of an impaired cellular response to insulin. Nevertheless, this effect is less pronounced than the endocrine changes seen with cigarette smoking. The person using the nicotine patch is also not exposed to the toxic components of the cigarette smoke.

REFERENCES

1. Fiore MC, Jaén CR, Baker TB, et al. Treating Tobacco Use and Dependence: 2008 Update. Clinical Practice Guideline. Rockville, MD, U.S. Department of Health and Human Services. Public Health Service, 2008. Available at: *http://bphc.hrsa.gov/buckets/treatingtobacco.pdf*. Accessed March 24, 2016.

2. U.S. Department of Health and Human Services. The Health Consequences of Smoking—50 Years of Progress: A Report of the Surgeon General. Atlanta, GA, U.S. Department of Health and Human Services, Centers for Disease Control and Prevention, National Center for Chronic Disease Prevention and Health Promotion, Office on Smoking and Health, 2014. Available at: *http://www.surgeongeneral.gov/library/reports /50-years-of-progress/exec-summary.pdf*. Accessed April 29, 2016.

3. American Diabetes Association. Standards of medical care in diabetes—2016. Diabetes Care 2016;39(Suppl 1):S1–S106.

4. Willi C, Bodenmann P, Ghali WA, Faris PD, Cornuz J. Active smoking and the risk of type 2 diabetes: a systematic review and meta-analysis. JAMA 2007;298:2654–2664.

5. Pan A, Wang Y, Talaei M, Hu FB, Wu T. Relation of active, passive, and quitting smoking with incident type 2 diabetes: a systematic review and meta-analysis. Lancet Diabetes Endocrinol 2015;3(12):958–967.

6. Mills AM, Rhodes KV, Follansbee CW, Shofer FS, Prusakowski M, Bernstein ST. Effect of household children on adult ED smokers' motivation to quit. Am J Emerg Med 2008;26:757–762.

7. Benowitz NL. Nicotine addiction. N Engl J Med 2010;362:2295–2303.

8. Kotz D, Viechtbauer W, Simpson C, Van schayck OC, West R, Sheikh A. Cardiovascular and neuropsychiatric risks of varenicline: a retrospective cohort study. Lancet Respir Med 2015;3(10):761–768.

9. Centers for Disease Control and Prevention. Current cigarette smoking among adults—United States, 2005–2013. Morbid Mortal Wkly Rep 2014;63(47):1108–1112. Available at: *http://www.cdc.gov/mmwr /preview/mmwrhtml/mm6347a4.htm*. Accessed April 29, 2016.

10. U.S. Preventive Services Task Force. Behavioral and pharmacologic treatments to help adults quit smoking: U.S. Preventive Services Task Force Recommendation Statement. Ann Intern Med 2015;163:1–40.

77

SCHIZOPHRENIA

A Thousand Worms Inside My Body.............Level I

Leigh Anne Nelson, PharmD, BCPP

LEARNING OBJECTIVES

After completing this case study, the reader should be able to:

- Identify the target symptoms of schizophrenia.

- Manage an acutely psychotic patient with appropriate pharmacotherapy.

- Manage the adverse effects of antipsychotics.

- Discuss the role of second-generation antipsychotics in the treatment of schizophrenia.

PATIENT PRESENTATION

▨ Chief Complaint

"I want to see my lawyer."

▨ HPI

This is the first inpatient admission for Anita Gonzalez, a 32-year-old woman who was brought to the psychiatric hospital by the police. Earlier today she was brought to the Crisis Center by a friend in her apartment building after the landlord threatened to call the police since Anita was creating a disturbance. At the Crisis Center, Anita became increasingly agitated and suspicious; the police were called; however, she left before being evaluated by staff. The patient apparently has been delusional and believes people sneak into her room at night when she is asleep and place a thousand worms inside her body. She also believes that she is being raped by passing men on the street. She is quite preoccupied about having massive wealth. She claims to have bought some gold and left it at the grocery store. She believes that her ideas have been given to a Cuban communist who has had plastic surgery to look like her and is using her identification to take possession of all of her property. She states that she is having difficulty getting her property back.

Apparently, the precipitating event today that eventually resulted in her hospitalization was that she created a disturbance at a local fast-food restaurant, claiming that she owned it. Because of the disturbance, police were called, and she subsequently was sent here on an order of protective custody. According to the patient, she bought a hamburger and sat down to eat it, and for some reason, somebody called the police and charged her with illegal trespassing. She claims that 6 years ago she was raped by a relative of a sister and broke her hip in the process. She states that her feet were cut off because she would not do what her impostors wanted her to do, and her feet were subsequently sent back to her from Central America and were reattached.

Her speech is quite rambling. She speaks of having been part of an experiment in Monterey, Mexico, in which 38 eggs were taken from her body, and children were produced from them and then killed by the government. She claims that she has worms in her that are the type that kill dogs and horses and says that they have been put there by the government. She also claims that at one time she had transmitters in her backbone and that it took 3 years to have them taken out by the government. She claims to have had surgery in the past, and the surgeon did not know what he was doing and took out her gallbladder and put it in the intestines, where it exploded. The patient also states that on one occasion a physician was removing the snakes from her abdominal cavity, and the snakes killed the doctor and a nurse. She also claims that she worked as a surgeon herself before 1963.

▨ Past Psychiatric History

Denies any prior hospitalization for mental health problems. Denies any illicit drug or alcohol use. Smokes two packs of cigarettes per day.

▨ PMH

Medical records indicate that she did have gallbladder surgery (cholecystectomy) 2 months ago.
There is no record of her ever being raped or having a broken hip.
No further medical history is known.

▨ Family Psychiatric History

The patient claims that her alleged family is not really her family and that she is not sure who her family is.

▨ Meds

None noted

▨ All

Penicillin → rash

▨ Legal/Social Status

Divorced; heterosexual; lives in an apartment alone; employment history unknown

▨ Mental Status Examination

The patient is a white female of Hispanic ethnicity, modestly dressed, with some disarray. She is morbidly obese. Her hair is black and unwashed. She is alert, oriented, and in no acute distress. Her speech is clear, constant, and pressured, with many grandiose delusions and illogical thoughts. She is quite rambling, going from one subject to the other without interruption. Her affect is mood-congruent, her mood is euphoric, and there is a marked degree of grandiosity. Her thought processes are quite illogical, with markedly delusional thinking. There is no current evidence of auditory hallucinations, and she denies visual hallucinations. She denies any suicidal or homicidal ideation, but she is quite verbal and pressured in her thought content, verbalizing a great deal about the things that have been taken away from her illegally by people impersonating her. She has marked delusional symptoms with paranoid ideation prominent. Her memory (immediate, recent, and remote) is fair. Her cognition and concentration are adequate. Her intellectual functioning is within the average range. Insight and judgment are markedly impaired.

▨ Review of Systems

Reports occasional GI upset; complains that worms are inside her stomach; otherwise negative

PE

VS

BP 140/85 mm Hg, P 80 bpm, RR 17, T 37.1°C; Wt 97 kg; Ht 5'3"

Skin

Scratches on both hands

HEENT

PERRLA; EOMI; fundi benign; throat and ears clear; TMs intact

Neck

Supple, no nodes; normal thyroid

Lungs

CTA & P

CV

RRR, normal S_1 and S_2

Abd

(+) BS, nontender

Ext

Full ROM, pulses 2+ bilaterally

Neuro

A & O × 3; reflexes symmetric; toes downgoing; normal gait; normal strength; sensation intact; CNs II–XII intact

Labs

See Tables 77-1 to 77-3.

TABLE 77-1 Laboratory Values

Na 140 mEq/L	Hgb 14.6 g/dL	WBC $11.0 \times 10^3/mm^3$	AST 34 IU/L	Ca 9.6 mg/dL
K 3.9 mEq/L	Hct 45.7%	Neutros 66%	ALT 22 IU/L	Phos 5.1 mg/dL
Cl 104 mEq/L	RBC $4.7 \times 10^6/mm^3$	Lymphs 24%	Alk phos 89 IU/L	TSH 4.5 µIU/mL
CO_2 22 mEq/L	MCV 90.2 µm^3	Monos 8%	GGT 38 IU/L	RPR negative
BUN 19 mg/dL	MCH 31 pg	Eos 1%	T. bili 0.9 mg/dL	Serum alcohol <10 mg/dL
SCr 1.1 mg/dL	MCHC 34.5 g/dL	Basos 1%	Alb 3.6 g/dL	Urine pregnancy (–)
Glu 100 mg/dL		Plt $232 \times 10^3/mm^3$	T. chol 208 mg/dL	

Urinalysis

Color yellow
appearance slightly
   cloudyglucose (–)
bilirubin (–)
ketones, trace
SG 1.025
blood (–)
pH 6.0
protein (–)
nitrites (–)
leukocyte esterase (–)

Urine drug screen

Amphetamines (–)
Barbiturates (–)
Benzodiazepines (–)
Cannabinoids (–)
Cocaine (–)
Opiates (–)
PCP (–)
Oxycodone (–)

TABLE 77-2 Antipsychotic Treatment Recommendations

Recommendation	APA 2004 (commentary 2009)	IPAP 2005	PORT 2009
First Episode	SGA	SGA	SGA (except clozapine and olanzapine), FGA
Second Episode	SGA, FGA, clozapine	SGA	SGA, FGA

TABLE 77-3 Recommended Monitoring Parameters for Patients Receiving SGA

Parameter	Baseline	4 WEEKS	8 WEEKS	12 WEEKS	Quarterly	Annually
Personal/Family History	X					
Weight (BMI)	X	X	X	X	X	
Blood Pressure	X			X		X
Fasting Plasma Glucose	X			X		X
Fasting Lipid Profile	X			X		X
Waist Circumference	X					X
Tardive Dyskinesia Evaluation	X					X
Hematologic Profile*	X					X
CV Status**	X					X

* Desirable for all SGA but required for clozapine according to a strict monitoring protocol.

** ECG if > 40 years or h/o CV disease.

■ **Assessment**

Psychiatric diagnosis: schizophrenia, first episode, currently in acute episode

Medical diagnoses: S/P cholecystectomy; obesity; tobacco use disorder

QUESTIONS

Problem Identification

1.a. Create a list of the patient's drug therapy problems.

1.b. What information (signs, symptoms, laboratory values) indicates the presence or severity of an acute exacerbation of schizophrenia?

Desired Outcome

2. What are the goals of pharmacotherapy in this case?

Therapeutic Alternatives

3.a. What nondrug therapies might be useful for this patient?

3.b. What pharmacotherapeutic options are available for the treatment of this patient?

Optimal Plan

4.a. What drug, dosage form, dose, schedule, and duration of therapy are best for this patient?

4.b. What alternatives would be appropriate if the initial therapy fails or cannot be used?

Outcome Evaluation

5. What clinical and laboratory parameters are necessary to evaluate the therapy for achievement of the desired therapeutic outcome and to detect or prevent adverse effects?

Patient Education

6. What information should be provided to the patient to enhance adherence, ensure successful therapy, and minimize adverse effects?

■ SELF-STUDY ASSIGNMENTS

1. Perform a literature search regarding weight gain with each of the second-generation antipsychotics currently marketed. Which ones are more likely to cause weight gain? Which ones are less likely to cause weight gain?

2. Perform a literature search regarding QTc changes with both first- and second-generation antipsychotics. Which antipsychotics are more likely to alter the QTc interval?

3. Review the pharmacoeconomic literature for the second-generation antipsychotics. For your geographic area, compare costs for the average daily (monthly for long-acting injectable [LAI]) doses of haloperidol (oral and LAI formulation), clozapine (oral and rapid-dissolving formulation), olanzapine (oral, rapid-dissolving formulation, and LAI formulation), risperidone (oral, rapid-dissolving formulation, and LAI formulation), aripiprazole (oral, rapid-dissolving formulation, and LAI formulations), quetiapine (oral), ziprasidone (oral), paliperidone (oral and LAI formulations), asenapine (oral), iloperidone (oral), lurasidone (oral), brexpiprazole (oral), and cariprazine (oral).

CLINICAL PEARL

A benzodiazepine (eg, lorazepam) may be used during the initiation of an antipsychotic to minimize agitation or aggression and allow time for the antipsychotic to take effect. For management of acute agitation or aggression, the addition of lorazepam may also allow lower dosages of the antipsychotic to be used and help prevent antipsychotic-induced side effects such as extrapyramidal symptoms (eg, dystonia).

REFERENCES

1. Velligan DI, Weiden PJ, Sajatovic M, et al. The Expert Consensus Guideline Series: adherence problems in patients with serious and persistent mental illness. J Clin Psychiatry 2009;7:1–48.

2. Castle DJ, Buckley PF. Schizophrenia, 2nd ed. Oxford, UK, Oxford University Press, 2015.

3. Lehman AF, Lieberman JA, Dixon LB, et al. American Psychiatric Association Practice Guidelines; Work Group on Schizophrenia. Practice guideline for the treatment of patients with schizophrenia, 2nd ed. Am J Psychiatry 2004;161(2 Suppl):1–56.

4. Dixon LB, Perkins B, Calmas C. Guideline Watch (September 2009): practice guideline for the treatment of patients with schizophrenia. Psychiatry Online. Available at: *http://psychiatryonline.org/pb/assets /raw/sitewide/practice_guidelines/guidelines/schizophrenia-watch.pdf*. Accessed March 23, 2016.

5. Buchanan RW, Kreyenbuhl J, Kelly DL, et al. The 2009 schizophrenia PORT psychopharmacological treatment recommendations and summary statements. Schizophr Bull 2010;36:71–93.

6. World Federation of Societies of Biological Psychiatry Guidelines of Biological Treatment of Schizophrenia. World J Biol Psychiatry 2005;6(3):132–191.

7. Lieberman JA, Stroup TS, McEvoy JP, et al., for the Clinical Antipsychotic Trials of Intervention Effectiveness (CATIE) Investigators. Effectiveness of antipsychotic drugs in patients with chronic schizophrenia. N Engl J Med 2005;353:1209–1223.

8. American Psychiatric Association. Schizophrenia spectrum and other psychotic disorders. In: Diagnostic and Statistical Manual of Mental Disorders, 5th ed. Washington, DC, American Psychiatric Association, 2013:87–122.

9. American Diabetes Association, American Psychiatric Association, American Association of Clinical Endocrinologists, and North American Association for the Study of Obesity. Consensus Development Conference on Antipsychotic Drugs and Obesity and Diabetes. Diabetes Care 2004;27:596–601.

ADDITIONAL RESOURCES

1. Sharma T, Mockler D. The cognitive efficacy of atypical antipsychotics in schizophrenia. J Clin Psychopharmacol 1998;18(Suppl 1):12S–19S.

2. Gopalakrishna G, Aggarwal A, Lauriello J. Long-acting injectable aripiprazole: how might it fit in our tool box? Clin Schizophr Relat Psychoses 2013;7(2):87–92. doi:10.3371/CSRP.GOAG.043013.

3. Citrome L. Paliperidone Palmitate—review of efficacy, safety and cost of new second-generation depot antipsychotic medication. Int J Clin Pract 2011;65:189–210.

4. Citrome L. A review of the pharmacology, efficacy and tolerability of recently approved and upcoming oral antipsychotics: an evidence-based medicine approach. CNS Drugs 2013;27(11):879–911.

5. Clinical Pharmacology Research Institute at Indiana University. Flockhart DA. P450 drug interaction: abbreviated "clinically relevant" table. Available at: *http://medicine.iupui.edu/clinpharm/ddis/table.asp*. Accessed March 25, 2016.

6. Preskorn SH. Clinically important differences in the pharmacokinetics of the ten newer atypical antipsychotics: part 2. Metabolism and elimination. J Psychiatr Pract 2012;18:361–366.

78

MAJOR DEPRESSION

A Life Worth Living . . . . Level I

Brian L. Crabtree, PharmD, BCPP

Lydia E. Weisser, DO, MBA

LEARNING OBJECTIVES

After completing this case study, the reader should be able to:

- Identify the signs and symptoms of depression.

- Develop a pharmacotherapy plan for a patient with depression.

- Compare side-effect profiles of various antidepressant drugs.

- Discuss pharmacoeconomic considerations that must be taken into account when selecting antidepressant therapy.

PATIENT PRESENTATION

■ Chief Complaint

"I don't know if I can handle this anymore."

■ HPI

Geneva Flowers is a 41-year-old woman who is referred by her family physician to an outpatient mental health clinic. She complains of feeling down and sad, with crying spells, trouble sleeping, increased eating, impaired concentration, and fatigue. She has not worked in over 2 months and has used up her vacation and sick leave from work.

She went through treatment for alcohol use disorder over a year ago. Things were going fairly well for her after her treatment and she remarried approximately 8 months ago. Arguments with her teenage sons about family issues and past incidents have made her increasingly depressed over the past few months. Her older son, 17, moved out to live with his father. Her younger son, 12, moved to live with his paternal grandparents.

She divorced the boys' father after approximately 10 years of marriage when she discovered that he was having an affair with another woman. She left her second husband after approximately 2 years because of problems involving his children that caused increasing conflict with her then-husband. Without a second income in the household, she accumulated large credit card debts. She began drinking and soon developed a pattern of using alcohol to relieve stress. Just before entering alcoholism treatment, there was a sexual fondling incident involving one of her son's friends while the friend was visiting her son at her house, but she was amnestic for the incident the next day. Her present husband, her third, has been supportive of her, but she feels guilty about her failed previous marriages and her sons, worries about her debt, and has become more despondent. She has taken a leave of absence from her job as an administrative assistant at an elementary school.

The patient sought treatment for depression 3 months ago from her family physician, who prescribed mirtazapine. Her spirits have not improved, and she says the medication made her gain weight. Because of vague references that the physician believed could possibly indicate suicidal ideas, she has been referred for psychiatric evaluation.

■ PMH

Childhood illnesses: she has had all of the usual childhood illnesses. She was hospitalized at age 3 for bacterial meningitis but knows of no residual effects.

Adult illnesses: no current nonpsychiatric adult illnesses; no previous psychiatric treatment.

Trauma: fractured arm due to bicycle accident at age 9, otherwise unremarkable.

Surgeries: Hx childbirth by C-section; tonsillectomy at age 6.

Travel: no significant travel history.

Diet: no dietary restrictions. Despite not having much of an appetite, reports eating more since taking mirtazapine.

Exercise: no regular exercise program.

Immunizations: no personal records of childhood vaccinations; had tetanus booster 9 years ago; does not remember when she had most recent influenza immunization.

■ FH

Father is deceased, had coronary artery disease, but ultimately died of colon cancer. Mother has well-controlled HTN. A sister has depression and anxiety, takes antidepressant medication (patient does not know its name). A second sister committed suicide.

■ SH

High school graduate; works as an administrative assistant but on leave for approximately 2 months. Married approximately 8 months, two previous divorces. Lived with husband and sons until sons moved out in the last few weeks. Health insurance is through the school district where she is employed; includes adjusted copay on prescriptions. Reports heavy credit card debt. Attended church regularly in the past (Protestant), but not recently. Attends AA weekly.

Denies drinking alcohol since chemical dependence treatment. Denies smoking. Drinks three to four cups of caffeinated coffee per day; usually drinks iced tea with evening meal; drinks colas as leisure beverage. Used marijuana a few times after high school, denies use in more than 10 years; denies present or past use of other illicit substances.

■ Meds

Mirtazapine 30 mg PO QHS (started on mirtazapine 15 mg PO QHS approximately 3 months ago)

Ortho-Novum 1/35-28, one PO daily; has not taken for 2 months

St. John's wort 300 mg PO TID for the past 2 weeks at suggestion of husband (purchased at health food store)

Acetaminophen 1000–1500 mg PO PRN headaches, two or three times a week

Uses OTC antihistamines and decongestants for colds or allergies; none in recent months

■ All

NKDA

■ ROS

General appearance: pt c/o feeling tired much of the time

HEENT: wears contact lenses; no tinnitus, ear pain, or discharge; no c/o nasal congestion; Hx of dental repair for caries

Chest: no Hx of asthma or other lung disease

CV: reports occasional feelings of "pounding heart"; no Hx of heart disease

GI: reports infrequent constipation; takes MOM PRN; has gained 9 lb in last 2 months

GU: has regular menses; LMP ended a week ago

Neuromuscular: occasional headaches, worse over the past few months; no syncope, vertigo, weakness or paralysis, numbness or tingling

Skin: no complaints

■ Physical Examination

Performed by nurse practitioner

Gen

Overweight WF, slightly unkempt

VS

BP 132/78 mm Hg, P 88 bpm, RR 22, T 36.9°C; Wt 187 lb, Ht 5′8″

Skin

Normal skin, hair, and nails

HEENT

PERRLA; EOM intact, no nystagmus. Fundus—disks sharp, no retinopathy; no nasal discharge or nasal polyps; TMs gray and shiny bilaterally; minor accumulation of cerumen.

Neck/Lymph Nodes

Supple without thyromegaly or lymphadenopathy

Chest/Lungs

Frequent sighing during examination, but no tachypnea or SOB; chest CTA

Breasts

No masses, tenderness, or discharge

Heart

RRR without murmur

Abd

Soft, nontender; (+) BS; no organomegaly

Genit/Rect

Deferred

Ext

Unremarkable

Neuro

CN: EOM intact, no nystagmus, no weakness of facial or tongue muscles. Casual gait normal. Finger-to-nose normal.

Motor: normal symmetric grip strength. DTRs 2+ and equal.

Sensory: intact bilaterally.

Mental Status

When seen in the clinic, the patient is pale and appears moderately overweight, dressed in casual slacks and sweater. Grooming is fair and without makeup. She speaks slowly, often not responding to questions for approximately 30 seconds before beginning answers. She describes depressed mood and lack of energy and says she feels no pleasure in life. Her husband is good to her, but she feels everyone else she loves has left her. She has no social contacts other than occasional visits by her parents. She spends most of her time in bed. She feels worthless and blames herself for her problems. She feels particularly anguished about the incident with her son's friend even though she does not remember it. She is often anxious and worries about the future. She wonders if her sons love her and if they will ever return. She worries how she will repay her financial debts. Her speech is logical, coherent, and goal-oriented. She denies suicidal intent but says the future seems dim to her, and she wonders sometimes if life is worth living. She admits she sometimes wishes she could just go to sleep and not wake up. She denies hallucinations. Paranoid delusions, FOI, IOR, and LOA are absent. There is no dysarthria or anomia.

■ Labs (Collected 11:45 AM)

Na 139 mEq/L	Hgb 14.0 g/dL	AST 34 IU/L
K 4.2 mEq/L	Hct 46.2%	ALT 42 IU/L
Cl 102 mEq/L	MCV 92 μm³	GGT 38 IU/L
CO$_2$ 24 mEq/L	MCH 29 pg	T. bili 0.8 mg/dL
BUN 12 mg/dL	Plt 234 × 10³/mm³	T. prot 7.0 g/dL
SCr 0.9 mg/dL	WBC 7.3 × 10³/mm³	Alb 4.4 g/dL
Glu 98 mg/dL	Segs 49%	CK 57 IU/L
Ca 9.5 mg/dL	Bands 1%	T$_4$ 8.6 mcg/dL
Mg 1.7 mEq/L	Lymphs 42%	T$_3$ uptake 29%
Uric acid 4.0 mg/dL	Monos 2%	TSH 2.8 mIU/L
	Eos 6%	

■ UA

Glucose (–); ketones (–); pH 5.8; SG 1.016; bilirubin (–); WBC 1/hpf, protein (–), amorphous—rare, epithelial cells 1/hpf; color yellow; blood (–), RBC 0/hpf; mucus—rare; bacteria—rare; casts 0/lpf; appearance clear

■ Assessment

Major depressive disorder, single episode, with melancholic features

■ Plan

Refer for support group, psychotherapy; begin antidepressant medication

QUESTIONS

Problem Identification

1.a. Create a list of this patient's drug therapy problems.

1.b. What signs, symptoms, and laboratory values indicate the presence and severity of depression in this patient?

1.c. What factors in the family history support a diagnosis of depression?

1.d. Is there anything in the patient's medication history that could cause or worsen depression?

Desired Outcome

2. What are the goals of pharmacotherapy in this case?

Therapeutic Alternatives

3.a. What nonpharmacologic treatments are important in this case? Should nonpharmacologic treatments be tried before beginning medication?

3.b. What pharmacotherapeutic options are available for the treatment of depression?

Optimal Plan

4.a. What drug regimen (drug, dosage, schedule, and duration) is best for this patient?

4.b. How should the patient be advised about the herbal therapy, St. John's wort?

4.c. What alternatives would be appropriate if the patient fails to respond to initial therapy?

Outcome Evaluation

5. What clinical and laboratory parameters are necessary to evaluate the therapy for efficacy and adverse effects?

Patient Education

6. What information should be provided to the patient to enhance adherence, ensure successful therapy, and minimize adverse effects?

■ CLINICAL COURSE: ALTERNATIVE THERAPY

Mrs Flowers understands that she must stop the St. John's wort she has been taking because of an interaction with her prescribed mirtazapine and Ortho-Novum, but she wonders if it would have been helpful if she had started it when she first began feeling depressed. See Section 19 in this Casebook for questions about the use of St. John's wort for treatment of depression.

■ SELF-STUDY ASSIGNMENTS

1. The selective serotonin reuptake inhibitor (SSRI) antidepressants are commonly used and have the same serotonin reuptake pharmacology; contrast the agents in this class, considering relative side effects, dosing, and drug interactions.

2. Compare other antidepressants with SSRIs with regard to adverse effects and relative advantages and disadvantages.

3. Discuss the role of combination drug therapy in the treatment of depression, including the use of drugs not usually classified as antidepressants.

4. Review the medical literature and evaluate the scientific evidence for the efficacy of St. John's wort in the treatment of depression.

CLINICAL PEARL

Although SSRIs are of one pharmacologic class, they are not of one chemical class. Therefore, failure to respond to one SSRI does not reliably predict failure to respond to others.

REFERENCES

1. American Psychiatric Association. Depressive disorders. In: Diagnostic and Statistical Manual of Mental Disorders, 5th ed. Washington, DC, American Psychiatric Association, 2013:155–188.

2. Teter CJ, Kando JC, Wells BG. Major depressive disorder. In: DiPiro JT, Talbert RL, Yee GC, et al, eds. Pharmacotherapy: A Pathophysiologic Approach, 9th ed. New York, NY, McGraw Hill, 2014:1047–1066.

3. Cuijpers P, Dekker J, Hollon SD, Anderson G. Adding psychotherapy to pharmacotherapy in the treatment of depressive disorders in adults: a meta-analysis. J Clin Psychiatry 2009;70:1219–1229.

4. Linde K, Kriston L, Rucker G, et al. Efficacy and acceptability of pharmacological treatments for depressive disorders in primary care: systematic review and network meta-analysis. Ann Fam Med 2015;13:69–79.

5. Spina E, Santoro V, D'Arrigo C. Clinically relevant pharmacokinetic drug interactions with second-generation antidepressants: an update. Clin Ther 2008;30:1206–1227.

6. Perry PJ. Pharmacotherapy for major depression with melancholic features: relative efficacy of tricyclic versus selective serotonin reuptake inhibitor antidepressants. J Affect Disord 1996;39:1–6.

7. Bishop JR, Stevenson JM, Burghardt KJ. Pharmacogenetics in mental health. In: Johnson JA, Ellingrod VL, Kroetz DL, Kuo GM, eds. Pharmacogenomics: Application to Patient Care, 3rd ed. Lenexa, KS, American College of Clinical Pharmacy, 2015:115–134.

79

BIPOLAR DISORDER

Up All Night . . . . Level II

Jason M. Noel, PharmD, BCPP

LEARNING OBJECTIVES

After completing this case study, the reader should be able to:

• Given a description of a patient case, identify and assess the symptoms of an acute episode of bipolar disorder.

• Recommend appropriate pharmacotherapy for patients with acute mania.

• Generate parameters for monitoring anticonvulsant therapy for bipolar disorder.

• Identify the pharmacotherapeutic options for treating the subtypes of bipolar disorder.

PATIENT PRESENTATION

▓ Chief Complaint

"I am trying to keep the evil spirits away!"

▓ HPI

Tyler Clemens is a 28-year-old man brought by the police to the Crisis Center for an emergency evaluation. According to neighbors who called the police, the patient has been acting increasingly strange. The lights in the house are left on all night, and loud music is played at all hours. Last evening, he dug a trench around his front yard with an electric lawn edger and filled it with various herbal plants. This evening, he hung wreaths and horseshoes on his front door and threw many of his belongings into his yard and the street. When approached by neighbors, he apparently began screaming and preaching at them. When the police arrived, they found the patient standing naked on the dining room table in his front yard preaching. When the police approached, he began throwing garlic cloves at them and screaming, "I refuse to let you all curse me in my own home." He became increasingly hostile during the arrest shouting, "You can't do this – I have rights!" He then tried to bite one of the officers.

PMH

Manic episodes first occurred while he was in college, leading to psychiatric admissions at ages 21 and 23 for acute mania. Patient was treated with haloperidol and lithium, with adequate response and discharged on both occasions after about a month. Adherence to outpatient treatment has been inconsistent, with several documented missed appointments and prescription refills.

He also receives outpatient treatment for migraine headaches and shift work disorder.

Patient Interview

Patient is disheveled with pungent body odor. He is pacing the room, waving his hands in the air and preaching in an elated, loud, sing-songy voice. He is wearing a dirty t-shirt and jeans. When asked how he felt, he stated, "Playful, with intense clarity, sharp, spiffy, and clean." He then became hostile and angry, insisting that he be discharged before sunrise or he would "be tormented by the demons forever." He claims to have witnessed spirits that attached themselves to various people and that now control their thoughts and actions. He spoke in long run-on sentences with many political, religious, and sexual references. He was very difficult to interrupt. For example, at one point he stated, "Can't you see, or are you an idiot?! I am being persecuted by the evil spirits I must stop them now and if you don't get that, you're an idiot."

When asked about his sleep, he angrily replied, "Would you sleep at a time like this? If I sleep, this whole town will be taken over! I cannot allow that to happen." The patient stated that he has not been eating and has not taken his lithium in several days because, "Lithium is of the ground, the underworld. The Lord will sustain me." When his interviewers challenged him on these beliefs, he suspected them of being part of plot to undermine his mission. When told that he might need to be in the hospital so we can help him with his problems, he screamed, "You can't help me! You're nonbelievers."

Abnormal Involuntary Movements

Excessive eye blinking and mild grimacing; unclear whether abnormal (patient states this is the "demon blood trying to take over my body"). He is bothered by it in that to him, it represents his "sinful nature."

FH

Father has a history of depression; paternal grandmother was placed in an "asylum" for hysteria secondary to childbirth. Mother and brother have type 2 diabetes.

SH

Recently fired from his job as a nursing assistant at a local hospital, where he worked the night shift on a "7 on/7 off" schedule. Patient states that he drinks "only occasionally," but he was noted to be intoxicated, with a BAC 0.14%, on a previous admission.

Meds

Haloperidol 5 mg PO daily
Lithium carbonate 600 mg PO twice daily
Acetaminophen/butalbital/caffeine two tablets PO as needed for headaches
Modafinil 200 mg PO at 9 PM for shift work disorder

All

NKDA

ROS

Migraine headaches about twice a month, no aura, (+) nausea and photophobia. Occasional GI upset with no clear relationship to meals or time of day; frequent loose stools.

Physical Examination

VS

BP 118/73 mm Hg, P 83 bpm, RR 16, T 37.1°C; Wt 94 kg, Ht 5'2"

HEENT

PERRLA; EOMI; fundi benign; throat and ears clear; TMs intact; rapid eye blinking and facial grimacing (may indicate early tardive dyskinesia)

Skin

Psoriasis evident on both elbows

Neck

Supple, bite mark, no nodes

Lungs

CTA & P

CV

RRR; S_1, S_2 normal; no MRG

Abd

(+) BS, nontender

Ext

Full ROM, pulses 2+ bilaterally

Neuro

A & O × 3; reflexes symmetric; toes downgoing; normal gait; normal strength; sensation intact; CNs II–XII intact

Labs

See Table 79-1.

TABLE 79-1	Lab Values			
Na 141 mEq/L	Hgb 14.6 g/dL	WBC 12.0 × 10³/mm³	AST 32 IU/L	Ca 9.7 mg/dL
K 3.8 mEq/L	Hct 45.7%	Neutros 67%	ALT 21 IU/L	Phos 5.3 mg/dL
Cl 103 mEq/L	RBC 4.73 × 10⁶/mm³	Lymphs 23%	Alk phos 87 IU/L	TSH 4.1 µIU/mL
CO₂ 24 mEq/L	MCV 90.2 µm³	Monos 7%	GGT 46 IU/L	RPR: neg
BUN 19 mg/dL	MCH 31 pg	Eos 2%	T. bili 0.9 mg/dL	Lithium 0.1 mEq/L
SCr 1.1 mg/dL	MCHC 34.4 g/dL	Basos 1%	Alb 3.7 g/dL	
Glu 89 mg/dL	Plt 256 × 10³/mm³		T. chol 218 mg/dL	

UA

Color yellow; appearance slightly cloudy; glucose (–), bili (–), ketones trace; SG 1.025, blood (–), pH 6.0, protein (–), nitrites (–), leukocyte esterase (–)

Diagnoses

Bipolar I disorder, Current episode manic, With psychotic features
Migraine headaches
Shift work disorder

QUESTIONS

Problem Identification

1.a. List the manic symptoms present in this patient based on DSM-5 diagnostic criteria for his bipolar disorder diagnosis.

1.b. Identify possible triggers for this patient's acute episode.

1.c. What data in this case can be used to assess the severity of the current episode.

1.d. Create a list of this patient's drug therapy problems.

Desired Outcome

2. List the subjective and objective parameters that can be used to determine response to treatment.

Therapeutic Alternatives

3.a. What nondrug therapies might be useful for this patient?

3.b. What feasible pharmacotherapeutic alternatives are available for treatment of bipolar disorder? Specify whether they are appropriate for acute mania.

Optimal Plan

4.a. What drug, dosage form, dose, schedule, and duration of therapy are best for this patient?

4.b. What alternatives would be appropriate if the initial therapy fails or cannot be used?

Outcome Evaluation

5. Which clinical and laboratory parameters are necessary to evaluate response to therapy and to detect or prevent adverse effects?

Patient Education

6. What information should be provided to the patient to enhance adherence, ensure successful therapy, and minimize adverse effects?

■ SELF-STUDY ASSIGNMENTS

1. Perform a literature search and explore the anticonvulsants that are not specifically approved for use in bipolar disorder (eg, gabapentin, oxcarbazepine, and topiramate) in the treatment of bipolar disorder.

2. Standardized rating scales are often used in clinical trials and occasionally in clinical practice to quantify the presence of symptoms in people with psychiatric disorders and drug-induced movement disorders. Perform a Web search for each of the following rating scales. For each scale, determine the symptom domains measured, the overall score ranges, and severity score cutoff ranges (e.g., mild, moderate, and severe).

Mania:

Young Mania Rating Scale (YMRS)

Depression

Hamilton Depression Rating Scale (HAM-D)

Montgomery–Åsberg Depression Rating Scale (MADRS)

Movement Disorders

Abnormal Involuntary Movement Scale (AIMS)

Dyskinesia Identification System: Condensed User Scale (DISCUS)

CLINICAL PEARL

When a patient admitted with acute mania is taking activating drugs such as antidepressants or stimulants, those drugs should be tapered and withdrawn. In some patients, antidepressants and stimulants may activate mania or increase the rate of cycling, and potentially delay response to antimanic/mood stabilizers.

REFERENCES

1. Bipolar and Related Disorders [Internet]. In: Diagnostic and Statistical Manual of Mental Disorders, 5th ed. Arlington, VA, American Psychiatric Association; 2013. Available at: *http://dx.doi.org/10.1176 /appi.books.9780890425596.dsm03*. Accessed March 30, 2016.

2. Hirschfeld RM, Baker JD, Wozniak P, et al. The safety and early efficacy of oral-loaded divalproex versus standard-titration divalproex, lithium, olanzapine, and placebo in the treatment of acute mania associated with bipolar disorder. J Clin Psychiatry 2003;64:841–846.

3. Calabrese JR, Sullivan JR, Bowden CL, et al. Rash in multicenter trials of lamotrigine in mood disorders: clinical relevance and management. J Clin Psychiatry 2002;63:1012–1019.

4. Suppes T, Dennehy E, Hirschfeld R, et al. The Texas Implementation of Medication Algorithms. J Clin Psychiatry 2005;66:870–886.

5. Perlis R, Ostacher M, Patel J, et al. Predictors of recurrence in bipolar disorder: primary outcomes from the Systematic Treatment Enhancement Program for Bipolar Disorder (STEP-BD). Am J Psychiatry 2006;163:217–224.

6. Yatham L, Kennedy S, Parikh S, et al. Canadian Network for Mood and Anxiety Treatments (CANMAT) and International Society for Bipolar Disorders (ISBD) collaborative update of CANMAT guidelines for the management of patients with bipolar disorder: update 2013. Bipolar Disorders 2012;15(1):1–44.

7. NICE. Bipolar disorder: assessment and management. NICE Clinical Guideline 2014. Available at: *nice.org.uk/guidance/cg185.*

8. Hirschfeld R, Bowden C, Gitlin M, et al. Practice guideline for the treatment of patients with bipolar disorder (revision). Am J Psychiatry 2002;159(4 Suppl):1–50. Available at: *http://dx.doi.org/10.1176 /foc.1.1.64.* Accessed April 19, 2016.

9. McElroy SL, Keck PE, Tugrul KC, et al. Valproate as a loading treatment in acute mania. Neuropsychobiology 1993;27:146–149.

10. Sachs GS, Nierenberg AA, Calabrese JR, et al. Effectiveness of adjunctive antidepressant treatment for bipolar depression. N Engl J Med 2007;356:1711–1722.

11. Goodwin GM, Bowden CL, Calabrese JR. A pooled analysis of 2 placebo-controlled 18-month trials of lamotrigine and lithium maintenance in bipolar I disorder. J Clin Psychiatry 2004;65:432–441.

80

GENERALIZED ANXIETY DISORDER

Nervous Neddie . . . . Level I

Sarah T. Melton, PharmD, BCPP, BCACP, CGP, FASCP

Cynthia K. Kirkwood, PharmD, BCPP

LEARNING OBJECTIVES

After completing this case study, the reader should be able to:

- Identify target symptoms associated with generalized anxiety disorder (GAD).

- Construct pharmacotherapeutic goals for GAD.

- Recommend appropriate pharmacotherapy and duration of treatment for the acute, continuation, and maintenance phases of GAD.

- Develop a plan to educate patients and consult with providers about the pharmacotherapy used in the treatment of GAD.

- Develop a monitoring plan for a patient treated for GAD based on the treatment regimen.

PATIENT PRESENTATION

■ Chief Complaint

"I am so worried all the time that I can't do anything else. I need some serious help."

■ HPI

Ned Johnson is a 55-year-old man who presents to his family physician with complaints of severe irritability, feelings of "being on edge," and inability to fall asleep at night. He states that he always feels tense and exhausted with constant muscle tension and body aches. He was laid off from his job as a manager at a building supply store 9 months ago. Over the past year, he has had difficulty concentrating when filling out job application forms, and his mind often "goes blank" when talking with people. His irritability has impacted his relationship with his wife, and he is worried that she will leave him. He has developed frequent abdominal pain and daily episodes of diarrhea. He constantly worries about the lack of financial resources, his wife losing her job, and his relationship with his wife. He is afraid that he and his wife will lose their house and cars. He states that he cannot control his constant worry and that his anxiety has increased in intensity over the past 6 months. He denies having obsessive–compulsive thoughts or behaviors or symptoms of panic disorder. He recently went to the emergency department because he was so worried about multiple issues in his life that he could not eat or sleep for 2 days. He was given an IM injection of hydroxyzine and sent home with a prescription for hydroxyzine 25-mg capsules orally four times daily as needed for anxiety. He stopped this medication last week secondary to constipation and decreased urinary flow. He tried kava kava from a herbal store a few months ago.

It was not effective, and he discontinued it after 2 weeks because of severe abdominal pain.

■ PMH

Records from the family physician indicate frequent visits over the past 9 months for insomnia, headaches, abdominal pain, and diarrhea. He has been treated with buspirone for anxiety for the past 6 months.

After a recent visit to the ED, he was prescribed hydroxyzine to be taken up four times daily as needed for anxiety.

Past psychiatric history is significant for episode of depression and alcohol abuse when he was 33 years old, that was treated with fluoxetine. He took the fluoxetine for 2 weeks and discontinued it secondary to insomnia.

■ FH

Father, 80 years old, on "nerve medication" for several years. Mother deceased at age 73 from breast cancer with history of major depression and alcohol abuse. Patient has one sister who has been treated with multiple medications in the past for anxiety and depression and was treated for benzodiazepine abuse 5 years ago.

■ SH

Married for 25 years; no children; high school graduate; past tobacco user (quit 5 years ago with 40 pack-year history); past alcohol abuse (has been sober for 10 years and attends Alcoholics Anonymous on a weekly basis); little exercise because of time constraints; drinks four to five cups of coffee per day, and three to four Mountain Dew soft drinks throughout the day. He admits to occasional marijuana use when his anxiety is "out of control." (Note: marijuana is not legal for medical or recreational use in his state.) He does not have any prescription drug coverage at this time.

■ Meds

Buspirone 30 mg PO BID for anxiety
Phenylephrine 10 mg PO QID PRN nasal congestion
Loperamide 2 mg PO Q 6 H PRN diarrhea

■ All

Sulfa (hives); codeine (nausea)

■ ROS

Positive only for paresthesias and mild diaphoresis; negative for dizziness, palpitations, SOB, chest pain

■ Physical Examination

Gen

Nervous, well-groomed man sitting on examination table; cooperative; oriented × 3

VS

BP 125/85 mm Hg, P 90 bpm, RR 18, T 36.5°C; Wt 90 kg, Ht 5'11"

Skin

Clammy; no rashes, lesions, or track marks

HEENT

EOMI; PERRLA; fundi benign; ear and nose clear; dentition intact; tonsils 1+

Neck/Lymph Nodes

Supple, no lymphadenopathy; thyroid symmetric and of normal size

Lungs/Chest

Symmetric chest wall movement; BS equal bilaterally; no rub; clear to A & P

CV

RRR, normal S_1 and S_2, no MRG

Abd

Symmetric; NTND; normal BS; no organomegaly or masses

Genit/Rect

Deferred

MS/Ext

Average frame; normal bones, joints, and muscles

Neuro

CNs II–XII intact; motor and sensory grossly normal; coordination intact

MSE

Appearance and behavior: well groomed, fair eye contact, wringing hands, and bouncing legs
Speech: well spoken and coherent with normal rate and rhythm
Mood: anxious, worried about everything in his life, and concerned that he is very sick
Affect: full
Thought processes: linear, logical, and goal-directed
Thought content: negative for suicidal or homicidal ideations, obsessions/compulsions, delusions, or hallucinations
Memory: 3/3 at 0 minutes, 2/3 at 5 minutes; spelled "world" backward
Abstractions: good
Judgment: good by testing
Insight: fair
Score on Hamilton Anxiety Scale = 34 points (see Appendix A)

■ Labs

Na 142 mEq/L	Hgb 14.0 g/dL
K 4.3 mEq/L	Hct 38%
Cl 105 mEq/L	TSH 3 mIU/L
CO_2 28 mEq/L	AST 23 IU/L
BUN 15 mg/dL	ALT 20 IU/L
SCr 0.9 mg/dL	Alk phos 23 IU/L
Glu 80 mg/dL	Vit D 25-OH 51 ng/mL

■ ECG

NSR; rate 88 bpm

■ Urine Toxicology Screen

Positive for 9-carboxy-THC

■ Assessment

GAD

QUESTIONS

Problem Identification

1.a. Create a list of the patient's drug therapy problems.

1.b. Is there anything in the patient's medication history that could cause or worsen anxiety?

1.c. What information (signs, symptoms, and laboratory values) indicates the presence or severity of GAD?

Desired Outcome

2. What are the goals of pharmacotherapy in this case?

Therapeutic Alternatives

3.a. What nondrug therapies might be useful for this patient?

3.b. What feasible pharmacotherapeutic alternatives are available for the treatment of GAD?

Optimal Plan

4.a. What drug, dosage form, dose, schedule, and duration of therapy are best for this patient?

4.b. What pharmacotherapeutic alternatives would be appropriate if the optimal plan fails or cannot be used?

Outcome Evaluation

5. What clinical and laboratory parameters are necessary to evaluate the therapy for achievement of the desired therapeutic outcome and to detect or prevent adverse effects?

Patient Education

6. What information should be provided to the patient to enhance adherence, ensure successful therapy, and minimize adverse effects?

■ CLINICAL COURSE: ALTERNATIVE THERAPY

Mr Johnson is still worried about both the side effects of prescription drugs to treat his anxiety and whether he will be able to afford them. He states that he has read a lot of information about kava that "it really works for anxiety." Mr Johnson says, "Maybe I was just using a bad product last time I tried it and that's why it didn't help much and hurt my stomach. Should I get a better product and try it again?" Please see Section 19 of this Casebook for questions about the use of kava kava for the treatment of GAD.

■ SELF-STUDY ASSIGNMENTS

1. Perform a literature search to review the role of atypical antipsychotics in the treatment of GAD. Write a summary of the controlled trials that evaluated the use of atypical antipsychotics in GAD as adjunctive agents or monotherapy.

2. Individuals with GAD may misuse alcohol, cannabis, or other substances in an effort to ameliorate their anxiety. Review and summarize the recommendations put forth by the International Psychopharmacology Algorithm Project on treating patients with GAD and a history of or current substance abuse.

3. Many patients with mental illness do not have prescription drug insurance coverage and this impacts the choice of pharmacotherapy. Using this case example, go to a Web-based patient assistance program and document how you would go about helping this patient obtain a first-line agent that he otherwise would not be able to afford (eg, escitalopram, duloxetine, venlafaxine extended-release capsules).

CLINICAL PEARL

With effective pharmacotherapy available for the acute and long-term therapy of GAD, the treatment goal for anxiety is remission. Many patients exhibit treatment response but still have anxiety symptoms and social and functional impairment. Remission is a more rigorous treatment goal that requires a HAM-A score of ≤7 or reduction of at least 70% in baseline levels of symptoms.

REFERENCES

1. Hamilton M. Hamilton Anxiety Scale. In: Guy W, ed. ECDEU Assessment Manual for Psychopharmacology. Rockville, MD, U.S. Department of Health, Education, Welfare, 1976:193–198.
2. Baldwin DS, Anderson IM, Nutt DJ, et al. Evidence-based pharmacological treatment of anxiety disorders, post-traumatic stress disorder and obsessive–compulsive disorder: a re-vision of the 2005 guidelines from the British Association for Pharmacology. J Psychopharmacol 2014;28:403–439.
3. Davidson JR, Zhang W, Connor KM, et al. A psychopharmacological treatment algorithm for generalized anxiety disorder (GAD). J Psychopharmacol 2010;24:3–26.
4. Zhang Y, Huang G, Yang S, Liang W, Zhang L, Wang C. Duloxetine in treating generalized anxiety disorder in adults: a meta-analysis of published randomized, double-blind, placebo-controlled trials. Asia Pac Psychiatry 2015. doi:10.1111/appy.12203.
5. Bandelow B, Sher L, Bunevicius R, et al. Guidelines for the pharmacological treatment of anxiety disorders, obsessive–compulsive disorder and posttraumatic stress disorder in primary care. Int J Psychiatry Clin Pract 2012;16:77–84.
6. Frampton JE. Pregabalin: a review of its use in adults with generalized anxiety disorder. CNS Drugs 2014;28:835–854.
7. Maneeton N, Maneeton B, Woottiluk P, et al. Quetiapine monotherapy in acute treatment of generalized anxiety disorder: a systematic review and meta-analysis of randomized controlled trials. Drug Des Devel Ther 2016;10:259–276.
8. Sarris J, LaPorte E, Schweitzer I. Kava: a comprehensive review of efficacy, safety, and psychopharmacology. Aust N Z J Psychiatry 2011;45:27–35.

APPENDIX A

The results of the HAM-A Scale (ECDEU version)[1] for this patient:

Mark and score as follows: 0, not present; 1, mild; 2, moderate; 3, severe; 4, very severe

Anxious mood

___4___ Worries, anticipation of the worst, fearful anticipation, irritability

Tension

___3___ Feelings of tension, fatigability, startle response, moved to tears easily, trembling, feelings of restlessness, inability to relax

Fears

___1___ Of dark, of strangers, of being left alone, of animals, of traffic, of crowds

Insomnia

___4___ Difficulty in falling asleep, broken sleep, unsatisfying sleep and fatigue on waking, dreams, nightmares, night terrors

Intellectual

___3___ Difficulty in concentration, poor memory

Depressed mood

___1___ Loss of interest, lack of pleasure in hobbies, depression, early waking, diurnal swing

Somatic (muscular)

___3___ Pains and aches, twitchings, stiffness, myoclonic jerks, grinding of teeth, unsteady voice, increased muscular tone

Somatic (sensory)

___1___ Tinnitus, blurring of vision, hot and cold flushes, feelings of weakness, pricking sensation

Cardiovascular symptoms

___2___ Tachycardia, palpitations, pain in chest, throbbing of vessels, fainting feelings, sighing, dyspnea

Respiratory symptoms

___1___ Pressure or constriction in chest, choking feelings, sighing, dyspnea

Gastrointestinal symptoms

___3___ Difficulty in swallowing, wind, abdominal pain, burning sensations, abdominal fullness, nausea, vomiting, borborygmi, looseness of bowels, loss of weight, constipation

Genitourinary symptoms

___2___ Frequency of micturition, urgency of micturition, amenorrhea, menorrhagia, development of frigidity, premature ejaculation, loss of libido, impotence

Autonomic symptoms

___3___ Dry mouth, flushing, pallor, tendency to sweat, giddiness, tension, headache, raising of hair

Behavior at interview

___3___ Fidgeting, restlessness or pacing, tremor of hands, furrowed brow, strained face, sighing or rapid respiration, facial pallor, swallowing, etc.

Total score: ___34___

81

OBSESSIVE–COMPULSIVE DISORDER

Five Is the Magic Number........................Level I

Cynthia K. Kirkwood, PharmD, BCPP

Sarah T. Melton, PharmD, BCPP, BCACP, CGP, FASCP

LEARNING OBJECTIVES

After completing this case study, the reader should be able to:

- Identify target symptoms associated with obsessive–compulsive disorder (OCD).

- Construct goals of pharmacotherapy for OCD.

- Develop an appropriate plan and duration of therapy for the management of OCD.

- Counsel patients and consult with providers about the pharmacotherapy used for OCD.

- Develop a monitoring plan for a patient treated for OCD based on the treatment regimen.

PATIENT PRESENTATION

■ Chief Complaint

"I am so afraid that I'm going to hurt my child."

■ HPI

Sonya Reed is a 30-year-old woman presenting to her family physician accompanied by her mother after threatening to overdose on Benadryl. The patient has complaints of anxiety and feelings of unease that were increasing in severity over the past 2 weeks to the point that she had thoughts of killing herself. She reports having intrusive thoughts of throwing her 2-year-old child down the stairs. Because these thoughts are becoming more frequent, she feels she is a bad mother and may actually harm her child. She recently started checking all appliances in the house multiple times during the day to make sure they are turned off because she fears starting a fire that will injure the child. At first, she incessantly checked on the toddler but now is beginning to avoid the child because of her fears. She states that she knows that these thoughts are irrational. She is concerned because the checking behavior consumes 2–3 hours each day. She stopped going out with the child last week because she has to check and recheck the car seat safety belts so often that she usually does not make it to her destination. She also reports rubbing her arm in multiples of five to feel some relief from the overwhelming anxiety that develops throughout the day from the intrusive thoughts. She states that she has tried to hide this behavior from her parents, but it has become so time-consuming and distressful that she felt the only way out was to overdose. She now regrets ever thinking about killing herself.

■ PMH

$G_2P_1A_1$—normal spontaneous vaginal delivery

Obesity

Kidney stone at age 25 years

Dental surgery 2 months ago

■ PPH

No hospitalizations or outpatient psychiatric treatment, but she recalls from childhood doing strange counting rituals while lying in bed or watching TV. She has always felt a need to "control things."

■ FH

Father, 68 years old, with history of major depression. Mother, 65 years old, with multiple sclerosis. Older brother is a "perfectionist" and has to have everything "just right."

■ SH

Divorced for 7 years and recently broke up with boyfriend of 2 years about a month ago; degree in hotel restaurant management and works part-time at a local hotel; denies tobacco use but admits to occasional alcohol use. After her son was born, she had excessive worrying that the baby was starving because he was not getting enough breast milk. She does not have prescription coverage.

■ Meds

Multivitamin, one PO daily

Acetaminophen 500 mg PO PRN headaches (patient uses one to two times per month)

Diphenhydramine 25 mg PO PRN insomnia (patient uses three to four times per month)

■ All

Sulfa (hives), adhesive bandages

■ ROS

Unremarkable except patient reports that she feels she is "going insane" and has guilt over her obsessions. Patient denies fatigue, change in appetite, sleep pattern, difficulty concentrating, and crying spells. No palpitations or dyspnea.

■ Physical Examination

Gen

Anxious, obese woman sitting on examination table rubbing her arm up and down, cooperative, oriented × 3

VS

BP 120/75 mm Hg, P 90 bpm, RR 19, T 36.5°C; Wt 80.3 kg, Ht 5′4″

Skin

Left arm red and slightly inflamed from elbow to wrist; no rashes, lesions, or track marks. Warm to touch

HEENT

EOMI; PEERLA; fundi benign; ear and nose clear; dentition intact; tonsils 1+

Neck/Lymph Nodes

Supple, no lymphadenopathy; thyroid symmetric and of normal size

Lungs/Chest

Symmetric chest wall movement, BS equal bilaterally, no rub; clear to A & P

Breasts

Normal, expecting menstruation

CV

RRR, normal S_1 and S_2, no MRG

Abd

Symmetric; NT/ND; normal BS; no organomegaly or masses

Gyn

Normal hair distribution and external genitalia; normal urethra; parous cervix with no lesions or discharge; uterus normal; no adnexal masses or tenderness

MS/Ext

Small frame; normal bones, joints, muscles

Neuro

CNs II–XII intact; motor and sensory grossly normal; coordination intact; no tremor

MSE

Appearance and behavior: well groomed, poor eye contact, rubbing arm up and down in a slow methodical manner
Speech: well spoken, coherent with normal rate and rhythm
Mood: anxious, worried that she is a "bad mother"
Affect: anxious, frightened
Thought processes: linear, logical, and goal-directed
Thought content: negative for suicidal or homicidal ideations; positive for obsessions about harming her child; compulsions including checking and rubbing arm in multiples of five; denies delusions and hallucinations
Memory: 3/3 at 0 minutes, 3/3 at 5 minutes (ball, pencil, chair); spelled "world" backward
Abstractions: fair
Judgment: good by testing
Insight: good
Score on Yale–Brown Obsessive Compulsive Scale = 30 points

■ **Labs**

Na 140 mEq/L	Hgb 15.0 g/dL
K 3.7 mEq/L	Hct 40%
Cl 107 mEq/L	TSH 2.8 mIU/L
CO_2 28 mEq/L	AST 28 IU/L
BUN 14 mg/dL	ALT 25 IU/L
SCr 0.8 mg/dL	Alk phos 42 IU/L
Glu 75 mg/dL	HCG negative

■ **ECG**

NSR; rate 88 bpm

■ **Urine Toxicology Screen**

Negative

■ **Drug Levels**

Acetaminophen 10 mcg/mL

■ **Assessment**

OCD

■ **Plan**

Start paroxetine 20 mg PO daily

QUESTIONS

Problem Identification

1.a. Create a list of the patient's drug therapy problems.

1.b. What information (signs, symptoms, and laboratory values) indicates the presence or severity of OCD?

Desired Outcome

2. What are the goals of pharmacotherapy for OCD in this case?

Therapeutic Alternatives

3.a. What are the most appropriate nonpharmacologic therapies for this patient?

3.b. What pharmacotherapeutic alternatives are available for the treatment of OCD?

Optimal Plan

4.a. What drug, dosage form, dose, schedule, and duration of therapy are best for this patient?

4.b. What pharmacotherapeutic alternatives would be appropriate if the optimal plan fails?

4.c. When is a patient with OCD considered to be "treatment-refractory?" What other pharmacologic alternatives are available if this patient is determined to be refractory to standard pharmacotherapy?

Outcome Evaluation

5. Which clinical and laboratory parameters are necessary to evaluate the therapy for achievement of the desired therapeutic outcomes and to detect or prevent adverse effects?

Patient Education

6. What information should be provided to the patient to enhance adherence, ensure successful therapy, and minimize adverse effects?

■ FOLLOW-UP QUESTIONS

1. When is a decrease in the Y-BOCS score considered clinically significant?

2. If this patient had presented to the physician desiring to become pregnant after 6 months of pharmacotherapy, what would your recommendations be regarding pharmacotherapy?

■ SELF-STUDY ASSIGNMENTS

1. Prepare a grid contrasting the pros and cons of each SSRI in the management of OCD.

2. Perform a literature search and write a short paper describing the symptoms of hoarding disorder and the association with OCD. How is this disorder treated?

3. Discuss the pharmacotherapeutic agents used to augment antidepressant monotherapy in the treatment of OCD in patients who have a partial response.

4. Visit the Web site for the International OCD Foundation and review the patient brochure "What You Need to Know about Obsessive–Compulsive Disorder," especially the section on children and teens with OCD.

CLINICAL PEARL

Higher dosages of antidepressant medication than those typically used for depression are often required to obtain antiobsessional effects. A response to pharmacotherapy may not occur until a therapeutic dose has been maintained for at least 10–12 weeks.

REFERENCES

1. Goodman WK, Price LH, Rasmussen SA, et al. The Yale–Brown Obsessive Compulsive Scale I. Development, use, and reliability. Arch Gen Psychiatry 1989;46:1006–1011.

2. American Psychiatric Association. Practice Guideline for the Treatment of Patients with Obsessive–Compulsive Disorder. Arlington, VA, American Psychiatric Association, 2007. Available at: *http://psychiatryonline.org/pb/assets/raw/sitewide/practice_guidelines/guidelines/ocd.pdf*. Accessed March 30, 2016.

3. Koran LM, Simpson HB. Guideline watch (March 2013): Practice guideline for the treatment of patients with obsessive–compulsive disorder. Available at: *http://psychiatryonline.org/pb/assets/raw/sitewide/practice_guidelines/guidelines/ocd-watch.pdf*. Accessed March 30, 2016.

4. Fineberg NA, Reghunandanan S, Simpson HB, et al. Obsessive-compulsive disorder (OCD): practical strategies for pharmacological and somatic treatment in adults. Psychiatry Res 2015;227:114–125.

5. Baldwin DS, Anderson IM, Nutt DJ, et al. Evidence-based pharmacological treatment of anxiety disorders, post-traumatic stress disorder, and obsessive–compulsive disorder: a revision of the 2005 guidelines from the British Association for Psychopharmacology. J Psychopharmacol 2014;28:403–439.

6. Matsunaga H, Nagata T, Hayashida K, Ohya K, Kiriike N, Stein DJ. A long-term trial of the effectiveness and safety of atypical antipsychotic agents in augmenting SSRI-refractory obsessive–compulsive disorder. J Clin Psychiatry 2009;70:863–868.

7. ACOG Practice Bulletin. Clinical management guidelines for obstetrician–gynecologists number 92, April 2008 (replaces practice bulletin number 87, November 2007). Use of psychiatric medications during pregnancy and lactation. Obstet Gynecol 2008;111:1001–1020.

8. Alwan S, Friedman JM, Chambers C. Safety of selective serotonin reuptake inhibitors in pregnancy: review of the evidence. CNS Drugs 2016. doi:10.1007/s40263-016-0338-3.

9. Reefhuis J, Devine O, Friedman JM, Louik C, Honein MA. Specific SSRIs and birth defects: Bayesian analysis to interpret new data in the context of previous reports. BMJ 2015;351:h3190. doi:10.1136/bmj.h3190.

10. Berle JO, Spigset O. Antidepressant use during breastfeeding. Curr Womens Health Rev 2011;7:28–34.

82

INSOMNIA

Poor Adherence and Poor Sleep . . . . Level II

Mollie Ashe Scott, PharmD, BCACP, CPP

Amy M. Lugo, PharmD, BCPS, BC-ADM, FAPhA

LEARNING OBJECTIVES

After completing this case study, the reader should be able to:

- Identify the psychosocial, disease-related, and drug-induced causes of insomnia.

- Explain the impact of poor medication adherence on chronic illnesses.

- Educate a patient regarding nonpharmacologic treatments for insomnia.

- Design a therapeutic plan for the treatment of insomnia.

PATIENT PRESENTATION

■ Chief Complaint

"I can't sleep."

■ HPI

Jenny Moore is a 42-year-old woman who is referred by her family medicine physician to a Pharmacotherapy Clinic for medication therapy management for insomnia. She receives help paying for her medications from medication assistance programs. She reports that she is unable to sleep at all during the week and then sleeps all day on Sunday. Ms Moore is currently taking temazepam 30 mg daily at bedtime that was recently increased from 15 mg. She is also experiencing depression due to an abusive relationship with her boyfriend as well as lack of current employment. Her most recent Patient Heath Questionnaire-9 (PHQ-9) result was 20. She admits to being nonadherent to her medication regimen. She reports that she is no longer able to see her psychiatrist due to cost of the visits.

■ PMH

Insomnia for many years
COPD
Depression
Migraine headaches
GERD
Allergic rhinitis

■ FH

Mother is alive and well and lives nearby. Father died of an MI at age 65.

■ SH

Single, lives with her abusive boyfriend. Unemployed, but receives some money from her mother. She smokes approximately five cigarettes per day, but has smoked up to two ppd in the past. She denies alcohol use. She sees a deacon at her church for counseling. She receives medication assistance for several of her medications from a local agency.

■ Medications

Temazepam 30 mg PO QHS PRN sleep
Fluticasone/salmeterol DPI 250/50, one inhalation BID
Albuterol MDI, two puffs Q 6 H PRN SOB
Tiotropium Handihaler, one inhalation daily
Citalopram 20 mg PO Q AM
Olanzapine 3 mg/fluoxetine 25 mg PO Q PM
Sumatriptan 100 mg PO PRN migraine
Atenolol 25 mg PO Q AM for migraine prophylaxis
Dexlansoprazole 60 mg PO Q AM
Ibuprofen 200–400 mg PO Q 6 H PRN pain
Tramadol 50 mg PO Q 6 H PRN pain
Pseudoephedrine 30 mg PO Q 6 H PRN allergies

■ Allergies

NKDA

■ ROS

Patient reports that she does not sleep during the week and only sleeps on Sunday. She reports poor sleep hygiene, because she reads and watches television in bed. She drinks six to eight cups of coffee throughout the day and really does not pay attention to how late she eats or exercises. Patient reports difficulty going to sleep and staying asleep, and reports having had this problem for several years. Additionally, the temazepam does not seem to help much. She has a long history of depression but has never been hospitalized. She currently denies a "blue mood" or any thoughts of suicide, and her PHQ-9 score today is 20. She is prescribed citalopram and the combination olanzapine/fluoxetine to help with her depressive symptoms. Her COPD is secondary to a long history of smoking but is currently controlled on tiotropium, fluticasone/salmeterol, and albuterol PRN. She has experienced migraine headaches for several years and uses sumatriptan and ibuprofen PRN and atenolol daily for prophylaxis. Her GERD, which she experiences when she is supine, is currently controlled on dexlansoprazole. She has runny nose, congestion, and itchy eyes in the spring.

■ Physical Examination (From the Last Visit With Her PCP)

Gen

Obese woman in NAD who looks her stated age

VS

BP 125/80 mm Hg, P 76 BPM, RR 16, T 37°C; Wt 105 kg; Ht 5′6″

Skin

Normal skin color and turgor, no lesions noted

HEENT

Normocephalic, PERRLA, EOMI

Neck/Lymph Nodes

Supple with normal size thyroid, (–) adenopathy

Lungs

CTA bilaterally

CV

Normal S_1, S_2; no MRG

Abd

NTND, no HSM

Genit/Rect

Deferred. Last PAP smear was WNL 6 months ago.

Ext

No C/C/E; normal muscle bulk and tone; muscle strength 5/5 and equal in all extremities; normal pulses

Neuro

Oriented to person, place, and time; CN II–XII intact; Mini-Mental State Examination results: 30/30

■ Labs

Na 140 mEq/L	Hgb 14 g/dL	AST 34 IU/L	*Lipid panel*
K 4.2 mEq/L	Hct 43%	ALT 32 IU/L	TC 212 mg/dL
Cl 105 mEq/L	RBC 4.7×10^6/mm³	LDH 112 IU/L	LDL 135 mg/dL
CO₂ 28 mEq/L	Plt 262×10^3/mm³	GGT 47 IU/L	HDL 45 mg/dL
BUN 11 mg/dL	WBC 6.2×10^3/mm³	T. bili 0.3 mg/dL	TG 160 mg/dL
SCr 0.8 mg/dL	TSH 3.9 mIU/L	T. prot 7.1 g/dL	
Glu 82 mg/dL	Free T₄ 4.1 ng/dL	Alb 4.0 g/dL	

■ Assessment

1. Insomnia uncontrolled with temazepam, poor sleep hygiene

2. Depression

3. Migraine headaches

4. COPD, currently controlled

5. GERD, currently controlled

6. Nonadherence

7. Allergic rhinitis

8. Obesity

9. Health maintenance

QUESTIONS

Problem Identification

1.a. Create a drug-related problem list for the patient.

1.b. Which information (signs, symptoms, laboratory values) indicates the presence or severity of insomnia?

1.c. Could any of the patient's problems have been caused by drug therapy?

1.d. What additional information is needed to satisfactorily assess this patient's insomnia?

Desired Outcome

2. What are the goals of pharmacotherapy in this case?

Therapeutic Alternatives

3.a. What nonpharmacologic therapies might be useful for this patient's insomnia?

3.b. What feasible pharmacotherapeutic alternatives are available for treatment of insomnia?

3.c. What economic, psychosocial, cultural, and ethical considerations are applicable to this patient?

Optimal Plan

4.a. What drug, dosage form, dose, schedule, and duration of therapy are best for this patient's insomnia?

4.b. What alternatives would be appropriate if the initial therapy fails or cannot be used?

Outcome Evaluation

5. Which clinical and laboratory parameters are necessary to evaluate the therapy for achievement of the desired therapeutic outcome and to detect or prevent adverse effects?

Patient Education

6. What information should be provided to the patient to enhance adherence, ensure successful therapy, and minimize adverse effects?

■ FOLLOW-UP QUESTION

1. What other medication adjustments should be made at this time?

■ SELF-STUDY ASSIGNMENTS

1. Discuss clinical pharmacy interventions that can improve medication adherence.

2. Explain important monitoring parameters for patients receiving atypical antipsychotics.

CLINICAL PEARL

Patients with underlying depression frequently have insomnia, and poor medication adherence to antidepressants can exacerbate sleep disorders.

REFERENCES

1. Morin A, Jarvis C, Lynch A. Therapeutic options for sleep-maintenance and sleep-onset insomnia. Pharmacotherapy 2007;27:89–110.

2. National Sleep Foundation. Healthy sleep tips. Available at: *http://www.sleepfoundation.org/article/sleep-topics/healthy-sleep-tips*. Accessed March 29, 2016.

3. Maness DL, Khan M. Nonpharmacologic management of chronic insomnia. Am Fam Physician 2015;92:1058–1064.

4. The American Geriatrics Society 2015 Beers Criteria Update Expert Panel. American Geriatrics Society 2015 Updated Beers Criteria for Potentially Inappropriate Medication Use in Older Adults. The American Geriatrics Society 2015 Beers Criteria Update Expert Panel. J Am Geriatr Soc 2015;63:2227–2246.

5. US Food and Drug Administration Center for Drug Evaluation and Research. Sleep Disorder (Sedative–Hypnotic) Drug Information. Available at: *http://www.fda.gov/Drugs/DrugSafety/PostmarketDrugSafetyInformationforPatientsandProviders/ucm101557.htm*. Accessed April 22, 2016.

6. U.S. Food and Drug Administration. FDA Drug Safety Communication: FDA warns of next-day impairment with sleep aid Lunesta (eszopiclone) and lowers recommended dose. Available at: *http://www.fda.gov/Drugs/DrugSafety/ucm397260.htm*. Accessed May 1, 2016.

7. Melatonin. Natural Medicines [database online]. Stockton, CA, Therapeutic Research Center; 2016. Accessed April 22, 2016.

8. Patel KV, Aspesi AV, Evoy KE. Suvorexant: a dual orexin receptor antagonist for the treatment of sleep onset and sleep maintenance insomnia. Ann Pharmacother 2015;49:477–483.

9. Hanlon JT, Semla TP, Schmader KE. Alternative medications for medications in the use of high-risk medications in the elderly and potentially harmful drug–disease interactions in the elderly quality measures. J Am Geriatr Assoc 2015;63:e8–e18.

10. Kripke DF, Langer RD, Kline LE. Hypnotics' association with mortality or cancer: a matched cohort study. BMJ Open 2012. doi:10.1136/bmjopen-2012-000850.

83

TYPE 1 DIABETES MELLITUS AND KETOACIDOSIS

Disconnected . . . . Level II

Holly S. Divine, PharmD, BCACP, CGP, CDE, FAPhA

Carrie L. Isaacs, PharmD, CDE

LEARNING OBJECTIVES

After completing this case study, the reader should be able to:

- Recognize signs and symptoms of diabetic ketoacidosis (DKA).

- Determine laboratory parameters for the diagnosis and monitoring of DKA.

- Identify anticipated fluid and electrolyte abnormalities associated with DKA and their treatment.

- Recommend appropriate insulin therapy for treating DKA.

- Identify therapeutic decision points in DKA treatment and provide parameters for altering therapy at those points.

PATIENT PRESENTATION

■ Chief Complaint

"I felt weak and nauseated during softball practice. I checked my blood glucose and it read 'HI.'"

■ HPI

Mary McGee is a 21-year-old woman with a history of type 1 diabetes, diagnosed 3 years ago. She is a college senior at the local university where she also plays softball. She started using an insulin pump approximately 6 months ago.

She noticed she was unusually tired and short of breath at the beginning of her practice and then began feeling weak and nauseated. She was also very thirsty during practice. Her softball coach said she seemed "a little confused." He advised her to check her blood glucose and it read (HI). She checked her insulin pump and noticed the pump had become disconnected. She is unsure how long she has been without insulin. She vomited two times since shortly thereafter and was transported via EMS to the ED.

■ PMH

Type 1 DM diagnosed 3 years ago

■ FH

Parents are alive and healthy. One twin sister who also has type 1 DM.

■ SH

College student; no tobacco, alcohol, or illicit drug use

■ Meds

NovoLog 100 U/mL, per insulin pump
Basal rates:
    0.6 units/hour 0000–0300
    0.9 units/hour 0300–0700
    0.8 units/hour 0700–1100
    0.7 units/hour 1100–1730
    0.8 units/hour 1730–0000
Correction factor: 1 U:40 mg/dL >120 mg/dL
Insulin:carbohydrate ratios:
    1:10 insulin:carbohydrate before breakfast
    1:15 insulin:carbohydrate before lunch and dinner
Glucagon injection kit, as needed

■ Allergies

NKDA

■ ROS

Complains of blurry vision, lethargy, shortness of breath, nausea, polyuria, and polydipsia. Denies constipation, diarrhea, and headache.

■ Physical Examination

Gen

WDWN Caucasian female appearing her stated age, with deep respirations, ketones on her breath, and slurred speech; slightly confused, but responds appropriately to questions

VS

BP 101/72 mm Hg, P 123 bpm, RR 32, T 37.0°C; Wt 56 kg, Ht 5'6"

Skin

Unremarkable

HEENT

PERRLA, EOMI; mucous membranes are dry

Neck/Lymph Nodes

Supple without lymphadenopathy or thyromegaly

Lungs

CTA, Kussmaul respirations

CV

S_1 and S_2 are normal without S_3, S_4, murmur or rub; RRR

Abd

NT/ND

Genit/Rect

Deferred

MS/Ext

No edema, pulses 2+ throughout, mild calluses

Neuro

A & O × 3; DTRs 2+ throughout; feet with normal sensation and vibration

■ Labs

Na 136 mEq/L	WBC $15.0 \times 10^3/mm^3$
K 4.8 mEq/L	RBC $4.61 \times 10^6/mm^3$
Cl 101 mEq/L	Hgb 14.2 g/dL
CO_2 10 mEq/L	Hct 40.7%
BUN 23 mg/dL	Platelets $239 \times 10^3/mm^3$
SCr 1.4 mg/dL	Ketones positive
Glu 479 mg/dL	

■ ABG

pH 7.26; $PaCO_2$ 21 mm Hg; PaO_2 128 mm Hg; HCO_3 7.1 mEq/L; O_2 sat 97%

■ UA

(+) Ketones; (+) glucose

■ Chest X-Ray

Normal

■ ECG

Sinus tachycardia

■ Assessment

DKA precipitated by insulin deficiency

QUESTIONS

Problem Identification

1.a. What signs, symptoms, and laboratory findings indicate the presence and severity of DKA in this patient?

1.b. What are the precipitating risk factors for DKA, and which of those risk factors are present in this patient?

1.c. What are the diagnostic criteria for DKA?

1.d. What problems need to be addressed in DKA besides hyperglycemia?

Desired Outcome

2. What are the goals of therapy for this patient?

Therapeutic Alternatives

3. What therapies are available to correct the metabolic derangements of DKA?

Optimal Plan

4. Design a pharmacotherapeutic plan to resolve this patient's DKA.

Outcome Evaluation

5.a. What monitoring is necessary for the therapeutic plan that you developed for the patient?

5.b. If the blood glucose does not fall by at least 10% in the first hour, what is the appropriate next therapeutic step? What changes in the therapeutic regimen should be considered when the blood glucose drops below 200 mg/dL?

5.c. At what point is the DKA considered to be resolved, and when can IV insulin therapy be converted to subcutaneous therapy?

5.d. Outline a plan for converting the patient from IV to subcutaneous insulin after resolution of the DKA.

Patient Education

6. What additional counseling or interventions should occur with this patient regarding prevention of future DKA?

■ SELF-STUDY ASSIGNMENTS

1. What does the ADA state about DKA and hyperosmolar hyperglycemic state (HHS) in patients with type 2 DM? Compare these two disorders with respect to prevention, precipitating causes, signs and symptoms, pathophysiology, and treatment.

2. Investigate other causes of DKA, such as illness, and write a sick day management plan for this patient.

CLINICAL PEARL

DKA is the second most common complication seen with insulin pump therapy. Young persons who have recurrent DKA should be evaluated for psychological problems, including eating disorders, as a potential contributing factor.

REFERENCES

1. Kitabchi AE, Umpierrez GE, Miles JM, Fisher JN. Hyperglycemic crises in adult patients with diabetes. Diabetes Care 2009;32:1335–1343.
2. Wilson JF. In clinic. Diabetic ketoacidosis. Ann Intern Med 2010;152:ITC 1–1 to ITC 1–16.
3. American Diabetes Association Standards of Medical Care in Diabetes-2016. Diabetes Care 2016;39(Suppl 1):S1–S112.
4. American Association of Clinical Endocrinologists and American College of Endocrinology—Clinical Practice Guidelines for Developing a Diabetes Mellitus Comprehensive Care Plan-2015. Endocr Pract 2015;21(Suppl 1):1–87.
5. Duhon B, Attridge RL, Franco-Martinez AC, Maxwell PR, Hughes DW. Intravenous sodium bicarbonate therapy in severely acidotic diabetic ketoacidosis. Ann Pharmacother 2013;47:970–975.
6. Potti LG, Haines ST. Continuous subcutaneous insulin infusion therapy: a primer on insulin pumps. J Am Pharm Assoc 2009;49:e1–e17.
7. Scheiner G, Sobel RJ, Smith DE, et al. Insulin pump therapy: guidelines for successful outcomes. Diabetes Educ 2009;35(Suppl 2):29S–41S.

84

TYPE 2 DIABETES MELLITUS: NEW ONSET

The Candy Man................................ Level II

Nicole C. Pezzino, PharmD

Scott R. Drab, PharmD, CDE, BC-ADM

Deanne L. Hall, PharmD, CDE, BCACP

LEARNING OBJECTIVES

After completing this case study, the reader should be able to:

- Recognize the signs, symptoms, and risk factors associated with type 2 diabetes mellitus (DM).

- Identify the comorbidities in type 2 DM associated with insulin resistance (metabolic syndrome).

- Compare the pharmacotherapeutic options in the management of type 2 DM including mechanism of action, contraindications, and side effects.

- Describe the role of self-monitoring of blood glucose (SMBG), and identify factors to enhance patient adherence.

- Develop a patient-specific pharmacotherapeutic plan for the treatment and monitoring of type 2 DM.

PATIENT PRESENTATION

■ Chief Complaint

"My vision has been blurred lately and it seems to be getting worse."

■ HPI

Alfonso Giuliani is a 68-year-old man who presents to his family physician's office complaining of periodic blurred vision for the past month. He further complains of fatigue and lack of energy that prohibits him from working in his garden.

■ PMH

HTN × 18 years
Dyslipidemia × 8 years
Gouty arthritis × 16 years with complicated course of uric acid urolithiasis
Hypothyroidism × 15 years
Overweight × 25 years

■ FH

Diabetes present in mother. Immigrated to the United States with his mother and sister after their father died suddenly from unknown causes at age 45. One younger sibling died of breast cancer at age 48.

■ SH

Retired candy salesman, married × 46 years with three children. No tobacco use. Drinks one to two glasses of homemade wine with meals. He reports adherence with his medications.

■ Meds

Lisinopril 20 mg PO once daily
Allopurinol 300 mg PO once daily
Levothyroxine 0.088 mg PO once daily

■ All

NKDA

■ ROS

Occasional polydipsia, polyphagia, fatigue, weakness, and blurred vision. Denies chest pain, dyspnea, tachycardia, dizziness or light-headedness on standing, tingling or numbness in extremities, leg cramps, peripheral edema, changes in bowel movements, GI bloating or pain, nausea or vomiting, urinary incontinence, or presence of skin lesions.

■ Physical Examination

Gen

The patient is a centrally obese, Caucasian man who appears to be restless and in mild distress

VS

BP 124/76 mm Hg without orthostasis, P 80 bpm, RR 18, T 37.2°C; Wt 77 kg, Ht 66″; BMI 27.4 kg/m^2

Skin

Dry with poor skin turgor; no ulcers or rash

HEENT

PERRLA; EOMI; TMs intact; no hemorrhages or exudates on funduscopic examination; mucous membranes normal; nose and throat clear w/o exudates or lesions

Neck/LN

Supple; without lymphadenopathy, thyromegaly, or JVD

CV

RRR; normal S_1 and S_2; no S_3, S_4, rubs, murmurs, or bruits

Lungs

CTA

Abd

Soft, NT, central obesity; normal BS; no organomegaly or distention

Genit/Rect

Normal external male genitalia

Ext

Normal ROM and sensation; peripheral pulses 2+ throughout; no lesions, ulcers, or edema

Neuro

A & O × 3, CN II–XII intact; DTRs 2+ throughout; feet with normal vibratory and pinprick sensation (5.07/10 g monofilament)

Labs

Na 141 mEq/L	Ca 9.9 mg/dL	A1C 7.8%
K 4.0 mEq/L	Phos 3.2 mg/dL	*Fasting lipid profile*
Cl 96 mEq/L	AST 21 IU/L	T. chol 280 mg/dL
CO_2 22 mEq/L	ALT 15 IU/L	HDL 27 mg/dL
BUN 24 mg/dL	Alk phos 45 IU/L	LDL 193 mg/dL
SCr 1.1 mg/dL	T. bili 0.9 mg/dL	Trig 302 mg/dL
Random Glu 202 mg/dL		

UA

(–) Ketones, (–) protein, (–) microalbuminuria

Assessment

1. Elevated random glucose and A1C, diagnostic for type 2 DM, new onset

2. Dyslipidemia requiring treatment

3. HTN apparently well controlled

4. Overweight

5. Gouty arthritis; patient claims not to have had an acute attack in over 3 years; will obtain a uric acid level to evaluate

6. Hypothyroidism; will obtain a thyroid panel to evaluate

Clinical Course

The patient returned to clinic 3 days later for lab work, which revealed: TSH 1.8 mIU/L, free T_4 1.2 ng/dL, UA 1.2 mg/dL, and FBG 157 mg/dL

QUESTIONS

Problem Identification

1.a. What risk factors for type 2 DM are present in this patient?

1.b. What information (signs, symptoms, and laboratory values) supports the diagnosis of type 2 DM?

1.c. What information indicates the presence of insulin resistance?

1.d. Create a list of this patient's drug therapy problems.

Desired Outcome

2.a. What are the desired goals for the treatment of this patient's diabetes?

2.b. Considering his other medical problems, what other treatment goals should be established?

Therapeutic Alternatives

3.a. What nonpharmacologic therapies might be useful in the management of this patient?

3.b. What feasible pharmacotherapeutic alternatives are available for the treatment of this patient's DM? Identify the factors that will influence your choice of initial therapy.

Optimal Plan

4.a. Outline a complete pharmacotherapeutic plan to manage this patient's current problems including drug, dosage form, dose, schedule, and rationale for your selections.

4.b. What changes in therapy would you recommend if your initial plan fails to achieve adequate glycemic control?

Outcome Evaluation

5.a. What clinical and laboratory parameters will you monitor to evaluate glycemic efficacy and to detect or prevent adverse effects?

5.b. The patient's physician suggested that he obtain a blood glucose meter for self-testing. What are the healthcare provider's responsibilities with respect to patients and SMBG?

5.c. Identify at least four potential situations in which the information provided by SMBG would be useful to patients and healthcare providers.

5.d. What factors should be considered in the selection of an appropriate blood glucose meter?

Patient Education

6.a. What information should be provided to the patient about diabetes and its treatment to enhance adherence, ensure successful therapy, minimize adverse effects, and prevent future complications?

6.b. How would you educate the patient regarding how and when to check his blood glucose?

■ CLINICAL COURSE: ALTERNATIVE THERAPY

While discussing Mr Giuliani's diagnosis with him, he states that his neighbor with diabetes told him that she just follows her diabetic diet and takes cinnamon and something called "alip acid" and does not have to take any prescriptions for her blood sugar. He also says that he has read about fish oil being used for diabetes. Mr Giuliani asks if he should start any of those to help get his blood sugar under control. See Section 19 in this Casebook for questions about the use of fish oil, cinnamon, and alpha-lipoic acid for treatment of diabetes.

■ FOLLOW-UP QUESTIONS

1. Which nonprescription products could be recommended for patients to use in treating hypoglycemic episodes?

2. List several potential sources of error in SMBG.

3. When starting patients on insulin, the use of combination oral antihyperglycemic agents and insulin offers several advantages over switching entirely to insulin:

   (a) What are the advantages of adding insulin to existing therapies with oral agents?

   (b) List an appropriate method of starting insulin therapy to adequately control fasting hyperglycemia in patients on combination oral agents.

■ SELF-STUDY ASSIGNMENTS

1. Describe how you would evaluate and monitor this patient's quality of life.

2. Characterize the relationship between insulin resistance and the risk for ASCVD.

3. Prepare a list of medications that have been associated with increasing blood glucose. Provide literature evidence on the strength of the association with each medication.

4. Review the literature and conduct a comparative review of the efficacy of inhaled insulin therapy relative to the insulin products commercially available for subcutaneous injection.

CLINICAL PEARL

Approximately 29 million Americans have diabetes, and approximately one-third are undiagnosed. Approximately 1.4 million Americans are diagnosed with diabetes every year, providing further evidence that diabetes is a major public health threat of epidemic proportions. Excess caloric intake, low physical activity, and increasing levels of obesity are the main contributors to the increased incidence.

REFERENCES

1. American Diabetes Association. Standards of Medical Care in Diabetes—2016. Diabetes Care 2016;39(1 Suppl):S1–S112.
2. Bloomgarden ZT. Insulin resistance: current concepts. Clin Ther 1998;20:216–231.
3. American College of Endocrinology and American Association of Clinical Endocrinologists. Clinical Practice Guidelines for Developing a Diabetes Mellitus Comprehensive Care Plan—2015. Endocr Pract 2015;21(Suppl 1).
4. American College of Endocrinology and American Association of Clinical Endocrinologists. Consensus Statement on the Comprehensive Type 2 Diabetes Management Algorithm—2016 Executive Summary. Endocr Pract 2016;22(No 1).
5. American College of Cardiology/American Heart Association. 2013 ACC/AHA Guideline on the Treatment of Blood Cholesterol to Reduce Atherosclerotic Cardiovascular Risk in Adults. Circulation [published corrections] 2014;129(25 Pt B):2889–2934.
6. Avandia Prescribing Information. Research Triangle Park, NC, GlaxoSmithKline, May, 2011.
7. Inzucchi SE, Bergenstahl RM, Buse JB, et al. Management of hyperglycemia in type 2 diabetes: a patient-centered approach: position statement of the American Diabetes Association (ADA) and the European Association for the Study of Diabetes (EASD). Diabetes Care 2012;35(6):1364–1379.
8. Inzucchi SE, Bergenstahl RM, Buse JB, et al. Management of hyperglycemia in type 2 diabetes: a patient-centered approach: position statement of the American Diabetes Association (ADA) and the European Association for the Study of Diabetes (EASD): update to a Position Statement of the ADA and EASD for the Study of Diabetes. Diabetes Care 2015;38:140–149.
9. Cho TM, Wideman RD, Kieffer TJ. Clinical application of glucagon-like peptide 1 receptor agonists for the treatment of type 2 diabetes mellitus. Endocrinol Metab 2013;28:262–274.
10. Zinmann B, Wanner C, Lachin JM, et al. Empagliflozin, cardiovascular outcomes, and mortality in type 2 diabetes. N Engl J Med 2015;373:2217–2128.

85

TYPE 2 DIABETES MELLITUS: EXISTING DISEASE

Establishing Optimal Control . . . . Level II

Sharon B. S. Gatewood, PharmD, FAPhA

Margaret A. Robinson, PharmD

LEARNING OBJECTIVES

After completing this case study, the reader should be able to:

- Identify the goals of therapy for the treatment of type 2 diabetes mellitus (DM).

- Discuss the risk factors and comorbidities associated with type 2 DM.

- Compare options for drug therapy management of type 2 DM, including mechanisms of action, combination therapies, comorbidities, and patient-friendly treatment plans.

- Develop an individualized drug therapy management plan, including dosage regimens, therapeutic endpoints, and monitoring parameters.

- Provide patient education regarding medications and the importance of adhering to the treatment plan, monitoring the disease state, maintaining blood glucose control, and seeking advice from healthcare providers when necessary.

PATIENT PRESENTATION

■ Chief Complaint

"I have had diabetes for about six months and would like to have my blood sugar tested. I think that my blood sugar is running low because I have a terrible headache."

■ HPI

Sarah Martin is a 45-year-old woman who comes to the pharmacy for a diabetes education class taught by the pharmacist. She would like for the pharmacist to check her blood sugar before the class begins. She was diagnosed with type 2 DM about 6 months ago. She had been attempting to control her disease with diet and exercise, but had no success. Her physician started her on metformin 1000 mg twice daily with food about 3 months ago. She has gained 10 lb over the past year. She monitors her blood sugar once a day, and her results have ranged from 215 to 280 mg/dL. Her fasting blood sugars have averaged 200 mg/dL.

■ PMH

Type 2 DM × 6 months
HTN × 17 years
Bipolar disorder × 25 years
Dyslipidemia × 12 years
Morbid obesity × 20 years

■ FH

Father has a history of HTN, dyslipidemia, and bipolar disorder. Mother has a history of dyslipidemia and hypothyroidism. Brother has DM thought to be secondary to alcoholism.

■ SH

Has been married for 23 years. She has two children who are teenagers and one child in college. She works as a sales associate in the electronics department of a local mass merchandiser. She denies any use of tobacco products after stopping smoking 10 years ago, but does drink alcohol occasionally (three beers or glasses of wine per week).

■ Meds

Metformin 1000 mg PO BID with food
Lisinopril 20 mg PO once daily
Zyprexa 5 mg PO QHS
Carbamazepine ER 200 mg PO BID
Lorazepam 1 mg PO TID PRN
Fluoxetine 20 mg PO Q AM
Pravastatin 40 mg PO once daily

■ All

Penicillin—hives

ROS

Complains of nocturia, polyuria, and polydipsia on a daily basis. Denies nausea, constipation, diarrhea, signs or symptoms of hypoglycemia, paresthesias, and dyspnea.

Physical Examination

Gen

WDWN severely obese, white woman in NAD

VS

BP 154/90 mm Hg, P 98 bpm, RR 18, T 37.0°C; Wt 109 kg, Ht 5′8″, waist circ 38 in

HEENT

PERRLA, EOMI, R & L fundus exam without retinopathy

Neck/Lymph Nodes

No LAN

Lungs

CTA & P

CV

RRR, no m/r/g

Abd

NT/ND

Genit/Rect

Deferred

MS/Ext

Carotids, femorals, popliteals, and right dorsalis pedis pulses 2+ throughout; left dorsalis pedis 1+; feet show mild calluses on MTPs

Neuro

DTRs 2+ throughout, feet with normal sensation (5.07 monofilament) and vibration

Labs

Na 138 mEq/L	Ca 9.4 mg/dL	*Fasting lipid profile*
K 3.7 mEq/L	Phos 3.3 mg/dL	T. chol 244 mg/dL
Cl 103 mEq/L	AST 16 IU/L	LDL 141 mg/dL
CO₂ 31 mEq/L	ALT 19 IU/L	HDL 58 mg/dL
BUN 16 mg/dL	Alk phos 62 IU/L	Trig 225 mg/dL
SCr 0.9 mg/dL	T. bili 0.4 mg/dL	TC/HDL ratio 4.2
Glu (random) 243 mg/dL	A1C 10.0%	

UA

1+ protein, (+) microalbuminuria

Assessment

The patient reports that she exercises at most once a week and her diet is difficult to maintain due to being busy with her children's schedules and having an erratic eating schedule at both work and home. Her glycemic control has worsened from an A1C of 8.9% 6 months ago. She has had a moderate weight gain of 10 lb over the past year. Her blood pressure and cholesterol are not at goal on the current drug therapy. Her bipolar disorder is controlled on the current drug therapy. When the patient is in a depression or manic phase, she tends to use food to "treat" the symptoms.

QUESTIONS

Problem Identification

1.a. What are this patient's drug therapy problems?

1.b. What findings indicate poorly controlled diabetes in this patient?

Desired Outcome

2.a. What are the goals of treatment for type 2 DM in this patient?

2.b. What individual patient characteristics should be considered in determining the treatment goals?

Therapeutic Alternatives

3.a. What nonpharmacologic interventions should be recommended for this patient's drug therapy problems?

3.b. What pharmacologic interventions could be considered for this patient's drug therapy problems?

Optimal Plan

4. What pharmacotherapeutic regimen would you recommend for each of the patient's drug therapy problems?

Outcome Evaluation

5. What parameters should be monitored to evaluate the efficacy and possible adverse effects associated with the optimal regimens you selected?

Patient Education

6. What information should be given to the patient regarding DM, HTN, dyslipidemia, bipolar disorder, obesity, and her treatment plan to increase adherence, minimize adverse effects, and improve outcomes?

■ FOLLOW-UP QUESTION

1. What alternative therapies might be appropriate if the initial plan for diabetes treatment fails?

■ SELF-STUDY ASSIGNMENTS

1. Discuss the phenomenon known as the metabolic syndrome and the role that insulin resistance is postulated to play in its sequelae.

2. Explore and discuss the importance of monitoring postprandial blood glucose levels and its impact on overall glucose control, A1C levels, and progression of diabetes complications.

3. Research the various blood glucose monitors available, and compare, among available monitors, the features that meet the needs of individual patients and improve adherence to testing regimens.

4. Research new therapies for diabetes and discuss their potential role in the management of patients with type 2 DM.

5. Keep a food diary, including carbohydrate counting for each meal, and exercise log for 1 week. Evaluate and discuss your experience from the viewpoint of a patient with type 2 DM.

6. Investigate continuous blood glucose monitoring systems (CGMS) technology, and discuss the role of CGMS in a patient with type 2 DM.

7. Research and compare current insulin pumps in the market. Discuss the role of insulin pump therapy in a patient with type 2 DM and what patient characteristics make or eliminate the patient as an insulin pump candidate.

CLINICAL PEARL

Although metformin is considered the first-line therapy for a patient with type 2 DM, not all patients with type 2 DM are appropriate candidates for metformin. Metformin has several contraindications, and patients generally must have good renal, hepatic, cardiac, and respiratory function to be considered a candidate for metformin therapy. Thus, a thorough assessment of the patient's comorbid conditions must be made. Early initiation of insulin therapy in patients who do not meet target goals is recommended.

REFERENCES

1. American Diabetes Association. Standards of Medical Care in Diabetes—2016. Diabetes Care 2016;39(1 Suppl):S1–S109.
2. Stone NJ, Robinson J, Lichtenstein AH, et al. 2013 ACC/AHA guideline on the treatment of blood cholesterol to reduce atherosclerotic cardiovascular risk in adults: a report of the American College of Cardiology/American Heart Association Task Force on Practice Guidelines. J Am Coll Cardiol 2014;63:2889–2934.
3. James PA, Oparil S, Carter BL, et al. 2014 evidence-based guideline for the management of high blood pressure in adults: report from the panel members appointed to the Eighth Joint National Committee (JNC 8). JAMA 2014;311:507–520.
4. National Heart Lung and Blood Institute. The Practical Guide: Identification, Evaluation, and Treatment of Overweight and Obesity in Adults. U.S. Department of Health and Human Services. National Institutes of Health, 2000. NIH Publication No. 00-4084.
5. Haupt DW. Differential metabolic effects of antipsychotic treatments. Eur Neuropsychopharmacol 2006;16:S149–S155.
6. Koski RR. Practical review of oral antihyperglycemic agents for type 2 diabetes mellitus. Diabetes Educ 2006;32(2):869–876.
7. Inzucchi SE, Bergenstal RM, Buse JB, et al. Management of hyperglycemia in type 2 diabetes, 2015: a patient-centered approach. Update to a position statement of the American Diabetes Association and the European Association for the Study of Diabetes. Diabetes Care 2015;38:140–149.
8. Jamerson K, Weber MA, Bakris GL, et al. ACCOMPLISH Trial Investigators. Benazepril plus amlodipine or hydrochlorothiazide for hypertension in high-risk patients. N Engl J Med 2008;359:2417–2428.
9. Pepine CJ, Handberg EM, Cooper-DeHoff RM. A calcium antagonist vs a noncalcium antagonist hypertension treatment strategy for patients with coronary artery disease: The International Verapamil-Trandolapril Study (INVEST): a randomized control trial. JAMA 2003;290:2805–2816.
10. Edwards SJ, Smith CJ. Tolerability of atypical antipsychotics in the treatment of adults with schizophrenia or bipolar disorder: a mixed treatment comparison of randomized controlled trials. Clin Ther 2009;31:1345–1359.

86

HYPERTHYROIDISM: GRAVES DISEASE

Gland Central. . . . . Level II

Kristine S. Schonder, PharmD

LEARNING OBJECTIVES

After completing this case study, the reader should be able to:

- Describe the signs, symptoms, and laboratory parameters associated with hyperthyroidism, and relate them to the pathophysiology of the disease.

- Select and justify appropriate patient-specific initial and follow-up pharmacotherapy for patients with hyperthyroidism.

- Develop a plan for monitoring the pharmacotherapy for hyperthyroidism.

- Provide appropriate education to patients receiving drug therapy for hyperthyroidism.

PATIENT PRESENTATION

Chief Complaint

"My heart feels like it is racing, and I feel jittery."

HPI

Carrie Gibson is a 23-year-old woman who presents to her PCP with complaints of palpitations and a fine tremor. The palpitations started a few months ago and would come and go until the past week when they began occurring more frequently, almost daily. She denies CP. She reports that she began noticing a fine tremor approximately 3 weeks ago. She also reports loose stools and a 5-kg weight loss over the past 6 months, despite a good appetite and food intake. She feels hot all of the time and sweats a lot. She further states that she has been losing her hair recently and that she is more irritable than usual.

PMH

She has been healthy up to this point with no medical conditions. She reports having had "the flu" last November, but states that she did not seek medical attention at that time.

FH

Father has HTN; mother had a history of Graves disease and passed away 1 year ago from breast CA at age 53. Her oldest sister is 32 years of age and has breast CA; she has two other sisters, ages 29 and 25, and one brother, age 27, all of whom are healthy. Her aunt (mother's sister) and grandmother both had Graves disease.

SH

She smokes 1.5 ppd × 5 years and drinks alcohol socially on the weekends ("a few drinks on Fridays and Saturdays").

TABLE 86-1	Lab Values			
Na 140 mEq/L	Hgb 12.8 g/dL	RDW 10.2%	AST 14 IU/L	Total T$_4$ 24 mcg/dL
K 4.1 mEq/L	Hct 38.4%	WBC 4.8 × 10^3/mm^3	ALT 16 IU/L	Free T$_4$ 4 ng/dL
Cl 98 mEq/L	RBC 3.08 × 10^6/mm^3	Polys 72%	T. bili 0.2 mg/dL	TSH 0.02 mIU/L
CO$_2$ 23 mEq/L	Plt 298 × 10^3/mm^3	Lymphs 27%	Amylase <30 IU/L	T$_3$ resin uptake 35%
BUN 9 mg/dL	MCV 86.4 μm^3	Monos 1%	Ca 9.5 mg/dL	Total T$_3$ 550 ng/dL
SCr 0.6 mg/dL	MCH 27.1 pg	Basos 2%	Mg 2.0 mEq/L	Free thyroxine index 28.7
Glu 78 mg/dL	MCHC 31.8 g/dL		Phos 3.7 mg/dL	

■ Meds

Drospirenone/ethinyl estradiol daily

■ All

None

■ ROS

She reports no visual changes, CP, or dyspnea. She has occasional N/V/D.

■ Physical Examination

Gen

Patient is a thin, tanned WF in NAD. She appears anxious and has a fine motor tremor in her hands.

VS

BP 136/80 mm Hg, P 120 bpm, RR 18, T 38.1°C; Wt 48 kg, Ht 5′6″

Skin

Hair is fine and sparse in the temporal area

HEENT

PERRL, EOMI, (+) lid lag, no proptosis (no ophthalmoplegia) or periorbital edema

Neck/Lymph Nodes

Supple, (+) smooth, symmetrically enlarged thyroid (approximately twice the normal size), prominent pulsations in neck vessels

Lungs

CTA bilaterally, no wheezes or rales

CV

Regular rhythm, tachycardic without murmurs; (–) bruits

Abd

Soft, NT/ND; (+) hyperactive BS; no HSM or masses. Aortic pulsations palpable.

Rect

Guaiac (–) stool

Ext

Normal pulses bilaterally, no calf tenderness. No cyanosis. Fingernails and toenails are flaking. Thumbnails have prominent ridges.

Neuro

A & O × 3; fine tremor with outstretched hands; hyperreflexia at knees; no proximal muscle weakness

■ Labs

See Table 86-1.

■ ECG

NSR, with HR of 120 bpm

■ Assessment

A 23-year-old woman with goiter, probable hyperthyroidism. Most likely cause is Graves disease.

QUESTIONS

Problem Identification

1.a. Create a list of the patient's drug therapy problems.

1.b. What signs, symptoms, and laboratory values indicate the presence or severity of hyperthyroidism?

Desired Outcome

2. What are the goals of pharmacotherapy for this patient?

Therapeutic Alternatives

3.a. What nondrug therapies might be useful for this patient?

3.b. What feasible pharmacotherapeutic alternatives are available for the treatment of Graves disease?

Optimal Plan

4. What drug, dosage form, dose, schedule, and duration of therapy are best for this patient?

Outcome Evaluation

5. What clinical and laboratory parameters are necessary to evaluate thyroid replacement therapy to achieve euthyroidism and prevent adverse effects?

Patient Education

6. What information should be provided to the patient to enhance adherence, ensure successful therapy, and minimize adverse effects?

■ CLINICAL COURSE

The patient is started on the treatment you recommended and returns for a 6-month follow-up visit. She reports that she has noticed marked improvement in her symptoms. The palpitations and tremor have both resolved. She states that she missed her last menses and is concerned that she may be pregnant. The following vital signs and laboratory results are obtained:

VS: BP 124/70 mm Hg, P 88 bpm, RR 16, T 37.2°C

Hgb 12.5 g/dL	WBC 5.8 ×10³/mm³	AST 18 IU/L
Hct 37.5%	Polys 65%	ALT 16 IU/L
MCV 85.6 μm³	Lymphs 30%	T. bili 0.2 mg/dL
MCH 26.5 pg	Monos 2%	Total T₄ 14.2 mcg/dL
MCHC 30.9 g/dL	Basos 2%	TSH <0.17 mIU/L
RDW 9.4%	Basos 1%	hCG 2637 mIU/mL

Total T_4 14.2 mcg/dL

■ FOLLOW-UP QUESTIONS

1. What changes to the patient's treatment for Graves disease, if any, would you suggest at this point?

2. What other interventions would you recommend for this patient?

■ SELF-STUDY ASSIGNMENTS

1. Develop a monitoring protocol for the pharmacotherapy of hyperthyroidism.

2. Design a systematic approach for a patient counseling technique for the drug therapy of hyperthyroidism.

CLINICAL PEARL

Ophthalmopathy associated with Graves disease can produce significant morbidity in patients and can cause blindness in severe cases that affect the optic nerve or cornea. Graves ophthalmopathy is thought to be an autoimmune disorder mediated by autoreactive T lymphocytes and cytokine release. The most common symptoms include diplopia, photophobia, tearing, and pain. Correction of the underlying hyperthyroidism can improve symptoms of Graves ophthalmopathy in most cases. However, symptoms can temporarily worsen with radioactive iodine treatment, until the hyperthyroidism is corrected. Severe cases of Graves ophthalmopathy should be treated with systemic or intraocular glucocorticoids. Alternative therapies include orbital radiotherapy and other immunomodulating drugs, such as cyclosporine and rituximab. Surgery is reserved for the most severe cases or those refractory to steroids.

REFERENCES

1. Bahn RX, Burch HB, Cooper DS, et al. Hyperthyroidism and other causes of thyrotoxicosis: management guidelines of the American Thyroid Association and American Association of Clinical Endocrinologists. Thyroid 2011;21(6):593–646.

2. Brent GA. Graves' disease. N Engl J Med 2009;358(24):2594–2605 [correction: N Engl J Med 2008;359;1407–1409].

3. Bahn RS, Burch HS, Cooper DS, et al. The role of propylthiouracil in the management of Graves' disease in adults: report of a meeting jointly sponsored by the American Thyroid Association and the Food and Drug Administration. Thyroid 2009;19(7):673–674.

4. Wiersinga WM. Smoking and thyroid. Clin Endocrinol 2013;79:145–151.

5. Bartalena L, Tanda ML. Graves' ophthalmopathy. N Engl J Med 2009;360(10):994–1001.

6. Stagnaro-Green A, Abalovich M, Alexander E, et al. Guidelines of the American Thyroid Association for the Diagnosis and Management of Thyroid Disease during pregnancy and postpartum. Thyroid 2011;21(10):1081–1125.

7. American College of Obstetricians and Gynecologists. Smoking cessation during pregnancy. Committee opinion no. 471. Obstet Gynecol 2010;116(5):1241–1244.

87

HYPOTHYROIDISM

Trying to Have a Baby Is Making Me Tired! . . . . . . Level II

Michael D. Katz, PharmD

LEARNING OBJECTIVES

After completing this case study, the reader should be able to:

- Recognize the signs, symptoms, and associated complications of mild and overt hypothyroidism.

- Identify the goals of therapy for hypothyroidism.

- Develop an appropriate treatment and monitoring plan for thyroid replacement based on individual patient characteristics.

- Select an appropriate product for thyroid replacement therapy.

- Properly educate a patient taking thyroid replacement therapy.

PATIENT PRESENTATION

■ Chief Complaint

"We are trying so hard to have a baby. Maybe that's why I'm so tired all the time … too much pressure."

■ HPI

Vickie Greene is a 31-year-old African-American woman who presents with her husband Eric (age 33) to the Endocrinology Clinic after being referred by her OB-GYN based on the results of some recent blood work. The Greenes have been trying to have a baby for almost 2 years, without Vickie becoming pregnant. The infertility workup done by the OB-GYN showed that Eric had a normal sperm count and sperm motility, and that Vickie had no anatomical abnormalities of her reproductive tract and no evidence of endometriosis. Vickie's serum sex hormone and gonadotropin levels were all normal. The couple is contemplating in vitro fertilization, but wants to make sure that there are no hormone-related causes of her infertility. Vickie says that for the past few months she has felt increasingly fatigued, which she attributes to the stress of her unsuccessful attempts to become pregnant. She wonders if she is becoming depressed. She also notes that for the past few months, she has had more difficulty concentrating at work, and she has "gained a few pounds." Over the past 6 months, Vickie has noticed that her periods are a little heavier than normal and are somewhat more irregular. She notes that 2 years ago, she attended a local health fair that provided a variety of laboratory tests. The result of her TSH at that time was 4.2 mIU/L. Her PCP at that time felt that the TSH value was within the normal range and required no follow-up.

■ PMH

Infertility × 2 years
Iron deficiency anemia as a teenager

■ FH

Father, age 55, has mild COPD; mother, age 54, has type 2 DM, HTN; she has one sister, age 32, who has hypothyroidism. No history of sickle cell trait or disease.

SH

Married × 6 years, first marriage for both. No history of STDs. Works as an immigration attorney for a private firm. Social drinker in past but has not used alcohol since attempting to become pregnant; (–) tobacco or illicit drug use.

Meds

MiraLAX PO daily PRN constipation
Seasonale one PO daily (stopped 2 years ago)
$FeSO_4$ 300 mg PO daily
Calcium carbonate 500 mg PO twice daily
Acetaminophen 325–650 mg PO PRN headache, body aches

All

Skin rash from sulfa drug

ROS

(+) Fatigue that she attributes to stress, (+) occasional insomnia, (+) constipation relieved with MiraLAX; (+) occasional headaches relieved with nonaspirin pain reliever; (–) tinnitus, vertigo, or infections; (–) urinary symptoms; (+) dry skin

Physical Examination

Gen

Well-appearing African-American woman in NAD

VS

BP 112/74 mm Hg, P 64 bpm, RR 12, T 36.8°C; Wt 62 kg, Ht 5'7"

Skin

Slightly dry-appearing skin; (–) rashes or lesions

HEENT

PERRLA, EOMI; (–) sinus tenderness; TMs appear normal

Neck/Lymph Nodes

(–) Thyroid nodules, possible slight thyroid enlargement; (–) lymphadenopathy, (–) carotid bruits

Lungs/Thorax

CTA

Breasts

(–) Lumps/masses

CV

RRR, normal S_1, S_2; (–) S_3 or S_4

Abd

NT/ND, (–) organomegaly

Neuro

A & O × 3; CN II–XII intact; DTRs 2+, symmetric

GU

Deferred given recent extensive w/u by OB-GYN

Labs (Fasting)

Na 138 mEq/L	Hgb 13.1 g/dL	Anti-TPO antibody +
K 4.2 mEq/L	Hct 39.2%	TSH 9.8 mIU/L
Cl 98 mEq/L	WBC 6.8 ×10³/mm³	Free T_4 0.72 ng/dL
CO_2 25 mEq/L	MCV 89 μm³	T. chol 212 mg/dL
BUN 8 mg/dL	Ca 9.6 mg/dL	LDL chol 142 mg/dL
SCr 0.7 mg/dL	Mg 2.0 mEq/L	HDL chol 45 mg/dL
Glu 98 mg/dL	PO_4 3.8 mg/dL	TG 125 mg/dL
	Albumin 4.0 g/dL	
	AST 22 IU/L	
	ALT 19 IU/L	
	T. bili 0.4 mg/dL	
	Alk phos 54 IU/L	

Assessment

A 31-year-old woman with infertility, fatigue, other nonspecific symptoms, and an elevated TSH level, suggestive of hypothyroidism

QUESTIONS

Problem Identification

1.a. Identify this patient's drug therapy problems.

1.b. What information (signs, symptoms, and laboratory values) indicates the presence of hypothyroidism?

1.c. Could hypothyroidism be a cause of her infertility?

1.d. List examples of medications that are known to cause hypothyroidism. Could any of the patient's complaints have been caused by drug therapy?

1.e. What was the significance, if any, of her previous TSH of 4.2 mIU/L?

Desired Outcome

2. What are the goals of pharmacotherapy in this case?

Therapeutic Alternatives

3.a. What nondrug therapies might be useful for this patient?

3.b. What feasible pharmacotherapeutic alternatives (including complementary/alternative medicine products) are available for the treatment of hypothyroidism?

Optimal Plan

4. What drug, dosage form, dose, schedule, and duration of therapy are best for this patient?

Outcome Evaluation

5. Which clinical and laboratory parameters are necessary to evaluate the therapy for achievement of the desired therapeutic outcome and to detect or prevent adverse effects?

Patient Education

6. What information should be provided to the patient to enhance adherence, ensure successful therapy, and minimize adverse effects?

■ FOLLOW-UP QUESTIONS

1. How should this patient's elevated LDL cholesterol be managed now? What if her cholesterol continues to be elevated after she becomes euthyroid?

2. What changes in her thyroid therapy might be necessary if she does become pregnant?

3. Evaluate this patient's continued need for iron and calcium. Should they be discontinued? If not, what potential problems (if any) might be expected once thyroid replacement therapy is started?

■ SELF-STUDY ASSIGNMENTS

1. Review the effects of untreated hypothyroidism during pregnancy on both mother and baby.

2. Research information on the US bioequivalence testing of levothyroxine (LT_4) products. How does US bioequivalence testing of LT_4 products differ from that of other oral products? Does LT_4 bioequivalence ensure therapeutic equivalence? Is there a consensus regarding the substitution of LT_4 product?

3. Review the factors that may alter LT_4 dose requirements, including drug interactions.

CLINICAL PEARL

Pregnant women who are receiving LT_4 replacement must undergo monthly monitoring of the TSH level to assure adequate replacement. The majority of such women will require an increase of their LT_4 dose during pregnancy to assure adequate replacement for both mother and fetus.

REFERENCES

1. Aoki Y, Belin RM, Clickner R, Jeffries R, Phillips L, Mhafey KR. Serum TSH and total T4 in the United States population and their association with participant characteristics. National Health and Nutrition Examination Survey (NHANES 1999–2002). Thyroid 2007;17:1211–1123.

2. Canaris GJ, Manowitz NR, Mayor G, Ridgway EC. The Colorado thyroid disease prevalence study. Arch Intern Med 2000;160:526–534.

3. Stagnaro-Green A, Pearce E. Thyroid disorders in pregnancy. Nat Rev Endocrinol 2012;8:650–658.

4. Poppe K, Velkeniers B, Glinoer D. The role of thyroid autoimmunity in fertility and pregnancy. Nat Clin Pract Endocrinol Metab 2008;4:394–405.

5. Laurberg P, Andersen S, Carle A, et al. The TSH upper reference limit: where are we at? Nat Rev Endocrinol 2011;7:232–239.

6. Almandoz JP, Gharib H. Hypothyroidism: etiology, diagnosis and management. Med Clin North Am 2012;96:203–221.

7. Blakesley V, Awni W, Locke C, Ludden T, Granneman GR, Braverman LE. Are bioequivalence studies of levothyroxine sodium formulations in euthyroid volunteers reliable? Thyroid 2004;14:191–200.

8. Carr D, McLeod DT, Parry G, Thornes HM. Fine adjustment of thyroxine replacement dosage: comparison of the thyrotropin releasing hormone test using a sensitive thyrotropin assay with measurement of free thyroid hormones and clinical assessment. Clin Endocrinol 1988;28:325–333.

9. Dong BJ, Hauck WW, Gambertoglio JG, et al. Bioequivalence of generic and brand-name levothyroxine products in the treatment of hypothyroidism. JAMA 1997;277:1205–1213.

10. Mayor GH, Orlando T, Kurtz NM. Limitations of levothyroxine bioequivalence evaluation: an analysis of an attempted study. Am J Ther 1995;2:417–432.

11. Grozinsky-Glasberg S, Fraser A, Nahashoni E, Weizman A, Leibovici L. Thyroxine triiodothyronine combination therapy versus thyroxine monotherapy for clinical hypothyroidism: a meta-analysis of randomized controlled trials. J Clin Endocrinol Metab 2006;91:2592–2599.

12. Franklyn KA. The thyroid—too much and too little across the ages: the consequences of subclinical thyroid dysfunction. Clin Endocrinol 2013;78:1–8.

13. Stagnaro-Green A, Abalovich M, Alexander E, et al. Guidelines of the American Thyroid Association for the Diagnosis and Management of Thyroid Disease during pregnancy and postpartum. Thyroid 2011;21:1081–1125.

14. De Groot L, Abalovich M, Alexander EK, et al. Management of thyroid dysfunction during pregnancy and postpartum: an Endocrine Society clinical practice guideline. J Clin Endocrinol Metab 2012;97:2543–2565.

15. Reid SM, Middleton P, Cossich MC, et al. Interventions for clinical and subclinical hypothyroidism pre-pregnancy and during pregnancy. Cochrane Database Syst Rev 2013;5:CD007752. doi:10.1002/14651858. CD007752.pub3.

88

CUSHING SYNDROME

A Tale of Two Glands. . . . . Level II

Andrew Y. Hwang, PharmD

Steven M. Smith, PharmD, MPH, BCPS

John G. Gums, PharmD, FCCP

LEARNING OBJECTIVES

After completing this case study, the reader should be able to:

• Recognize and differentiate the signs, symptoms, and laboratory changes associated with the various forms of Cushing syndrome.

• Recognize the biochemical, anatomic, and emotional changes that can occur with Cushing syndrome.

• Recommend appropriate treatment regimens for patients with Cushing syndrome.

• Suggest appropriate adjunctive pharmacotherapy to other healthcare providers for patients with Cushing disease.

• Provide patient counseling on proper dosing, administration, and adverse effects of treatment for Cushing disease.

PATIENT PRESENTATION

■ Chief Complaint

"I have been tired and weak lately, and I've noticed some swelling in my legs recently."

■ HPI

Susan Taylor is a 31-year-old woman who presents to her family physician complaining of fatigue, weakness, and edema. She also reports weight gain (50 lbs over 2 years) and depression with insomnia.

■ PMH

Patient has been healthy with no other major medical illnesses, except seasonal allergic rhinitis. She had two healthy children by uncomplicated vaginal deliveries.

FH

Mother is alive at age 54 with type 2 DM; father is living at age 56 with HTN. She has two sisters: one is healthy and the other has depression.

SH

Patient does not smoke, and drinks occasionally. She is a photographer. Children are ages 6 and 3.

Meds

Lessina PO once daily as directed
Nasonex two sprays in each nostril once daily PRN allergic symptoms
Unisom SleepTabs PO Q HS PRN sleep
Advil one to two tablets PO Q 6 H PRN headache

All

Sulfa—rash

ROS

(+) For fatigue, weakness, occasional back pain, and weight gain; also reports episodes of sadness, depressed mood, and insomnia; skin bruises easily; occasional headache, blurred vision, and heartburn; no CP, wheezing, or SOB. Normal menstruation with regular periods.

Physical Examination

Gen

WDWN obese, cushingoid-appearing white woman in NAD

VS

BP 165/86 mm Hg, HR 85 bpm, RR 14/min, T 37.0°C; Wt 82.1 kg, Ht 5′3″

Skin

Thin skin with some bruising and scratches; purple striae visible on abdomen

HEENT

Rounded face; moderate facial hair; PERRLA; EOMI; funduscopic exam shows normal retinal background, optic cup-to-disk ratios 0.4; visual fields appear to be grossly intact; OP moist and pink

Neck/Lymph Nodes

Supple; (+) JVD at 30° (7 cm); (–) bruits, adenopathy, or thyromegaly

Chest

CTA bilaterally

Breasts

No lumps or masses

CV

RRR, no MRG

Abd

Obese, soft, NT, (–) masses or organomegaly

Genit/Rect

Guaiac (–); normal external genitalia; no masses

MS/Ext

Appears to have decreased strength bilaterally; DTR 1–2+ and symmetric throughout all four extremities; 2+ pitting pedal edema bilaterally; pedal pulses palpable with moderate intensity

Neuro

Oriented × 3; flat affect; CNs II–XII intact

Labs

Na 138 mEq/L	Hgb 13.4 g/dL	AST 9 IU/L	TSH 2.33 mIU/L
K 3.3 mEq/L	Hct 38.5%	ALT 7 IU/L	A1C 7.1%
Cl 105 mEq/L	RBC 4.0 × 10⁶/mm³	Alk phos	*Fasting lipid profile*
CO_2 25 mEq/L	Plt 264 × 10³/mm³	180 IU/L	T. chol 261 mg/dL
BUN 12 mg/dL	WBC 14.5 × 10³/mm³	T. bili	HDL 62 mg/dL
SCr 0.9 mg/dL		0.5 mg/dL	LDL 120 mg/dL
Glu 160 mg/dL		Alb 4.5 g/dL	Trig 396 mg/dL
		UA 5.6 mg/dL	

Assessment

Probable Cushing syndrome of unknown etiology requiring further evaluation by an endocrinologist

Clinical Course

The patient was seen by an endocrinologist for further evaluation. Baseline 24-hour UFC was 356 and 362 mcg on separate days. A midnight salivary cortisol concentration was 0.54 mcg/dL. An overnight 1-mg DST showed a plasma cortisol concentration of 9.2 mcg/dL. Plasma ACTH concentrations on 2 consecutive days at 1:00 PM were 103 and 110 pg/mL. A CRH stimulation test revealed a baseline plasma cortisol of 10.4 mcg/dL and ACTH of 108 pg/mL, with an increase to a plasma cortisol of 13.5 mcg/dL and ACTH of 187 pg/mL following CRH administration. An MRI revealed an enlarged pituitary gland; the same finding was seen on a focused repeat MRI. There was no focal inhomogeneity that would suggest an isolated adenoma (ie, the tumor cannot be localized).

The risks and benefits of all the treatments were explained to Ms Taylor. She preferred to undergo radiation treatments rather than exploratory-type surgery. She indicated that she would like to have more children and would prefer to try other treatments prior to surgery.

QUESTIONS

Problem Identification

1.a. Create a list of this patient's drug therapy problems.

1.b. What information (signs, symptoms, laboratory values) indicates the presence or severity of Cushing syndrome?

1.c. What information (presentation, history, laboratory values, imaging) can be used to identify the most likely etiology of Cushing syndrome?

Desired Outcome

2. What are the goals of pharmacotherapy in this case?

Therapeutic Alternatives

3.a. What nondrug therapies might be useful for this patient?

3.b. What feasible pharmacotherapeutic alternatives are available for the treatment of Cushing disease?

Optimal Plan

4.a. What drug, dosage form, dose, schedule, and duration of therapy are best for treating this patient's Cushing disease?

4.b. What adjunctive pharmacotherapy may be required if the therapy identified above is successful?

Outcome Evaluation

5. What clinical and laboratory parameters are necessary to evaluate the therapy for achievement of the desired therapeutic outcome and to detect or prevent adverse events?

Patient Education

6. What information should be provided to the patient to enhance adherence, ensure successful therapy, and minimize adverse events?

■ FOLLOW-UP QUESTIONS

1. What advantages does measuring late-night salivary cortisol have over measuring late-night serum cortisol concentrations?

2. What changes, if any, should be made to the treatment of allergic rhinitis?

■ CLINICAL COURSE

The patient received radiation therapy with adjuvant pharmacotherapy to reduce cortisol levels. Given that it may take several months for therapy to normalize cortisol levels, several other interventions were initiated to ameliorate the complications of Cushing disease. She received hydrochlorothiazide 25 mg daily for hypertension, pioglitazone 30 mg daily for elevated blood glucose, rosuvastatin 5 mg daily for dyslipidemia, and escitalopram 10 mg daily for depression. A DXA scan revealed a Z-score of –2.4 standard deviations at the hip and –2.6 vertebrally. Accordingly, she received a diagnosis of steroid-induced osteoporosis. One month following initiation of the above agents, she presented to her physician for follow-up. She reported increased weakness, leg cramps, and palpitations. Lab work revealed a serum potassium concentration of 2.7 mEq/L.

3. What pharmacologic therapy would you recommend to reduce her risk of fracture?

4. What medication changes would you suggest at this time?

■ SELF-STUDY ASSIGNMENTS

1. Many of the tests used in the differential diagnosis of Cushing syndrome require drug therapy (eg, DST, CRH). Create a table to assist healthcare providers in performing these tests correctly (include possible adverse events, timing, critical values, and evaluation of the results).

2. Compare the retail costs in your area for each of the pharmacotherapeutic alternatives for the treatment of Cushing syndrome. Write a brief summary of your findings, and describe whether this information would cause you to change your recommendation for the initial drug therapy for this patient.

3. Describe methods that may be used to minimize drug-induced Cushing syndrome.

CLINICAL PEARL

Most patients with Cushing disease are treated with transsphenoidal surgery because of its high cure rate (80–90%). Pharmacotherapy is usually used as adjunctive therapy rather than primary therapy.

REFERENCES

1. Newell-Price J, Bertagna X, Grossman AB, Nierman LK. Cushing syndrome. Lancet 2006;367:1605–1617.

2. Sharma ST, Nieman LK, Feelders RA. Cushing syndrome: epidemiology and developments in disease management. Clin Epidemiol 2015;7:281–293.

3. Nieman LK, Biller BMK, Findling JW, et al. Treatment of Cushing Syndrome: an Endocrine Society Clinical Practice Guideline. J Clin Endocrinol Metab 2015;100:2807–2831.

4. Lacroix A, Feelders RA, Stratakis CA, Nieman LK. Cushing syndrome. Lancet 2015;386(9996):913–927.

89

ADDISON DISEASE

I May Look Great, But I Don't Feel Well . . . . Level II

Cynthia P. Koh-Knox, PharmD

Zachary A. Weber, PharmD, BCPS, BCACP, CDE

LEARNING OBJECTIVES

After completing this case study, the reader should be able to:

- Recognize the clinical presentation, symptoms, and laboratory changes associated with Addison disease.

- Optimize pharmacologic and nonpharmacologic therapy for patients with Addison disease and comorbid conditions.

- Provide education and counseling to patients and family members about Addison disease and the proper administration, side effects, and adverse effects of corticosteroids and mineralocorticoids, and the importance of adherence to therapy.

- Provide counseling and education about common side effects associated with high and low cortisol serum concentrations.

- Compare corticosteroids with respect to relative glucocorticoid and mineralocorticoid potencies.

PATIENT PRESENTATION

■ Chief Complaint

"I've noticed that over the past six months, my son's skin is getting darker, and he has been more lethargic, somewhat withdrawn, and sleeping more. I have also noticed that he has been making some poor choices, in terms of friends and activities."

■ HPI

Gregory Waters is a 19-year-old man who is brought to the ED by his mother after she finds him crying, confused, and disoriented. His mother states that she has recently noticed that he has not had the same level of energy, and has been complaining about not being able to run and play basketball with his friends at the park. She has also noticed he has been hanging out with a different group of friends, and she is concerned he may be involved in some abhorrent activities and may not be taking his medications appropriately.

PMH

Type 1 DM × 7 years
Hypothyroidism × 3 years

FH

Mother, 52 years old, has HTN; father, 54 years old, has hypothyroidism; sister, 24 years old, has both HTN and type 1 DM

SH

Denies use of alcohol, tobacco, or illicit drugs; lives with his mother

Meds

Lantus 24 units subcutaneously at bedtime
NovoLog 1:15 scale carbohydrate counting ratio, subcutaneously with meals
Levothyroxine 100 mcg PO daily

All

NKDA

ROS

Increased tanning of the skin noted over the past 6 months. Increased fatigue, nausea, and a 2.5-kg weight loss over the past month.

Physical Examination

Gen

Alert, somewhat disoriented and confused

VS

BP 84/47 mm Hg, HR 91 bpm, RR 16/min, T 36.2°C; Wt 62.5 kg, Ht 5′4″

Skin

Warm, dry, and intact. Slightly tanned color

HEENT

Normocephalic; oral mucosa moist. PERRL. EOMI

Neck

No JVD. Nontender. No thyroid nodularity

Lungs

CTA. Respirations are nonlabored

CV

Normal rate and rhythm. No murmurs. Normal perfusion. No edema

Abd

Soft, NT/ND. Normal BS

MS/Ext

No CCE; normal ROM

Neuro

Alert, somewhat disoriented

Psych

Somnolent, but cooperative

Labs (Fasting, Drawn at 10:15 AM)

Na 116 mEq/L	Hgb 14.2 g/dL	AST 111 IU/L	T. chol 168 mg/dL
K 4.9 mEq/L	Hct 43.8%	ALT 59 IU/L	Trig 120 mg/dL
Cl 99 mEq/L	RBC 4.88 ×	Alk phos	Fe 93 mcg/dL
CO_2 26 mEq/L	$10^6/mm^3$	75 IU/L	TSH 25.8 mIU/L
BUN 14 mg/dL	Plt 244 × $10^3/mm^3$	GGT 63 IU/L	Free T_4 0.41 ng/dL
SCr 0.9 mg/dL	WBC 3.6 × $10^3/mm^3$	LDH 173 IU/L	Cortisol 0.4 mcg/dL
Glu 140 mg/dL	Neutros 41%	T. bili 1.1 mg/dL	ACTH 2003 pg/mL
Ca 9.2 mg/dL	Lymphos 43%	D. bili 0.5 mg/dL	A1C 8.2%
Phos 5.1 mg/dL	Monos 13%	T. prot 7.3 g/dL	
Uric acid	Eos 2%	Alb 4.1 g/dL	
4.1 mg/dL	Basos 1%		

Reference range for cortisol: AM 8–25 mcg/dL, PM 4–20 mcg/dL; ACTH 0–130 pg/mL

UA

Clear, pale yellow, SG 1.020, pH 6.8

Other

CT scan negative; ECG normal

Assessment

1. Primary adrenal insufficiency, most likely due to an autoimmune disease

2. Hypothyroidism with an elevated TSH, likely secondary to nonadherence to prescribed levothyroxine regimen

3. Type 1 DM with an elevated A1C, likely secondary to nonadherence to prescribed insulin regimen

QUESTIONS

Problem Identification

1.a. Create a list of the patient's drug therapy problems.

1.b. What information (signs, symptoms, and laboratory values) indicates the presence or severity of Addison disease?

Desired Outcome

2. What are the goals of pharmacotherapy in this case?

Therapeutic Alternatives

3.a. What nondrug therapies might be useful for this patient?

3.b. What feasible pharmacotherapeutic alternatives are available for the treatment of Addison disease?

3.c. What psychosocial considerations are applicable to this patient?

Optimal Plan

4. What drug, dosage form, dose, schedule, and duration of therapy are best for this patient?

Outcome Evaluation

5. Which clinical and laboratory parameters are necessary to evaluate the response to therapy and to detect or prevent adverse effects?

Patient Education

6. What information should be provided to the patient to enhance adherence, ensure successful therapy, and minimize adverse effects?

■ SELF-STUDY ASSIGNMENTS

1. Review the signs and symptoms of an acute adrenal crisis, and describe the treatment.

2. Differentiate the glucocorticoids with respect to duration of activity, glucocorticoid potency, and mineralocorticoid potency.

3. Differentiate the biologic functions of cortisol and aldosterone.

4. Explain why the skin becomes pigmented in adrenal insufficiency.

5. Identify drugs that may precipitate acute adrenal insufficiency or adrenal crisis.

CLINICAL PEARL

Although rare, a decrease in insulin requirements and unexplained hypoglycemia in patients with type 1 DM may be initial signs of Addison disease.[4,7]

REFERENCES

1. Baker SJ, White K. Addison's Disease Owner Manual. Available at: *http://www.addisons.org.uk/info/manual/adshgguidelines.pdf.* Accessed December 2, 2015.

2. Abdel-Motleb M. The neuropsychiatric aspect of Addison's disease: a case report. Innov Clin Neurosci 2012 Oct;9(10):34–36. Available at: *http://www.ncbi.nlm.nih.gov/pmc/articles/PMC3508960/.* Accessed December 2, 2015.

3. Kordonouri O, Maguire AM, Knip M, et al. Other complications and associated conditions with diabetes in children and adolescents. Ped Diab 2009;10(Suppl 12):204–210.

4. Michels A, Michels, N. Addison disease: early detection and treatment principles. Am Fam Phys 2014;89(7):563–568.

5. Chakera AJ, Vaidya B. Addison disease in adults: diagnosis and management. Am J Med 2010;123:409–413.

6. Reisch N, Arlt W. Fine tuning for quality of life: 21st century approach to treatment of Addison's Disease. Endocrinol Metab Clin N Am 2009;38:407–418.

7. Petersen KS, Rushworth RL, Clifton PM, et al. Recurrent nocturnal hypoglycaemia as a cause for morning fatigue in treated Addison's disease—a favourable response to dietary management: a case report. BMC Endocr Disord 2015;15:61. Published online 24 Oct 2015.

8. Arlt W. The approach to the adult with newly diagnosed adrenal insufficiency. J Clin Endocrinol Metab 2009;94(4):1059–1067.

9. Gagliardi L, Nenke AM, Tilenka RJ, et al. Continuous subcutaneous hydrocortisone infusion therapy in Addison's disease: a randomized, placebo-controlled clinical trial. J Clin Endocrinol Metab 2014;99:4149–4157.

10. Elbelt U, Hahner S, Allolio B. Altered insulin requirement in patient with type 1 diabetes and primary adrenal insufficiency receiving standard glucocorticoid replacement therapy. Eur J Endocrinol 2009;160:919–924.

90

HYPERPROLACTINEMIA

The Missing Period . . . . Level I

Amy Heck Sheehan, PharmD

Karim Anton Calis, PharmD, MPH, FASHP, FCCP

LEARNING OBJECTIVES

After completing this case study, the reader should be able to:

- Recognize the signs and symptoms of hyperprolactinemia.

- Recommend appropriate treatment options for hyperprolactinemia.

- Design a plan to monitor the response to the pharmacologic treatment of hyperprolactinemia.

PATIENT PRESENTATION

■ Chief Complaint

"I haven't had my period for almost a year."

■ HPI

Susan Oliver is a 31-year-old woman with a history of oligomenorrhea (menstrual cycle every 2–6 months) since menarche at age 14. She presents to her gynecologist after 11 months of amenorrhea and a small amount of milky discharge from her left breast, which she first noticed 1–2 months ago. The patient and her husband would like to have a baby, but she is concerned that she may be unable to have children. The patient states that she and her husband have not used birth control for more than 1 year, and she has had several negative home pregnancy tests.

■ PMH

GERD
Seasonal allergies
Depression

■ FH

Father died at age 58 from an AMI; mother (age 62) has type 2 DM and HTN. Patient has two brothers (ages 33 and 35) who are alive and well.

■ SH

The patient is employed as an administrative assistant. She does not smoke and has less than one drink of alcohol per month. She has been married for 5 years and lives with her husband and two stepdaughters (ages 7 and 9).

■ Meds

Omeprazole 20 mg PO daily
Desloratadine 5 mg PO daily
Fluoxetine 20 mg PO daily
Prenatal vitamins one tablet PO daily
Acetaminophen 500 mg PO PRN

All

Codeine (hives)

ROS

Galactorrhea of the left breast and amenorrhea for 11 months as described in the HPI. No visual defects. No active GERD or migraine symptoms.

Physical Examination

Gen

The patient is a WDWN white woman in NAD

VS

BP 124/71 mm Hg, P 72 bpm, RR 13, T 37.1°C; Wt 72 kg, Ht 5′8″

Skin

Normal, intact, warm, and dry

HEENT

PERRLA, EOMI, normal funduscopic exam, normal visual fields

Neck/Lymph Nodes

Normal thyroid, no lymphadenopathy

Lungs/Chest

CTA & P

Breasts

Galactorrhea of left breast, no masses

CV

RRR, S_1 and S_2 normal, no MRG

Abd

Soft, nontender, no organomegaly, (+) bowel sounds

GU

LMP 11 months ago, normal pelvic exam and Pap smear

MS/Ext

Normal ROM, no edema, pulses 2+ throughout

Neuro

A & O × 3, bilateral reflexes intact, normal gait, CNs II–XII intact

Labs

Na 138 mEq/L	AST 23 IU/L	TSH 2.1 mIU/L
K 4.0 mEq/L	ALT 31 IU/L	T_3 111 ng/dL
Cl 101 mEq/L	Alk phos 110 IU/L	Total T_4 7.5 mcg/dL
CO_2 25 mEq/L	T. bili 0.5 mg/dL	Free T_4 1.3 ng/dL
BUN 13 mg/dL		Serum β-HCG negative
SCr 0.8 mg/dL		FSH 12 IU/L
Glu 89 mg/dL		

Serum prolactin on 3 separate days: 133, 159, and 142 mcg/L

Other Test Results

DXA T-score –0.90 at the lumbar spine (no previous DXA results)
MRI of the pituitary gland revealed an 8-mm pituitary adenoma

Assessment

Hyperprolactinemia due to a microprolactinoma

QUESTIONS

Problem Identification

1.a. List this patient's drug therapy problems.

1.b. What signs, symptoms, and laboratory values indicate the presence of hyperprolactinemia?

1.c. Could this patient's hyperprolactinemia be drug-induced?

Desired Outcome

2. What are the goals of treatment for a woman with hyperprolactinemia?

Therapeutic Alternatives

3.a. What nondrug therapies can be considered for the treatment of hyperprolactinemia?

3.b. What pharmacotherapeutic options are available for the treatment of hyperprolactinemia in this woman?

Optimal Plan

4. What medication regimen would you recommend for this patient?

Outcome Evaluation

5.a. What clinical and laboratory parameters are necessary to monitor the patient's response to therapy?

5.b. If the initial therapy you recommend is effective, how soon can the patient hope to become pregnant?

Patient Education

6. What information should be provided to the patient to enhance adherence, optimize therapy, and minimize adverse effects?

■ CLINICAL COURSE

The patient was started on the regimen you recommended, and she returned to the clinic 4 weeks later complaining of significant nausea and abdominal pain that was temporally associated with medication administration. Serum prolactin concentrations measured 10 minutes apart were 140, 151, and 137 mcg/L. Galactorrhea and amenorrhea were unchanged.

■ FOLLOW-UP QUESTIONS

1. Identify the possible reasons for the patient's poor initial response to therapy.

2. Given the new patient information, what alternative therapies should be considered?

3. How long will this patient require drug treatment for the prolactinoma?

■ SELF-STUDY ASSIGNMENTS

1. Review the available information on the safety of dopamine agonist pharmacotherapy in pregnant women. If this patient eventually becomes pregnant, should a dopamine agonist be continued throughout the pregnancy?

2. Research information on the use of hormone replacement therapy in patients with hyperprolactinemia. Is this patient a candidate for hormone replacement therapy? Why or why not?

3. Describe the treatment of hyperprolactinemia in the presence of a macroadenoma. How would the management of hyperprolactinemia be different if the patient were diagnosed with a macroprolactinoma instead of a microprolactinoma?

CLINICAL PEARL

Although dopamine agonists are the mainstay of therapy for hyperprolactinemia, approximately 5–10% of patients do not respond to these agents because of poor compliance, suboptimal dosing, or the presence of a treatment-resistant prolactinoma.

REFERENCES

1. Melmed S, Casanueva FF, Hoffman AR, et al. Diagnosis and treatment of hyperprolactinemia: an Endocrine Society clinical practice guideline. J Clin Endocrinol Metab 2011;96:273–288.

2. Glezer A, Bronstein MD. Prolactinomas. Endocrinol Metab Clin N Am 2015;44:71–78.

3. Webster J, Piscitelli G, Polli A, et al. A comparison of cabergoline and bromocriptine in the treatment of hyperprolactinemic amenorrhea. N Engl J Med 1994;331:904–909.

4. Colao A, Abs R, Barcena DG, et al. Pregnancy outcomes following cabergoline treatment: extended results from a 12-year observation study. Clin Endocrinol 2008;68:66–71.

5. Molitch ME. Management of the pregnant patient with a prolactinoma. Eur J Endocrinol 2015;172:R205–R213.

6. Klibanski A. Prolactinomas. N Engl J Med 2010;362:1219–1226.

WOMEN'S HEALTH (GYNECOLOGIC DISORDERS)

91

PREGNANCY AND LACTATION

Pregnant at This Age?........................ Level II

Lisa R. Garavaglia, PharmD, BCPS

LEARNING OBJECTIVES

After completing this case study, the reader should be able to:

- Describe each FDA pregnancy category using the U.S. Food and Drug Administration Drug Classification System and the new Pregnancy and Lactation Labeling Rule (PLLR).[1]

- Determine the factors (clinical vs pharmacologic) that should be considered when treating a pregnant or lactating patient.

- List the risks and benefits associated with medication use during pregnancy for hypertension, depression, and mechanical heart valve requiring chronic anticoagulation for thromboembolism prophylaxis.

- Identify alternative therapies that are considered safe during pregnancy for the treatment of depression and hypertension, and for thromboembolism prophylaxis in a patient with a mechanical heart valve.

- Design a pharmacotherapeutic plan for a pregnant patient with depression, hypertension, and a mechanical heart valve including treatment options, appropriate monitoring, and therapeutic goals.

- Educate a patient on the treatment options, benefits, risks, and monitoring of antidepressants, antihypertensives, and anticoagulants during pregnancy.

PATIENT PRESENTATION

■ Chief Complaint

"I have been nauseated and vomiting for the past week. I took a pregnancy test yesterday, and it was positive! How am I going to handle a pregnancy at this age? Plus, I am taking a lot of different medications. Could I have harmed my baby?"

■ HPI

Laurel Livingston is a 44-year-old woman who reports experiencing two to three episodes of nausea per day with vomiting occasionally in the evenings. Her GI symptoms began about 2 weeks ago and have remained consistent, preventing her from going to work. Around the same time that her GI symptoms began, she started having frequent, painful urination, and was diagnosed with a UTI.

She is on day 5 of 7 of antibiotic treatment with nitrofurantoin. She states that she feels "run down" all the time and needs to start feeling better soon, or she will lose her job. In addition, she is extremely concerned about her "blood thinner" medication, remembering that she could not take it with her previous three pregnancies. Due to the death of her brother 5 years ago, Laurel was prescribed an antidepressant and is currently stable (no depressive episodes for the past 3 years). She eats well, exercises, and admits stopping her birth control due to weight gain.

■ PMH

Depression
Mechanical prosthetic heart valve
Hypothyroidism
Hypertension

■ FH

Mother alive and well; father died of pancreatic cancer at the age of 67. Patient has one sister, age 45, who is alive and well; brother died in car accident 5 years ago at the age of 32.

■ SH

Married, mother of two daughters, ages 10 and 13 (both healthy), and one son, 6 years old with cerebral palsy. She is a physical therapist at the local community hospital. She runs three times a week and follows a strict low-fat diet. She was a smoker (one pack per day) but is currently tobacco-free and occasionally drinks a glass of wine or alcoholic beverage on the weekends. She has no prior history of thromboembolism.

■ Medications

Paroxetine 20 mg PO once daily
Levothyroxine 125 mcg PO once daily
Warfarin 7.5 mg PO once daily
Lisinopril 10 mg PO once daily
Nitrofurantoin 100 mg PO twice daily × 7 days

■ Allergies

NKDA

■ ROS

(+) Nausea/vomiting × 2 weeks; fatigue; weight loss

■ Physical Examination

Gen

WDWN concerned female

VS

BP 160/90 mm Hg, P 76 bpm, RR 17, T 36.3°C; Wt 82 kg, Ht 5′8″

Skin

Warm, dry, no eruptions, boils, or lesions

HEENT

WNL

Neck/Lymph Nodes

No adenopathy, no thyromegaly, supple

Lungs

CTA bilaterally

Breasts

Tender to palpation; no masses

CV

Mechanical click systolic murmur, Grade 2/4

ABD

Soft, NT, (+) BS; no masses, no bruits

Genit/Rect

Pelvic exam confirms pregnancy; stool heme/guaiac (–)
Urine (–) for protein/glucose

Ext

(–) CCE; pulses intact

Neuro

Normal sensory and motor levels

■ Labs

Urinalysis: culture negative (no growth)
Ultrasound: confirmed pregnancy

Na 138 mEq/L	Hgb 13 g/dL	Blood type: O–
K 4 mEq/L	Hct 40%	PT/INR 10.0 seconds/3.0
Cl 102 mEq/L	WBC $8.0 \times 10^3/mm^3$	Random glucose 100 mg/dL
CO_2 27 mEq/L	Plt $345 \times 10^3/mm^3$	
BUN 10 mg/dL	TSH 1.45 mIU/L	
SCr 0.9 mg/dL		

■ Assessment

A 44-year-old pregnant woman presenting with nausea, vomiting, and fatigue, who is concerned about the safety of her medications during pregnancy.

QUESTIONS

Problem Identification

1. Create a list of the patient's potential drug therapy problems (now that she is pregnant). Be sure to include the information that indicates the severity of this patient's problems: FDA's pregnancy category, new labeling rules, and information regarding fetal malformations or risks associated with each of the patient's medications.

Desired Outcome

2. What are the goals of therapy for this patient's preexisting disease states/conditions (hypertension, depression, mechanical heart valve requiring anticoagulation, and hypothyroidism) during her pregnancy?

Therapeutic Alternatives

3.a. What are the benefits and risks of treating this patient's depression and hypertension and in providing anticoagulation for thromboembolism prophylaxis in light of the patient's mechanical heart valve?

3.b. What pharmacotherapeutic alternatives may be used to manage the patient's depression, hypertension, and anticoagulation for her heart valve?

Optimal Plan

4.a. The physician decided to prescribe labetalol for the patient's hypertension and enoxaparin for anticoagulation. What dose, schedule, and duration are the best for this patient for each of these medications?

4.b. The patient has been asymptomatic for more than a year and has agreed to discontinue her antidepressant. What are your recommendations for stopping the medication?

Outcome Evaluation

5. What clinical and laboratory parameters are necessary to evaluate the therapy for achievement of the desired therapeutic outcomes for the patient's hypertension and anticoagulation therapy and to detect or prevent medication-related adverse effects?

Patient Education

6. What information should be provided to the patient to enhance adherence to the medication, ensure successful therapy, and minimize adverse effects?

■ CLINICAL COURSE

The patient returns to your office 4 weeks after she delivers her healthy baby boy. She reports that her clinical symptoms of depression have intensified postpartum and would like to know if she should reinitiate her antidepressant, and if so, at what dose.

■ FOLLOW-UP QUESTIONS

1. Based on the American College of Obstetricians and Gynecologists (ACOG) guidelines, what would you recommend to the patient?

2. What is the Pregnancy and Lactation Labeling Rule?

CLINICAL PEARLS

Electronic resources for information related to fetal and neonatal effects in pregnancy and lactation include Reprotox (*www.reprotox.org*) and TERIS (*http://depts.washington.edu/terisweb*). There are also postmarketing pregnancy exposure registries available through the U.S. Food and Drug Administration Pregnancy Labeling Task Force. Alternatively, there is General Practice Research Database (GPRD) that can be utilized as data sources for investigating drug exposure during pregnancy.

REFERENCES

1. U.S. Food and Drug Administration. Pregnancy and lactation labeling (drug) final rule. Available at: *http://www.fda.gov/Drugs/DevelopmentApprovalProcess/DevelopmentResources/Labeling/ucm093307.htm*. Accessed April 16, 2016.

2. Koren G, Nordeng H. Antidepressant use during pregnancy: the benefit–risk ratio. Am J Obstet Gynecol 2012:157–163.

3. Pearlstein T. Depression during Pregnancy. Best Pract Res Clin Obstet Gynaecol 2015;29:754–764.

4. Yonkers KA, Wisner K, Stewart DE, et al. The management of depression during pregnancy: a report from the American Psychiatric Association and the American College of Obstetricians and Gynecologists. Gen Hosp Psychiatry 2009;31:403–413.

5. Buhimschi C, Weiner C. Medications in pregnancy and lactation Part 1. Teratology. Obstet Gynecol 2009;113:166–188.

6. American College of Obstetricians and Gynecologists. Report of the American College of Obstetricians and Gynecologists' Task Force on Hypertension in Pregnancy: Hypertension in pregnancy. Obstet Gynecol 2013;122:1122–1131.

7. Buhimschi C, Weiner C. Medications in pregnancy and lactation Part 2. Drugs with minimal or unknown human teratogenic effect. Obstet Gynecol 2009;113:417–432.

8. Bates SM, Greer IA, Middeldrop S, Veenstra DL, Prabulos AM, Vandvik PO. VTE, Thrombophilia, Antithrombotic Therapy, and Pregnancy: Antithrombotic Therapy and Prevention of Thrombosis, 9th ed: American College of Chest Physicians Evidence-Based Clinical Practice Guidelines. Chest 2012;141(2 Suppl):e691S–e736S. doi:10.1378/chest.11-2300.

9. Nishimura RA, Otto CM, Bonow RO, et al. 2014 AHA/ACC guidelines for the management of patients with valvular heart disease: executive summary: a report of the American College of Cardiology/American Heart Association Task Force on Practice Guidelines. J Am Coll Cardiol 2014;63:2438–2488.

10. Kaplan MM. Management of thyroxine during pregnancy. Endocr Pract 1996;2:281–286.

11. Marik PE, Plante LH. Venous thromboembolic disease and pregnancy. N Engl J Med 2008;359:2025–2033.

92

CONTRACEPTION

Babies Aren't Us Yet............................ Level II

Julia M. Koehler, PharmD, FCCP

Jennifer R. Guthrie, MPAS, PA-C

LEARNING OBJECTIVES

After completing this case study, the reader should be able to:

- Discuss the absolute and relative contraindications to the use of hormonal contraceptives.

- Discuss the advantages and disadvantages of the various forms of contraceptives, including both oral and nonoral hormonal formulations as well as intrauterine devices.

- Compare and contrast the marketed contraceptive options and be able to select the best product for an individual patient.

- Develop strategies for managing the possible side effects of oral contraceptives (OCs) and prepare appropriate alternative treatment plans.

- Provide specific patient education on the administration and expected side effects of selected hormonal contraceptives.

PATIENT PRESENTATION

Chief Complaint

"My fiancé and I are getting married soon, and we're not ready for kids just yet."

HPI

Macy Madison is a 25-year-old graduate student who presents to the women's health clinic for contraceptive counseling. She and her fiancé, Fritz, are planning to be married in approximately 4 months. Macy states that she and Fritz have been in a monogamous sexual relationship for the past 3 years, and that their primary method of contraception has been via the inconsistent use of male condoms. She is here today to be evaluated for the use of contraceptives. The patient states she began menses at age 14, with irregular cycles of 25–36 days in length. Her last menses was 2 weeks ago. The patient states she has heard about contraceptive options that "decrease your number of periods," and she wants to know more about those options, and if they would be okay for her to try.

PMH

Migraine headaches without aura or focal neurologic symptoms, well controlled for the past 12 months on prophylactic therapy; no history of HTN, dyslipidemia, or heart disease

FH

Mother, age 56, has HTN and osteoporosis and is postmenopausal. Grandmother died from complications of breast cancer, which was diagnosed at age 60. Father, age 58, has osteoarthritis, hypothyroidism, HTN, and dyslipidemia. Grandfather died at age 74 of MI.

SH

Currently lives in a house on campus, which she rents with three other graduate students. Once she and Fritz are married, they plan to rent an apartment together until she finishes graduate school. She admits to occasional social use of alcohol ("a few drinks at parties on the weekends"). Otherwise, she denies regular alcohol use during the week. Denies tobacco and illicit drug use.

Meds

Propranolol LA 160 mg PO once daily for migraine prophylaxis
Naproxen 220 mg, one to two tablets PO Q 8 H PRN mild menstrual cramps

All

NKDA

ROS

Denies excessive vaginal bleeding or significant pelvic pain with menses. Menstrual periods are the most irregular during mid-term and final exam times. Migraine headaches are not accompanied by aura or focal neurologic symptoms, and have been well controlled on prophylactic medication. (Patient states she has not had a migraine for more than 12 months; however, prior to being placed on propranolol for migraine prophylaxis, she reported experiencing menstrual-related headaches in addition to frequent migraines.) No history of STIs. No history or current symptoms of depression or anxiety. Immunizations up to date.

Physical Examination

Gen

Thin, well-developed female in NAD

VS

BP 112/70 mm Hg, P 66 bpm, RR 14, T 37°C; Wt 59 kg, Ht 5′7″, BMI 20.4 kg/m²

Skin

Warm, dry, and without rashes; mild facial acne; normal pigmentation

HEENT

Deferred

Neck/Lymph Nodes

Supple without lymphadenopathy or thyromegaly

Lungs

CTA, no wheezing

CV

RRR; no MRG

Breasts

Symmetric in size without nodularity or masses, nontender; nipples appear normal, everted and without discharge

Abd

Soft, NT, no masses or organomegaly

Genit/Rect

Normal-appearing external genitalia without lesions; uterus ante-verted, mobile, and without masses or tenderness; no cervical motion tenderness; ovaries palpable, of normal size, and without tenderness; rectal exam not performed

MS/Ext

Normal ROM; normal muscle strength; no peripheral edema

Neuro

A & O × 3; CN II–XII intact and without focal deficits of sensation or strength; normal mood and affect

■ Labs

Negative Pap test and UPT

■ Assessment

A young, generally healthy, sexually active female with history of migraine headache disorder that has been well controlled with pro-phylactic medication is requesting a contraceptive for birth control and regulation of menses

QUESTIONS

Problem Identification

1.a. Create a list of the patient's potential drug therapy problems.

1.b. What medical problems are absolute contraindications to hor-monal contraceptive use, and do any of those conditions apply to this patient?

1.c. What medical problems are relative contraindications to hormonal contraceptive use, and do any of these apply to this patient?

1.d. What other information should be obtained before creating a pharmacotherapeutic plan?

Desired Outcome

2. What are the goals of pharmacotherapy in this case?

Therapeutic Alternatives

3. What pharmacotherapeutic alternatives are available for preven-tion of pregnancy in this patient, and what are the advantages or disadvantages of each?

Optimal Plan

4. What contraceptive method, dose, and schedule are best for this patient?

Outcome Evaluation

5. What clinical and laboratory parameters are necessary to evalu-ate the therapy for efficacy and adverse effects?

Patient Education

6. What information should be provided to the patient to enhance adherence, ensure successful therapy, and minimize adverse effects?

■ CLINICAL COURSE

Macy returns to the clinic in 2 months complaining of worsening acne and breakthrough bleeding.

■ FOLLOW-UP QUESTIONS

1. What medical conditions can be the cause of breakthrough bleeding?

2. If breakthrough bleeding is not caused by an underlying medical condition, how can it be managed?

3. What recommendations can be made to address this patient's complaint of worsening acne?

■ SELF-STUDY ASSIGNMENTS

1. Compare the costs of each method of birth control and prepare a report that contains your conclusions as to which method pro-vides the best efficacy at the most reasonable cost.

2. Visit a pharmacy and review the various home pregnancy tests; determine how you would counsel a patient to use each one, and evaluate them for ease of use.

CLINICAL PEARL

Oral, transdermal, transvaginal, injectable, and implantable hor-monal contraceptives, as well as intrauterine devices and most barrier contraceptives (with the exception of latex and synthetic condoms), do not protect against the acquisition of STIs. Thus, it is important to properly educate patients who are sexually active about the importance of taking necessary precautions to minimize their risk for acquiring an STI, regardless of the type of hormonal contraceptive used.

REFERENCES

1. Hatcher RA, Trussell J, Nelson AL, Cates W Jr, Kowal D, Policar M. Contraceptive Technology, 20th revised ed. New York, Ardent Media Inc, 2011.

2. U.S. Preventive Services Task Force. USPSTF A and B Recommendations. Available at: *http://www.uspreventiveservicestaskforce.org/Page/Name/uspstf-a-and-b-recommendations/#more*. Accessed April 12, 2016.

3. Centers for Disease Control and Prevention. US Medical Eligibility Criteria for Contraceptive Use, 2010. Adapted from the World Health Organization medical eligibility criteria for contraceptive use, 4th ed. MMWR 2010;59:1–86. Available at: *http://www.cdc.gov/mmwr/preview/mmwrhtml/rr5904a1.htm*. Accessed April 12, 2016.

4. Schoenen J, Sándor PS. Headache with focal neurological signs or symptoms: a complicated differential diagnosis. Lancet Neurol 2004;3:237–245.

5. Centers for Disease Control and Prevention. U.S. Selected Practice Recommendations for Contraceptive Use, 2013: adapted from the World Health Organization selected practice recommendations for contraceptive use, 2nd ed. MMWR 2013;62:1–60. Available at: *http://www.cdc.gov/mmwr/preview/mmwrhtml/rr6205a1.htm*. Accessed April 12, 2016.

6. Dinger J, Bardenheuer K, Heinemann K. Cardiovascular and general safety of a 24-day regimen of drospirenone-containing combined oral contraceptives: final results from the International Active Surveillance Study of Women Taking Oral Contraceptives. Contraception 2014;89:253–263.

7. Vinogradova Y, Coupland C, Hippisley-Cox J. Use of combined oral contraceptives and risk of venous thromboembolism: nested case–control studies using the QResearch and CPRD databases. BMJ 2015;350:h2135. doi:10.1136/bmj.h2135.

8. Vercellini P, Frontino G, De Giorgi O, Pietropaolo G, Pasin R, Crosignani PG. Continuous use of an oral contraceptive for endometriosis-associated recurrent dysmenorrhea that does not respond to a cyclic pill regimen. Fertil Steril 2003;80:560–563.

9. ACOG Committee on Practice Bulletins—Gynecology. ACOG practice bulletin. No. 73: use of hormonal contraception in women with co-existing medical conditions. Obstet Gynecol 2006;107:1453–1472.

10. Machado RB, Pereira AP, Coelho GP, Neri L, Martins L, Luminoso D. Epidemiological and clinical aspects of migraine in users of combined oral contraceptives. Contraception 2010;81:202–208.

11. ACOG Committee on Practice Bulletins—Gynecology. ACOG practice bulletin. No. 131: screening for cervical cancer. Obstet Gynecol 2012;120:1222–1238.

12. ACOG Committee on Gynecologic Practice. Well-woman visit. Committee Opinion No 534. American College of Obstetricians and Gynecologists. Obstet Gynecol 2012;120:421–424.

13. American Cancer Society. American Cancer Society recommendations for early breast cancer detection in women without breast symptoms. Available at: *http://www.cancer.org/cancer/breastcancer/moreinformation/breastcancerearlydetection/breast-cancer-early-detection-acs-recs*. Accessed April 12, 2016.

93

EMERGENCY CONTRACEPTION

Forget Me Not................................ Level II

Emily C. Papineau, PharmD, BCPS

LEARNING OBJECTIVES

After completing this case study, the reader should be able to:

- Describe the advantages and disadvantages of the various options for emergency contraception.

- Discuss the possible side effects and contraindications of the various forms of emergency contraceptives, including both oral and nonoral options.

- Provide patient education regarding the use of emergency contraception.

PATIENT PRESENTATION

■ Chief Complaint

"I forgot to restart my birth control pill pack. I have gone 9 days without a 'real' pill. I'm not ready to be pregnant yet!"

■ HPI

Olivia Furtel is a 19-year-old woman who presents to the Family Medicine Clinic in a panic. She states that she typically throws out the last week of pills in her pack, "since they are not 'real' pills anyway," and she forgot to start her new pill pack on time. She had intercourse with her husband 2 days ago and wants to know what she should do to avoid pregnancy.

■ PMH

Seasonal allergies

■ FH

Mother, age 47, with type 2 diabetes. Father, age 45, with hypertension. Maternal grandmother, age 69, with COPD.

■ SH

Denies smoking
Enjoys an occasional glass of wine
Married × 1 year—mutually monogamous relationship

■ Meds

Cetirizine 10 mg PO once daily × 5 years
Aviane (ethinyl estradiol 20 mcg/levonorgestrel 0.1 mg) 1 tablet PO once daily × 2 years

■ All

NKDA

■ ROS

Patient is a nulligravida woman whose menstrual periods are regular with the use of the combined oral contraceptive pill. She denies any breakthrough bleeding or spotting with routine use. She is tolerating the contraceptive pill well.

■ Physical Examination

Gen

WDWN female appearing anxious

VS

BP 106/70 mm Hg, P 60 bpm, RR 13, T 37°C; Wt 53.5 kg, Ht 5'5", BMI 19.6 kg/m^2

Skin

Clear

Exam

Deferred; she had a complete examination 3 months ago that was normal

■ Labs

3 months ago

Negative Pap smear

1 year ago

Tests negative for *Chlamydia*, gonorrhea, syphilis, and HIV

■ Assessment

Healthy, sexually active female who missed two doses of her combined oral contraceptive pill, extending her pill-free interval >7 days. Emergency contraceptive options to prevent pregnancy should be discussed.

QUESTIONS

Problem Identification

1. Identify the patient's drug therapy problem.

Desired Outcome

2. What are the goals of pharmacotherapy in this case?

Therapeutic Alternatives

3.a. What pharmacotherapeutic options are available for emergency contraception for this patient, and what are the advantages or disadvantages of each?

3.b. What contraindications exist to the use of emergency contraception, and do they apply to this patient?

Optimal Plan

4. Recommend an appropriate emergency contraceptive method and dose for this patient.

Outcome Evaluation

5. What clinical and laboratory parameters are necessary to evaluate the efficacy of the therapy?

Patient Education

6.a. Counsel the patient regarding how the emergency contraceptive regimen works, how to take it, and what side effects may occur.

6.b. Explain to the patient how she will know if the emergency contraception regimen was effective.

6.c. Instruct the patient on when emergency contraception may be warranted, should she need to use it in the future.

6.d. Instruct the patient when she should reinitiate her combined oral contraceptive regimen.

6.e. Counsel the patient regarding how she can minimize the need for emergency contraception in the future.

■ CLINICAL COURSE

A few weeks later, Ms Furtel calls into the clinic to report that she started her period and is not pregnant. She states that she is thankful for the advice provided to her.

■ SELF-STUDY ASSIGNMENTS

1. For other forms of hormonal contraception, such as the patch, the ring, progestin-only pills and injectables, create a table identifying when emergency contraception may be needed if these methods are not used appropriately.

2. Identify strategies to minimize the hormone-free interval with the use of hormonal contraception and thereby diminish the potential need for emergency contraception.

3. For patients not using hormonal contraception, identify additional scenarios for which emergency contraception may be utilized.

4. Explain how BMI may influence efficacy of emergency contraceptive products.

CLINICAL PEARL

Although not FDA-approved for this purpose, a copper IUD may also be used as emergency contraception within the first 120 hours after unprotected intercourse.

REFERENCES

1. Centers for Disease Control and Prevention. U.S. Selected Practice Recommendations for Contraceptive Use, 2013: Adapted from the World Health Organization Selected Practice Recommendations for Contraceptive Use, 2nd ed. MMWR Recomm Rep 2013;62:1–60. Available at: *http://www.cdc.gov/mmwr/preview/mmwrhtml/rr6205a1.htm*. Accessed April 29, 2016.

2. American College of Obstetricians and Gynecologists. ACOG Practice Bulletin No. 152: emergency contraception. Obstet Gynecol 2015;126(3):e1–11.

3. Shrader SP, Hall LN, Ragucci KR, Rafie S. Updates in hormonal emergency contraception. Pharmacotherapy 2011;31:887–895.

4. Zieman M, Hatcher RA, Allen AZ. Managing Contraception for Your Pocket, 13th ed. Tiger, Georgia: Bridging the Gap Foundation, 2015.

5. Ulipristal prescribing information. Morristown, NJ: Watson Pharma, Inc, 2010. Revised March 2015.

6. American College of Obstetricians and Gynecologists. Committee Opinion No. 539: adolescents and long-acting reversible contraception: implants and intrauterine devices. Obstet Gynecol 2012;120:983–988.

7. Baird DT. Emergency contraception: how does it work? Reprod Biomed Online 2009;18(1):32–36.

8. Centers for Disease Control and Prevention. U.S. Medical Eligibility Criteria for Contraceptive Use, 2010: Adapted from the World Health Organization Medical Eligibility Criteria for Contraceptive Use, 4th ed. MMWR Recomm Rep 2010;59:1–86. Available at: *http://www.cdc.gov/mmwr/preview/mmwrhtml/rr5904a1.htm?s_cid=rr5904a1_e*. Accessed April 29, 2016.

9. Rafie S, McIntosh J, Gardner DK, et al. Over-the-counter access to emergency contraception without age restriction: an opinion of the Women's Health Practice and Research Network of the American College of Clinical Pharmacy. Pharmacotherapy 2013;33:549–557.

10. American Academy of Pediatrics. Policy statement: emergency contraception. Pediatrics 2012;130:1174–1182.

94

PREMENSTRUAL DYSPHORIC DISORDER

A Gloomy Girl . . . . Level II

Larissa N. H. Bossaer, PharmD, BCPS

LEARNING OBJECTIVES

After completing this case study, the reader should be able to:

- Differentiate between the clinical presentation and diagnosis of premenstrual syndrome (PMS) and premenstrual dysphoric disorder (PMDD).

- Identify the desired therapeutic outcomes for patients with PMDD.

- Design an appropriate therapeutic plan for a patient with PMDD.

- Design an appropriate monitoring plan for a patient with PMDD, taking into account patient-specific factors (Table 94-1).

- Educate patients and other healthcare professionals about PMDD and therapeutic options.

PATIENT PRESENTATION

■ Chief Complaint

"I think my boss may fire me if I don't get some help."

■ HPI

Gloria Gray, a 29-year-old woman, is an established patient at the Family Physician clinic who returns with complaints of bloating, breast tenderness, angry outbursts, irritability, depression, and fatigue. She has kept a record of her symptoms over the past 3 months, and it appears that her symptoms occur during the last week of her menstrual cycle each month. During this time, she really has a difficult time at work in particular. She gets angry easily and yells at coworkers. She feels very fatigued during this time, which causes her to lose focus and fall behind on her work. She is really concerned that she may lose her job. In addition, even though her husband has been very patient with her during these episodes, she can tell that it is really negatively affecting their relationship because they argue more frequently. She has tried over-the-counter ibuprofen and Midol Teen Formula, but these agents helped only minimally. Her symptoms typically resolve within the first few days of her menses. She says that she is depressed about her current situation, and she would really like some help. On an additional note, she states that she and her husband are not ready to have children as they previously thought. She says that there has just been too much stress in their lives lately, so she is interested in taking birth control. She and her husband use condoms, but they want to take every precaution at this time to effectively prevent pregnancy.

TABLE 94-1 **Item Content of the Daily Record of Severity of Problems (DRSP)[3]**

1.a. Felt depressed, sad, "down," or "blue"
1.b. Felt hopeless
1.c. Felt worthless or guilty
  2. Felt anxious, tense, "keyed up," or "on edge"
3.a. Had mood swings (eg, suddenly felt sad or tearful)
3.b. Was more sensitive to rejection or my feelings were easily hurt
4.a. Felt angry, irritable
4.b. Had conflicts or problems with people
  5. Had less interest in usual activities (eg, work, school, friends, and hobbies)
  6. Had difficulty concentrating
  7. Felt lethargic, tired, fatigued, or had a lack of energy
8.a. Had increased appetite or overate
8.b. Had cravings for specific foods
9.a. Slept more, took naps, found it hard to get up when intended
9.b. Had trouble getting to sleep or staying asleep
10.a. Felt overwhelmed or that I could not cope
10.b. Felt out of control
11.a. Had breast tenderness
11.b. Had breast swelling, felt "bloated," or had weight gain
11.c. Had headache
11.d. Had joint or muscle pain

At work, at school, at home, or in daily routine, at least one of the problems noted above caused reduction of productivity or inefficiency.
At least one of the problems noted above interfered with hobbies or social activities (eg, avoid or do less).
At least one of the problems noted above interfered with relationships with others.

■ PMH

Migraines without aura
Irritable bowel syndrome

■ FH

Mother has dyslipidemia. Father has irritable bowel syndrome.

■ SH

Married for 4 years. No children. Previous smoker 10 years ago, but no current tobacco use. She drinks alcohol socially on the weekends. She works full-time as a professor at a small community college.

■ Meds

Metamucil one teaspoonful of powder in 8 oz of water daily
Propranolol 20 mg Q 6 H
Sumatriptan 100 mg PRN migraine headache, may repeat × one dose
Women's multivitamin daily

■ All

NKDA

■ Physical Examination

Gen

Tearful, petite female

VS

BP 108/66 mm Hg, P 55 bpm, RR 17, T 98.3°F; Wt 112 lb, Ht 5′6″

Skin

Normal; intact; warm and dry

HEENT

PERRLA; EOMI; moist mucous membranes; TMs intact

Neck/Lymph Nodes

Supple without evidence of JVD, lymphadenopathy, or thyromegaly

Lungs/Thorax

CTA & P

Breasts

Symmetric; no lumps or masses; nipples without discharge; tender to touch

CV

RRR without MRG

Abd

Soft, NT/ND; +BS; no masses

Genit/Rect

Normal pelvic exam and pap smear

Ext

Normal ROM; pulses 2+; No CCE

Neuro

A & O × 3; CN II–XII intact; DTRs 2+

■ Labs

Na 141 mEq/L	Ca 9.2 mg/dL	*Fasting lipid profile*	WBC $6 \times 10^3/mm^3$
K 3.5 mEq/L	AST 20 IU/L	T. chol 190 mg/dL	Hgb 13 g/dL
Cl 104 mEq/L	ALT 17 IU/L	TG 120 mg/dL	Hct 39%
CO_2 27 mEq/L	Alb 3.9 g/dL	LDL 95 mg/dL	MCV 92.8 μm^3
Glu 81 mg/dL	TSH 0.74 mIU/L	HDL 71 mg/dL	MCH 31.7 pg
BUN 14 mg/dL			MCHC 34.2 g/dL
SCr 0.9 mg/dL			Plt $249 \times 10^3/mm^3$

■ Assessment

1. PMDD
2. Desire for contraception
3. Migraines without aura, currently well controlled
4. Irritable bowel syndrome, currently well controlled

QUESTIONS

Problem Identification

1.a. Create a list of the patient's drug therapy problems.

1.b. What symptoms in the patient's clinical presentation indicate PMDD?

1.c. How does this patient's clinical presentation differ from that of a patient suffering from PMS? What are the diagnostic differences between PMS and PMDD?

Desired Outcome

2. What are the desired therapeutic outcomes in this patient with regard to PMDD?

Therapeutic Alternatives

3.a. What nondrug therapies might be useful for a patient with PMDD?

3.b. What feasible pharmacotherapeutic alternatives are available for treatment of PMDD?

Optimal Plan

4. What drug(s), dosage form, dose, schedule, and duration of therapy is/are best for this patient?

Outcome Evaluation

5. What clinical and laboratory parameters are necessary to evaluate the therapy for achievement of the desired therapeutic outcome and to detect or prevent adverse effects?

Patient Education

6. What information should be provided to the patient to enhance adherence, ensure successful therapy, and minimize adverse effects?

■ SELF-STUDY ASSIGNMENTS

1. Develop a patient educational handout that outlines the differences between PMS and PMDD and provides resources for patients to get more information on PMDD.

2. List diseases that mimic the symptoms of PMDD that must be ruled out before the diagnosis of PMDD can be confirmed in a patient.

3. Discuss how migraine headaches and irritable bowel syndrome may be affected by the menstrual cycle.

CLINICAL PEARL

PMDD and PMS are similar in many ways, but they differ in diagnostic criteria and severity. While up to 80% of women experience PMS, only up to 8% of women suffer from PMDD. PMDD is classified as a psychiatric disorder. Therefore, it is important to differentiate PMDD from PMS in order to appropriately treat patients who suffer from the disease.

REFERENCES

1. American Psychiatric Association. Desk Reference to the Diagnostic Criteria from DSM-5. Washington, DC, American Psychiatric Publishing, 2013:100–101.

2. Futterman LA, Rapkin AJ. Diagnosis of premenstrual disorders. J Reprod Med 2006;51:349–358.

3. Endicott J, Nee J, Harrison W. Daily record of severity of problems (DRSP): reliability and validity. Arch Women Ment Health 2006;9:41–49.

4. Jang SH, Kim DI, Choi MS. Effects and treatment methods of acupuncture and herbal medicine for premenstrual syndrome/premenstrual dysphoric disorder: systematic review. BMC Complement Altern Med 2014;14:11. doi:10.1186/1472-6882-14-11.

5. Kroll R, Rapkin AJ. Treatment of premenstrual disorders. J Reprod Med 2006;51:359–370.

6. Biggs WS, Demuth RH. Premenstrual syndrome and premenstrual dysphoric disorder. Am Fam Physician 2011;84:918–924.

7. Marjoribanks J, Brown J, O'Brien PM, Wyatt K. Selective serotonin reuptake inhibitors for premenstrual syndrome. Cochrane Database Syst Rev 2013;6:CD001396. doi:10.1002/14651858.CD001396.

8. Lopez LM, Kaptein AA, Helmerhorst FM. Oral contraceptives containing drospirenone for premenstrual syndrome. Cochrane Database Syst Rev 2012;2:CD006586. doi:10.1002/14651858.CD006586.

9. American College of Obstetricians and Gynecologists. Noncontraceptive uses of hormonal contraceptives. Obstet Gynecol 2010;115:206–218. doi:10.1097/AOG.0b013e3181cb50b5.

10. U.S. Food and Drug Administration. FDA Drug Safety Communication: updated information about the risk of blood clots in women taking birth control pills containing drospirenone. Available at: *http://www.fda.gov/Drugs/DrugSafety/ucm299305.htm*. Accessed April 12, 2016.

11. Freeman EW, Halbreich U, Grubb GS, et al. An overview of four studies of a continuous oral contraceptive (levonorgestrel 90 mcg/ethinyl estradiol 20 mcg) on premenstrual dysphoric disorder and premenstrual syndrome. Contraception 2012;85:437–445.

95

ENDOMETRIOSIS

Persistent Pelvic Pain .... Level II

Connie K. Kraus, PharmD, BCACP

LEARNING OBJECTIVES

After completing this case study, the reader should be able to:

- Identify the signs and symptoms associated with endometriosis.

- Compare and contrast the benefits and risks associated with various hormonal medications used for the treatment of endometriosis-associated pelvic pain.

- Determine a treatment approach for this case taking into account other health issues and potential health benefits.

- Discuss possible side effects associated with treatment for endometriosis.

PATIENT PRESENTATION

■ Chief Complaint

"Although the pain associated with my menstrual period is better, the naproxen upsets my stomach, and I am still having pain in my lower abdomen at other times during the month."

■ HPI

Lisbeth Anderson is a 30-year-old woman who was diagnosed with endometriosis 3 months ago based on a history of dysmenorrhea, intermittent pain with defecation, and past history of dyspareunia. She presents to the nurse practitioner today for evaluation and management of continued endometriosis-related pain despite treatment with naproxen.

■ PMH

S/P deep vein thrombosis 4 years ago after a flight to Southeast Asia; treated for 6 months with warfarin; no recurrence
G1P1A0; one healthy male child aged 2 years

■ FH

Mother (aged 57 years) has a history of endometriosis, no other health conditions; father (aged 58 years) has hypertension and elevated cholesterol; one female sibling (aged 25 years) is healthy

■ SH

Patient is a freelance photographer. She has one child. She is single; currently not sexually active. She does not smoke and consumes no more than two alcohol-containing beverages per week. She exercises 30 minutes most days of the week.

■ Meds

Naproxen 250 mg three times daily with food at first sign of menses for 5–7 days was begun at previous visit
Multivitamin one daily

■ All

NKDA

■ ROS

(+) For moderate pain in pelvic region, (–) for constipation, menstrual periods occur at regular intervals of 29 days

■ Physical Examination

Gen

WDWN female in NAD

VS

BP 115/70 mm Hg, P 65 bpm, RR 15, T 37°C; Wt 72 kg, Ht 5'11"; patient has maintained same weight prepregnancy and postpregnancy

Skin

No lesions

HEENT

WNL

Neck/Lymph Nodes

Supple, no bruits, no adenopathy, no thyromegaly

Lungs/Thorax

CTA bilaterally

Breasts

Supple; no masses

CV

RRR, normal S_1 and S_2

Abd

Soft; patient states, at baseline, she experiences pain that averages a "4" on a 0–10 pain scale (with 10 being the worst possible pain), (+) BS; no masses noted

Genit/Rect

Pelvic exam: (+) adnexal pain elicited and rated at "6" on a 10-point scale, no masses

MS/Ext

Pulses intact

Neuro

Normal sensory and motor levels

■ Labs

Na 135 mEq/L	*Fasting lipid profile*
K 3.8 mEq/L	T. chol 140 mg/dL
Cl 104 mEq/L	LDL 55 mg/dL
CO_2 25 mEq/L	HDL 65 mg/dL
BUN 10 mg/dL	Trig 100 mg/dL
SCr 0.6 mg/dL	
Random Glu 89 mg/dL	

■ Other

PAP smear: Normal

Chlamydia/gonorrhea: Negative

UPT: Negative

■ Assessment

A 30-year-old woman with recent diagnosis of endometriosis with chronic pelvic pain and has partial relief from dysmenorrhea with naproxen. Because of naproxen-related side effects and pain at other times besides during menses, she would like to consider hormonal treatment options.

QUESTIONS

Problem Identification

1.a. What are the patient's current medication-related problems?

1.b. What information indicates the severity of this patient's problems?

Desired Outcome

2. What are the goals of therapy for this patient's endometriosis pain?

Therapeutic Alternatives

3.a. What nondrug therapies might be useful for the treatment of pain associated with endometriosis?

3.b. What pharmacotherapeutic options are available for the treatment of pain associated with endometriosis?

3.c. What are the potential risks and benefits of the various treatment options for this patient?

3.d. Are there any treatments contraindicated in this patient?

Optimal Plan

4. What drug, dosage form, dose, schedule, and duration are best for this patient?

Outcome Evaluation

5. What clinical and laboratory parameters are necessary to evaluate the therapy for achievement of the desired therapeutic outcome and to detect or prevent adverse effects?

Patient Education

6. What information should be provided to the patient to enhance adherence to the medication, ensure successful therapy, and minimize adverse effects?

■ CLINICAL COURSE

The patient returns to her nurse practitioner 6 months after starting medroxyprogesterone acetate 150 mg intramuscular injections every 3 months. She reports that her pelvic pain is better controlled with an overall average rating pain of "1" on the 10-point scale. She states that she had intermittent spotting initially, but now has no menstrual periods.

■ FOLLOW-UP QUESTIONS

1. What is the optimal length of time for a patient to continue on medroxyprogesterone acetate injections for the treatment of endometriosis-related chronic pelvic pain?

2. Are there other options that this patient could select to achieve similar results with the same or better side-effect profile?

3. Would your recommendation change if this patient had risk factors for osteopenia or osteoporosis?

4. Would your recommendation change if this patient had indicated an interest in having another child in the next 1–2 years?

■ SELF-STUDY ASSIGNMENTS

1. Research complementary therapies that have been studied for the relief of endometriosis, and compare the evidence for their efficacy with standard treatments.

2. Review the contraindications of the various contraceptive agents used for the treatment of endometriosis.

CLINICAL PEARL

Pharmacologic treatment of endometriosis may be useful for decreasing pain. Pharmacotherapeutic agents that mimic pregnancy or menopause are the cornerstone of treatment. All of these agents have comparable efficacy in treating pain but have different side-effect profiles. Treatment with hormonal therapy does not improve fertility, which can also be a potential consequence of the disease.

REFERENCES

1. Flower A, Liu JP, Lewith G, Little P, Li Q. Chinese herbal medicine for endometriosis. Cochrane Database Syst Rev 2012;(5):CD006568. doi:10.1002/14651858.CD006568.pub3.

2. Luciano DE, Luciano AA. Management of endometriosis-related pain: an update. Women's Health 2011;7(5):585–590.

3. Falcone T, Lebovic DI. Clinical management of endometriosis. Obstet Gynecol 2011;118:691–705.

4. Wong AYK, Tang LCH, Chin RKH. Levonorgestrel-releasing intrauterine system (Mirena) and Depot medroxyprogesterone acetate (Depoprovera) as long-term maintenance therapy for patients with moderate and severe endometriosis: a randomized, controlled trial. Aust N Z J Obstet Gynaecol 2010;50:273–279.

5. Walch K, Unfried G, Huber J, et al. Implanon® versus medroxyprogesterone acetate: effects on pain scores in patients with symptomatic endometriosis—a pilot study. Contraception 2009;70:29–34.

6. Brown J, Pan A, Hart RJ. Gonadotrophin-releasing hormone analogues for pain associated with endometriosis. Cochrane Database Syst Rev 2010;(12):CD008475. doi:10.1002/14651858.CD008475.pub2.

7. ESHRE Endometriosis Guideline Development Group. Management of women with endometriosis. 2013:1–97. Available at: *https://www.eshre.eu/guidelines-and-legal/guidelines/endometriosis-guideline.aspx*. Accessed April 15, 2016.

8. Ferro S, Gillott DJ, Venturini, Remorgida V. Use of aromatase inhibitors to treat endometriosis-related pain symptoms: a systematic review. Reprod Biol Endocrinol 2011;9(89):1–10.

9. Hatcher RA, Trussell J, Nelson AL, Cates W Jr, Kowal D, Policar M. Contraceptive Technology, 20th ed. Contraceptive Technology Communications, Inc, 2011.

10. Department of Reproductive Health, World Health Organization. Medical Eligibility Criteria for Contraceptive Use, 5th ed. 2015. Available at: *http://www.who.int/reproductivehealth/publications/family_planning/Ex-Summ-MEC-5/en/.* Accessed April 15, 2016.

96

MANAGING MENOPAUSAL SYMPTOMS

A Hot Topic.................................... Level II

Nicole S. Culhane, PharmD, FCCP, BCPS

LEARNING OBJECTIVES

After completing this case study, the reader should be able to:

- Identify the signs and symptoms associated with menopause.

- List the risks and benefits associated with hormone therapy (HT), and identify appropriate candidates for HT.

- Differentiate between topical and systemic forms of HT.

- Recommend nonpharmacologic therapy for menopausal symptoms.

- Identify alternative, nonhormonal therapies for women unable to take HT.

- Design a comprehensive pharmacotherapeutic plan for a patient on HT including treatment options and monitoring.

- Determine the desired therapeutic outcomes for a patient taking HT.

- Educate patients on the treatment options, benefits, risks, and monitoring of HT.

PATIENT PRESENTATION

■ Chief Complaint

"I have been having hot flashes for the past few months, and I just can't take it anymore."

■ HPI

Emma Peterson is a 50-year-old woman who reports experiencing two to three hot flashes per day, occasionally associated with insomnia. She also states she is awakened from sleep about two to three times per week needing to change her bed clothes and linens. Her symptoms began about 3 months ago, and over that time they have worsened to the point where they have become very bothersome. She states that her mother was prescribed a pill for this, but she is hesitant to take the same thing because she heard on the news

and from friends that the medication may not be safe. She also does not want to "get her period back" if possible. Successfully treated for depression in the past, she is currently controlled on paroxetine therapy. She exercises three times a week and tries to follow a low-cholesterol diet.

■ PMH

Depression
GERD
HTN
Hypothyroidism

■ FH

Mother died of stroke at age 67; father died of lung cancer at age 62. Patient has one brother, 52, and one sister, 48, who are alive and well, but both with HTN.

■ SH

Married, mother of two healthy daughters, ages 21 and 25. She is an RN in a neighboring physician's office. She walks on her treadmill three times a week and is trying to follow a dietitian-designed low-cholesterol diet. She does not smoke and occasionally drinks a glass of red wine with dinner.

■ Meds

Hydrochlorothiazide 25 mg PO once daily
Omeprazole 20 mg PO once daily
Paroxetine 20 mg PO once daily
Synthroid 0.075 mg PO once daily

■ All

NKDA

■ ROS

(+) Hot flashes, occasional night sweats and insomnia, vaginal dryness. (–) weight gain, constipation. LMP 12 months ago.

■ Physical Examination

Gen

WDWN female in NAD

VS

BP 128/86 mm Hg, P 78 bpm, RR 15, T 36.4°C; Wt 76.2 kg, Ht 5′6″

Skin

Warm, dry, no lesions

HEENT

WNL

Neck/LN

Supple, no bruits, no adenopathy, no thyromegaly

Lungs/Thorax

CTA bilaterally

Breasts

Supple; no masses

CV

RRR, normal S_1 and S_2; no MRG

Abd

Soft, NT/ND, (+) BS; no masses

Genit/Rect

Pelvic exam normal except (+) mucosal atrophy; stool guaiac (–)

Ext

(–) CCE; pulses intact

Neuro

Normal sensory and motor levels

■ Labs

Na 136 mEq/L	Hgb 12.7 g/dL	Ca 9.3 mg/dL	*Fasting lipid profile*
K 3.9 mEq/L	Hct 39.3%	AST 32 IU/L	T. chol 190 mg/dL
Cl 104 mEq/L	WBC $6.5 \times 10^3/mm^3$	ALT 30 IU/L	LDL 132 mg/dL
CO_2 25 mEq/L	Plt $208 \times 10^3/mm^3$	TSH 2.46 mIU/L	HDL 50 mg/dL
BUN 10 mg/dL		FSH 87.8 mIU/mL	Trig 180 mg/dL
SCr 0.7 mg/dL		UPT (–)	
Random Glu 98 mg/dL			

■ Other

Pap smear and mammogram: Normal

■ Assessment

A 50-year-old symptomatic postmenopausal woman considering HT versus other treatment options

QUESTIONS

Problem Identification

1.a. Create a list of the patient's drug therapy problems.

1.b. What information (signs, symptoms, and laboratory values) indicates the presence or severity of this patient's problems as she begins menopause?

Desired Outcome

2. What are the goals of therapy for this patient's menopausal symptoms?

Therapeutic Alternatives

3.a. What nondrug therapies might be useful for this patient?

3.b. What are the benefits and risks of HT for this patient?

3.c. What pharmacotherapeutic *hormonal* therapies are available for the treatment of menopause?

3.d. What *nonhormonal* alternatives may be used to manage menopausal symptoms?

Optimal Plan

4. What drug, dosage form, dose, schedule, and duration are best for this patient?

Outcome Evaluation

5. What clinical and laboratory parameters are necessary to evaluate the therapy for achievement of the desired therapeutic outcome and to detect or prevent adverse effects?

Patient Education

6. What information should be provided to the patient to enhance adherence to the medication, ensure successful therapy, and minimize adverse effects?

■ CLINICAL COURSE

The patient returns to her physician after taking HT for 1 year. She reports that her hot flashes, night sweats, and occasional insomnia have significantly decreased and would like to know if she should continue taking the HT regimen and if so, for how long.

■ FOLLOW-UP QUESTIONS

1. What is the optimal dose and length of time for a patient to continue on HT?

2. How should HT be discontinued after successful treatment?

3. Would your recommendation for HT change if the patient had been complaining of genital symptoms only? Why or why not?

4. Would your recommendation for HT change if this patient were to have had significant risk factors for CAD or a personal history of breast cancer? Why or why not?

5. How would you respond to the patient if she asked you about taking bioidentical HT?

■ CLINICAL COURSE: ALTERNATIVE THERAPY

Because Mrs Peterson is considering stopping her HT because of her family history of breast cancer but still desires some relief from hot flushes, she asks for additional information on other alternatives. She has heard that black cohosh should not be used in women with breast cancer, but she has a friend who also has a family history of breast cancer who has been on black cohosh for about 9 months on the recommendation of her physician, although the friend must have a checkup with lab tests every 6 months. Mrs Peterson asks if black cohosh or soy would be an appropriate option to help keep her hot flushes under control. See Section 19 in this Casebook for questions about the use of black cohosh for managing menopausal symptoms.

■ SELF-STUDY ASSIGNMENTS

1. Research nonhormonal therapies that have been studied for the relief of menopausal symptoms and compare the scientific evidence of their efficacy to traditional hormonal medications.

2. Review the results of the Women's Health Initiative (WHI) study from 2002 and the 2007 reanalysis of the WHI results regarding the impact of HT on cardiovascular disease related to age and duration of HT use. Provide a summary of the overall findings regarding HT and cardiovascular risk and breast cancer risk.

CLINICAL PEARL

Women should receive a thorough history and physical exam, including assessing CAD and breast cancer risk factors, before HT is considered. If a woman does not have any contraindications to HT, including CAD or significant CAD risk factors, and also does not have a personal history of breast cancer, short-term HT would be an appropriate therapy option as it remains the most effective treatment for vasomotor symptoms and vulvovaginal atrophy.

REFERENCES

1. Goff DC Jr, Lloyd-Jones DM, Bennett G, et al. 2013 ACC/AHA guideline on the assessment of cardiovascular risk. A report of the American College of Cardiology/American Heart Association Task Force on practice guidelines. Circulation 2014;129:S49–S73.

2. Cosman F, deBeur SJ, LeBoff MS, et al. A clinician's guide to the prevention and treatment of osteoporosis. Osteoporosis Int 2014;25:2359–2381.

3. The 2012 hormone therapy position statement of the North American Menopause Society. Menopause 2012;19:257–271.

4. Hulley S, Grady D, Bush T, et al. Randomized trial of estrogen plus progestin for secondary prevention of coronary heart disease in postmenopausal women. Heart and Estrogen/progestin Replacement Study (HERS) Research Group. JAMA 1998;280:605–613.

5. Rossouw JE, Anderson GL, Prentice RL, et al. Writing Group for the Women's Health Initiative Investigators. Risks and benefits of estrogen plus progestin in healthy postmenopausal women: principal results from the Women's Health Initiative randomized controlled trial. JAMA 2002;288:321–333.

6. Rossouw JE, Prentice RL, Manson JE, et al. Postmenopausal hormone therapy and risk of cardiovascular disease by age and years since menopause. JAMA 2007;297:1465–1477.

7. Anderson GL, Limacher M, Assaf AR, et al. Effects of conjugated equine estrogen in postmenopausal women with hysterectomy: the Women's Health Initiative randomized controlled trial. JAMA 2004;291:1701–1712.

8. Nonhormonal management of menopause-associated vasomotor symptoms: 2015 position statement of The North American Menopause Society. Menopause 2015;22:1–18.

9. Cheema D, Coomarasamy A, El-Toukhy T. Non-hormonal therapy of postemenopausal vasomotor symptoms: a structured evidence-based review. Arch Gynecol Obstet 2007;276:463–469.

10. Leach MJ, Moore V. Black cohosh (*Cimicifuga* spp.) for menopausal symptoms. Cochrane Database Syst Rev 2012;9:CD007244. doi:10.1002/14651858.CD007244.pub2.

97

ERECTILE DYSFUNCTION

Where There's a Pill, There's a Way.............Level III

Cara Liday, PharmD, CDE

LEARNING OBJECTIVES

After completing this case study, the reader should be able to:

- Recognize risk factors associated with development of erectile dysfunction (ED).
- Provide brief descriptions of the advantages and disadvantages of the common therapies available for treating ED.
- Compare and contrast the benefits and risks of the available PDE-5 inhibitors.
- Provide appropriate patient education on administration and expected side effects of selected treatment modalities for ED.

PATIENT PRESENTATION

Chief Complaint

"My sex life just isn't what it used to be...."

HPI

Peter Johnson is a 63-year-old man who presents to his PCP with the above complaint. On questioning, he states that for the last year he has been able to achieve only partial erections that are insufficient for intercourse. He does not notice nocturnal penile tumescence. He feels that the problem is leading to a strained relationship with his wife, and he is interested in trying an herbal product or "nutritional supplement" for help.

PMH

Type 2 DM × 14 years
HTN
HF (NYHA class II)
Dyslipidemia

FH

Father deceased at age 72 of cancer; mother alive with HTN

SH

Married for 38 years; no history of marital problems; does not smoke or drink alcohol; walks for 30 minutes 5 days per week

Meds

Insulin glargine 60 U SC at bedtime
Metformin 1000 mg PO BID
Lisinopril 40 mg PO once daily
Carvedilol 25 mg PO BID
Furosemide 20 mg PO every morning
Atorvastatin 40 mg PO once daily
ASA 81 mg PO once daily

All

NKDA

ROS

Denies significant life stressors, fatigue, nocturia, urgency, or symptoms of prostatitis. Complains of occasional nocturia, numbness in his feet, and difficulty achieving and maintaining erections. Occasionally has transient edema in his ankles, and many of his toenails are brittle and yellowing.

Physical Examination

Gen
Alert, well-developed, cooperative man in NAD

VS
BP 136/78 mm Hg, P 60 bpm, RR 18, T 37.2°C; Wt 120 kg, Ht 5'11"

Skin
Warm, dry; no lesions

HEENT
NC/AT; EOMI; PERRLA; funduscopic examination shows no arteriolar narrowing, hemorrhages, or exudates

Neck/Lymph Nodes
Supple without JVD, lymphadenopathy, masses, or goiter

Lungs/Chest
Clear to A & P bilaterally

CV
RRR; normal S_1 and S_2; no MRG

Abd

Soft, obese; NTND; normal bowel sounds; no masses or organomegaly

Genit/Rect

Normal scrotum, testes descended; NT w/o masses; penis without discharge or curvature; slightly enlarged prostate

MS/Ext

Muscle strength 5/5 throughout; full ROM in all extremities; pulses 2+ throughout; no edema present; multiple toenails with yellow discoloration and thickening

Neuro

CNs II–XII intact; DTRs 2+ and equal bilaterally. No sensory/motor deficits; reduced sensation in extremities bilaterally with vibratory and monofilament testing.

■ Labs

Na 139 mEq/L	Hgb 16.0 g/dL	Ca 9.5 mg/dL	*Fasting lipid profile*
K 3.9 mEq/L	Hct 50%	Mg 1.8 mEq/L	T. chol 192 mg/dL
Cl 102 mEq/L	AST 35 IU/L	A1C 8.5%	HDL 41 mg/dL
CO_2 24 mEq/L	ALT 18 IU/L	Testosterone 700 ng/dL	LDL 94 mg/dL
BUN 12 mg/dL		TSH 1.54 mIU/L	TG 129 mg/dL
SCr 1.0 mg/dL		BNP 79 pg/mL	VLDL 19 mg/dL
Glu (fasting) 166 mg/dL			

■ UA

SG 1.00; pH 5.1; leukocyte esterase (–); nitrite (–); protein 100 mg/dL; ketones (–); urobilinogen normal; bilirubin (–); blood (–); albumin/Cr ratio 18 mg/g

■ Assessment

A 63-year-old male with ED, hypertension, HF, dyslipidemia, poor long-term control of type 2 diabetes, and probable diagnosis of onychomycosis

QUESTIONS

Problem Identification

1.a. Create a list of the patient's drug therapy problems.

1.b. What risk factors for ED are present in this patient?

1.c. What are the etiologies of ED, and what is this patient's most likely etiology?

1.d. Could any of the patient's problems have been caused by drug therapy?

Desired Outcome

2. What are the goals of therapy in this case?

Therapeutic Alternatives

3.a. What nondrug therapies are available for the treatment of ED?

3.b. What pharmacologic alternatives are available for the treatment of ED?

Optimal Plan

4. What therapy is most appropriate and effective for initial treatment of this patient? If drug therapy is indicated, list the drug, dosage form, dose, schedule, and duration of therapy.

Outcome Evaluation

5. What clinical parameters are necessary to evaluate the therapy for achievement of the desired therapeutic outcome and to detect or prevent adverse effects?

Patient Education

6. What information should be provided to the patient to enhance compliance, ensure successful therapy, and minimize adverse effects?

■ CLINICAL COURSE

Mr Johnson was referred to his cardiologist for exercise treadmill testing. It was determined that he may safely resume sexual activity at this time. He is to call immediately if he has significant SOB or chest pain during or after intercourse.

■ SELF-STUDY ASSIGNMENTS

1. If therapy for onychomycosis is desired, what medication would be optimal, and how would the addition of this agent change your treatment of the patient's ED?

2. β-Blockers are typically associated with an increased incidence of ED. Determine why nebivolol may have a lower incidence of ED and may possibly improve erectile function.

3. Discuss the possible benefits of using a PDE-5 inhibitor in patients with symptomatic benign prostatic hyperplasia (BPH).

4. Evaluate the incidence of women's sexual dysfunction and options for therapy in this population.

CLINICAL PEARL

Patients with cardiovascular (CV) disease have a greater risk of developing ED. In addition, the presence of ED in otherwise healthy individuals may indicate an increased risk of subsequent CV disease. The development of ED may precede the onset of CV symptoms by 3 years or more. Providers should use this opportunity to screen or treat CV disease appropriately.

REFERENCES

1. Corona G, Mondaini N, Ungar A, Razzoli E, Rossi A, Fusco F. Phosphodiesterase type 5 (PDE5) inhibitors in erectile dysfunction: the proper drug for the proper patient. J Sex Med 2011;8:3418–3432.

2. Mola JR. Erectile dysfunction in the older adult male. Urol Nurs 2015;35:87–93.

3. Hatzimouratidis K, Eardley I, Giuliano F, Moncada I, Salonia A. Guidelines on male sexual dysfunction: erectile dysfunction and premature ejaculation. European Association of Urology Website. *http://uroweb.org/guideline/male-sexual-dysfunction/*. Updated 2015. *http://uroweb.org/wp-content/uploads/14-Male-Sexual-Dysfunction_LR1.pdf*. Accessed November 10, 2015.

4. Tsertsvadze A, Fink HA, Yazdi F, et al. Oral phosphodiesterase-5 inhibitors and hormonal treatments for erectile dysfunction: a systematic review and meta-analysis. Ann Intern Med 2009;151:650–661.

5. Consumer Updates. Hidden risks of erectile dysfunction "treatments" sold online. US Food and Drug Administration. Available at: *www.fda.gov/ForConsumers/ConsumerUpdates/ucm048386.htm*. Accessed November 10, 2015.

6. Nehra A, Jackson G, Miner M, et al. The Princeton III Consensus recommendations for the management of erectile dysfunction and cardiovascular disease. Mayo Clin Proc 2012;87:766–778.

98

BENIGN PROSTATIC HYPERPLASIA

Trouble with Dribbles...........................Level II

Kathryn Eroschenko, PharmD

Kevin W. Cleveland, PharmD, ANP

LEARNING OBJECTIVES

After completing this case study, the reader should be able to:

- Recognize the clinical manifestations of benign prostatic hyperplasia (BPH) and lower urinary tract symptoms (LUTS) secondary to BPH.

- Differentiate between obstructive and irritative symptoms in patients with BPH.

- Recommend appropriate pharmacotherapeutic treatment for BPH.

- Identify and manage drug interactions associated with BPH pharmacotherapy.

- Recognize when surgical therapies should be considered for patients with BPH.

- Understand how some drugs can exacerbate BPH symptoms.

PATIENT PRESENTATION

■ Chief Complaint

"I'm up four to five times a night feeling that I have to urinate, and then when I get to the bathroom all I do is dribble. I'm very lightheaded when I stand up, and sometimes I don't make it to the bathroom in time. I have a girlfriend now, but I am finding it difficult to be intimate with her. Also, going to the bathroom all night is really impacting my love life."

■ HPI

Jimmy McCracken is a 65-year-old man with a long-standing history of UTIs. He has a history of urosepsis requiring hospitalization. He is being evaluated because of complaints of worsening urinary hesitancy, nocturia, and dribbling. He also has a new complaint of ED.

■ PMH

HTN
Laminectomy 10 years ago
BPH with urge incontinence
Chronic UTIs
Type 2 DM
Allergy to cat dander
ED
Obesity
Osteoarthritis

■ FH

Educated through the 12th grade. Father died of massive MI at age 78; mother died of natural causes at age 91.

■ SH

Worked for 35 years in a grocery store; retired 7 years ago. Married once. Wife deceased 6 months ago (stroke); one daughter, two granddaughters. Lives alone but is socially active. Recently started dating a 60-year-old woman he met online through a senior dating website. Patient would like information on current prescription medications used to treat BPH symptoms but is not opposed to treating current symptoms with natural products if possible. Used smokeless tobacco × 35 years; heavy ETOH in the past, occasional glass of wine now.

■ ROS

In conversation, he is alert, friendly, and courteous. He has no c/o dyspepsia, dysphagia, abdominal pain, hematemesis, or visible blood in the stool.

■ Meds

Metformin 1000 mg PO BID
Terazosin 10 mg PO once daily
Amitriptyline 25 mg PO at bedtime (insomnia)
Metoprolol succinate 50 mg PO once daily
Ibuprofen 800 mg PO BID
Claritin-D 24-hour one tablet PO daily (allergy to cats)

■ All

NKDA; allergic to cat dander

■ Physical Examination

Gen

White male in NAD; well-kept appearance; A & O × 3

VS

BP 110/60 mm Hg, P 65 bpm, RR 18, T 37°C; Wt 115.2 kg, Ht 6'0"

Skin

Vertical scars on neck and lower back from laminectomies

HEENT

PERRLA; EOMI; TMs WNL; nose and throat clear w/o exudate or lesions

Neck/Lymph Nodes

Supple w/o LAD or masses; thyroid in midline

Lungs/Thorax

CTA, distant sounds

CV

RRR w/o murmurs

Abd

Soft, NTND w/o masses or scars; (+) BS

Genit/Rect

Testes ↓↓, penis circumcised w/o DC; guaiac (+) stool

MS/Ext

Neurovascular intact; distal pulses 1–2+

Neuro

DTRs 2+; CNs II–XII grossly intact

■ Labs

See Table 98-1.

TABLE 98-1 | Item Lab Values

Na 136 mEq/L	Hgb 12.6 g/dL	WBC 5.6 × 10³/mm³	AST 12 IU/L	Ca 8.5 mg/dL
K 4.1 mEq/L	Hct 37.9%	Neutros 75%	ALT 16 IU/L	Phos 3.5 mg/dL
Cl 103 mEq/L	MCV 92.5 μm³	Lymphs 16%	Alk phos 55 IU/L	Uric acid 3.5 mg/dL
CO$_2$ 41 mEq/L	MCH 30.8 pg	Monos 5%	LDH 121 units/L	T$_4$ 7.3 mcg/dL
BUN 9 mg/dL	MCHC 33.3 g/dL	Eos 3%	T. bili 0.6 mg/dL	TSH 1.04 mIU/L
SCr 0.7 mg/dL	Plt 191 × 10³/mm³	Basos 1%	T. prot 6.1 g/dL	A1C 7%
Glu 120 mg/dL			T. chol 146 mg/dL	PSA 4.5 ng/mL

■ UA

Color straw; appearance clear; SG 1.010; pH 6.5; glucose (–); bilirubin (–); ketones (–); blood (–); urobilinogen 0.2 mg/dL; nitrite (–); leukocyte esterases (–); epithelial cells—occasional per hpf; WBC—occasional per hpf; RBC—none seen; bacteria—trace; amorphous—none seen; crystals—1+ calcium oxalate; mucus—none seen. Culture not indicated.

■ GU Consult

Patient treated for UTI 2 weeks ago with Cipro 250 mg PO Q 12 H × 3 days. Urine clear; negative for glucose. Bladder examination with ultrasound revealed postvoid residual estimate of 200 mL. Prostate approximately 35 g, benign. AUA Symptom Score = 20. Uroflowmetry (Q_{max}) = 8 mL/s.

■ Assessment

BPH with urge incontinence
ED
Symptomatic hypotension
Normocytic anemia possibly secondary to UGI bleed

QUESTIONS

Problem Identification

1.a. Create a list of the patient's drug therapy problems.

1.b. Describe the natural history and epidemiologic characteristics of BPH.

1.c. Which complaints are consistent with obstructive symptoms of BPH? Which are consistent with irritative symptoms?

1.d. What steps are recommended in the initial evaluation of all patients presenting with BPH (Fig. 98-1)?

1.e. What other medical conditions should be ruled out before treating this patient for BPH?

Desired Outcome

2. What are the goals of pharmacotherapy in this case?

Therapeutic Alternatives

3. What are the treatment alternatives for BPH?

Patient Name: _____ DOB: _____ ID: _____ Date of assessment: _____

Initial Assessment ( ) Monitor during: _____ Therapy ( ) after: _____ Therapy/surgery ( ) _____

AUA BPH Symptom Score

	Not at all	Less than 1 time in 5	Less than half the time	About half the time	More than half the time	Almost always	
1. Over the past month, how often have you had a sensation of not emptying your bladder completely after you finished urinating?	0	1	2	3	4	5	
2. Over the past month, how often have you had to urinate again less than two hours after you finished urinating?	0	1	2	3	4	5	
3. Over the past month, how often have you found you stopped and started again several times when you urinated?	0	1	2	3	4	5	
4. Over the past month, how often have you found it difficult to postpone urination?	0	1	2	3	4	5	
5. Over the past month, how often have you had a weak urinary stream?	0	1	2	3	4	5	
6. Over the past month, how often have you had to push or strain to begin urination?	0	1	2	3	4	5	
	None	1 time	2 times	3 times	4 times	5 or more times	
7. Over the past month, how many times did you most typically get up to urinate from the time you went to bed at night until the time you got up in the morning?	0	1	2	3	4	5	
						Total Symptom Score	

FIGURE 98-1. The American Urologic Association (AUA) symptom index for benign prostatic hyperplasia (BPH). *(Reprinted with permission from BPH, Main Report: Roehrborn CG, McConnell JD, Barry MJ, et al. AUA Guideline on the Management of Benign Prostatic Hyperplasia. American Urological Association Education and Research, Inc., © 2003.)*

Optimal Plan

4. What drug, dosage form, dose, schedule, and duration of therapy are best for this patient?

Outcome Evaluation

5. What clinical and laboratory parameters are necessary to evaluate the therapy for achievement of the desired therapeutic outcome and to detect or prevent adverse effects?

Patient Education

6. What information should be provided to the patient to enhance compliance, ensure successful therapy, and minimize adverse effects?

■ CLINICAL COURSE: ALTERNATIVE THERAPY

As the pharmacist in the team, you perform a literature search on the use of saw palmetto for BPH. You discover that there are reports of the dietary supplement both improving and worsening symptoms of ED. In addition, your readings indicate that saw palmetto should really only be used by patients with mild-to-moderate BPH. Based on this information, you do not recommend use of saw palmetto for the patient's BPH symptoms. However, because the patient is requesting information on natural products you search for alternative dietary supplements that may provide some benefit for this patient's BPH without contributing to ED. Would *Pygeum africanum* be a reasonable option to consider? For questions related to the use of *P. africanum* for the treatment of BPH, please see Section 19 of this Casebook.

■ CLINICAL COURSE

Mr McCracken's blood pressure increased to 130/80 mm Hg, and the BPH and ED symptoms improved remarkably after your recommendations were implemented. Over the ensuing weeks, he continued to experience occasional urgency and hesitancy. Use of an anticholinergic agent was recommended as an additional therapy to help with his continued symptoms. However, Mr McCracken did not want to take multiple medications, and 6 months later he opted for laser prostatectomy. This procedure was successful in alleviating his symptoms.

■ SELF-STUDY ASSIGNMENTS

1. Compare the efficacy of saw palmetto (*Serenoa repens*) to finasteride and α$_1$-antagonists for the treatment of BPH.

2. Compare treatment options for ED in patients with BPH. Identify the risks and potential benefits of using α$_1$-antagonists and 5α-reductase inhibitors in treating comorbid ED and BPH.

3. Identify the BPH patient subpopulation that would benefit the most from finasteride/dutasteride therapy.

4. Perform a literature search for evidence that supports the use of phosphodiesterase type 5 inhibitors and α$_1$-antagonists as combination therapy for BPH/ED.

5. Perform a literature search for the use of phosphodiesterase type 5 inhibitors as monotherapy for LUTS secondary to BPH.

CLINICAL PEARL

Physiologic measurements such as postvoid residuals, uroflowmetry, and pressure-flow studies often do not correlate well with the patient's perception of BPH symptom severity.

REFERENCES

1. Miner M, Rosenberg MT, Perelman MA. Treatment of lower urinary tract symptoms in benign prostatic hyperplasia and its impact on sexual function. Clin Ther 2006;28:13–25.

2. Kaminetsky JC. Comorbid LUTS and erectile dysfunction: optimizing their management. Curr Med Res Opin 2006;22:2407–2506.

3. McVary KT, Roehrborn CG, Avins AL, et al. Update on AUA guideline on the management of benign prostatic hyperplasia. J Urol 2011;185(5):1793–1803.

4. Hollingsworth J, Wilt T. Lower urinary tract symptoms in men. BMJ 2014;349:g4474. doi:10.1136/bmj.g4474.

5. Narayan P, Evans CP, Moon T. Long-term safety and efficacy of tamsulosin for the treatment of lower urinary tract symptoms associated with benign prostatic hyperplasia. J Urol 2003;170(Pt 1):498–502.

6. Sarma AV, Wei JT. Clinical practice. Benign prostatic hyperplasia and lower urinary tract symptoms. N Engl J Med 2012;19:367(3):248–257.

7. Greco KA, McVary KT. The role of combination medical therapy in benign prostatic hyperplasia. Int J Impot Res 2008;20(Suppl 3): S33–S43.

8. Van Asseldonk B, Barkin J, Elterman D. Medical therapy for benign prostatic hyperplasia: a review. Can J Urol 2015;22(Suppl 1):7–17.

9. Donatucci CF, Brock GB, Goldfischer ER, et al. Tadalafil administered once daily for lower urinary tract symptoms secondary to benign prostatic hyperplasia: a 1-year, open-label extension study. BJU Int 2011;107(7):1110–1116.

10. Tacklind J, MacDonald R, Rutks I, Stanke JU, Wilt TJ. Serenoa repens for benign prostatic hyperplasia. Cochrane Database Syst Rev 2012(Dec 12);12:CD001423.

99

URINARY INCONTINENCE

Bladder Matters.............................. Level II

Mary W. L. Lee, PharmD, BCPS, FCCP

Roohollah R. Sharifi, MD, FACS

LEARNING OBJECTIVES

After completing this case study, the reader should be able to:

- Differentiate among overactive bladder syndrome, stress urinary incontinence, overflow urinary incontinence, and functional urinary incontinence.

- Recommend appropriate nondrug therapy for the management of overactive bladder syndrome.

- Determine when anticholinergic drugs should be recommended for the management of overactive bladder syndrome.

- Compare and contrast muscarinic receptor selectivity, lipophilicity, and pharmacokinetic properties of commonly used antimuscarinic agents for the management of overactive bladder syndrome and discuss the clinical implications of these properties.

- Explain how concomitant medications may exacerbate overactive bladder syndrome.

- Recommend medication options for patients who poorly tolerate initial anticholinergic therapy for overactive bladder syndrome.

PATIENT PRESENTATION

Chief Complaint

"I can't seem to control my urine. I feel like I have to urinate all the time. However, when I do go to the bathroom, I often pass only a small amount of urine. Sometimes I wet myself. I was started on a medication for my leaking a few weeks ago, but it doesn't seem to be working."

HPI

Susan Jones is an 83-year-old woman with urinary urgency, frequency, and incontinence. She reports soiling her underwear at least one to three times during the day and night and has resorted to wearing panty liners or changing her underwear several times a day. The patient has curtailed much of her volunteer work and social activities because of this problem. Urinary leakage is not worsened by laughing, coughing, sneezing, carrying heavy objects, or walking up and down stairs. She does not report wetting herself without warning. She has been taking Detrol LA 2 mg PO daily for the past month with no improvement in her voiding symptoms, and she complains of new-onset constipation, confusion, and difficulty remembering routine tasks.

PMH

HTN for many years, treated with medications for 10 years. Dyslipidemia for 5 years, controlled with a low-cholesterol diet, weight control, regular exercise, and medication. Menopausal; stopped ovulating at age 52; no longer has hot flashes. Has difficulty falling asleep and often has sleepless nights. She has no history of spinal or pelvic surgery.

FH

Noncontributory

SH

Nonsmoker; social drinker; married

Meds

Hydrochlorothiazide 25 mg PO once daily with supper
Pravastatin 40 mg PO at bedtime
Diovan (valsartan) 160 mg PO every morning
Detrol LA 2 mg PO daily
Sominex (diphenhydramine) 15 mg PO at bedtime as needed
Amitriptyline 50 mg PO at bedtime as needed

All

NKDA

ROS

Complains of urinary incontinence that has not responded to Detrol LA and feeling bloated and constipated

Physical Examination

Gen

WDWN female

VS

BP 135/84 mm Hg, P 90 bpm, RR 16, T 37°C; Wt 65 kg, Ht 5'2"

Skin

No rashes, wounds, or open sores

HEENT

PERRLA; EOMI; no AV nicking or hemorrhages

Neck/Lymph Nodes

No palpable thyroid masses; no lymphadenopathy

Pulm

Clear to A & P

Breasts

Normal; no lumps

CV

Regular S_1, S_2; (+) S_4; (–) S_3, murmurs, or rubs

Abd

Soft, NTND: (+) bowel sounds

Genit/Rect

Genital examination shows atrophic vaginitis consistent with menopausal status. Perineal sensation and anal sphincter tone are normal.

Pelvic examination shows no uterine prolapse and a mild degree of cystocele. Cervix is normal. No pelvic, adnexal, or uterine masses found.

External hemorrhoids; heme (–) stool.

Ext

Normal; equal motor strength in both arms and legs

Neuro

Although alert, the patient is not oriented to correct month, day, or year. CNs II–XII grossly intact; DTRs 3/5 bilaterally; negative Babinski. When asked to recall a series of five objects after 5 minutes, the patient had difficulty and could only recall one object.

Labs

Na 145 mEq/L	Hgb 12 g/dL
K 4.2 mEq/L	Hct 37%
Cl 105 mEq/L	Plt 400 × 10³/mm³
CO_2 28 mEq/L	WBC 5.0 × 10³/mm³
BUN 15 mg/dL	
SCr 1.0 mg/dL	
Glu 100 mg/dL	

UA

No bacteria; no WBC

Other

Using an ultrasonic bladder scan, a residual urine volume was measured after the patient voided. No residual urine was found. The bladder was then filled with 300 mL of saline. The patient felt the first desire to void at 100 mL. The catheter was removed. The patient was asked to cough in different positions. No stress urinary incontinence was demonstrated. The patient voided the entire volume of saline that was instilled.

Assessment

Overactive bladder with symptoms of urinary urgency, frequency, and incontinence, which has not responded to Detrol LA 2 mg PO daily for 1 month. Patient is also having new-onset constipation, confusion, and forgetfulness, which are probably related to Detrol LA. Will evaluate carefully and consider alternative medication options.

QUESTIONS

Problem Identification

1.a. Create a list of the patient's drug therapy problems.

1.b. What information (signs, symptoms, medical history, laboratory values, and other test results) suggests the presence or severity of urge incontinence?

1.c. Differentiate urge incontinence from stress incontinence, overflow incontinence, and functional incontinence.

1.d. Define overactive bladder syndrome.

1.e. In addition to the medications the patient is currently taking, what other drugs could exacerbate the symptoms of overactive bladder syndrome?

Desired Outcome

2. What are the goals of pharmacotherapy in this case?

Therapeutic Alternatives

3.a. What nondrug therapies might be useful for this patient?

3.b. What pharmacotherapeutic options are available for the treatment of overactive bladder? Compare and contrast antimuscarinic agents for the treatment of overactive bladder syndrome.

3.c. What are the possible consequences of persistent CNS adverse effects of anticholinergic agents in this patient?

Optimal Plan

4. Which anticholinergic agents have a low potential to cause constipation and CNS adverse effects? Describe the physicochemical or pharmacokinetic characteristics of these agents that contribute to this favorable profile.

Outcome Evaluation

5. What clinical and laboratory parameters are necessary to evaluate the therapy for achievement of the desired therapeutic outcome and to detect or prevent adverse effects?

Patient Education

6. What information should be provided to the patient to enhance compliance, ensure successful therapy, and minimize adverse effects?

CLINICAL COURSE

Assume that the physician stopped Detrol LA and started the patient on darifenacin 7.5 mg daily by mouth. After 3 weeks of the new medication regimen, the patient returns to the clinic. Although her voiding symptoms, confusion, and forgetfulness have resolved, the constipation has worsened. She complains of feeling bloated all the time. She says that she cannot tolerate this and wants different drug treatment.

FOLLOW-UP QUESTIONS

1. Explain how constipation could have worsened because of darifenacin.

2. What alternative medication would you recommend for this patient to manage her voiding symptoms with a low potential for causing constipation and CNS adverse effects?

3. Why should medications with anticholinergic effects be used cautiously in elderly patients?

SELF-STUDY ASSIGNMENTS

1. Patients have been classified as extensive versus poor metabolizers of tolterodine. Describe the characteristics of these patients and the clinical implications of this patient classification.

2. Botulinum toxin has been reported to be effective for relieving symptoms of overactive bladder. Explain how it is administered and the adverse effects associated with its use.

3. Mirabegron and anticholinergic agents work by different mechanisms to improve symptoms of overactive bladder syndrome. Is there published evidence that documents the value of a combination of these agents for treating this disorder?

CLINICAL PEARL

A uroselective antimuscarinic agent generally exerts systemic clinical effects. This is because M_3 receptors may predominate in the detrusor muscle of the bladder, but M_3 receptors are not organ specific. M_3 receptors are also located in the colon and salivary glands. Therefore, antagonism of M_3 receptors may relieve symptoms of overactive bladder, but may also produce dose-related undesirable anticholinergic adverse effects including constipation and dry mouth.

REFERENCES

1. Latini JM, Giannantoni A. Pharmacotherapy of overactive bladder: epidemiology and pathophysiology of overactive bladder. Expert Opin Pharmacother 2011;12(7):1017–1027.

2. Abraham N, Goldman HB. An update on the pharmacotherapy for lower urinary tract dysfunction. Expert Opin Pharmacother 2015;16:79–93.

3. Gormley EA, Lightner DJ, Faraday M, Vasavada SP. Diagnosis and treatment of overactive bladder (non-neurogenic) in adults: AUA/SUFU Guideline amendment. J Urol 2015;193:1572–1580.

4. Marinkovic SP, Rovner ES, Moldwin RM, Stanton SL, Gillen LM, Marinkovic CM. The management of overactive bladder syndrome. BMJ 2012(Apr 17);344:e2365.

5. Shamilyan T, Wyman JF, Ramakrishnan R, Sainfort F, Kane RL. Benefits and harms of pharmacologic treatment of urinary incontinence in women. Ann Intern Med 2012;156:861–874.

6. Glavind K, Chancellor M. Antimuscarinics for the treatment of overactive bladder: understanding the role of muscarinic subtype selectivity. Int Urogynecol J 2011;22:907–917.

7. Chancellor M, Boone T. Anticholinergics for overactive bladder therapy: central nervous system effects. CNS Neurosci Ther 2012;18(2):167–174.

8. Oefelein MG. Safety and tolerability profiles of anticholinergic agents used for the treatment of overactive bladder. Drug Saf 2011;34(9):733–749.

9. Baldwin CM, Keating GM. Transdermal oxybutynin. Drugs 2009;69:327–337.

10. Leone, RMU, Cardozo L, Ferrero S, et al. Mirabegron in the treatment of overactive bladder. Expert Opin Pharmacother 2014;15:873–887.

100

SYSTEMIC LUPUS ERYTHEMATOSUS

Sometimes, It's Lupus . . . . Level II

Nicole Paolini Albanese, PharmD, CDE, BCACP

LEARNING OBJECTIVES

After completing this case study, the reader should be able to:

- Discuss the clinical presentation of SLE, including its complications.

- Design appropriate therapy for the treatment of SLE and the complications of antiphospholipid syndrome (APS) and iron deficiency anemia.

- Construct a monitoring plan for SLE, including disease activity, drug efficacy, and drug toxicity.

- Recommend appropriate therapy for the treatment of SLE during pregnancy.

PATIENT PRESENTATION

■ Chief Complaint

"My knees are killing me, I'm tired all the time, and I've got horrible pain in my stomach."

■ HPI

Ann Baker is a 32-year-old woman who has been having knee pain on and off for about 2 years. She has been to the doctor a few times since then with the same complaint. Workups showed no radiologic changes to the knees, and the doctor settled on a diagnosis of early arthritis. She was not evaluated by a rheumatologist. Despite scheduled APAP and ibuprofen throughout the day, the pain has not decreased much. The pain seems to be cyclical; it is very bad for a period of weeks, and then it wanes over time. It is also worse in the summer. She thinks the rashes she gets now and then on her face and arms have something to do with the pain, since the rash happens around the same time of a bad flare-up. No matter how much sleep she gets, it does not seem to be enough; a couple of sleep medications later, she is no better than before she tried them. She has also noticed a darkening of her stool over the past couple of months.

■ PMH

Knee pain × 2 years
HTN × 1 year
Depression × 3 years
Fatigue × 1 year

■ FH

Father alive in his mid-60s; has HTN and dyslipidemia. Mother alive in her mid-60s; has asthma and seasonal allergies.

■ SH

Employed as a travel agent; married 5 years; occasional EtOH use and no current or past tobacco use. On inquiry, Ms Baker states she and her husband are trying to conceive.

■ Meds

Hydrochlorothiazide 12.5 mg PO once daily
Amlodipine 5 mg PO once daily
Fluoxetine 20 mg PO once daily
Ibuprofen 800 mg PO four times daily
Acetaminophen 500 mg PO three times daily
Past meds: Zolpidem 10 mg PO at bedtime and ramelteon 8 mg PO at bedtime (stopped using both after inefficacy)

■ All

NKDA

■ ROS

(+) Fatigue, rash; (–) fever, chills, peripheral edema, or alopecia

■ Physical Examination

Gen

Tired-looking woman in moderate pain.
Pain scale: Presently 6/10; per patient, her worst pain is 10/10; her best score is 0/10.

VS

BP 136/82 mm Hg, P 74 bpm, RR 17, T 38°C, Wt 59 kg, Ht 5′4″

Skin

Warm, moist to touch, slight red, scaly rash on forearms and across both cheekbones but sparing the nasolabial folds

HEENT

PERRLA; EOMI

Neck/Lymph Nodes

Supple without adenopathy

Lungs/Thorax

CTA; no rales/rhonchi

CV

RRR; S_1 and S_2 heard

Abd

Tender, nondistended; (+) bowel sounds; (+) stool guaiac

Ext

Peripheral pulses intact; no edema
Joint examination: (–) bony proliferation, synovitis, crepitus, muscle atrophy, or deformities; no limitations on range of motion

Neuro

A & O × 3; CN II–XII intact; Babinski negative

▓ Labs

Na 136 mEq/L	Hgb 10.0 g/dL	RF titer 1:40
K 4.7 mEq/L	Hct 31%	Anti-CCP antibody (–)
Cl 105 mEq/L	WBC 7.2 × 10³/mm³	ANA titer 1:320 (rim pattern)
CO_2 25 mEq/L	Plt 250 × 10³/mm³	C3 50 mg/dL
BUN 13 mg/dL	Fe 35 mcg/dL	C4 10 mg/dL
SCr 0.8 mg/dL	TIBC 455 mcg/dL	Lupus anticoagulant (+)
Uric acid 5.5 mg/dL	Ferritin 8 ng/mL	Anticardiolipin Ab (+)
Glucose 82 mg/dL	ESR 66 mm/hour	dsDNA Ab (+)

▓ UA

(–) WBC, RBC, RBC casts; (+) microalbuminuria; (–) protein

▓ Radiologic Joint Evaluation

(–) Patellar or tibial fracture, (–) displacement, (–) fragments, (–) ligament damage, no evident soft tissue damage

▓ Assessment

Mild-to-moderate SLE with biomarkers for APS; iron deficiency anemia possibly secondary to NSAID use; possible NSAID-associated gastropathy

QUESTIONS

Problem Identification

1.a. What information (signs, symptoms, and laboratory values) indicates the development of SLE?

1.b. What information (signs, symptoms, and laboratory values) indicates the development of iron deficiency anemia?

Desired Outcome

2.a. What are the goals of pharmacotherapy for SLE in this patient?

2.b. What are the goals of pharmacotherapy for APS in this patient?

2.c. What are the goals of pharmacotherapy for iron deficiency anemia in this patient?

Therapeutic Alternatives

3.a. What nondrug suggestions can you make to this patient for the treatment of SLE?

3.b. What pharmacotherapeutic options are available for the treatment of SLE in this patient?

3.c. What options are available for prophylaxis of thrombotic events due to APS?

3.d. Is this patient a candidate for belimumab therapy? Why or why not?

Optimal Plan

4.a. What is the optimal regimen for SLE in this patient, and are there any concerns with this regimen if she were to conceive?

4.b. What is your choice for prophylaxis against thrombotic events due to APS?

4.c. What are your recommendations for treating this patient's iron deficiency anemia and NSAID-associated gastropathy?

4.d. Should any changes be made in this patient's antihypertensive therapy?

Outcome Evaluation

5. What clinical and laboratory parameters are necessary to evaluate the therapy for achievement of the desired therapeutic outcome and to detect or prevent adverse events?

Patient Education

6. What information can be provided to the patient to minimize future relapses, ensure successful therapy, and minimize adverse events?

▓ FOLLOW-UP QUESTIONS

1. What can this patient do to increase the chances of having a successful pregnancy?

2. If your initial medication regimen does not work, what is the next step in treating this patient?

▓ SELF-STUDY ASSIGNMENTS

1. How do B lymphocyte stimulator antagonists work, and where do they fit in with the pharmacotherapeutic management of SLE?

2. Devise a comprehensive patient education plan for women with SLE who wish to start a family.

CLINICAL PEARL

Because UV light exacerbates SLE, drugs that induce photosensitivity should be avoided in patients with the disease.

REFERENCES

1. Giles I, Rahman A. How to manage patients with systemic lupus erythematosus who are also antiphospholipid antibody positive. Best Pract Res Clin Rheumatol 2009;23(4):525–537.

2. Lateef A, Petri M. Managing lupus patients during pregnancy. Best Pract Res Clin Rheumatol 2013;27(3):435–447.

3. Guidelines for referral and management of systemic lupus erythematosus in adults. American College of Rheumatology Ad Hoc Committee on Systemic Lupus Erythematosus Guidelines. Arthritis Rheum 1999;42(9):1785–1796.

4. Sciascia S, Hunt BJ, Talavera-Garcia E, Lliso G, Khamashta MA, Cuadrado MJ. The impact of hydroxychloroquine treatment on pregnancy outcome in women with antiphospholipid antibodies. Am J Obstet Gynecol 2015. doi:10.1016/j.ajog.2015.09.078.

5. Manzi S, Sanchez-Guerrero J, Merrill JT, et al. Effects of belimumab, a B lymphocyte stimulator-specific inhibitor, on disease activity across multiple organ domains in patients with systemic lupus erythematosus: combined results from two phase III trials. Ann Rheum Dis 2012;71(11):1833–1838.

6. Alarcon GS, McGwin G, Bertoli AM, et al. Effect of hydroxychloroquine on the survival of patients with systemic lupus erythematosus:

data from LUMINA, a multiethnic US cohort (LUMINA L). Ann Rheumatic Dis 2007;66(9):1168–1172.

7. Mekinian A, Lazzaroni MG, Kuzenko A, et al. The efficacy of hydroxy-chloroquine for obstetrical outcome in anti-phospholipid syndrome: data from a European multicenter retrospective study. Autoimmun Rev 2015;14(6):498–502.

8. Andreoli L, Fredi M, Nalli C, et al. Pregnancy implications for systemic lupus erythematosus and the antiphospholipid syndrome. J Autoimmun 2012;38(2–3):J197–J208.

9. Duran-Barragan S, McGwin G, Jr., Vila LM, Reveille JD, Alarcon GS. Angiotensin-converting enzyme inhibitors delay the occurrence of renal involvement and are associated with a decreased risk of disease activity in patients with systemic lupus erythematosus—results from LUMINA (LIX): a multiethnic US cohort. Rheumatology (Oxford) 2008;47(7):1093–1096.

101

ALLERGIC DRUG REACTION

Return of the 3-Day Itch . . . . Level II

Lynne M. Sylvia, PharmD

LEARNING OBJECTIVES

After completing this case study, the reader should be able to:

- Interpret drug allergy information (eg, timing of the reaction, signs, and symptoms) to identify the likelihood of an IgE-mediated reaction.

- Assess the potential for cross-sensitivity between penicillins and carbapenems.

- Differentiate desensitization from graded challenge dosing procedures and identify patients who are appropriate candidates for each procedure.

- Select appropriate antibiotic therapy for a patient with multiple antibiotic allergies.

PATIENT PRESENTATION

▓ Chief Complaint

"My cough is back and I feel like I did when I was admitted two weeks ago."

▓ HPI

Alan Adams is a 55-year-old man with a history of COPD who presents today to the pulmonary clinic for a follow-up visit. Two weeks ago, he presented to the ER complaining of a 3-day history of tiredness and a cough productive of greenish sputum. Sputum cultures at that time revealed *Pseudomonas aeruginosa* sensitive to aztreonam and cefepime with intermediate sensitivity to piperacillin–tazobactam and tobramycin. Due to his multiple antibiotic allergies, the patient underwent desensitization to cefepime. He was subsequently treated for 7 days with IV cefepime without incident. He was discharged from the hospital to his home 2 weeks ago. He has had four admissions this year for COPD and pneumonia.

▓ PMH

COPD × 17 years

Chronic empyema secondary to bronchial pleural fistulae with chest tube placement 7 months ago

Right upper lobe abscess secondary to *Candida* and *Aspergillus*; S/P upper lobe lobectomy 11 years ago

HTN × 10 years

S/P MI 15 years ago

▓ SH

Lives with his mother; he is unemployed. He has a 40 pack-year smoking history. Admits to occasional alcohol use; denies use of recreational drugs.

▓ Meds

Albuterol MDI two puffs Q 6 H PRN

Ipratropium MDI two puffs Q 6 H

Aspirin 325 mg PO once daily

Amlodipine 10 mg PO once daily

Prednisone 20 mg PO daily (initiated as 60 mg PO daily during previous hospital admission; plan was to taper the dose and discontinue therapy within 2 weeks of hospital discharge)

▓ All

Ampicillin–sulbactam: facial edema, tongue swelling, and periorbital edema

Ceftazidime: urticarial rash on chest and face with shortness of breath

Codeine: nausea, pruritus

▓ ROS

(+) Fatigue, fever, sore throat, shortness of breath, and cough with thick sputum; (–) nausea, vomiting, diarrhea, chills, or chest pain

▓ Physical Examination

Gen

A 55-year-old Caucasian man appearing older than his stated age in moderate respiratory distress. He is lethargic and hard of hearing.

VS

BP 100/60 mm Hg, P 85 bpm, RR 16, T 39°C; Wt 52 kg, Ht 5′5″

Skin

Dry scaly skin; no tenting

HEENT

PERRLA, EOM intact, dry mucous membranes

Neck/Lymph Nodes

(–) Bruits, (–) lymphadenopathy

Lungs/Thorax

(+) Diffuse crackles at the left base; wheezes throughout with poor breath sounds

CV

Normal S_1 and S_2, RRR, (–) MRG

Abd

Distended with (+) bowel sounds; (–) hepatosplenomegaly

Genit/Rect

Deferred

Ext

(+) Clubbing; (−) cyanosis or edema; poor muscle tone

▌ Labs

Na 137 mEq/L	Hgb 14.8 g/dL	WBC $17 \times 10^3/mm^3$
K 3.7 mEq/L	Hct 44.6%	Neutros 72%
Cl 96 mEq/L	RBC $5.36 \times 10^6/mm^3$	Bands 5%
CO_2 29 mEq/L	Plt $244 \times 10^3/mm^3$	Eos 4%
BUN 22 mg/dL	MCV 83.2 μm^3	Lymphs 11%
SCr 1.0 mg/dL	MCHC 33.2 g/dL	Monos 8%
Glu 119 mg/dL		Basos 0%

▌ ABG

pH 7.44, PaO_2 55 mm Hg, $PaCO_2$ 38 mm Hg, O_2 sat 90%

▌ Chest X-Ray

Haziness in the left lower lobe S/P right upper lobe resection

▌ Sputum Gram Stain

Pending

▌ Sputum Cultures

Pending

▌ Blood Cultures

Pending

▌ Assessment

1. HCAP
2. Multiple allergies to antibiotics
3. COPD
4. HTN
5. S/P MI

QUESTIONS

Problem Identification

1.a. Based on the patient's allergy history, how should his allergies to ampicillin–sulbactam and ceftazidime be categorized—as minor, moderate, or severe?

1.b. What additional information would be helpful to fully assess the patient's risk of hypersensitivity reactions to β-lactam antibiotics?

1.c. What additional information would be helpful to assess whether the patient experiences true hypersensitivity versus pseudoallergy to codeine?

Desired Outcome

2. What are the goals for the treatment of pneumonia in this case?

▌ CLINICAL COURSE

The patient is admitted to the hospital from the pulmonary clinic. He is started on DuoNebs (albuterol 3 mg/3 mL and ipratropium 0.5 mg/3 mL) by nebulizer 3 mL Q 2 H PRN, guaifenesin with

---

TABLE 101-1	Initial Empiric Treatment for HCAP and HAP in Patients with Risk Factors for Drug-Resistant Pathogens[a]

Combination antibiotic therapy
Antipseudomonal cephalosporin (cefepime, ceftazidime)
Or
Antipseudomonal carbapenem (imipenem or meropenem)
Or
β-Lactam/β-lactamase inhibitor (piperacillin–tazobactam)
Plus
Antipseudomonal fluoroquinolone (ciprofloxacin or levofloxacin) Or Aminoglycoside
Plus
Linezolid or vancomycin

[a]American Thoracic Society and the Infectious Diseases Society of America. Guidelines for the management of adults with hospital-acquired, ventilator-associated, and health care-associated pneumonia. Am J Respir Crit Care Med 2005;171:388–416.

codeine (100 mg/10 mg per 5 mL) PO Q 4 H PRN, acetaminophen 325–650 mg PO Q 4 H PRN, and prednisone 40 mg PO once daily. While cultures are pending, the medical resident reviews this patient's recent hospital course, the cultures and sensitivities obtained 2 weeks ago, and the hospital's guidelines for treating HCAP. Consideration is given to initiating empiric therapy with meropenem 500 mg IV Q 6 H, ciprofloxacin 400 mg IV Q 12 H, and vancomycin 750 mg IV Q 24 H. Prior to writing these orders, the medical resident asks for your advice on the initiation of meropenem in this patient.

Therapeutic Alternatives

3.a. The initial empiric regimens currently recommended for HCAP are summarized in Table 101-1. Both cefepime and aztreonam are alternatives to meropenem in these multidrug regimens. Based on this patient's history, are cefepime and aztreonam safe alternatives to meropenem for empiric therapy of HCAP? (See Fig. 101-1 for the chemical structures of cefepime and ceftazidime.)

3.b. If a multidrug regimen including cefepime was chosen for empiric therapy, would this patient require another course of desensitization prior to initiation of full-dose cefepime therapy?

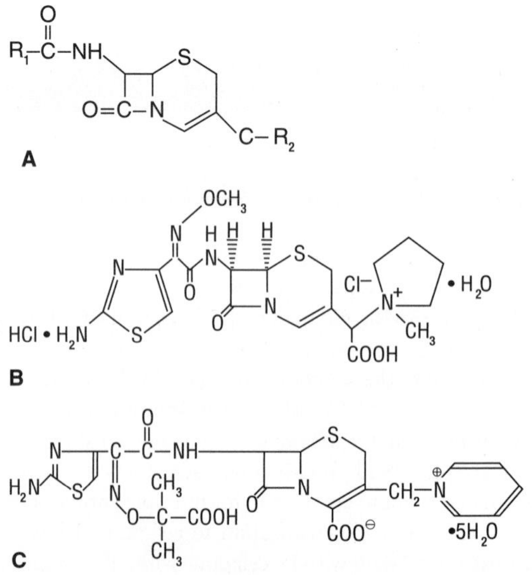

FIGURE 101-1. Chemical structures of cefepime and ceftazidime. *A.* Basic cephalosporin structure. *B.* Cefepime. *C.* Ceftazidime.

Optimal Plan

4. Assess the risk of a hypersensitivity cross-reaction to meropenem in this patient. Based on your review of the literature, determine which of the following courses of action is best: (a) initiation of full-dose meropenem therapy; (b) desensitization to meropenem prior to initiating full treatment doses; or (c) graded challenge dosing of meropenem prior to initiating full treatment doses. Substantiate your position on the most appropriate course of action based on evidence from the literature.

Outcome Evaluation

5. In patients who undergo desensitization and/or graded challenge dosing, what clinical and laboratory parameters should be evaluated during and after these procedures to detect or prevent allergic events?

Patient Education

6. What information should be provided to the patient about his drug allergies to minimize allergic events in the future?

■ SELF-STUDY ASSIGNMENTS

1. Define the following terms: CAP, HAP, HCAP, and VAP. Differentiate the initial empiric regimens for each of these types of pneumonia.

2. Develop a care map for patients allergic to penicillin for whom a carbapenem is ordered. Outline the process by which the clinician would determine the most appropriate course of action for these patients. Be specific to the type of allergy to the penicillin (ie, maculopapular rash vs Stevens–Johnson syndrome vs anaphylactic reaction).

3. Apply the concepts of graded challenge dosing and desensitization (see the section "Clinical Pearl") to the issue of β-lactam hypersensitivity. Develop criteria describing those patients with history of β-lactam hypersensitivity who would be appropriate candidates for graded challenge dosing versus desensitization to structurally related antibiotics.

CLINICAL PEARL

A graded challenge dose (test dosing) involves the cautious administration of a medication to a patient. Graded challenge doses of a medication are often recommended for patients who have history of hypersensitivity to a structurally related medication and the risk of a cross-reaction is deemed unlikely. Unlike desensitization, graded challenge dosing does not alter the body's immune response to an antigenic medication.

REFERENCES

1. Lieberman P, Nicklas RA, Oppenheimer J, et al. The diagnosis and management of anaphylaxis practice parameter: 2010 update. J Allergy Clin Immunol 2010;126:480.e1–480.e42.

2. Solensky R. Drug hypersensitivity. Med Clin North Am 2006;90:233–260.

3. Romano A, Di Fonso M, Viola M, et al. Selective hypersensitivity to piperacillin. Allergy 2000;55:787.

4. Pichichero ME. Cephalosporins can be prescribed safely for penicillin-allergic patients. J Fam Pract 2006;55:106–112.

5. Kelkar PS, Li JT. Cephalosporin allergy. N Engl J Med 2001;345:804–809.

6. Win PH, Brown H, Zankar A, et al. Rapid intravenous cephalosporin desensitization. J Allergy Clin Immunol 2005;116:225–228.

7. Solensky R. Drug desensitization. Immunol Allergy Clin North Am 2004;24:425–443.

8. Prescott WA, Kusmierski KA. Clinical importance of carbapenem hypersensitivity in patients with self-reported and documented penicillin allergy. Pharmacotherapy 2007;27(1):137–142.

9. Romano A, Viola M, Gueant-Rodriguez RM, et al. Imipenem in patients with immediate hypersensitivity to penicillins. N Engl J Med 2006;354:2835–2837.

10. Romano A, Viola M, Gueant-Rodriguez RM, et al. Brief communication: tolerability of meropenem in patients with IgE-mediated hypersensitivity to penicillins. Ann Intern Med 2007;146:266–269.

11. Atanaskovic-Markovic M, Gaeta F, Medjo B, et al. Tolerability of meropenem in children with IgE-mediated hypersensitivity to penicillins. Allergy 2008;63:237–240.

12. Gaeta F, Valluzzi RL, Alonzi C, et al. Tolerability of aztreonam and carbapenems in patients with IgE-mediated hypersensitivity to penicillins. J Allergy Clin Immunol 2015;135:972–976.

13. Wilson DL, Owens RC, Zuckerman JB. Successful meropenem desensitization in a patient with cystic fibrosis. Ann Pharmacother 2003;37:1424–1428.

102

SOLID ORGAN TRANSPLANTATION

Kidney—Don't Fail Me Now!....................Level III

Kristine S. Schonder, PharmD

LEARNING OBJECTIVES

After completing this case study, the reader should be able to:

- Develop a patient-specific therapeutic plan for acute cellular rejection following solid organ transplantation.

- Assess a transplant medication regimen for potential drug interactions and develop a plan to resolve any identified interactions.

- Describe possible adverse effects of immunosuppressive medications and prophylactic medications for solid organ transplant recipients and develop a plan to resolve these effects.

- Counsel a transplant recipient on the importance of medication adherence and implement mechanisms to enhance adherence.

PATIENT PRESENTATION

■ Chief Complaint

"I have pain over my kidney transplant, my legs are swollen, and my urine output is decreased."

■ HPI

Brent Salston is a 42-year-old man who presents to the renal transplant clinic for evaluation of the above complaints. He states the symptoms began about 1 week ago and have gotten progressively worse.

■ PMH

6 months S/P living kidney transplant from his wife
ESRD secondary to IgA nephropathy
HTN
Gout
Peripheral neuropathy, diagnosed 2 weeks ago by PCP

■ FH

Mother is alive with hypertension; father deceased from kidney disease. Two aunts and sister also have kidney disease. He is married with two children, Sarah and Justin, who are alive and well.

■ SH

He drinks beer occasionally with friends, but not since his transplant. He has no history of smoking or IVDA.

■ ROS

He has pain over his kidney and bilateral edema in his lower extremities. He reports mild pain and tingling in lower extremities. Urine output has decreased from baseline.

■ Meds

Tacrolimus 4 mg PO BID (last dose taken last night at 8:00 PM)
Mycophenolate mofetil 1000 mg PO BID
Dapsone 100 mg PO daily
Valganciclovir 900 mg PO daily
Aspirin 81 mg PO once daily
Metoprolol XL 100 mg PO daily
Amlodipine 10 mg PO daily
Magnesium chloride 64 mg PO BID
Allopurinol 100 mg PO daily
Carbamazepine 200 mg PO BID, started 2 weeks ago by PCP for neuropathy

■ All

Sulfa (rash)

■ Physical Examination

Gen

WDWN man in NAD

VS

BP 169/92 mm Hg, P 66 reg, RR 14, T 37.4°C; Wt 87 kg (previous Wt 85 kg 2 weeks ago), Ht 5′10″

Skin

Warm and dry

HEENT

PERRLA; EOMI

Chest

CTA & P

CV

Normal S_1 and S_2; no MRG

Abd

Tenderness over kidney allograft; incisional wound healed; liver size normal

Ext

3+ pitting edema in LE; 2+ DP pulses bilaterally. No cyanosis.

Neuro

A & O × 3; CN II–XII intact; DTRs 2+ throughout

■ Labs

At 8:00 AM today (fasting):

Na 141 mEq/L	Hgb 12.2 g/dL	Ca 8.9 mg/dL
K 5.4 mEq/L	Hct 36.6%	Phos 2.3 mg/dL
Cl 104 mEq/L	RBC 5.1×10^6/mm³	Mg 1.1 mg/dL
CO₂ 23 mEq/L	Plt 289×10^3/mm³	Uric acid 6.8 mg/dL
FBS 78 mg/dL	WBC 1.9×10^3/mm³	FK <2 ng/mLᵃ
BUN 39 mg/dL	Polys 68%	
(last was 20 mg/dL)	Lymphs 27%	
SCr 2.5 mg/dL	Monos 2%	
(last was 1.1 mg/dL)	Eos 1%	
	Basos 2%	

ᵃTacrolimus whole blood concentration (therapeutic range, 5–20 ng/mL).

■ Renal Biopsy

Moderate acute cellular rejection (Banff 2A)

■ Assessment

Acute rejection of kidney allograft, hyperkalemia, leukopenia

QUESTIONS

Problem Identification

1.a. Create a list of the patient's drug therapy problems.

1.b. Which signs, symptoms, and laboratory values indicate rejection of the kidney allograft?

1.c. What are the potential causes of hyperkalemia in this patient?

1.d. What are the potential causes of leukopenia in this patient?

1.e. What are the potential causes of the other medical problems in this patient?

Desired Outcome

2. What are the goals of pharmacotherapy in this case?

Therapeutic Alternatives

3.a. What nonpharmacologic therapies and education might be useful for this patient?

3.b. What pharmacotherapeutic alternatives are available for the treatment of kidney allograft rejection?

3.c. What pharmacotherapeutic alternatives are available for treating hyperkalemia in this patient?

3.d. What pharmacotherapeutic alternatives are available for treating leukopenia in this patient?

Optimal Plan

4.a. What drug, dosage form, dose, schedule, and duration of therapy are best to treat this patient's kidney allograft rejection?

4.b. What alternatives would be appropriate if the initial therapy fails or cannot be used?

4.c. Design a pharmacotherapeutic plan to treat this patient's hyperkalemia, leukopenia, and other medical problems.

Outcome Evaluation

5. What clinical and laboratory parameters are necessary to evaluate the response to therapy and to detect or prevent adverse effects?

Patient Education

6. What information should be provided to the patient to enhance adherence, ensure successful therapy, and minimize adverse effects?

■ CLINICAL COURSE

The patient receives the treatment you recommended for acute cellular rejection. The rejection episode resolves and renal function returns to baseline levels. He is now presenting 3 months later for a routine follow-up appointment.

Meds

Tacrolimus 7 mg PO BID (last dose taken last night at 8:00 PM)
Prednisone 15 mg PO once daily
Mycophenolate mofetil 1000 mg PO BID
Dapsone 100 mg PO daily
Valganciclovir 900 mg PO daily
Aspirin 81 mg PO daily
Metoprolol XL 100 mg PO daily
Amlodipine 10 mg PO daily
Furosemide 40 mg daily
Magnesium chloride 128 mg PO BID
Allopurinol 100 mg PO daily

The patient's PCP decided to discontinue the carbamazepine and begin gabapentin 100 mg PO at bedtime and titrate the dose upward slowly over the next several months based on the patient's response. The patient began this treatment 1 day ago.

Labs (at 8:00 AM Today)

Na 139 mEq/L	Hgb 12.1 g/dL	Ca 9.1 mg/dL
K 4.8 mEq/L	Hct 36.3%	Phos 3.5 mg/dL
Cl 109 mEq/L	RBC 5.2×10^6/mm³	Mg 1.8 mg/dL
CO_2 25 mEq/L	Plt 278×10^3/mm³	FK 5.4 ng/mL
FBS 82 mg/dL	WBC 3.7×10^3/mm³	
BUN 19 mg/dL		
SCr 1.1 mg/dL		

■ FOLLOW-UP QUESTION

1. What changes, if any, should be made to the patient's drug regimen?

■ SELF-STUDY ASSIGNMENTS

1. Develop a pharmacotherapeutic plan for the different strategies to treat acute cellular rejection of the allograft in solid organ transplant recipients.

2. Design a systematic approach for patient education for a new solid organ transplant recipient focusing on immunosuppressive therapies, adverse effects and drug interactions, and strategies to manage patient compliance with a complicated regimen.

3. Formulate a pharmacotherapeutic plan for the management of hyperkalemia that identifies different strategies based on the onset and magnitude of hyperkalemia.

CLINICAL PEARL

Acute rejection can occur in up to 20% of kidney transplant recipients within the first 6 months after transplant. Although an abrupt rise in serum creatinine ≥30% over baseline can signal an acute rejection episode, a renal biopsy must be performed for a definitive diagnosis. The greatest risk factor for acute cellular rejection is a decrease in the level of immunosuppression. Treatment of acute rejection is typically based on the severity of the rejection episode.

REFERENCES

1. Kidney Disease: Improving Global Outcomes (KDIGO) Blood Pressure Work Group. KDIGO Clinical Practice Guideline for the Management of Blood Pressure in Chronic Kidney Disease. Kidney Int Suppl 2012;2(5):337–414. Available at: *http://www.kdigo.org/clinical_practice_guidelines/pdf/KDIGO_BP_GL.pdf*.
2. Weir MR, Burgess ED, Cooper JE, et al. Assessment and management of hypertension in transplant patients. J Am Soc Nephrol 2015;26(6):1248–1260.
3. Kidney Disease: Improving Global Outcomes (KDIGO) Transplant Work Group. KDIGO clinical practice guideline for the care of kidney transplant recipients. Am J Transplant 2009;9(Suppl 3):S1–S157.
4. Webster AC, Pankhurst T, Rinaldi F, Chapman RJ, Craig JC. Monoclonal and polyclonal antibody therapy for treating acute rejection in kidney transplant recipients: a systematic review of randomized trial data. Transplantation 2006;81:953–965.
5. Baia LC, Heilberg IP, Navi G, de Borst MH. Phosphate and FGF-23 homeostasis after kidney transplantation. Nat Rev Nephrol 2015;11:656–666.

103

OSTEOPOROSIS

A bone to pick with osteoporosis . . . . Level II

Emily C. Papineau, PharmD, BCPS

LEARNING OBJECTIVES

After completing this case study, the reader should be able to:

- Identify the risk factors for the development of osteoporosis and use the FRAX tool to assess risk of an osteoporotic fracture.

- Recommend appropriate nonpharmacologic measures for the prevention and treatment of osteoporosis.

- Recommend appropriate calcium supplementation required for the prevention and treatment of osteoporosis.

- Design an appropriate pharmacologic treatment regimen for the treatment of osteoporosis in postmenopausal women.

- Provide patient education regarding osteoporosis and its therapy.

PATIENT PRESENTATION

■ Chief Complaint

"I am anxious to get the results of my DXA scan. My mother is still undergoing rehabilitation in the nursing home after her hip fracture three weeks ago. I've heard osteoporosis can run in families, and I don't want to experience what she is going through."

■ HPI

Beverly Farland is a 65-year-old Caucasian woman with a history of COPD, hypothyroidism, and GERD. She presents to the family medicine clinic for her yearly physical and to discuss the results of her recent labs and DXA scan.

In an effort to become more active, she recently started walking around her neighborhood every day, but has to stop after 15 minutes because she is out of breath. She admits that she has a hard time remembering to take her medications faithfully. She states she uses her Combivent inhaler approximately twice a day and takes her medicines "most of the time."

■ PMH

Hypothyroidism × 5 years
COPD (GOLD 2) diagnosed one year ago and currently stable; no history of COPD exacerbations
Breast cancer with mastectomy of left breast and radiation therapy at age 45

Menopause at age 51
GERD

■ FH

Paternal history (+) for hypertension; father died in his sleep at age 80
Maternal history (+) for stroke and vascular disorders; hip fracture

■ SH

Married; G_2P_3; 1 ppd smoker; drinks occasionally

■ ROS

Reports vaginal dryness; has noticed that her height has decreased by 2″ since she was "in her prime;" reports shortness of breath with exercise; denies headache, chest pain, GI pain, or heartburn

■ Meds

Combivent Respimat 1 inhalation four times daily
Omeprazole 20 mg PO once daily × 1 year
Synthroid 75 mcg PO once daily × 5 years

■ All

NKDA

■ Physical Examination

Gen

WDWN Caucasian woman in NAD

VS

Today:
BP initially 158/96 mm Hg, Repeated at end of office visit 133/88 mm Hg, P 70 bpm, RR 18, T 37°C; Wt 53.5 kg, Ht 5′3″
1 month ago:
BP 130/82 mm Hg, P 66 bpm, RR 20, T 37°C; Wt 53.5 kg, Ht 5′3″

Skin

Fair complexion, color good, no lesions

HEENT

PERRLA; EOMI; eyes and throat clear; funduscopic exam reveals mild arteriolar narrowing, with AV ratio 1:3; no hemorrhages, exudates, or papilledema

Neck/Lymph Nodes

Supple, without obvious nodes; no JVD

Chest

Decreased breath sounds bilaterally; air movement decreased; no rales or rhonchi

Breasts

Mastectomy scar left breast; right breast normal

CV

RRR; no MRG

Abd

Soft, NT/ND, (+) BS

Genit/Rect

Deferred

MS/Ext

Good pulses bilaterally

Neuro

CN II–XII intact; DTRs 2+; sensory and motor levels intact

▨ Labs

Na 145 mEq/L	Ca 9.1 mg/dL
K 4.0 mEq/L	TSH 3.492 mIU/L
Cl 104 mEq/L	AST 32 IU/L
CO_2 25 mEq/L	ALT 27 IU/L
BUN 18 mg/dL	
SCr 1.1 mg/dL	
Glu 97 mg/dL	

▨ Other

DXA scan results from Hologic machine:

Lumbar spine 2 weeks ago reveals: L2–4 = 0.780 g/cm^2 (T score: –3.2 SD); right femoral neck = 0.52 g/cm^2 (T score: –2.8 SD)

X-ray of the spine 2 weeks ago shows a compression fracture on L3

CAT score of 12

▨ Assessment

1. Severe osteoporosis requiring initiation of therapy
2. Stable COPD Patient Group B (GOLD 2)
3. Hypothyroidism well controlled on current regimen

QUESTIONS

Problem Identification

1.a. Create a list of the patient's drug therapy problems.

1.b. What information (signs, symptoms, laboratory values, FRAX score) indicates the presence or severity of the patient's osteoporosis? What are the patient's risk factors for osteoporosis?

Desired Outcome

2. What are the goals of pharmacotherapy for osteoporosis in this case?

Therapeutic Alternatives

3.a. What nondrug therapies might be useful for this patient's osteoporosis?

3.b. What feasible pharmacotherapeutic alternatives are available for treatment of the osteoporosis?

Optimal Plan

4.a. What drug, dosage form, dose, schedule, and duration of therapy are best for treating this patient's osteoporosis?

4.b. What alternatives would be appropriate if the initial therapy fails or cannot be used?

Outcome Evaluation

5. Which clinical and laboratory parameters are necessary to evaluate the therapy for achievement of the desired therapeutic outcome and to detect or prevent adverse effects?

Patient Education

6. What information should be provided to the patient to enhance adherence, ensure successful therapy, and minimize adverse effects?

▨ SELF-STUDY ASSIGNMENTS

1. Create a list of medications associated with an increased risk for developing osteoporosis.
2. Investigate the new drugs and drug classes under development for the treatment of osteoporosis.
3. Develop an exercise plan to prevent osteoporosis.

CLINICAL PEARL

In elderly patients or those on acid-suppressive therapy, recommend calcium citrate instead of calcium carbonate, because this salt form does not require an acidic gastric pH for dissolution.

REFERENCES

1. Global Initiative for Chronic Obstructive Lung Disease. Global strategy for diagnosis, management and prevention of chronic obstructive pulmonary disease: updated 2016. Available at: http://goldcopd.org/global-strategy-diagnosis-management-prevention-copd-2016/. Accessed April 20, 2016.

2. The North American Menopause Society. Management of osteoporosis in postmenopausal women: 2010 position statement of The North American Menopause Society. Menopause 2010;17(1):25–54.

3. American Association of Clinical Endocrinologists Osteoporosis Task Force. AACE medical guidelines for clinical practice for the diagnosis and treatment of postmenopausal osteoporosis. Endocr Pract 2010;16:1–37.

4. Cosman F, de Beur SJ, LeBoff MS, et al. Clinician's guide to prevention and treatment of osteoporosis. Osteoporosis Int 2014;25:2359–2381.

5. Newcomb PA, Trentham-Dietz A, Hamptom JM. Bisphosphonates for osteoporosis treatment are associated with reduced breast cancer risk. Br J Cancer 2010;102:799–802.

6. Brown JP, Prince RL, Deal C, et al. Comparison of the effect of denosumab and alendronate on BMD and biochemical markers of bone turnover in postmenopausal women with low bone mass: a randomized, blinded, phase 3 Trial. J Bone Miner Res 2009;24:153–161.

7. Moyer VA. Menopausal hormone therapy for the primary prevention of chronic conditions: U.S. Preventive Services Task Force Recommendation Statement. Ann Intern Med 2013;158:1–34.

8. Tsai JN, Uihlein AV, Kumbhani, et al. Teriparatide and denosumab, alone or combined, in women with postmenopausal osteoporosis: the DATA study randomized trial. Lancet 2013;382:50–56. doi:10.1016/S0140-6736(13)60856-9.

9. Kendler DL, Roux C, Benhamou CL, et al. Effects of denosumab on bone mineral density and bone turnover in postmenopausal women transitioning from alendronate therapy. J Bone Miner Res 2010;25:72–81.

10. Adler RA, Fuleihan GE, Bauer DC, et al. Managing osteoporosis in patients on long-term bisphosphonate treatment: report of a Task Force of the American Society for Bone and Mineral Research. J bone Miner Res 2016;31:16–35.

104

RHEUMATOID ARTHRITIS

Joint Project . . . . Level II

Amie Brooks, PharmD, FCCP, BCACP, BCPS

LEARNING OBJECTIVES

After completing this case study, the reader should be able to:

- Identify signs and symptoms of rheumatoid arthritis (RA) and assess disease severity and prognosis.

- Recommend appropriate non pharmacologic therapy for adjunctive management of RA.

- Recommend evidence-based, patient-specific analgesic, anti-inflammatory, and disease-modifying drug therapy for patients with RA.

- Develop an evidence-based, patient-specific monitoring plan to assess disease progress and evaluate the safety and efficacy of medication therapy.

- Educate patients and their families about the medications used to treat RA.

PATIENT PRESENTATION

◼ Chief Complaint

"I am still very achy, I feel exhausted, and I am having a hard time getting going in the morning."

◼ HPI

Analise Schaefer is a 44-year-old African-American woman who presents to rheumatology clinic with complaints of generalized arthralgias, fatigue, and morning stiffness. She presented with similar symptoms 3 months ago, at which time she was started on naproxen and oral methotrexate. She reports a slight improvement in her symptoms relative to her visit 3 months ago.

◼ PMH

RA (moderate disease activity with features of poor prognosis) × 3 months
Latent tuberculosis infection

◼ FH

Father is alive and being treated for hypertension and osteoarthritis. Mother is alive and being treated for severe RA. Two siblings with no major health concerns.

◼ SH

Tax accountant; married for 15 years; heterosexual, sexually active, monogamous. Denies tobacco or illicit drug use. Drinks one to two glasses of wine per week.

◼ Meds

Naproxen 500 mg PO twice daily
Methotrexate 2.5 mg, six tablets (15 mg) PO once a week
Folic acid 1 mg PO once daily

Patient receives medications at a local community pharmacy. Medication profile indicates that she refills her medications on time the first of each month.

◼ All

Sulfonamides—hives

◼ ROS

Complains of swelling and pain in both hands; reports decreased ROM in hands and wrists; has morning stiffness every day for about 2 hours and fatigue daily during the afternoon hours; denies HA, chest pain, SOB, bleeding episodes, or syncope; no nausea, vomiting, diarrhea, loss of appetite, or weight loss.

◼ Physical Examination

Gen

Caucasian woman in moderate distress because of pain, swelling, and fatigue related to arthritis

VS

BP 118/76 mm Hg, P 82 bpm, RR 14, T 37.1°C; Wt 65 kg, Ht 5′6″

Skin

No rashes; normal turgor; no breakdown or ulcers; no subcutaneous nodules

HEENT

Normocephalic, atraumatic; moist mucous membranes; PERRLA; EOMI; pale conjunctiva bilaterally; TMs intact; no oral mucositis

Neck/Lymph Nodes

Neck supple, no JVD or thyromegaly; no thyroid bruit; no lymphadenopathy

Chest

CTA

Breasts

Deferred

CV

RRR; normal S_1, S_2; no MRG

Abd

Soft, NT/ND; (+) BS

Genit/Rect

Deferred

MS/Ext

Total of 16 tender and 16 swollen joints bilaterally
Hands: swelling and tenderness on palpation of second, third, fourth, and fifth PIP and MTP joints bilaterally; decreased grip strength, L > R (patient is left-handed)
Wrists: decreased ROM
Elbows: good ROM
Shoulders: decreased ROM (especially abduction) bilaterally
Hips: good ROM
Knees: good ROM, no pain bilaterally
Feet: no obvious swelling of MTP joints; full plantar flexion; reduced dorsiflexion; 2+ pedal pulses

TABLE 104-1	Lab Values		
Na 135 mEq/L	Hgb 10.8 g/dL	AST 15 IU/L	CK <20 IU/L
K 4.1 mEq/L	Hct 31%	ALT 12 IU/L	ANA negative
Cl 101 mEq/L	WBC 6.2 × 10³/mm³	Alk phos 56 IU/L	Wes ESR 60 mm/hour
CO₂ 22 mEq/L	Plt 356 × 10³/mm³	T. bili 0.8 mg/dL	RF (−)1:50
BUN 12 mg/dL	Ca 9.1 mg/dL	Alb 4.2 g/dL	Anti-CCP 70 EU
SCr 0.8 mg/dL	Urate 5.1 mg/dL	HBsAg (−)	aPTT 31 sec
Glu 103 mg/dL	TSH 0.74 mIU/L	Anti-HCV (−)	INR 1.0

Neuro

CN II–XII intact; muscle strength 4/5 UE, 4/5 LE, DTRs 2+ throughout

▇ Labs

See Table 104-1.

▇ UA

Normal

▇ Chest X-Ray

No fluid, masses, or infection; no cardiomegaly

▇ Hand X-Ray

Multiple erosions of MCP and PIP joints bilaterally; measurable joint space narrowing from previous x-ray 3 months ago

▇ DAS 28

7.0 reported 3 months ago; 6.2 today

▇ Assessment

A 44-year-old woman in moderate distress with RA not adequately controlled with current therapy. DAS exhibits high disease activity with features of poor prognosis although patient reports a slight improvement in symptoms over 3 months ago. Patient is adherent with current medication regimen.

QUESTIONS

Problem Identification

1.a. Create a list of the patient's medical and medication therapy problems.

1.b. Identify all relevant information (signs, symptoms, and laboratory values) to assess the presence and severity of RA.

1.c. Identify and list any additional information that is needed to assess the patient.

Desired Outcome

2. List the goals of therapy in this case.

Therapeutic Alternatives

3.a. Describe nonpharmacologic modalities that may be beneficial for this patient.

3.b. List and describe pharmacologic agents that are available for the treatment of RA.

3.c. Identify potential economic and psychosocial considerations applicable to this patient.

Optimal Plan

4. Provide the best pharmacological therapy (drug, dosage form, dose, schedule, and duration) recommendation for this patient. Include rationale for your recommendation.

Outcome Evaluation

5. Provide recommendations for a monitoring plan for this patient's disease and medication therapy including clinical (symptoms and physical findings) and laboratory parameters.

Patient Education

6. Identify key information that should be provided to the patient to enhance adherence, ensure successful therapy, and minimize adverse effects

▇ SELF-STUDY ASSIGNMENTS

1. Create a list of clinically significant drug interactions for NSAIDs and DMARDs, including methotrexate.

2. Compare the biologic agents used to treat RA with respect to drug class, route of administration, efficacy, contraindications, and side effects.

CLINICAL PEARL

Patients with RA are at increased risk for TB infection due to underlying immune dysfunction.[9] In most cases, TB infection in patients receiving immunosuppressant therapy has been attributed to reactivation of latent disease.[9,10] Reactivation of latent tuberculosis infection is a concern with all immunosuppressant therapy but has been specifically associated with corticosteroid use, all biologic agents (TNF-α antagonists, IL-1 and IL-6 receptor inhibitors, B cell-depleting agents, T cell costimulation inhibitors), and some nonbiologic agents (tofacitinib and leflunomide).[9–11]

REFERENCES

1. Aletaha D, Neogi T, Silman A, et al. 2010 rheumatoid arthritis classification criteria. Arthritis Rheum 2012;62:2569–2581.

2. Fransen J, van Riel PLCM. The disease activity score and the EULAR response criteria. Rheum Dis Clin North Am 2009;35:745–757.

3. Singh JA, Saag KG, Bridges SL, et al. 2015 American College of Rheumatology guideline for the treatment of rheumatoid arthritis. Arthritis Rheumatol 2016;68:1–26.

4. Niewold TB, Harrison MJ, Paget SA. Anti-CCP antibody testing as a diagnostic and prognostic tool in rheumatoid arthritis. QJM 2007;193–201.

5. Singh JA, Christensen R, Wells GA, et al. Biologics for rheumatoid arthritis: an overview of Cochrane reviews (Protocol). Cochrane Database of Systematic Reviews 2009, Issue 2. Art. No.: CD007848. doi:10.1002/14651858.CD007848.

6. Curtis JR, Patkar N, Xie A, et al. Risk of serious bacterial infections among rheumatoid arthritis patients exposed to tumor necrosis factor alpha antagonists. Arthritis Rheum 2007;56:1125–1133.

7. Saag KG, Teng GG, Patkar NM, et al. American College of Rheumatology 2008 recommendations for the use of nonbiologic and biologic disease-modifying antirheumatic drugs in rheumatoid arthritis. Arthritis Care Res 1008;59:762–784.

8. O'Dell JR, Mikuls TR, Taylor TH, et al. Therapies for active rheumatoid arthritis after methotrexate failure. N Engl J Med 2013;369(4):307–318.

9. Carmona L, Hernández-García C, Vadillo C, et al. EMECAR Study Group. Increased risk of tuberculosis in patients with rheumatoid arthritis. J Rheumatol 2003;30:1436–1439.

10. Gòmez-Reino JJ, Carmona L, Angel Descalzo M. Biobadaser Group. Risk of tuberculosis in patients treated with tumor necrosis factor antagonists due to incomplete prevention of reactivation of latent infection. Arthritis Rheum 2007;57:756–761.

11. Keane J, Gershon S, Wise RP, et al. Tuberculosis associated with inflix-imab, a tumor necrosis factor alpha-neutralizing agent. N Engl J Med 2001;345:1098–1104.

105

OSTEOARTHRITIS

The Tolls of Labor............................. Level II

Christopher M. Degenkolb, PharmD, BCPS

LEARNING OBJECTIVES

After completing this case study, the reader should be able to:

- Describe the most common signs and symptoms of osteoarthritis (OA).

- Design an appropriate pharmacotherapeutic regimen for treating OA, taking into account a patient's other medical problems and drug therapy.

- Incorporate potential adjunctive therapies (pharmacologic, non-pharmacologic, and alternative) into the regimen of a patient with OA.

- Assess and evaluate the efficacy of an analgesic regimen for a patient with OA, and formulate an alternative plan if the regimen is inadequate or causes unacceptable toxicity.

PATIENT PRESENTATION

Chief Complaint

"What can I take to help this pain? This medication only takes the edge off!"

HPI

Ray Kansella is a 74-year-old man who comes in to see his PCP today complaining of right knee and right hip pain for the past 10 years since he retired from an assembly plant. He often did very heavy lifting in his job and put a lot of strain on his back and legs; now the patient feels he is paying the price for all of his hard work. Mr Kansella wakes up every morning very stiff, and his right knee cracks when he gets up out of bed. The cracking in the joint goes away after he finishes his breakfast, but the aching in his knee and hip persists and chronically bothers him. He has been taking Norco and Tylenol Extra Strength for the past several months on a scheduled basis with only minimal benefit. He reports not being sure of what medications he has tried in the past; all he knows is that whatever he is taking is not really helping. He reports adherence to all medications prescribed to him. His PCP is now asking for your recommendation on a pain management regimen for this patient given his past medical and medication history.

PMH

OA × 10 years
HTN × 20 years
Obesity × 15 years
Seizure disorder × 12 years (last seizure was 5 years ago)
CKD × 5 years

PSH

Appendectomy 35 years ago

FH

Father died at age 68 due to myocardial infarction
Mother died at age 81 of CVA
One brother (still living) with whom patient is not close

SH

Retired and has good insurance plan and a steady pension from his company
Denies tobacco use
Occasional EtOH (two to three beers on weekends)

Meds

Amlodipine 10 mg PO daily in AM
Lisinopril 10 mg PO daily in AM
Metoprolol 50 mg PO BID
Hydrocodone/APAP 7.5 mg/325 mg two tablets PO Q 6 H PRN pain
Acetaminophen 500 mg one tablet PO Q 6 H PRN pain
Levetiracetam 1000 mg PO BID

All

NKDA; reports allergy to egg products

ROS

Positive for pain and stiffness in the right knee and right hip; has low back pain with occasional shooting and aching pains radiating to the buttocks and groin area; negative for headache, neck stiffness, joint swelling, or erythema; no SOB or palpitations; has not had a bowel movement in the past 5 days.

Physical Examination

Gen

Well-developed, obese, Caucasian male with moderate pain, otherwise in NAD

VS

BP 148/89 mm Hg, P 68 bpm, RR 18, T 37.1°C; Ht 5′9″, Wt 225 lb, pain 6/10. No orthostatic changes

Skin

Warm, dry, intact

HEENT

NC/AT; PERRLA; funduscopic exam reveals sharp disks; mild A-V nicking, but no hemorrhages or exudates; no scleral icterus; TMs intact; mucous membranes moist; poor dentition with gingival erythema; no lateral deviation of tongue; no pharyngeal edema or erythema

Neck/Lymph Nodes

Supple; no thyromegaly or lymphadenopathy; no carotid bruits

Lungs

CTA

CV

Distant heart sounds, normal S_1 and S_2; PMI at fifth ICS/MCL; RRR; no MRG; no JVD or HJR

Abd

Obese, soft, nontender; no guarding; diminished BS; unable to assess liver size on palpation

Genit/Rect

Prostate gland normal; normal sphincter tone; guaiac (–) stool in rectal vault

MS/Ext

Back pain radiating to right buttock with straight leg raising at 60°; right hip pain with flexion >90° and with internal and external rotation >45°; right hip tender to palpation; right knee (+) crepitus; no swelling or edema; good pedal pulses

Neuro

Oriented × 3; normal affect; appears at times to alternate between apathy and anger/frustration; CN II–XII intact; DTRs equal bilaterally except for slightly diminished Achilles reflexes bilaterally; no focal deficits; gait impaired secondary to hip and knee pain; Babinski's downgoing

■ Labs

Na 135 mEq/L	Hgb 11.8 g/dL	AST 38 IU/L
K 4.7 mEq/L	Hct 34.5%	Alk phos 96 IU/L
Cl 98 mEq/L	WBC $6.5 \times 10^3/mm^3$	T. prot 7.4 g/dL
CO_2 26 mEq/L	Plt $286 \times 10^3/mm^3$	Alb 4.2 g/dL
BUN 18 mg/dL	MCV 85.3 μm^3	Phos 4.5 mg/dL
SCr 1.9 mg/dL	MCH 28.4 pg	ESR 18 mm/hour
Glu 99 mg/dL	MCHC 34.5 g/dL	Ca 11.2 mg/dL

■ UA

SG 1.011; pH 6.5; WBC (–), RBC (–), leukocyte esterase (–), nitrite (–), 2+ protein; microscopic examination reveals two to five epithelial cells/hpf and no bacteria.

■ X-Rays

Lumbar spine: advanced degenerative changes at L3–4 and at L4–5.
Right hip: moderate degenerative changes with some spurring of the femoral head and slight decrease in joint space.
Right knee: moderate degenerative changes; no effusion.

■ Assessment

1. Pain secondary to moderate-to-severe OA of the lumbar spine, right hip, and right knee
2. Obesity (150% of IBW, BMI = 33.2 kg/m²)
3. HTN
4. CKD
5. Seizure disorder

QUESTIONS

Problem Identification

1.a. Create a list of the patient's drug therapy problems.

1.b. What information (symptoms, signs, and laboratory values) indicates the presence or severity of the primary problem?

1.c. What additional information is needed to satisfactorily assess this patient's major medical problems?

Desired Outcome

2. What are the goals of pharmacotherapy for each of this patient's drug-related problems?

Therapeutic Alternatives

3.a. What nondrug therapies might be useful for this patient?

3.b. What feasible pharmacotherapeutic alternatives are available for treatment of this patient's OA?

Optimal Plan

4.a. What drug, dosage form, schedule, and duration of therapy are best for treating this patient's OA?

4.b. What alternatives would be appropriate if the initial therapy fails or cannot be used?

Outcome Evaluation

5. What clinical and laboratory parameters are necessary to evaluate the therapy for achievement of the desired therapeutic outcome and to detect or prevent adverse effects?

Patient Education

6. What information should be provided to the patient to enhance adherence, ensure successful therapy, and minimize adverse effects?

■ FOLLOW-UP QUESTIONS

1. Evaluate the acetaminophen dosing given what the patient reports taking on a daily basis. What are the risks of the current regimen and how can these risks be minimized?

2. The patient tells you that he wants his physician to inject a drug into his knee in order to alleviate the pain. What are the therapeutic options for injection into joints to treat OA, and when would you consider recommending this route of administration?

3. The physician is unsure of the dosing of this patient's levetiracetam for treating a seizure disorder. Is this current dose appropriate, and are there any considerations you should emphasize to the physician regarding monitoring of this medication?

4. Clinicians often rely on equianalgesic charts to convert from one opioid to another. What are some of the risks of relying too much on these dosing parameters, and how should you account for differences among the opioid medications?

■ CLINICAL COURSE: ALTERNATIVE THERAPY

While discussing multiple treatment options with Mr Kansella, he says, "This may seem silly, but I have a neighbor a couple years older than me who was getting some pretty bad arthritis in both knees a few years ago. He says he hardly has any pain anymore because he's taking these glucosamine and chondroitin pills. He even started back to golfing! Is there any way those could help me with my pain?" See Section 19 of this Casebook for questions regarding the use of glucosamine and chondroitin in osteoarthritis.

■ SELF-STUDY ASSIGNMENTS

1. Many patients who deal with pain and osteoarthritis often turn to unproven methods to control their pain. Research some of these unproven methods online and try to find active ingredients to determine if these are unsafe to recommend for patients with complex medication regimens.

2. Evaluate this patient's CKD. What stage of CRI does this patient have, and what is the most likely etiology of his renal disease? Prepare a paper describing some of the complications of long-standing kidney disease and how such complications should be managed.

CLINICAL PEARL

About 27 million Americans have OA, which is the most common joint disorder. It is a chronic debilitating condition associated with pain that affects activities of daily living. Current treatment guidelines have variable recommendations published by different organizations. Managing patient's pain can maintain mobility and improve quality of life. Although use of long-acting opioids for OA is not a first-line option, it may be a necessary therapy in certain circumstances. Therefore, it is important to dose cautiously with the lowest effective dose and monitor patient closely for side effects. Adjunctive therapies may always be considered to limit dose escalation of opioid analgesics.

REFERENCES

1. Hochberg MC, Altman RD, April KT, et al. American College of Rheumatology. American College of Rheumatology 2012 recommendations for the use of non-pharmacologic and pharmacologic therapies in osteoarthritis of the hand, hip, and knee. Arthritis Care Res (Hoboken) 2012;64:465–474.

2. American Academy of Orthopaedic Surgeons (AAOS). American Academy of Orthopaedic Surgeons clinical practice guideline on treatment of osteoarthritis of the knee. 2nd ed. Available at: http://www.aaos.org/cc_files/aaosorg/research/guidelines/treatmentofosteoarthritisoftheknee-neeguideline.pdf. Accessed March 29, 2016.

3. McAlindon TE, Bannuru RR, Sullivan MC, et al. OA Research Society International (OARSI) guidelines for the non-surgical management of knee osteoarthritis. Osteoarthritis Cartilage 2014;22:363–388.

4. Machado GC, Maher CG, Ferreira PH, et al. Efficacy and safety of paracetamol for spinal pain and osteoarthritis: systematic review and meta-analysis of randomized placebo controlled trials. BMJ 2015;350:h1225. doi:10.1136/bmj.h1225.

5. Chou R, Fanciullo GJ, Fine PG, et al. Clinical guidelines for the use of chronic opioid therapy in chronic non-cancer pain. J Pain 2009;10:113–130.

6. McPherson ML. Demystifying Opioid Conversion Calculations, 1st ed. Bethesda, MD: American Society of Health-System Pharmacists, 2010.

7. Hunter DJ. Viscosupplementation of osteoarthritis of the knee. N Engl J Med 2015;372:1040–1047.

8. U.S. Food and Drug Administration (FDA). FDA Drug Safety Communication: Prescription acetaminophen products to be limited to 325 mg per dosage unit; boxed warning will highlight potential for severe liver failure. January 13, 2011. Available at: http://www.fda.gov/Drugs/DrugSafety/ucm239821.htm. Accessed March 28, 2016.

106

GOUT AND HYPERURICEMIA

The King of Oktoberfest .... Level II

Erik D. Maki, PharmD, BCPS

LEARNING OBJECTIVES

After completing this case study, the reader should be able to:

- Identify major risk factors for developing gout in a given patient, including drugs that may contribute to or cause this disorder.

- Develop a pharmacotherapeutic plan for a patient with acute gouty arthritis that includes individualized drug selection and assessment of the treatment for efficacy or toxicity.

- Identify patients in whom maintenance therapy for gout and hyperuricemia is warranted.

- Identify medications not used primarily for gout that may have a beneficial effect on serum uric acid (SUA) levels.

PATIENT PRESENTATION

▓ Chief Complaint

"My toe is on fire."

▓ HPI

Roy Huff is a 78-year-old man who presents to the ED complaining of significant toe pain. Mr Huff states, "I think I'm paying the price for my fun at Oktoberfest." He reports having spent the weekend indulging on beer and sausage at the local Oktoberfest festival. In the early hours of Monday morning (approximately 3 hours ago), he awoke to sudden excruciating pain in his right big toe. Over the past hour, this toe has become red, swollen, and so painful that he cannot walk. He has not experienced any trauma or injuries. He also denies having experienced these symptoms previously.

▓ PMH

HTN
PUD
Obesity

▓ SH

The patient typically drinks "a can of beer or two" daily but drank significantly on Friday, Saturday, and Sunday. He does not smoke or use illicit drugs.

▓ Meds

Chlorthalidone 25 mg PO daily, started 1 month ago
Omeprazole 20 mg PO daily

▓ All

NKDA

ROS

Other than feeling somewhat dehydrated from all of his drinking, the patient has no major complaints prior to this ED visit. No chest pain, nausea/vomiting, or respiratory symptoms. Bowel habits are normal. He has no prior history of arthritic symptoms or joint problems.

Physical Examination

Gen

A healthy-appearing, obese, white man in acute distress

VS

BP 120/60 mm Hg, P 110 bpm, RR 19, T 37.5°C; Wt 88 kg, Ht 5′6″

Skin

Poor skin turgor. No rashes or other dermatologic abnormalities.

HEENT

PERRLA, dry mucous membranes, throat/ears clear of redness or inflammation

Neck/Lymph Nodes

Negative for lymph node swelling or masses

Lungs/Thorax

Clear to auscultation bilaterally, symmetric movement with inspiration

CV

Tachycardic, normal rhythm, normal S_1 and S_2

Abd

Obese, but soft, nontender; positive bowel sounds in all quadrants.

Genit/Rect

Deferred

MS/Ext

Erythematous, edematous right first metatarsophalangeal joint, which is very warm to touch; joint is exquisitely painful with patient relating the pain as currently a 10/10 (on a 1–10 scale with "0" being no pain and "10" being the worse pain the patient has ever suffered); no swelling of any other joints. No signs of tophi present

Neuro

A & O × 3; CN II–XII grossly intact, no focal neurologic deficits

Labs

Ankle and foot radiographs: negative for break or damage
Aspirated fluid from first metatarsophalangeal joint tap: >50 WBC/ hpf, containing negatively birefringent monosodium urate crystals

Na 145 mEq/L	Hgb 15.1 g/dL	WBC 12.8	*Fasting lipid*
K 3.5 mEq/L	Hct 45%	× 10³/mm³	*panel*
Cl 101 mEq/L	RBC 4.9 × 10⁶/mm³	Neutros 88%	HDL 50 mg/dL
CO₂ 23 mEq/L	Plt 210 × 10³/mm³	Bands 0%	Trig 190 mg/dL
BUN 40 mg/dL	MCV 81 μm³	Eos 1%	LDL 92 mg/dL
SCr 3.0 mg/dL	MCHC 35 g/dL	Lymphs 10%	T. chol 180 mg/dL
Glu 105 mg/dL	ESR 45 mm/hour	Monos 1%	
SUA 11.6 mg/dL		RF negative	

Assessment

1. Primary presentation of acute gouty arthritis

2. ARF secondary to dehydration and diuretic use

3. Probable ADR: drug-induced gout

4. Hypertension; currently well controlled

5. History of duodenal ulcer; on maintenance antisecretory therapy

QUESTIONS

Problem Identification

1.a. Create a list of the patient's drug therapy problems.

1.b. What patient information (symptoms, signs, and laboratory values) indicates the presence or severity of acute gouty arthritis?

1.c. What risk factors in this case could contribute to or cause gouty arthritis?

Desired Outcome

2. What are the goals of pharmacotherapy in this case?

Therapeutic Alternatives

3.a. What nondrug therapies may be useful for this patient?

3.b. What pharmacotherapeutic modalities are available for the treatment of acute gouty arthritis?

3.c. Should chronic treatment to decrease the patient's serum uric acid level be initiated at this time? Why or why not?

Optimal Plan

4.a. Considering the patient's information, what drug, dosage form, schedule, and duration of therapy are best in this case?

4.b. What agent would be best to treat the patient's hypertension assuming that his renal function normalizes?

Outcome Evaluation

5. Which clinical and laboratory parameters should be monitored to assess the efficacy of the pharmacotherapeutic plan and to prevent adverse effects?

Patient Education

6. What information should be provided to the patient to enhance adherence, ensure successful therapy, and avoid adverse effects?

■ CLINICAL COURSE

The patient responded to the therapy you recommended, and within 96 hours his pain has subsided significantly. Toe redness and swelling have decreased to near normal. Additionally, with fluids, his SCr has returned to baseline (0.8 mg/dL). After consultation with you, the patient's physician decides against maintenance therapy to decrease serum uric acid levels. The patient, remembering the severe pain this episode caused, follows your recommended lifestyle changes and is adherent to the new medication you recommended for his hypertension. At his 6-month follow-up appointment, he reports no more attacks of gout. He has lost 20 lbs and no longer drinks ethanol. His serum uric acid level has decreased to 6.9 mg/dL, and his BP is 130/80 mm Hg.

■ FOLLOW-UP QUESTIONS

1. At what point should maintenance therapy to decrease serum uric acid levels be considered?

2. If at some point maintenance therapy to decrease serum uric acid is begun, what additional therapy is needed to prevent acute flares?

■ SELF-STUDY ASSIGNMENTS

1. List antihyperuricemic agents that are available in the United States and their relative advantages and disadvantages. Describe new agents that are being studied for this indication and what clinical data support their use.

2. List medications that can either increase or decrease serum uric acid concentrations.

CLINICAL PEARL

Historically, colchicine was used for treatment of acute gout flares at doses of 0.6 mg Q 1–2 H until symptoms resolved or adverse GI symptoms developed (6 mg maximum). GI side effects were employed as a clinical endpoint for discontinuing the drug because these side effects tended to occur prior to the more severe adverse effects of colchicine-induced myopathy and myelosuppression. However, current recommendations are to use low-dose colchicine at a dose of 1.2 mg, followed in 1 hour with a single dose of 0.6 mg. For patients receiving prophylactic colchicine prior to the flare, it is recommended to wait 12 hours after treatment dosing before resuming prophylactic dosing.

REFERENCES

1. Khanna D, Fitzgerald JD, Khanna PP, et al. 2012 American College of Rheumatology guidelines for management of gout. Part 1: systematic nonpharmacologic and pharmacologic therapeutic approaches to hyperuricemia. Arthritis Care Res (Hoboken) 2012;64:1431–1446.
2. Wilson L, Nair KV, Saseen JJ. Comparison of New-Onset Gout in Adults Prescribed Chlorthalidone vs Hydrochlorothiazide for Hypertention. J Clin Hypertens (Greenwhich) 2014;16:864–868.
3. Khanna D, Khanna PP, Fitzgerald JD, et al. 2012 American College of Rheumatology guidelines for management of gout. Part 2: therapy and antiinflammatory prophylaxis of acute gouty arthritis. Arthritis Care Res (Hoboken) 2012;64:1447–1461.
4. Choi HK. A prescription for lifestyle change in patients with hyperuricemia and gout. Curr Opin Rheumatol 2010;22:166–172.
5. Zhang W, Doherty M, Bardin T, et al. EULAR evidence based recommendations for gout. Part II: Management. Report of a task force of the EULAR Standing Committee For International Clinical Studies Including Therapeutics (ESCISIT). Ann Rheum Dis 2006;65:1312–1324.
6. Jordan KM, Cameron JS, Snaith M, et al. British Society for Rheumatology and British Health Professionals in Rheumatology Guideline for the Management of Gout. Rheumatology 2007;46:1372–1374.
7. Taylor TH, Mecchella JN, Larson RJ, Kerin KD, Mackenzie TA. Initiation of allopurinol at first medical contact for acute attacks of gout: a randomized clinical trial. Am J Med 2012;125:1126–1134.
8. Neogi T. Clinical practice: gout. N Engl J Med 2011;364:443–452.
9. James PA, Oparil S, Carter BL, et al. 2014 evidence-based guideline for the management of high blood pressure in adults: Report from the panel members appointed to the eighth joint national committee (JNC 8). JAMA 2014;311:507–520.
10. Wolff ML, Cruz JL, Vanderman AJ, Brown JN. The effect of angiotensin II receptor blockers on hyperuricemia. Ther Adv Chronic Dis 2015;6:339–346.

107

GLAUCOMA

Silent Blindness.................................Level III

Brian McMillan, MD

Ashlee McMillan, PharmD, BCACP

LEARNING OBJECTIVES:

After completing this case study, the reader should be able to:

- Identify the importance of regular eye examinations and the early diagnosis of glaucoma.

- List the risk factors for developing open-angle glaucoma.

- Select and recommend agents from different pharmacologic classes when indicated and provide the rationale for drug selection, including combination products to increase adherence.

- Recommend conventional glaucoma therapy as well as other options in glaucoma management when indicated.

- Formulate basic ophthalmologic monitoring parameters used in glaucoma therapy.

- Counsel patients on medication regimens and proper ophthalmic administration technique.

- Discuss potential adverse drug reactions with patients to increase therapy adherence.

PATIENT PRESENTATION

◼ Chief Complaint

"My vision is closing down and I am having difficulty seeing cars at intersections while driving."

◼ HPI

Macy Connor is a 75-year-old woman who presents for follow-up of advanced POAG. She reports adherence with latanoprost nightly and timolol/brimonidine (Combigan) 2 times daily in the right eye and dorzolamide 3 times daily in the left eye. She feels that her vision in the left eye is beginning to blur, and she is having more difficulty seeing objects in the top part of her vision. She finds that she has to move her head more to see objects in her periphery. She denies eye pain, flashes or floaters. She is feeling more tired recently and just does not have the energy to do the things she used to do.

Mrs Connor was first diagnosed with POAG 20 years ago during a routine eye exam to update her eyeglass prescription. She had no visual disturbances at that time, and her best corrected vision was 20/20 OU. She was started on pilocarpine 1% 3 times daily in both eyes and developed brow ache and blurred vision. This was discontinued and she was started on timolol 0.5% twice daily in both eyes. Her highest IOP prior to treatment was 28 mm Hg, which improved to 22 mm Hg on timolol. Her eye pressure gradually increased requiring the addition of brimonidine 3 times daily and latanoprost nightly in both eyes. She underwent cataract surgery 2 years ago and experienced an IOP spike to 55 mm Hg and was given acetazolamide 250 mg PO 4 times daily for 5 days after surgery until her pressure improved back to baseline. She underwent trabeculectomy with mitomycin C on the left eye last year; dorzolamide 3 times daily was added when the IOP again began to increase.

◼ PMH

Hypertension, well controlled on lisinopril for 6 years

Kidney stones (occurred while taking acetazolamide)

Migraine headaches; well controlled on sumatriptan with 1–2 migraines per year

Depression; controlled with exercise and counseling only. Has never taken medications for depression

Myopia; corrected with glasses

Astigmatism; corrected with glasses

Pseudophakia; cataract surgery three years ago

◼ FH

Parents are both deceased; father had POAG requiring surgery and was blind in right eye; mother died of breast cancer; has one brother who is alive with myopia

◼ SH

Nonsmoker; drinks 1–2 glasses of wine per week

◼ ROS

Decreased energy with two falls in the last month at home. All other systems negative.

◼ Meds

Latanoprost 0.005% one drop nightly OD

Combigan 0.2%/0.5% one drop twice daily OD

Dorzolamide 2% one drop three times daily OS

Sumatriptan 25 mg PO as needed for headache

Lisinopril 20 mg PO once daily

◼ All

Penicillin – Rash

◼ Physical Examination

VS

BP 112/72, P 82, R 18, T 36.4°C

EYES

Visual Acuity: ODcc: 20/25; OScc: 20/60 (cc = with glasses)

Intraocular pressure: OD: 22; OS: 18

Central Corneal Thickness (CCT): OD: 515: OS: 510 (normal 540 μm)

Gonioscopy: Iridocorneal angle is open with ciliary body band visible OU (Open Angle)

Pupils: Equal round and reactive OU. No relative afferent pupillary defect (rAPD)

Extraocular Movements: Full OU

Slit Lamp Exam

Lids: Normal

Conjunctiva: 1+ injection OD, superior diffuse thick walled bleb

Cornea: Clear OU

Anterior chamber: Deep and quiet OU

Iris: Round and reactive OU, superior peripheral iridectomy OS

Lens: Posterior chamber intraocular lens OU

Vitreous: Normal

Optic nerve:

OD: Superior and inferior rim thinning with focal notch superiorly. Cup-to-Disk (C/D) ratio 0.85

OS: Superior rim loss, inferior rim thinning. Disk hemorrhage superior temporal disk C/D ratio 0.95 (normal C/D 0.25)

CN II-XII grossly intact

Humphrey Visual Fields:

OD: Good reliability, inferior arcuate depression; stable

OS: Good reliability, denser superior altitudinal defect splitting fixation, decreased foveal threshold

■ Assessment

1. Advanced POAG

   OD: Stable visual field, IOP slightly higher today

   OS: Dense visual field loss now affecting central vision. IOP improved from baseline; however, patient continues to progress

2. Pseudophakia—excellent result of cataract surgery

3. Myopia/Astigmatism

■ Plan

1. Right eye—Continue latanoprost nightly and Combigan 0.2%/0.5% twice daily and schedule for laser trabeculoplasty.

2. Left eye—Discontinue dorzolamide. Add latanoprost nightly and Combigan 0.2%/0.5% twice daily.

3. Follow-up in 1 month for IOP check. If pressure remains elevated OS, schedule for glaucoma drainage device.

QUESTIONS

Problem Identification

1.a. What evidence indicates that this patient has primary open-angle glaucoma (POAG)? See Figs. 107-1, 107-2, and 107-3.

1.b. Identify this patient's ophthalmic drug therapy problems.

1.c. What other drug therapy problems does the patient have?

1.d. What are this patient's risk factors for POAG?

1.e. Identify important information that indicates the severity of disease.

1.f. Which details of this patient's past medical history influence your therapy recommendations?

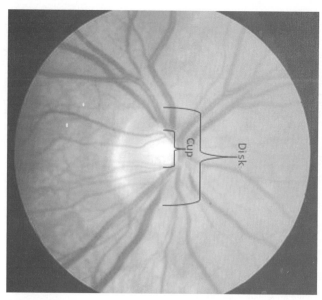

FIGURE 107-1. Normal optic nerve with cup/disk ratio (c/d) = 0.3.

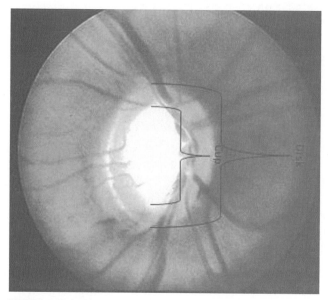

FIGURE 107-2. Abnormal, glaucomatous optic nerve with increased cup/disk ratio (c/d) = 0.8.

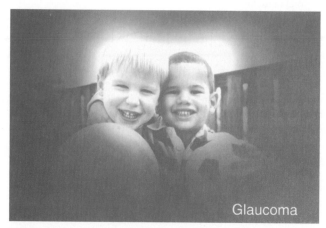

FIGURE 107-3. Simulated vision of patient with glaucoma. (Source: National Eye Institute, National Institutes of Health).

Desired Outcome

2. What are the goals of pharmacotherapy in this case?

Therapeutic Alternatives

3.a. If this patient were diagnosed today, what would be the optimal first-line pharmacologic therapy?

3.b. What pharmacologic classes and individual agents are available to treat glaucoma?

3.c. How can glaucoma medications be combined to improve patient adherence?

3.d. What surgical treatments might be useful for this patient?

3.e. During what phase of this patient's disease case are surgical treatments indicated?

Optimal Plan

4.a. Devise an optimal therapeutic regimen for this patient's glaucoma.

4.b. Which medications should be avoided in this patient?

Outcome Evaluation

5. What clinical and laboratory parameters are necessary to evaluate the therapy for achievement of the desired therapeutic outcome and to detect or prevent adverse effects?

Patient Education

6. What information should the patient receive about the disease of glaucoma, proper medication administration technique, and possible side effects of treatment?

■ SELF-STUDY ASSIGNMENTS

1. Perform a literature search on the reason why antimetabolites such as mitomycin C and 5-fluorouracil (5-FU) are used in glaucoma surgery. What is the mechanism of action of these antimetabolites in trabeculectomy pressure-lowering surgery?

2. Perform a literature search on memantine for treatment of glaucoma. Why is it not currently used as an adjunctive treatment? In what type of glaucoma could this medication be helpful?

CLINICAL PEARL

Glaucoma is a silent and generally slowly progressive optic neuropathy. Optimizing pharmacotherapy of glaucoma must consider systemic medical conditions, social and environmental factors that may limit adherence. Patients should be monitored regularly for disease progression because many patients with glaucoma continue to progress on treatment despite "normal pressures."

REFERENCES

1. Heijl A, Leske MC, Bengtsson B, et al. Reduction of intraocular pressure and glaucoma progression: results from the Early Manifest Glaucoma Trial. Arch Ophthalmol 2002;120:1268–1279.

2. Newman-Casey PA, Blachley T, Lee PP, et al. Patterns of glaucoma medication adherence over four years of follow up. Ophthalmology 2015;122:2010–2021.

3. Gordon MO, Beiser JA, Brandt JA, et al. The Ocular Hypertension Treatment Study. Baseline factors that predict the onset of primary open-angle glaucoma. Arch Ophthalmol 2002;120:714–720.

4. Drance S, Anderson DR, Schulzer M. Risk Factors for progression of visual field abnormalities in normal-tension glaucoma. Collaborative Normal-Tension Glaucoma Study. Am J Ophthalmol 2001;131:699–708.

5. Tielsch JM, Katz J, Sommer A, Quigley HA, Javitt JC. Family history and risk of primary open angle glaucoma. The Baltimore Eye Survey. Arch Ophthalmol 1994;112(1):69–73.

6. Kass MA, Kolker AE, Gordon M, et al. Acetazolamide and urolithiasis. Ophthalmology 1981;88;261–265.

7. Gross RL. Current medical management of glaucoma. In: Yanoff M, Duker J et al, eds. Ophthalmology. 3rd ed. Oxford, UK. Mosby–Elsevier 2009;1220–1225.

8. Katz LJ, Steinmann WC, Kabir A, et al. Selective laser trabeculoplasty versus medical therapy as initial treatment of glaucoma: a prospective randomized trial. J Glaucoma 2012;21;460–468.

9. Higginbotham EJ. Considerations in glaucoma therapy: fixed combination versus their component medications. Clin Ophthalmol 2010;4;1–9.

10. Zimmerman TJ, Kooner KS, Kandarakis AS, Ziegler LP. Improving the therapeutic index of topically applied ocular drugs. Arch Ophthalmol 1984;102:551–553.

108

ALLERGIC RHINITIS

Breathe in, Breathe out . . . . Level I

Jon P. Wietholter, PharmD, BCPS

LEARNING OBJECTIVES

After completing this case study, the reader should be able to:

- Recognize common signs and symptoms associated with allergic rhinitis.

- Educate patients on appropriate measures to limit or avoid exposure to specific antigens.

- Select an appropriate pharmacotherapeutic regimen for managing allergic rhinitis, focusing on specific symptoms.

- Educate patients with allergic rhinitis on appropriate medication use, including instillation technique for intranasal medications.

PATIENT PRESENTATION

▒ Chief Complaint

"I can't breathe! I feel congested around the clock and am constantly sneezing."

▒ HPI

James Joseph Patrick is a 19-year-old African-American man presenting to his family medicine clinic with complaints of severe congestion and persistent sneezing. He states that symptoms are at their worst immediately upon returning to his apartment every evening and that they started last August when he moved to his new apartment. Prior to this move, he noticed symptoms similar to these on a much more sporadic basis; since the move they have been bothering him every day, and he is having trouble sleeping.

He hasn't noticed a fever or a sore throat, but the symptoms are becoming unbearable. He is seeking advice on how to cope with and manage these symptoms.

■ PMH

Mild-persistent asthma (diagnosed when he was age 13)

■ FH

Father, age 44, with a history of asthma and allergic rhinitis. Mother, age 38, with a history of migraines. No siblings.

■ SH

Lives in an apartment close to his university and place of work; (–) tobacco, (–) illicit drugs, (+) alcohol use (primarily on weekends when partying with friends); has two cats that he adopted when he moved into his new apartment.

■ Meds

Diphenhydramine 25 mg PO Q HS (helps him sleep at night)
Albuterol MDI two puffs Q 6 H PRN (uses roughly one inhaler per year for asthma symptoms)
Fluticasone (Flovent HFA, 44 mcg/puff) two puffs twice daily for asthma

■ All

Penicillin (hives)

■ ROS

Denies headaches; no shortness of breath, wheezing, chest pain, or abdominal discomfort

■ Physical Examination

Gen

Young African-American male who appears tired and sounds congested. Although sneezing is a main complaint, he has not sneezed at all during this visit.

VS

BP 112/74 mm Hg, P 68 bpm, RR 18, T 36.9°C; Wt 175 lb, Ht 5′10″

Skin

Pale, turgor normal, no rashes or lesions

HEENT

NC/AT; PERRLA; EOMI; (–) periorbital edema or discoloration; TMs are intact; (+) swollen nasal mucous membranes and nasal turbinates with a pale, bluish hue and discharge down the posterior pharynx; (–) tenderness over frontal and maxillary sinuses; (–) oropharyngeal lesions; throat is non-erythematous

Neck/Lymph Nodes

No lymphadenopathy or thyromegaly

Chest

CTA bilaterally; no noticeable wheezing

CV

RRR without murmur or rub

Abd

Soft, nontender, (+) BS

Genit/Rect

Deferred

Ext

No erythema, pain, or edema; pulses 2+

Neuro

A & O × 3; CN: visual fields and hearing intact; 5/5 strength throughout

■ Labs

Na 136 mEq/L	Hgb 15.4 g/dL
K 3.9 mEq/L	Hct 45.3%
Cl 108 mEq/L	Plt 391 × 10³/mm³
CO₂ 28 mEq/L	WBC 4.5 × 10³/mm³
BUN 10 mg/dL	
SCr 0.7 mg/dL	
Glu 88 mg/dL	

Na 136 mEq/L Hgb 15.4 g/dL K 3.9 mEq/L Hct 45.3% Cl 108 mEq/L Plt 391×10^3/mm³ CO$_2$ 28 mEq/L WBC 4.5×10^3/mm³ BUN 10 mg/dL SCr 0.7 mg/dL Glu 88 mg/dL

■ Other

Peak expiratory flow (PEF): Patient states that readings are always >80% of personal best

■ Assessment

This is a 19-year-old man complaining of signs and symptoms consistent with moderate–severe persistent perennial allergic rhinitis

QUESTIONS

Problem Identification

1.a. Create a list of the patient's drug therapy problems.

1.b. What information (signs, symptoms, laboratory values) indicates the presence or severity of allergic rhinitis?

Desired Outcome

2. What are the treatment goals for allergic rhinitis in this case?

Therapeutic Alternatives

3.a. What nondrug therapies might be useful for this patient?

3.b. What feasible pharmacotherapeutic alternatives are available for treating this patient's allergic rhinitis?

Optimal Plan

4. What drug, dosage form, dose, schedule, and duration of therapy are best for this patient?

Outcome Evaluation

5. What clinical and laboratory parameters are necessary to evaluate the therapy for achievement of the desired therapeutic outcome and to detect or prevent adverse effects?

Patient Education

6. What information should be provided to a patient receiving an intranasal corticosteroid to enhance adherence, ensure successful therapy, and minimize adverse effects?

■ CLINICAL COURSE: ALTERNATIVE THERAPY

James' mother is quite concerned about drowsiness associated with prescription treatments for his symptoms because he has a tendency to nap when he is supposed to be doing homework. Mrs Patrick uses butterbur extract for migraine prophylaxis and has heard that it is effective for allergy symptoms; she asks about using the same product for James. See Section 19 of this Casebook for questions regarding the use of butterbur extract for allergy symptoms.

■ SELF-STUDY ASSIGNMENTS

1. Describe how the recommended treatment plan might differ if this was instead a 78-year-old patient or a 34-year-old pregnant patient.

2. Describe a situation where monotherapy with an antihistamine, a leukotriene receptor antagonist, or an oral decongestant would be appropriate or preferred for managing allergic rhinitis. Support your recommendations with efficacy and safety data.

CLINICAL PEARL

Prior to 2014, immunotherapy was only available via the subcutaneous route in the United States. Since then, sublingual versions have been approved (eg, grass pollen allergen extract and ragweed pollen allergen extract) that allow for an effective yet less invasive method of delivering immunotherapy.

REFERENCES

1. Wallace DV, Dykewicz MS, Bernstein DI, et al. Joint Task Force on Practice, American Academy of Allergy, Asthma & Immunology, American College of Allergy, Asthma and Immunology, Joint Council of Allergy, Asthma and Immunology. The diagnosis and management of rhinitis: an updated practice parameter. J Allergy Clin Immunol 2008;122(2 Suppl):S1–S84.

2. Roberts G, Xatzipsalti M, Borrego LM, et al. Paediatric rhinitis: position paper of the European Academy of Allergy and Clinical Immunology. Allergy 2013;68:1102–1116.

3. Wheatley LM, Togias A. Clinical practice. Allergic rhinitis. N Engl J Med 2015;372:456–463.

4. Brozek JL, Bousquet J, Baena-Cagnani CE, et al. Allergic rhinitis and its impact on asthma (ARIA) guidelines: 2010 revision. J Allergy Clin Immunol 2010;126(3):466–476.

5. Chan RY, Chien WT. The effects of two Chinese herbal medicinal formulae vs. placebo controls for treatment of allergic rhinitis: a randomised controlled trial. Trials 2014;15:261. http://www.trialsjournal.com/content/15/1/261. Accessed Dec. 11, 2015.

6. Choi SM, Park JE, Li SS, et al. A multicenter, randomized, controlled trial testing the effects of acupuncture on allergic rhinitis. Allergy 2013;68:365–374.

7. Devillier P, Dreyfus JF, Demoly P, Calderon MA. A meta-analysis of sublingual allergen immunotherapy and pharmacotherapy in pollen-induced seasonal allergic rhinoconjunctivitis. BMC Medicine 2014;12:71. Available at: http://www.biomedcentral.com/1741-7015/12/71.

8. De Castro G, Zicari AM, Indinnimeo L, et al. Efficacy of sublingual specific immunotherapy on allergic asthma and rhinitis in children's real life. Eur Rev Med Pharmacol Sci 2013;17:2225–2231.

9. Mosbech H, Canonica GW, Backer V, et al. SQ house dust mite sublingually administered immunotherapy tablet (ALK) improves allergic rhinitis in patients with house dust mite allergic asthma and rhinitis symptoms. Ann Allergy Asthma Immunol 2015;114:134–140.

109

CUTANEOUS REACTION TO DRUGS

A Case of TEN...............................Level III

Rebecca M. T. Law, BS Pharm, PharmD

LEARNING OBJECTIVES

After completing this case study, the reader should be able to:

- Understand the approach to identifying or ruling out a suspected drug-induced skin reaction.

- Recognize the signs and symptoms of drug-induced Stevens–Johnson syndrome (SJS) and toxic epidermal necrolysis (TEN).

- Name the drugs most commonly implicated in causing SJS and TEN.

- Determine an appropriate course of action for a patient with a suspected drug-induced skin reaction.

- Understand the treatment approach for a patient with TEN, including nonpharmacologic and pharmacologic therapies.

- Counsel patients with suspected drug-induced SJS or TEN about the nature of the reaction and necessary precautions, including which medications to avoid in the future.

- Identify patients with potentially serious skin reactions who should be referred for further medical evaluation and treatment.

PATIENT PRESENTATION

■ Chief Complaint

"My child has a blistering rash all over her body and is really sick!"

■ HPI

April Rayne is a 14-year-old Caucasian girl who presented to the ED with a high fever, vomiting, diarrhea, and a 3-day history of a skin rash. The rash is maculopapular with blisters and has spread to involve 75% of her body surface area. She had a UTI about 1.5 weeks ago and was prescribed a 7-day course of TMP/SMX. She adhered to the regimen; her urinary tract symptoms of dysuria and frequency and her abdominal discomfort resolved within 2–3 days. This was her first UTI. She continued to take the TMP/SMX as directed. Seven days after starting therapy, she noticed red spots on her arms and legs that began to spread over the whole body. The rash began to blister. She became febrile, and last night she began

vomiting and had two bouts of diarrhea. This morning her mother brought her to the ED and she was admitted to the ICU, where she was immediately intubated to protect her airway patency.

■ PMH

Unremarkable

■ FH

Parents A & W, no siblings

■ SH

April is a student who just began taking jazz classes about 2 months ago, which she really enjoys. She is not sexually active, does not smoke, and does not use alcohol. There have been no recent changes in diet or in her living environment.

■ Meds

Just completed a 7-day course of TMP/SMX. No additional drugs taken including OTCs, vitamins, herbals, or drugs of abuse. Not on oral contraceptives.

■ Meds in Hospital

For intubation: Ketamine 40 mg IV × 1, midazolam 1 mg IV × 1, propofol 120 mg IV × 1

For BP support: Dopamine IV infusion at 12 mcg/kg/min

■ All

NKDA

■ ROS

Skin is tender to the touch, with rash and blisters. Continues to have loose BM. Vomited × 1 in ED. Otherwise negative except for complaints noted above.

■ Physical Examination

Gen

Fairly anxious 14-year-old Caucasian girl looking acutely ill

VS

BP 90/50 mm Hg, HR 90, RR 25, T 40.1°C

Skin

Extensive maculopapular rash over 75% of BSA. Blisters involve over 30% of BSA and appear to still be spreading. Blisters have become confluent and result in detachment of the epidermis. Small blisters on discrete dark red purpuric macules symmetrically over face, hands, feet, limbs, and trunk with widespread erythema. Blisters and intensely red oozing erosions over lips (especially vermilion border), oral mucosa, and vaginal area. Some ruptured blisters on skin and some with necrotic centers. Positive Nikolsky's sign. Skin is tender to the touch.

HEENT

PERRLA, EOMI, fundi benign, TMs intact. Corneal abrasions but no blisters. Conjunctivitis with some debris collecting under eyelids. External nares clear. Blisters in oral cavity and ulceration on lower lip. Pharynx erythematous and blistering.

Chest

Upper airway congestion; debris and ulceration in mouth, throat, and epiglottis. (She was immediately intubated to protect airway patency.)

Cor

RRR without murmurs, rubs, or gallops; S_1 and S_2 normal

Abd

(+) BS, soft, nontender, no masses

Genitourinary

Blistering in vaginal area. Foley catheter inserted—urine output approximately 40–50 mL/hour

Rectal

Deferred

MS/Ext

Maculopapular rash and some blisters on arms and legs. Bilateral arthralgias and myalgias. Peripheral pulses present.

Neuro

Oriented × 3. No signs of confusion.

■ Labs

Na 140 mEq/L	Glucose 95 mg/dL	WBC 11 × 10³/mm³	Hgb 12 g/dL
K 4.0 mEq/L	BUN 9 mg/dL	PMNs 65%	Hct 31%
Cl 101 mEq/L	SCr 0.7 mg/dL	Bands 5%	Plt 239 ×
CO₂ 32 mEq/L	AST 15 IU/L	Eos 8%	10³/mm³
PO₄ 2.2 mg/dL	ALT 22 IU/L	Monos 1%	INR 1.24
T. protein 6.5 g/dL	LDH 120 IU/L	Basos 1%	aPTT 32.4 sec
Albumin 3.1 g/dL		Lymphs 20%	ESR 35 mm/hour
			RF negative

Urinalysis: No protein, ketones, blood, WBC, or bacteria.

■ Chest X-Ray

WNL

■ Clinical Course

Day 2 of Admission

Urine output still approximately 40–50 mL/hour; 1050 mL/previous 24 hours.

Day 3 of Admission

Histopathology of biopsy specimen from lesion on lip: Epidermal degeneration with intraepidermal vesiculation and subepidermal bullae. Mild perivascular lymphocytic infiltrate.

Direct immunofluorescence of biopsy specimen from lip lesion: Negative.

Swab from blisters on arm: Coagulase-negative *Staphylococcus*, *Pseudomonas aeruginosa*.

Blood cultures: Coagulase-negative *Staphylococcus*, sensitive to vancomycin.

Urine culture (mid-stream urine): No growth.

■ Assessment

This is a 14-year-old girl with TEN, likely drug-induced, who has probably developed secondary *Staphylococcus epidermidis* bacteremia

QUESTIONS

Problem Identification

1.a. Create a drug therapy problem list for this patient.

1.b. What signs and symptoms of TEN does this patient demonstrate?

1.c. Could the patient's signs and symptoms be caused by a drug?

1.d. What findings correlate with disease severity of TEN and a worse prognosis?

Desired Outcome

2. What are the treatment goals for this patient?

Therapeutic Alternatives

3.a. What nonpharmacologic alternatives are available for managing TEN in this patient?

3.b. What pharmacotherapeutic alternatives are available for managing this patient's TEN?

Optimal Plan

4. Design an optimal pharmacotherapeutic plan for TEN in this patient.

Outcome Evaluation

5. What efficacy and adverse effects monitoring is needed for the management strategies you recommended?

Patient Education

6. How would you inform this patient (and her caregivers) about her drug therapies?

■ SELF-STUDY ASSIGNMENTS

1. Differentiate among the various types, terminology, and manifestations of cutaneous drug reactions, including irritant drug reactions, fixed drug reactions, maculopapular skin reactions, photoallergic and phototoxic reactions, bullous reactions, morbilliform and urticarial reactions, pigmentation, lichenoid eruptions, SJS, TEN, drug hypersensitivity syndrome, and vasculitis.

2. If this patient had SJS, would the clinical presentation, disease course, and treatment differ from those of TEN? If so, how?

3. Obtain information on the anticonvulsants and NSAIDs that have been most commonly implicated in causing SJS/TEN.

4. Investigate the genetics of drug hypersensitivity, including associations with specific genetic markers (eg, HLA-B*5701 and HLA-B*1502 alleles).

CLINICAL PEARL

Aggressive and vigilant nondrug supportive therapies are vital to the effective management of TEN.

REFERENCES

1. Cohen V. Toxic epidermal necrolysis. eMedicine, updated October 21, 2015. Available at: *http://emedicine.–medscape.com/article/229698-overview*. Accessed March 7, 2016.
2. Croom DL. Dermatologic manifestations of Stevens–Johnson syndrome and toxic epidermal necrolysis. eMedicine, updated December 6, 2015. Available at: *http://emedicine.medscape.com/article/1124127-overview*. Accessed March 7, 2016.
3. Barron SJ, Del Vecchio MT, Aronoff SC. Intravenous immunoglobulin in the treatment of Stevens-Johnson syndrome and toxic epidermal necrolysis: a meta-analysis with meta-regression of observational studies. Int J Dermatol 2015;54:108–115.
4. Levi N, Bastuji-Garin S, Mockenhaupt M, et al. Medications as risk factors of Stevens–Johnson syndrome and toxic epidermal necrolysis in children: a pooled analysis. Pediatrics 2009;123(2):e297–e304.
5. Playe S, Murphy G. Recognizing adverse reactions to antibiotics. Emerg Med 2006;38(6):11–20.
6. Tilles SA. Practical issues in the management of hypersensitivity reactions: sulfonamides. South Med J 2001;94:817–824.
7. Roujeau JC, Kelly JP, Naldi L, et al. Medication use and the risk of Stevens–Johnson syndrome or toxic epidermal necrolysis. N Engl J Med 1995;333:1600–1607.
8. Mockenhaupt M, Viboud C, Dunant A, et al. Stevens–Johnson syndrome and toxic epidermal necrolysis: assessment of medication risks with emphasis on recently marketed drugs. The EuroSCAR-Study. J Invest Dermatol 2008;128:35–44.
9. Johnson KK, Green DL, Rife JP, et al. Sulfonamide cross-reactivity: fact or fiction? Ann Pharmacother 2005;39:290–301.
10. Strom BL, Schinnar R, Apter AJ, et al. Absence of cross-reactivity between sulfonamide antibiotics and sulfonamide nonantibiotics. N Engl J Med 2003;349:1628–1635.
11. Swanson L, Colven RM. Approach to the patient with a suspected cutaneous adverse drug reaction. Med Clin North Am 2015;99:1337–1348.
12. Wolkenstein P, Charue D, Laurent P, et al. Metabolic predisposition to cutaneous adverse drug reactions: Role in toxic epidermal necrolysis caused by sulfonamides and anticonvulsants. Arch Dermatol 1995;131(5):544–551. doi:10.1001/archderm.1995.01690170046006.
13. deShazo RD, Kemp SF. Allergic reactions to drugs and biologic agents. JAMA 1997;278:1895–1906.

110

ACNE VULGARIS

The Graduate..............................Level II

Rebecca M. T. Law, BS Pharm, PharmD

Wayne P. Gulliver, MD, FRCPC

LEARNING OBJECTIVES

After completing this case study, the reader should be able to:

- Understand risk factors and aggravating factors in the pathogenesis of acne vulgaris.

- Understand the treatment strategies for acne, including appropriate situations for using nonprescription and prescription medications and use of topical and systemic therapies.

- Educate patients with acne on systemic therapies.

- Monitor the safety and efficacy of selected systemic therapies.

PATIENT PRESENTATION

■ Chief Complaint

"I can't stand this acne!"

■ HPI

Elaine Morgan is an 18-year-old woman with a history of facial acne since age 15. One month ago, she completed a 3-month course of minocycline in combination with Differin (adapalene). Her acne has flared up again, and she has again presented to her family physician for treatment.

■ PMH

Has irregular menses as a result of polycystic ovary syndrome diagnosed 3 years ago, which has not required medical treatment. However, it has resulted in an acne condition that was initially quite mild; she responded well to nonprescription topical products. In the last 2 years, the number of facial lesions has increased despite OTC, and, later, prescription drug treatments. Initially her physician prescribed Benzamycin Gel (benzoyl peroxide 5%/erythromycin 3%), which was beneficial, but this had to be discontinued because of excessive drying. Differin XP (adapalene 0.3% gel) was used next, and it controlled her condition for about 6 months; then the acne worsened and oral antibiotics were added. Most recently, she has received two 3-month courses of minocycline over the past year. She has also noted some scarring and cysts in the last few months.

■ FH

Parents alive and well; two older brothers (ages 21 and 25). Father had acne with residual scarring.

■ SH

The patient is under some stress because she is graduating in a few weeks. She wants to do well in school so she will qualify for the best colleges. Both of her brothers graduated with honors. She has been sexually active for the past two months, and her boyfriend uses condoms.

■ Meds

None currently

■ All

NKDA

■ ROS

In addition to the complaints noted above, the patient has irregular menstrual periods and mild hirsutism

■ Physical Examination

Gen

Alert, moderately anxious teenager in NAD

VS

BP 110/70 mm Hg, RR 15, T 37°C; Wt 45 kg, Ht 5'2"

Skin

Comedones on forehead, nose, and chin. Papules and pustules on the nose and malar area. A few healing cysts on the chin. Superficial scars on malar area. Increased facial hair.

HEENT

PERRLA, EOMI, fundi benign, TMs intact

Chest

CTA bilaterally

Cor

RRR without MRG, S_1 and S_2 normal

Abd

(+) BS, soft, nontender, no masses

MS/Ext

No joint aches or pains; peripheral pulses present

Neuro

CN II–XII intact

■ Labs

Na 140 mEq/L	Hgb 13.0 g/dL	AST 21 IU/L	T. chol 170 mg/dL
K 3.7 mEq/L	Hct 38%	ALT 39 IU/L	LDL-C 90 mg/dL
Cl 100 mEq/L	Plt 300 ×	LDH 105 IU/L	Trig 90 mg/dL
CO$_2$ 25 mEq/L	10^3/mm^3	Alk phos 89 IU/L	HDL 45 mg/dL
BUN 12 mg/dL	WBC 7.0 ×	T. bili 1.0 mg/dL	DHEAS 221 mcg/dL
SCr 1.0 mg/dL	10^3/mm^3	Alb 3.9 g/dL	(6 μmol/L)
Glu 100 mg/dL		FSH 30 mIU/mL	Testosterone (free)
BUN 12 mg/dL		LH 150 mIU/mL	2.3 ng/mL
SCr 1.0 mg/dL			Prolactin 15 ng/mL

QUESTIONS

Problem Identification

1.a. Create a drug therapy problem list for this patient.

1.b. What signs and symptoms consistent with acne does this patient have?

1.c. How does polycystic ovary syndrome contribute to this patient's acne and other physical findings?

Desired Outcome

2. What are the treatment goals for this patient?

Therapeutic Alternatives

3. What feasible therapeutic alternatives are available for management of this patient's acne and hyperandrogenism?

Optimal Plan

4. What treatment regimen is best suited for this patient?

Outcome Evaluation

5. How would you monitor the therapy you recommended for efficacy and adverse effects?

Patient Education

6. How would you educate the patient about this treatment regimen to enhance compliance and ensure successful therapy?

■ CLINICAL COURSE

Two months later, the patient's acne is improving, but she has developed bloating, weight gain, and increased appetite, likely related to the therapy prescribed. She also reveals that her maternal grandmother and aunt both died of melanoma, and a friend told her that she should not be using her new therapy.

■ FOLLOW-UP QUESTION

1. What is the most appropriate course of action?

■ SELF-STUDY ASSIGNMENTS

1. Review the dysmorphic syndrome associated with acne.

2. Review the nonpharmacologic management of acne, including stress reduction and dietary changes.

CLINICAL PEARL

In females with acne, scarring + cysts + two courses of oral antibiotics means hormonal therapy and "consider isotretinoin."

REFERENCES

1. Williams HC, Dellavalle RP, Garner S. Acne vulgaris. Lancet 2012;379:361–372.

2. Eichenfield LF, Krakowski AC, Piggott C, et al. Evidence-based recommendations for the diagnosis and treatment of pediatric acne. Pediatrics 2013;131:S163–S186. Available at: http://pediatrics.aappublications.org/content/131/Supplement_3/S163.full. Accessed March 25, 2016.

3. Nast A, Dreno B, Bettoli V, et al. European evidence-based (S3) guidelines for the treatment of acne. J Eur Acad Dermatol Venereol 2012, 26(Suppl 1):1–29.

4. Asai Y, Baibergenova A, Dutil M, et al. Management of acne: Canadian clinical practice guideline. 2015. doi:10.1503/cmaj.140665. Early release November 16, 2015 at: http://www.cmaj.ca/content/188/2/118.full.pdf+html. Full guideline (Appendix 4) and other appendices available at: http://www.cmaj.ca/content/suppl/2015/11/16/cmaj.140665.DC1. Accessed March 26, 2016.

5. Mayo Clinic staff. Polycystic ovary syndrome (PCOS). Mayo Clinic Sept. 3, 2014. Available at: http://www.mayoclinic.org/diseases-conditions/pcos/basics/definition/con-20028841. Accessed March 16, 2016.

6. Gollnick H, Cunliffe W, Berson D, et al. Management of acne: a report from a Global Alliance to Improve Outcomes in Acne. J Am Acad Dermatol 2003;49(1 Suppl):S1–S37.

7. Law RM. The pharmacist's role in the treatment of acne. America's Pharmacist 2003;125:35–42.

8. Zaenglein AL, Pathy AL, Schlosser BJ, et al. Guidelines of care for the management of acne vulgaris. J Am Acad Dermatol 2016 74(5):945–973.

9. Thiboutot D, Gollnick H, Bettoli V, et al. New insights into the management of acne: an update from the Global Alliance to Improve Outcomes in Acne Group. J Am Acad Dermatol 2009;60(5 Suppl 1):S1–S50.

10. Tan J. Dapsone 5% gel: a new option in topical therapy for acne. Skin Therapy Letter 2012;17(8):1–3.

11. Society of Obstetricians and Gynaecologists of Canada: Position Statement: Diane-35 and Risk of Venous Thromboembolism (VTE). 19 February 2013. Available at: http://sogc.org/wp-content/uploads/2013/04/medDiane35VTE130219.pdf. Accessed March 25, 2016.

12. Chung JP, Yiu AK, Chung TK, et al. A randomized crossover study of medroxyprogesterone acetate and Diane-35 in adolescent girls with polycystic ovarian syndrome. J Pediatr Adolesc Gynecol 2014;27:166–171.

13. Karagas MR, Stukel TA, Dykes J, et al. A pooled analysis of 10 case-control studies of melanoma and oral contraceptive use. Br J Cancer 2002;86:1085–1092.

111

PSORIASIS

The Harried School Teacher . . . . Level II

Rebecca M. T. Law, BS Pharm, PharmD

Wayne P. Gulliver, MD, FRCPC

LEARNING OBJECTIVES

After completing this case study, students should be able to:

- Describe the pathophysiology and clinical presentation of plaque psoriasis.

- Discuss the appropriate use of topical, photochemical, and systemic treatment modalities including biologic response modifiers (BRMs) for psoriasis, based on disease severity.

- Compare the efficacy and adverse effects of systemic therapies for psoriasis, including first-line standard therapies (methotrexate, acitretin, cyclosporine), second-line therapies (azathioprine, hydroxyurea, sulfasalazine), and the BRMs (alefacept, adalimumab, etanercept, infliximab, and ustekinumab).

- Select appropriate therapeutic regimens for patients with plaque psoriasis based on disease severity and patient-specific considerations such as organ dysfunction.

- Educate patients with psoriasis about proper use of pharmacotherapeutic treatments, potential adverse effects, and necessary precautions.

PATIENT PRESENTATION

■ Chief Complaint

"Nothing is helping my psoriasis."

■ HPI

Gerald Kent is a 50-year-old man with a 25+ year history of psoriasis who presented to the outpatient dermatology clinic 2 days ago with another flare-up of his psoriasis. He was admitted to the inpatient dermatology service for a severe flare-up of plaque psoriasis involving his arms, legs, elbows, knees, palms, abdomen, back, and scalp (Fig. 111-1).

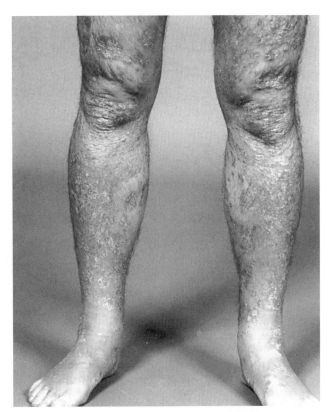

FIGURE 111-1. Example of severe plaque psoriasis involving the lower extremities in a male patient. *(Photo courtesy of Wayne P. Gulliver, MD.)*

He was diagnosed with plaque psoriasis at age 23. He initially responded to topical therapy with medium-potency topical corticosteroids, later to calcipotriol. He subsequently required photochemotherapy using psoralens with UVA phototherapy (PUVA) to control his condition. PUVA eventually became ineffective, and about 10 years ago, he was started on oral methotrexate 5 mg once weekly. Dosage escalations kept his condition under fairly good control for about 5 years. Flare-ups during that period were initially managed with SCAT (short-contact anthralin therapy), but they eventually became more frequent and lesions were more widespread despite increasing the methotrexate dose. A liver biopsy performed about 5 years ago showed no evidence of fibrosis, hepatitis, or cirrhosis.

After requiring two SCAT treatments in a 4-month period, along with methotrexate 25 mg once weekly orally (given as two doses of 12.5 mg 12 hours apart), a change in therapy was considered necessary at that time. Because he was receiving maximum recommended methotrexate doses and had already reached a lifetime cumulative methotrexate dose of 2.2 grams, he was changed to a cyclic regimen of cyclosporine microemulsion (Neoral) 75 mg twice daily for 3 months, followed by acitretin (Soriatane) 25 mg once daily with dinner for 3 months, and repeat. He found the acitretin drying, so after 6 months he was changed to his current regimen of only cyclosporine microemulsion 75 mg twice daily. Flare-ups had become infrequent and were again successfully managed by SCAT for over a year. However, in the last 6 months, he has already required two SCAT treatments for flare-ups, and this is his third flare-up.

■ PMH

One episode of major depressive illness triggered by the death of his first wife, which occurred 16 years ago (age 34). He was treated by his family physician who prescribed fluoxetine for 6 months. He has had no recurrences. He has no other chronic medical conditions and no other acute or recent illnesses.

FH

Parents alive and well. Father has HTN and Type 2 diabetes. Two older sisters and a younger brother. Younger brother was diagnosed with psoriasis about 5 years ago. No history of other immune disorders or malignancy.

SH

Patient is an elementary school teacher. He is currently a non-smoker but used to be a heavy smoker in his younger years (20s and 30s); social use of alcohol (glass of wine with dinner). He is married and has two children ages 10 and 12 with his second wife. There has been an increased workload for the past year because of layoffs at his school board.

Meds

Neoral 75 mg PO twice daily
Acetaminophen for occasional headaches

All

NKDA

ROS

Skin feels very itchy despite using a nonmedicated moisturizer TID. No joint aches or pains. No complaints of shortness of breath. Occasional nausea associated with a cyclosporine dose. Has been feeling jumpy and stressed because of tensions at work but does not feel depressed.

Physical Examination

Gen

Alert, mildly anxious 50-year-old Caucasian man in NAD

VS

BP 139/86, P 88, T 37°C; Wt 75 kg, Ht 5'9"

Skin

Confluent plaque psoriasis with extensive lesions on abdomen, arms, legs, back, and scalp. Thick crusted lesions on elbows, knees, palms, and soles. Lesions are red to violet in color, with sharply demarcated borders except where confluent, and are loosely covered with silvery-white scales. There are no pustules or vesicles. There are excoriations on trunk and extremities consistent with scratching.

HEENT

PERRLA, EOMI, fundi benign, TMs intact; extensive scaly lesions on scalp as noted

Neck/Lymph Nodes

No lymphadenopathy; thyroid non-palpable

Chest

CTA bilaterally

CV

RRR without MRG; S_1 and S_2 normal

Abd

(+) BS, soft, nontender, no masses; extensive scaly lesions and excoriations on skin as noted above in the Skin section

Genit

WNL

Rect

Deferred

MS/Ext

No joint swelling, increased warmth, or tenderness; skin lesions as noted above in Skin section; no nail involvement; peripheral pulses 2+ throughout

Neuro

A & O × 3; CN II–XII intact; DTRs 2+ toes downgoing

Labs

Na 139 mEq/L	Hgb 13.5 g/dL	AST 22 IU/L
K 4.0 mEq/L	Hct 35.0%	ALT 38 IU/L
Cl 102 mEq/L	Plt 255 × 10³/mm³	LDH 107 IU/L
CO₂ 25 mEq/L	WBC 6.0 × 10³/mm³	Alk phos 98 IU/L
BUN 14 mg/dL		T. bili 1.0 mg/dL
SCr 1.0 mg/dL		Alb 3.7 g/dL
Glu 98 mg/dL		Uric acid 4 mg/dL
		T. chol 180 mg/dL

QUESTIONS

Problem Identification

1.a. Create a list of this patient's drug therapy problems.

1.b. What signs and symptoms consistent with plaque psoriasis does this patient demonstrate?

1.c. What risk factors for developing psoriasis or experiencing a disease flare-up are present in this patient?

1.d. What comorbidities does this patient have?

1.e. Could the signs and symptoms be caused by any drug therapy he is receiving?

Desired Outcome

2. What are the goals of pharmacotherapy for this patient's plaque psoriasis?

Therapeutic Alternatives

3.a. What nonpharmacologic alternatives are available for managing the patient's psoriasis and its related symptoms?

3.b. What feasible pharmacotherapeutic alternatives are available for controlling the patient's disease and its related symptoms at this point?

Optimal Plan

4. What drug regimen is best suited for treating this flare-up of the patient's psoriasis and its related symptoms?

Outcome Evaluation

5. How should you monitor the therapy you recommended for efficacy and adverse effects?

Patient Education

6. What information should be provided to the patient to enhance compliance and ensure successful therapy?

■ SELF-STUDY ASSIGNMENTS

1. Perform a literature search to identify potential future therapies for psoriasis: topical therapies such as NSAIDs, protein kinase C inhibitors, methotrexate gel, an implantable 5-fluorouracil formulation; systemic therapies such as glucosamine, monoclonal antibodies, and cytokines.

2. Perform a literature search to review the current guidelines, opinions, and evidence regarding liver biopsies and long-term methotrexate use for patients with psoriasis.

CLINICAL PEARL

Provide patient-specific therapies and always consider any psychosocial effects, debilities, and comorbidities related to the patient's psoriasis.

REFERENCES

1. Menter A, Gottlieb A, Feldman SR, et al. Guidelines of care for the management of psoriasis and psoriatic arthritis. Section 1. Overview of psoriasis and guidelines of care for the treatment of psoriasis with biologics. J Am Acad Dermatol 2008;58:826–850.

2. Papp KA, Gulliver W, Lynde CW, Poulin Y (Steering Committee). Canadian Guidelines for the Management of Plaque Psoriasis. 1st Edition, June 2009. Available at: http://www.dermatology.ca/wp-content/uploads/2012/01/cdnpsoriasisguidelines.pdf. Accessed October 31, 2015.

3. Menter A, Korman NJ, Elmets CA, et al. 2009 guidelines of care for the management of psoriasis and psoriatic arthritis–Section 3. Guidelines of care for the management and treatment of psoriasis with topical therapies. J Am Acad Dermatol 2009;60:643–659.

4. Smith N, Weymann A, Tausk FA, et al. Complementary and alternative medicine for psoriasis: a qualitative review of the clinical trial literature. J Am Acad Dermatol 2009;61:841–856.

5. Menter A, Korman NJ, Elmets CA, et al. 2009 guidelines of care for the management of psoriasis and psoriatic arthritis–Section 4. Guidelines of care for the management and treatment of psoriasis with traditional systemic agents. J Am Acad Dermatol 2009;61:451–485.

6. Menter A, Korman NJ, Elmets CA, et al. 2009 guidelines of care for the management of psoriasis and psoriatic arthritis–Section 5. Guidelines of care for the treatment of psoriasis with phototherapy and photochemotherapy. J Am Acad Dermatol 2010;62:114–135.

7. Rosmarin DM, Lebwohl M, Elewski BE, et al. Cyclosporine and psoriasis: 2008 National Psoriasis Foundation Consensus Conference. J Am Acad Dermatol 2010;62:838–853.

8. Kalb RE, Strober B, Weinstein G, Lebwohl M. Methotrexate and psoriasis: 2009 National Psoriasis Foundation Consensus Conference. J Am Acad Dermatol 2009;60:824–837.

9. European S3-Guidelines on the systemic treatment of psoriasis vulgaris. Updated 2015. EDF in cooperation with EADV and IPC. Available at: http://www.euroderm.org/edf/index.php/edf-guidelines/category/5-guidelines-miscellaneous Accessed October 31, 2015.

10. Langley RG, Elewski BE, Lebwohl M, et al. Secukinumab in plaque psoriasis—results of two Phase 3 trials. N Engl J Med 2014;371;326–338. Available at: http://www.nejm.org/doi/pdf/10.1056/NEJMoa1314258.

11. Poulin Y, Langley RG, Teixeira HD, et al. Biologics in the treatment of psoriasis: clinical and economic overview. J Cutan Med Surg 2009:13(Suppl 2):S49–S57.

112

ATOPIC DERMATITIS

The Itch that Erupts when Scratched . . . . Level I

Rebecca M. T. Law, BS Pharm, PharmD

Poh Gin Kwa, MD, FRCPC

LEARNING OBJECTIVES

After completing this case study, students should be able to:

- Understand risk factors and aggravating factors in the pathophysiology of atopic dermatitis.

- Understand the treatment strategies for atopic dermatitis, including nonpharmacologic management.

- Educate patients and/or their caregivers about management of atopic dermatitis.

- Monitor the safety and efficacy of selected pharmacologic therapies.

PATIENT PRESENTATION

▧ Chief Complaint

As stated by the patient's mother, "My child constantly wants to scratch her skin, and she can't sleep well during the night."

▧ HPI

Julia Chan is a 3.5-year-old girl who just started attending daycare about 1 month ago. She did not want to go and still exhibits a lot of clinging behavior when her mother tries to leave; she still cries when her mother eventually does manage to leave. Her mother says that Julia's atopic dermatitis has flared up again. Julia has had atopic dermatitis since she was about 6 months old. It had been well controlled by topical corticosteroids and liberal use of moisturizers. Her recent flare-up began about 2–3 weeks ago. She has not been sleeping well and is constantly trying to scratch her skin at night. Her mother has been using 100% cotton sheets for her bed since she was an infant. She has sewn mittens on Julia's 100% cotton pajamas to prevent her from scratching, because she had previously caused excoriations from scratching, which then became infected. During the day, Julia constantly wants to scratch her skin but has been told to just "pat" the itchy area. The caregivers at the daycare center keep an eye on her scratching behavior as well but are not always able to prevent her from scratching herself. They also inform her mother that Julia likes to eat food shared by other children.

▧ PMH

Julia was breastfed from birth for a total of 8 weeks, when her mother decided to return to work. Julia was then cared for at home by a babysitter and fed cow's milk, with oatmeal cereal being introduced as the first solid food. She was fed some lemon meringue pie (made with egg white) once, and developed generalized hives, which led to the recognition that Julia has an egg allergy. This was confirmed by allergic skin testing. Julia's atopic dermatitis presented at 6 months of age. The parents have recently become aware that the babysitter left Julia alone a lot (sitting on the floor/carpet to play by herself). That was the major reason for sending Julia to a daycare center.

SH

Julia is the only child of a professional couple. Her father is an engineer and her mother is a litigation lawyer who often works long hours. The couple has a stressful lifestyle, and it appears that the stress is reflected in Julia's care. Sometimes Julia would be driven to one or another babysitter's homes at the last minute, when something urgent arises that the couple must attend to. There is very little family time. Unfortunately, their relatives do not live in the same city, and there is little social support for Julia on a day-to-day basis. The parents were hoping that the daycare center would be helpful, but so far that has proven to be another issue for Julia. She does not want to participate in activities there and has lots of temper tantrums. She does not play well with other children. Julia had been toilet trained but has now lost her toilet training and is using diapers again. Julia's mother started smoking again due to the recent stress; Julia keeps her up at night, and she is having difficulty dealing with Julia's multiple issues at home and at the daycare center.

FH

There is a strong family history of atopy. Julia's father has a severe allergy to shellfish, and her mother has a history of hay fever. Her father's sister has multiple food allergies. Her maternal grandmother had asthma. Her paternal first cousin had infantile eczema. Her maternal first cousin has a severe peanut allergy (generalized hives).

Meds

Hydrocortisone 1% cream applied to affected areas two to four times a day; although twice daily is her usual maintenance dose, she is currently using it three to four times a day

Vaseline ad lib

Diphenhydramine 0.5 teaspoonful PO at bedtime as needed (when skin is excessively itchy, to allow Julia to sleep)

Allergies

NKDA. Multiple food allergies: egg (hives, developed allergy as an infant), strawberries, raspberries, and tomatoes.

ROS

Not obtained

Physical Examination

Gen

Unhappy, cranky, thin, clinging girl who keeps sucking her thumb

VS

BP 98/50, HR 96, RR 18, T 37°C; Wt 12.2 kg (10th percentile), Ht 98 cm (38.6″; 50th percentile), head circumference 49.5 cm (19.5″; 50th percentile)

Skin

Generally dry. Eczematous skin lesions in flexure areas (behind ears, wrist joints, elbows, knees). Likely pruritic papules in flexure areas. Excoriations from scratching. Some bleeding seen but does not appear infected. Some cracking skin lesions seen behind the ears and knees. There are no lesions on the extensor parts of her body, no lesions on top of her nose, and no lesions in the diaper area.

The remainder of the physical exam was normal.

Labs

Na 135 mEq/L	Hgb 12.0 g/dL	WBC differential	AST 20 IU/L
K 4.0 mEq/L	Hct 35%	Neutros 50%	ALT 7 IU/L
Cl 102 mEq/L	Plt 230 × 10³/mm³	Bands 3%	IgE 300 IU/mL
CO_2 26 mEq/L	WBC 5.0 × 10³/mm³	Eosinophils 18%	D-dimer 90 ng/mL
BUN 8 mg/dL		Lymphs 27%	RAST elevated
SCr 0.2 mg/dL		Basophils 1%	INR 1.1
		Monos 1%	aPTT 30 s

Note: Reference ranges at age 3.5—BUN 8–20 mg/dL, SCr 0.2–0.8 mg/dL, AST 20–60 IU/L, ALT 0–37 IU/L, and IgE 0–25 IU/mL; WBC differential—neutros 20–65%, eos 0–15%, basos 0–2%, lymphs 20–60%, and monos 0–10%.

Swab of skin lesion where there is bleeding: No growth

Assessment

This is a 3.5-year-old child with an exacerbation of atopic dermatitis, likely stress-induced

QUESTIONS

Problem Identification

1.a. Create a drug therapy problem list for this patient.

1.b. What signs and symptoms of atopic dermatitis does this patient demonstrate?

1.c. What risk factors or aggravating factors may have contributed to the patient's atopic dermatitis flare?

1.d. Could the patient's signs and symptoms be caused by a drug?

Desired Outcome

2. What are the treatment goals for this patient?

Therapeutic Alternatives

3. What feasible nonpharmacologic and pharmacologic alternatives are available to manage this patient's pruritus and atopic dermatitis?

Optimal Plan

4. What treatment regimen is best suited for this patient?

Outcome Evaluation

5. What efficacy and adverse effects monitoring is needed for the management strategies you recommended?

Patient Education

6. How would you inform the patient's caregiver about the treatment regimen to enhance compliance and ensure successful therapy?

■ SELF-STUDY ASSIGNMENTS

1. Review the use of phototherapy for atopic dermatitis.

2. Discuss how an 8-month-old infant with atopic dermatitis might differ from a 3.5-year-old child (with respect to clinical presentation and treatment strategies).

CLINICAL PEARL

In atopic dermatitis, minimizing preventable risk factors such as stress, eliminating triggers, providing appropriate skin care, and controlling the itch are as important as pharmacologic treatment.

REFERENCES

1. National Institute of Arthritis and Musculoskeletal and Skin Diseases. Handout on Health: Atopic Dermatitis. US Department of Health and Human Services, 2013. NIH Publication No. 09–4272. http://www.niams.nih.gov/health_info/atopic_dermatitis/default.asp. Accessed Sept. 2, 2015.

2. Lynde C, Barber K, Claveau J, et al. Canadian practical guide for the treatment and management of atopic dermatitis. J Cutan Med Surg (incorporating Medical and Surgical Dermatology), published online June 28, 2005. http://www.springerlink.com/content/r5432000056r2748/fulltext.html. Accessed Sept. 2, 2015.

3. Kim BS. Atopic Dermatitis. Medscape eMedicine updated July 1, 2015. http://emedicine.medscape.com/article/1049085-overview. Accessed Aug. 29, 2015.

4. Eichenfield LE, Tom WL, Chamlin SI, et al. Guidelines of care for the management of atopic dermatitis. Section 1. Diagnosis and assessment of atopic dermatitis. J Am Acad Dermatol 2014;70:338–351.

5. Bieber T. Mechanisms of disease: atopic dermatitis. N Engl J Med 2008;358:1483–1494.

6. Sidbury R, Tom WL, Bergman JN, et al. Guidelines of care for the management of atopic dermatitis. Section 4: Prevention of disease flares and use of adjunctive therapies and approaches. J Am Acad Dermatol 2014; published online Sept. 25, 2014. http://dx.doi.org/10.1016/j.jaad.2014.08.038.

7. DaVeiga SP. Epidemiology of atopic dermatitis: a review. Allergy Asthma Proc 2012;23:227–234.

8. Koblenzer CS. Itching and the atopic skin. J Allergy Clin Immunol 1999;104(3 Pt 2):S109–S113.

9. Eichenfield LF, Tom WL, Berger TG, et al. Guidelines of care for the management of atopic dermatitis. Section 2. Management and treatment of atopic dermatitis with topical therapies. J Am Acad Dermatol 2014;71(1):116–132.

10. Eichenfield LF, Boguniewicz M, Simpson EL, et al. Translating atopic dermatitis management guidelines into practice for primary care providers. Pediatrics 2015;136(3), Sept. 2015. Published online at: www.pediatrics.org/cgi/doi/10.1542/peds.2014-3678. Accessed Aug. 27, 2015.

11. Sidbury R, Davis DM, Cohen DE, et al. Guidelines of care for the management of atopic dermatitis. Section 3. Management and treatment with phototherapy and systemic agents. J Am Acad Dermatol 2014;71:327–349.

12. van der Aa LB, Heymans HS, van Aalderen WM, Sprikkelman AB. Probiotics and prebiotics in atopic dermatitis: review of the theoretical background and clinical evidence. Pediatr Allergy Immunol 2010;21(2 Pt 2):e355–e367.

113

IRON DEFICIENCY ANEMIA

Wilbur Is Tired and His Stomach Hurts . . . . Level I

Robin L. Southwood, PharmD, CDE

LEARNING OBJECTIVES

After completing this case study, the reader should be able to:

- Recognize that certain drugs such as NSAIDs can cause chronic blood loss and iron deficiency anemia (IDA).

- Identify the signs, symptoms, and laboratory manifestations of IDA.

- Select appropriate iron therapies for the treatment of IDA.

- Understand the monitoring parameters for both short- and long-term treatment of IDA.

- Inform patients of the potential adverse effects of iron therapy.

- Educate patients about the importance of adherence to their iron therapy regimen.

PATIENT PRESENTATION

Chief Complaint

"I have belly pain and feel tired all the time."

HPI

Wilbur Cox is a 67 yo man who presents to your pharmacy with the above complaint. With further questioning, he relates the onset of his GI complaints shortly after he started self-medicating with ibuprofen 200 mg four tablets four times a day about 6 months ago for pain associated with "arthritis" in his right knee and ankle. His stomach pain has gotten progressively worse over the past few months. He describes this pain as a burning sensation that usually begins 30 minutes to 1 hour after meals and may or may not be relieved by antacid administration. Use of over the counter ranitidine as needed has likewise not provided much acute pain relief. Further questioning reveals a history of an ulcer approximately 5 years ago. You suggest that he stop taking ibuprofen and all other OTC NSAIDs and recommend that he use acetaminophen not more than 2 g per day if needed for pain. Additionally, you contact his primary care physician to make an appointment for Wilbur for further evaluation, and you let Wilbur know you will fax a brief note to his physician detailing the nature of your referral.

Clinical Course

Three days later, he is evaluated by his family physician, which provides the following additional information

PMH

OA of the knees and ankles
PUD 5 years ago
GI bleed—approximately 7 years ago
COPD × 10 years
HTN × 10 years

FH

Mother died in childbirth; father died of cancer at age 93

SH

Cigarette smoker—two ppd × 42 years. No alcohol; quit in 1990. He is married.

ROS

No fever or chills; (+) burning pain in stomach after meals; (−) heartburn; (+) melena; good appetite; has one daily BM; no significant weight changes over past 5 years; (+) dry mouth; (+) fatigue, tires easily; (−) paralysis, fainting, numbness, paresthesia, or tremor; headache only occasionally; has myopic vision; (−) tinnitus or vertigo; has hay fever in spring; (+) cough, sputum production (about one cup per day); (+) wheezing; denies chest pain, edema; (+) dyspnea and orthopnea; denies nocturia, hematuria, dysuria, or history of stones; (+) bilateral joint pain in both knees and ankles, worse on the right side, for over 5 years.

Meds

Lisinopril 10 mg PO daily
Tiotropium 18 mcg inhaled once daily
Formoterol 12 mcg inhaled Q 12 H
Ibuprofen 200 mg PO three or four tablets three or four times a day for knee and ankle pain
Antacids PO PRN for stomach pain
Prilosec OTC 20 mg PRN stomach pain

Allergies

Codeine (upset stomach)
Aspirin (upset stomach)

Physical Examination

Gen

WM in acute distress who appears his stated age

VS

BP 118/51 mm Hg, P 121 bpm, RR 22, T 36.2°C, pulse oximetry 90% in room air; Wt 78 kg, Ht 6′1″

Skin

Age- and sun-related lentigines and seborrheic keratoses noted

HEENT

PERRL; EOMI; conjunctivae are pale; mucous membranes pale and dry; normal funduscopic examination with no retinopathy noted; deviated nasal septum; no sinus tenderness; oropharynx clear

Neck/Lymph Nodes

Neck supple without masses; trachea midline; no thyromegaly, no JVD

Thorax

Breath sounds decreased bilaterally, increased anterior–posterior diameter, (+) rhonchi, pursed-lip breathing

CV

Tachycardia with a soft systolic murmur; PMI at fifth ICS, MCL; (–) bruits

Abd

Soft, tender to palpation; no masses or organomegaly; (+) BS

Genit/Rect

Normal external male genitalia; rectal examination (+) stool guaiac

MS/Ext

Slight knee joint enlargement, with pain and tenderness noted, and limited ROM of both knees and ankles, worse on right side; crepitation noted at the talus–tibia junction on dorsiflexion of the right foot; changes consistent with OA; strong pedal pulses bilaterally; no peripheral edema; pallor of the nail beds

Neuro

A & O × 3; DTR 2+; normal gait

Other

Peripheral blood smear: hypochromic, microcytic red blood cells (Fig. 113-1)

■ Labs

See Table 113-1.

■ Assessment

1. Severe IDA probably of GI origin, possibly secondary to NSAID-induced gastropathy
2. OA of both knees and ankles, worse on right side

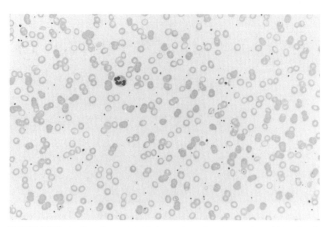

FIGURE 113-1. Blood smear with hypochromic, microcytic red blood cells (Wright–Giemsa ×330). *(Photo courtesy of Lydia C. Contis, MD.)*

3. COPD
4. HTN
5. FULL CODE status but patient does not wish to be left on a machine if there is no hope of recovery

■ Plan

Admit to hospital for further evaluation
Strict NPO
Infuse 4 units PRBCs
Begin D5% NS at 82 mL/hour continuous
Begin esomeprazole 40 mg IV daily
Morphine 2 mg IV Q 4 H as needed for pain
Consult GI service for suspected GI bleed
Sequential compression devices bilaterally for VTE prophylaxis

■ Clinical Course

The same day, the patient is seen by a gastroenterologist and undergoes both EGD and colonoscopy. Findings included severe gastritis with multiple bleeding lesions. Stool, blood, and biopsy tests for *Helicobacter pylori* were negative. Colonoscopy results were normal.

Final assessment: chronic, severe IDA secondary to bleeding gastric ulcer most likely secondary to NSAID therapy.

QUESTIONS

Problem Identification

1.a. What potential drug therapy problems does this patient have?

1.b. What signs, symptoms, and laboratory findings are consistent with the finding of IDA secondary to blood loss?

TABLE 113-1 Lab Values				
Na 138 mEq/L	Hgb 7.2 g/dL	WBC 10.7 × 10³/mm³	AST 10 IU/L	Ca 8.7 mg/dL
K 3.7 mEq/L	Hct 25%	Segs 61%	ALT 23 IU/L	Iron 4 mcg/dL
Cl 104 mEq/L	RBC 3.77 × 10⁶/mm³	Bands 2%	T. bili 0.3 mg/dL	TIBC 465 mcg/dL
CO₂ 27 mEq/L	MCV 66.2 μm³	Lymphs 23%	LDH 85 IU/L	Transferrin sat 1%
BUN 12 mg/dL	MCH 19 pg	Monos 10%	T. prot 6.3 g/dL	Ferritin 5 ng/mL
SCr 0.8 mg/dL	MCHC 28.7 g/dL	Eos 3%	Alb 3.7 g/dL	B₁₂ 680 pg/mL
Glucose 90 mg/dL	RDW 20.9%	Basos 1%	Folic acid 8.2 ng/mL	
	MPV 8.1 fL			
	Microcytosis 2+			
	Anisocytosis 1+			

Desired Outcome

2. What are the goals of pharmacotherapy for this patient's anemia?

Therapeutic Alternatives

3.a. What nondrug therapy may be effective for managing this anemia?

3.b. Discuss all of the oral and parenteral pharmacotherapeutic alternatives that could be used to treat this patient's anemia.

Optimal Plan

4. Outline an optimal pharmacotherapy plan for this patient.

Outcome Evaluation

5. What clinical and laboratory parameters are necessary to evaluate the therapy for achievement of the desired therapeutic outcome and to detect and prevent adverse effects?

Patient Education

6. What information should be provided to the patient to enhance compliance, ensure successful therapy, and minimize adverse effects?

■ CLINICAL COURSE

Mr Cox's hemoglobin and hematocrit increased after PRBCs to 12.6 g/dL and 40.8% by the second day of hospitalization. At that time, he was discharged on the treatment you recommended. For his OA, it is recommended that Wilbur be given a therapeutic trial of a nonacetylated salicylate such as choline magnesium trisalicylate along with acetaminophen up to two per day, if needed. A therapeutic trial of glucosamine can also be considered. Wilbur should be advised that NSAIDs, including those available over-the-counter, should be avoided because he is at high risk of a recurrent GI bleed that is related to both dose and length of NSAID therapy.

On his return to the clinic 1 month later for evaluation, he has no complaints of adverse effects from his medications. He indicates that he is fairly compliant with his iron therapy and is not experiencing any dose-limiting side effects. Stool exam for occult blood is negative. At that time, he is instructed to return in 2 more months. At that 3-month follow-up visit, his laboratory values continue to improve, and his next follow-up visit is scheduled in 3 more months. Laboratory values at 1, 3, and 6 months into therapy are shown in Table 113-2.

TABLE 113-2 Laboratory Test Values at 1, 3, and 6 Months			
Test (Units)	1 Month	3 Months	6 Months
RBC count (× 10^6/mm³)	4.1	4.2	4.8
Hgb (g/dL)	11.1	13.0	14.9
Hct (%)	36	40	47
MCV (μm³)	86	90	92
MCH (pg)	25	30	33
MCHC (g/dL)	31	34	36
RDW (%)	15.8	13.2	11.3
Serum iron (mcg/dL)	45	80	105
TIBC (mcg/dL)	489	491	500
Transferrin saturation (%)	9.0	19.0	21.0
Ferritin (ng/mL)	69	120	163
Stool guaiac	Negative	Negative	Negative

■ SELF-STUDY ASSIGNMENTS

1. Make a list of oral medications that should not be taken close to the time of iron administration; note the medications for which ferrous salts may interfere with their absorption.

2. Perform a literature search to determine the evidence supporting use of various sustained-release iron preparations, and determine the incremental cost of such products.

3. What monitoring steps should be incorporated into your pharmaceutical care plan to:
   (a) Check for recurrence of signs/symptoms of iron deficiency due to his chronic GI bleed?
   (b) Educate the patient concerning his risk of GI bleed associated with NSAID therapy and how he can minimize this risk?
   (c) Monitor for recurrence of signs and symptoms of gastropathy?
   (d) Monitor for efficacy of new treatments (such as acetaminophen or glucosamine) for his osteoarthritis?

4. Calculate the correct total dose of parenteral iron dextran (ie, total dose iron dextran) for this patient, and write a comprehensive order for its administration.

CLINICAL PEARL

In otherwise healthy patients, a transient increase in the reticulocyte count 3–10 days after beginning therapy can be used to confirm the correct diagnosis and treatment, and to rule out other causes of anemia.

Therapeutic doses of iron must be given for 3–6 months to ensure repletion of all iron stores; the serum ferritin is the best parameter for monitoring iron stores after correction of the hemoglobin and hematocrit.

REFERENCES

1. Zhu A, Kaneshiro M, Kaunitz JD. Evaluation and treatment of iron deficiency anemia: a gastroenterological perspective. Dig Dis Sci 2010;55:548–559.

2. Hershko C, Skikne B. Pathogenesis and management of iron deficiency anemia: emerging role of celiac disease, *Helicobacter pylori*, and autoimmune disease. Semin Hematol 2009;46:339–350.

3. Camaschella C. Iron-deficiency anemia. N Engl J Med 2015;372:1832–1843.

4. Lanza FL, Chan FK, Quigley EN. Practice Parameters Committee of the American College of Gastroenterology. Guidelines for the prevention of NSAID-related ulcer complications. Am J Gastroenterol 2009;104:728–738.

5. Hochberg MC, Altman RD, April KT, et al. American College of Rheumatology 2012 recommendations for the use of nonpharmacologic and pharmacologic therapies in osteoarthritis of the hand, hip, and knee. Arthritis Care Res 2012;64(4):465–474.

6. Laine L, Jensen DM. Management of patients with ulcer bleeding. Am J Gastroenterol 2012;107:345–360.

7. Auerbach M, Rodgers GM. Intravenous iron. N Engl J Med 2007;357:93–94.

8. Alleyne M, Horne MK, Miller JL. Individualized treatment for iron-deficiency anemia in adults. Am J Med 2008;121:943–948.

9. Auerbach M, Ballard H. Clinical use of intravenous iron: administration, efficacy, and safety. Hematology Am Soc Hematol Educ Program 2010;2010:338–347.

10. Avni T, Bieber A, Grossman A, Green H, Leibovici L, Gafter-Gvili A. The safety of intravenous iron preparations: systematic review and meta-analysis. Mayo Clin Proc 2015;90(1):12–23.

114

VITAMIN B$_{12}$ DEFICIENCY

Tongue Twister . . . . Level II

Jon P. Wietholter, PharmD, BCPS

LEARNING OBJECTIVES

After completing this case study, the reader should be able to:

- Recognize signs, symptoms, and laboratory abnormalities associated with vitamin B$_{12}$ deficiency anemia.

- Select an appropriate dosage regimen for treatment of anemia resulting from vitamin B$_{12}$ deficiency.

- Describe monitoring parameters for the initial and subsequent evaluations of patients with anemia caused by vitamin B$_{12}$ deficiency.

- Educate patients about appropriate vitamin B$_{12}$ therapy.

PATIENT PRESENTATION

▣ Chief Complaint

"I feel like I'm constantly tired and fatigued and my tongue is sore and swollen, making it extremely difficult for me to eat or drink anything."

▣ HPI

Aidan Joseph is a 65-year-old man who presents to your outpatient clinic with his wife. He claims that his fatigue and lethargy have been going on for years but have been worsening over the last 4–5 months to the point that he always feels tired. Additionally, he claims that over the last 2–3 weeks his tongue has become extremely painful and swollen and that he struggles to eat. His appetite has diminished because he tries to avoid eating anything that could worsen his pain, and he feels "fuller" more quickly than usual. On questioning, he also mentions a slight tingling and numbness in his feet that seems to worsen when finishing any physical activity. The patient has lost about 10 lb over the last 3 months, and he states that he feels like he is running a constant low-grade fever. His wife adds that she feels that he is becoming more confused, and this has been worsening over the last several years.

▣ PMH

COPD
Type 2 diabetes mellitus
Gout

▣ FH

Father alive (85 years old) with CAD, HTN, glaucoma, and type 2 DM
Mother deceased at age 75; had HTN, Alzheimer dementia, and CKD

▣ SH

Married for 42 years, lives with his wife; has two children (one son and one daughter) who are both healthy and live in the area; (+) tobacco, 1.5 ppd since age 24; (–) alcohol, (–) illicit drugs; is a retired pharmacist with good health insurance

▣ Meds

Docusate sodium 100 mg PO Q 12 H
Albuterol MDI two puffs Q 6 H PRN
Fluticasone/salmeterol 250/50 one puff Q 12 H
Tiotropium 18 mcg one puff daily
Metformin 1000 mg PO Q 12 H
Glyburide 5 mg PO daily
Colchicine 0.6 mg PO daily
Allopurinol 300 mg PO daily

▣ All

Penicillin (hives)
Levofloxacin (anaphylaxis)

▣ ROS

Complains of tongue pain and tingling sensation in his toes; (–) SOB, headache, chest pain, psychiatric abnormalities, polyuria, or polydipsia; denies any visual changes, constipation, diarrhea, or urinary retention

▣ Physical Examination

Gen

Elderly Caucasian male; moderately overweight in no acute distress with normal affect and speech; seems slightly irritated and exceptionally fatigued

VS

BP 123/87 mm Hg, P 106 bpm, RR 16, T 38.0°C; O$_2$ sat 94% on room air; Wt 92 kg, Ht 6′0″, BMI 27.4

Skin

Pale, turgor normal, no rashes or lesions

HEENT

PERRLA; EOMI; (–) photophobia; (+) red, smooth, swollen, sore tongue with loss of papillae; TMs appear normal

Neck

Supple; no masses, lymphadenopathy, or thyromegaly

Chest

Bilateral breath sounds; minor wheezing and rhonchi present on auscultation; (–) rales or orthopnea

CV

No discernible rhythm abnormality by auscultation; no murmurs or gallops; (+) tachycardia

Abd

Soft, nontender; mild splenomegaly; no masses; normal bowel sounds present

Rect

Deferred

Ext

No erythema, pain, or edema; normal pulses; (+) paresthesias; no joint redness or swelling; no limb weakness; reflexes intact

Neuro

A & O × 3; CN: visual fields and hearing intact; coordination intact; decreased pinprick in both lower extremities; decreased vibratory sensation in both lower extremities; decreased temperature sensation in both lower extremities; (–) ataxia, lightheadedness

■ Labs (All Fasting)

Na 136 mEq/L	Hgb 8.4 g/dL	AST 30 IU/L	Iron 124 mcg/dL
K 3.5 mEq/L	Hct 25.3%	ALT 24 IU/L	Ferritin 100 ng/mL
Cl 108 mEq/L	RBC 2.09 × 10^6/mm^3	Alk phos 79 IU/L	Transferrin 229 mg/dL
CO$_2$ 28 mEq/L	Plt 91 × 10^3/mm^3	T. bili 0.8 mg/dL	Antiparietal cell antibodies (–)
BUN 13 mg/dL	WBC 3.5 × 10^3/mm^3	D. bili 0.4 mg/dL	LDH 140 IU/L
SCr 1.0 mg/dL	MCV 121 μm^3	T. chol 153 mg/dL	B$_{12}$ 101 pg/mL
Glu 134 mg/dL	MCH 40 pg	Uric acid 4 mg/dL	Folate 12.3 ng/mL
A1C 6.8%	MCHC 33.2 g/dL		
TSH 3.4 mIU/L	Reticulocyte (corr) 0.7%		

■ Peripheral Blood Smear Morphology

Macro-ovalocytosis, hypersegmented granulocytes, large platelets, macrocytic red blood cells with megaloblastic changes (Fig. 114-1).

■ Assessment

1. Macrocytic anemia consistent with vitamin B$_{12}$ deficiency of unknown origin
2. Atrophic glossitis possibly associated with vitamin B$_{12}$ deficiency
3. Peripheral sensory neuropathy possibly associated with vitamin B$_{12}$ deficiency
4. COPD
5. Type 2 diabetes mellitus (controlled)
6. Gout

QUESTIONS

Problem Identification

1.a. Create a drug therapy problem list for this patient.

1.b. What information indicates the presence or severity of vitamin B$_{12}$ deficiency?

1.c. Could the vitamin B$_{12}$ deficiency have been caused by drug therapy? If so, should any changes be made to the patient's current drug regimen to aid in the treatment of his vitamin B$_{12}$ deficiency?

Desired Outcome

2. What are the pharmacotherapeutic goals in this case?

Therapeutic Alternatives

3.a. What nondrug therapies for vitamin B$_{12}$ deficiency might be useful for this patient?

3.b. What pharmacotherapeutic options are available for treating this patient's vitamin B$_{12}$ deficiency?

Optimal Plan

4. What drug, dosage form, dose, schedule, and duration of therapy are best for this patient?

Outcome Evaluation

5. What clinical and laboratory parameters are necessary to evaluate the therapy for achievement of the desired therapeutic outcome and to detect or prevent adverse effects?

FIGURE 114-1. Blood smear with enlarged hypersegmented neutrophils, one with eight nuclear lobes (*large arrow*) and macrocytes (*small arrows*) (Wright–Giemsa × 1650). (*Photo courtesy of Lydia C. Contis, MD.*)

Patient Education

6. What information should be provided to the patient to enhance compliance, ensure successful therapy, and minimize adverse effects?

■ FOLLOW-UP QUESTION

1. Mr Joseph returns to your clinic 3 months later reporting that he is feeling much less fatigued and is able to eat a more consistent diet but is still suffering from the tingling in his toes and a milder form of tongue soreness. What information can you give him regarding these remaining maladies?

■ SELF-STUDY ASSIGNMENTS

1. A serum vitamin B$_{12}$ level is no longer the most reliable laboratory test for evaluation of vitamin B$_{12}$ deficiency. Review the diagnostic tests that are becoming more common and provide a rationale for their increased use.

2. The anemia resulting from vitamin B$_{12}$ deficiency can be corrected by giving patients folic acid. Why then must we differentiate between the two common causes of macrocytic anemia (folic acid deficiency and vitamin B$_{12}$ deficiency) instead of simply treating all patients with folic acid?

CLINICAL PEARL

Pernicious anemia is a chronic illness arising from impaired absorption of vitamin B$_{12}$ due to a lack of intrinsic factor in gastric secretions. It garnered its name because it was universally fatal (pernicious is from the Latin word for violent death or destruction) due to a lack of available treatment options in the early stages of disease recognition. It can now be simply treated as any other vitamin B$_{12}$ deficiency and is a rather benign disease process if detected early.

REFERENCES

1. de Jager J, Kooy A, Lehert P, et al. Long term treatment with metformin in patients with type 2 diabetes and risk of vitamin B-12 deficiency: randomized placebo controlled trial. BMJ 2010;340:c2181.

2. Briani C, Dalla Torre C, Citton V, et al. Cobalamin deficiency: clinical picture and radiological findings. Nutrients 2013;5:4521–4539.

3. Dali-Youcef N, Andres E. An update on cobalamin deficiency in adults. QJM 2009;102:17–28.

4. Oberley MJ, Yang DT. Laboratory testing for cobalamin deficiency in megaloblastic anemia. Am J Hematol 2013;88:522–526.

5. Langan RC, Zawistoski KJ. Update on vitamin B$_{12}$ deficiency. Am Fam Physician 2011;83(12):1425–1430.

6. Liu Q, Li S, Quan H, Li J. Vitamin B$_{12}$ status in metformin treated patients: systematic review. PLOS ONE 2014;9(6):e100379. doi:10.1371/journal.pone.0100379.

7. Lewis JR, Barre D, Zhu K, et al. Long-term proton pump inhibitor therapy and falls and fractures in elderly women: a prospective cohort study. J Bone Miner Res 2014;29(11):2489–2497.

8. Smith AD, Refsum H. Vitamin B$_{12}$ and cognition in the elderly. Am J Clin Nutr 2009;89(Suppl):707S–711S.

9. Hankey GJ, Ford AH, Yi Q, et al. Effect of B vitamins and lowering homocysteine on cognitive impairment in patients with previous stroke or transient ischemic attack: a prespecified secondary analysis of a randomized, placebo-controlled trial and meta-analysis. Stroke 2013;44:2232–2239.

10. de Jager CA, Oulhaj A, Jacoby R, Refsum H, Smith AD. Cognitive and clinical outcomes of homocysteine-lowering B-vitamin treatment in mild cognitive impairment: a randomized controlled trial. Int J Geriatr Psychiatry 2012;27:592–600.

115

FOLIC ACID DEFICIENCY

More Wine, Anyone?...........................Level I

Jonathan M. Kline, PharmD, CACP, BCPS, CDE

Amber Nicole Chiplinski, PharmD, BCPS

LEARNING OBJECTIVES

After completing this case study, the reader should be able to:

- Recognize the signs, symptoms, and laboratory abnormalities associated with folic acid deficiency.

- Identify the confounding factors that may contribute to the development of folic acid deficiency (eg, medications, concurrent disease states, and dietary habits).

- Recommend an appropriate treatment regimen to correct anemia resulting from folic acid deficiency.

- Educate patients with folic acid deficiency regarding pharmacologic and nonpharmacologic interventions used to correct folic acid deficiency.

- Describe appropriate monitoring parameters for initial and subsequent monitoring of folic acid deficiency.

PATIENT PRESENTATION

Chief Complaint

"My stomach hurts and I have been throwing up today."

HPI

Laura Jones is a 43-year-old woman with a 1-day history of vomiting and mild abdominal pain. The pain radiates down to the lower abdominal quadrants bilaterally. She presents to the ED after experiencing some chest discomfort late in the day. She denies any fevers, chills, or similar pains in the past. She also complains of loose stools and chronic fatigue for the past 2–3 months.

PMH

Fibromyalgia
Celiac disease
Hypothyroidism
Osteopenia
History of endometriosis
Placenta previa—s/p TAH–BSO

FH

Mother positive for lupus; sister with Crohn disease; negative for DM, CAD, CVA, CA

SH

Married; (+) alcohol—three to four glasses of wine per day, increased recently from one to two glasses after her mother-in-law moved in; (+) smoking tobacco 0.5 ppd × 25 years, (–) recreational drug use; unemployed

Meds

Levothyroxine 100 mcg PO daily
Estradiol 0.05 mg/24 hour transdermal patch (Estraderm); replace twice weekly

All

Doxycycline—rash

ROS

(+) Generalized weakness; (–) dizziness; (–) weight gain or loss; (–) fever; (–) vision or hearing changes; (–) cough, chest pain, palpitations; (–) shortness of breath; (+) nausea/vomiting, abdominal pain, loose stools; (–) rectal bleeding; (–) nocturia or dysuria; (+) bilateral lower extremity weakness; (–) edema, rashes, or petechiae; (–) symptoms of depression or anxiety; (–) history of bleeding problems or VTE

Physical Examination

Gen

Caucasian female who appears generally ill, but nontoxic

VS

BP 135/90 mm Hg, P 82 bpm, RR 40, T 35.5°C

Skin

No petechiae, rashes, ecchymoses, or active lesions; decreased skin turgor

HEENT

Atraumatic/normocephalic; PERRLA, EOMI; conjunctivae pink, sclera white; TMs intact and reactive; nose is patent; tongue is large and erythematous; dry mucous membranes

Neck/Lymph Nodes

Normal ROM; no JVD, adenopathy, thyromegaly, or bruits

Lung/Thorax

Lungs CTA bilaterally

CV

RRR; no murmurs, gallops, or rubs

Abd

Soft, nondistended, with midepigastric and right flank and right lower quadrant tenderness; (+) bowel sounds

Genit/Rect

Deferred

MS/Ext

Lower extremities warm with 2+ bipedal pulses; no clubbing, cyanosis, or edema

Neuro

CN II–XII grossly intact; decreased muscle strength 3/5 bilaterally in upper and lower extremities; DTRs throughout

■ Labs

Na 138 mEq/L	Hgb 12.6 g/dL	AST 128 IU/L	Folate
K 4.2 mEq/L	Hct 37.2%	ALT 52 IU/L	2.8 ng/mL
Cl 102 mEq/L	RBC 3.78 × 10^6/mm^3	Alk phos	B_{12} 242 pg/mL
CO_2 21 mEq/L	Plt 217 × 10^3/mm^3	142 IU/L	
BUN 7 mg/dL	WBC 6.3 × 10^3/mm^3	GGT 288 IU/L	
SCr 0.52 mg/dL	MCV 120.4 μm^3	T. bili 2.1 mg/dL	
Glu 89 mg/dL	MCH 40.5 pg	Alb 3.4 g/dL	
Amylase 404 IU/L	MCHC 33.6 g/dL	TSH 2.06 mIU/L	
Lipase 679 IU/L	RDW 12.1%	T_4, free 1.2 ng/dL	

■ Assessment

Acute pancreatitis secondary to alcohol use
Dehydration
Macrocytic anemia secondary to folate deficiency

QUESTIONS

Problem Identification

1.a. Create a drug therapy problem list for this patient.

1.b. What signs, symptoms, and laboratory values indicate that this patient has anemia secondary to folate deficiency?

1.c. Could the patient's folate deficiency have been caused by drug therapy or comorbidity?

1.d. What additional information can be used to assess this patient's folate deficiency?

1.e. Why is it important to differentiate folate deficiency from vitamin B_{12} deficiency, and how is this accomplished?

Desired Outcome

2. What are the goals of pharmacotherapy for this patient's anemia?

Therapeutic Alternatives

3.a. What nondrug therapies may be used to correct this patient's folic acid deficiency?

3.b. What pharmacotherapeutic alternatives are available for treating this patient's anemia?

Optimal Plan

4. What are the most appropriate drug, dosage form, dose, schedule, and duration of therapy for resolving this patient's anemia?

Outcome Evaluation

5. What parameters should be used to evaluate the efficacy and adverse effects of folic acid replacement therapy in this patient?

Patient Education

6. What information would you provide to this patient about her folic acid replacement therapy?

■ SELF-STUDY ASSIGNMENTS

1. What are the advantages and disadvantages of folinic acid (leucovorin calcium) over standard folic acid, and why is this preferred folate supplement in patients receiving high-dose methotrexate?

2. List and compare the mechanism for how the following drugs can lead to folic acid deficiency: azathioprine, trimethoprim, and phenytoin.

3. What is the role of folic acid in the management of methanol ingestion?

CLINICAL PEARL

Unlike dietary folate, supplemented folic acid (pteroylglutamic acid) is absorbed even with abnormal function of GI mucosal cells. Likewise, persistent alcohol ingestion or the use of drugs affecting folic acid absorption, folate transport, or dihydrofolate reductase will not prevent a sufficient therapeutic response to oral supplementation.

REFERENCES

1. Arafah BM. Increased need for thyroxine in women with hypothyroidism during estrogen therapy. N Engl J Med 2001;344:1743–1749.

2. Malouf R, Grimley Evans J. Folic acid with or without vitamin B12 for the prevention and treatment of healthy elderly and demented people. Cochrane Database Syst Rev 2008;(4):CD004514. doi:10.1002/14651858.CD004514.pub2.

3. Snow CF. Laboratory diagnosis of vitamin B_{12} and folate deficiency: a guide for the primary care physician. Arch Intern Med 1999;159:1289–1298.

4. Hesdorffer CS, Longo DL. Drug-induced megaloblastic anemia. N Engl J Med 2015;373:1649–1658.

5. Presutti RJ, Cangemi JR, Cassidy HD, Hill DA. Celiac disease. Am Fam Physician 2007;76:1795–1802.

6. Seppa K, Sillanaukee P, Saarni M. Blood count and hematologic morphology in nonanemic macrocytosis: differences between alcohol abuse and pernicious anemia. Alcohol 1993;10:343–347.

7. Kaushansky K, Kipps TJ. Hematopoietic agents: growth factors, minerals, and vitamins. In: Brunton LL, Chabner B, Knollman B, eds. Goodman & Gilman's the Pharmacological Basis of Therapeutics, 12th ed. New York, NY, McGraw-Hill, 2011:1067–1100.

8. Rampersaud GC, Kauwell GP, Bailey LB. Folate: a key to optimizing health and reducing disease risk in the elderly. J Am Coll Nutr 2003;22:1–8.

9. Theisen-Toupal J, Horowitz G, Breu A. Low yield of outpatient serum testing: eleven years of experience. JAMA Intern Med 2014;174(10):1696–1697.

10. Selhub J, Morris MS, Jacques PF. In vitamin B12 deficiency, higher serum folate is associated with increased total homocysteine and methylmalonic acid concentrations. Proc Natl Acad Sci USA 2007;104:19995–20000.

116

SICKLE CELL ANEMIA

Engineering a Crisis..............................Level I

Sheh-Li Chen, PharmD, BCOP

LEARNING OBJECTIVES

After completing this case study, the reader should be able to:

- Recognize the clinical characteristics associated with an acute sickle cell crisis.

- Discuss the presentation of acute chest syndrome and treatment options.

- Recommend optimal analgesic therapy based on patient-specific information.

- Identify optimal endpoints of pharmacotherapy in sickle cell anemia patients.

- Recommend treatment that may reduce the frequency of sickle cell crises.

PATIENT PRESENTATION

■ Chief Complaint

"I can't breathe and my chest hurts."

■ HPI

Todd Jefferson is a 38-year-old African-American man with a history of sickle cell anemia who presents to the local community hospital ED with pain. On waking up three days prior to admission, he experienced a sudden onset of pain in his hands, legs, and lower back. He began taking oxycodone 15 mg every 4 hours at that time with minor pain relief. This morning he experienced a fever of 102°F, progressive shortness of breath, and priapism, which caused him to seek treatment at the ED. Patient acknowledged having sick contacts at his workplace.

■ PMH

Sickle cell anemia (hemoglobin SS disease) diagnosed before the age of 1 with approximately three to four crises per year requiring hospitalization
Acute chest syndrome 2 years ago that required intubation
Transfusion exchange with PRBC during the intubation admission
Several episodes of priapism, usually associated with sickle cell pain crisis

■ FH

Mother and father alive and well, both with sickle cell trait. Patient has one sister with sickle cell trait.

■ SH

Lives locally with his wife; currently works as chemical engineer. Reports no use of tobacco; occasional alcohol intake for social events.

■ ROS

Denies nausea, vomiting, or diarrhea. Cannot remember his last bowel movement but believes he has not had one in the last 3 days. Has had fever with some chills and sweats; no cough, nasal discharge, rashes, or skin lesions. Reports stuttering priapism with recurring episodes each lasting approximately 1 hour, with no intervention.

■ Meds

Folic acid 1 mg PO daily
Hydroxyurea 1000 mg PO BID
Oxycodone 15 mg PO Q 4 H PRN pain

■ All

Sulfa (reported rash when very young)
Codeine (nausea and dysphoria)

■ Physical Examination

Gen

Thin, well-developed, diaphoretic African-American man in acute distress

VS

BP 115/72 mm Hg, P 110 bpm, RR 20, T 38.5°C; 72 kg; O_2 sat is 84% in room air improving to 97% on 4 L O_2

HEENT

PERRL; EOMI; oral mucosa soft and moist; normal sclerae and funduscopic examination; no sinus tenderness

Skin

Normal turgor; no rashes or lesions

Neck

Supple; nontender, no lymphadenopathy or thyromegaly

CV

RRR; II/VI SEM; no rubs or gallops

Lungs

Crackles in both bases on auscultation; dullness to percussion

Abd

Voluntary guarding, mild distention, hypoactive bowel sounds, no palpable spleen; no hepatomegaly or masses

Genitourinary

Priapism evident

Ext

No edema; notable tenderness in right shoulder and elbow; mild erythema and inflammation is present

Neuro

A & O × 3; normal strength, reflexes intact

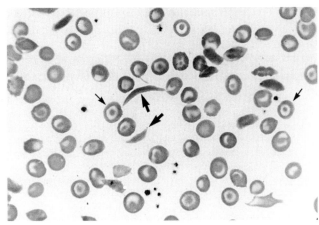

FIGURE 116-1. Peripheral blood with sickle cells (*large arrows*) and target cells (*small arrows*) (Wright–Giemsa ×1650). (*Photo courtesy of Lydia C. Contis, MD.*)

Labs

Na 143 mEq/L	Hgb 7.7 g/dL	AST 40 IU/L	Ca 8.8 mg/dL
K 4.2 mEq/L	Hct 20.8%	ALT 28 IU/L	Mg 1.9 mEq/L
Cl 112 mEq/L	Plt 480 × 10³/mm³	Alk phos 77 IU/L	Phos 3.9 mg/dL
CO₂ 28 mEq/L	MCV 110 μm³	LDH 1215 IU/L	(+) Anti-E red
BUN 50 mg/dL	Retic 18.2%	T. bili 5.0 mg/dL	cell antibody
SCr 1.4 mg/dL	WBC 18.2 × 10³/mm³	D. bili 0.8 mg/dL	
Glu 92 mg/dL	Segs 74%	Alb 3.4 g/dL	
	Bands 7.5%		
	Eos 1.5%		
	Lymphs 14%		
	Monos 3%		

Other

Arterial blood gas: pH 7.49, PaCO₂ 38, PaO₂ 72, bicarb 30, O₂ sat 96% on oxygen

Sputum culture: Mixed flora

Hgb electrophoresis: Hgb A₂ 3%; Hgb F 8%; Hgb S 89%

Peripheral blood smear: Sickle forms and target cells present (Fig. 116-1).

Chest X-Ray

This is a portable chest x-ray remarkable for diffuse interstitial infiltrates in both lung fields consistent with acute chest syndrome (Fig. 116-2). Cardiomegaly is also notable.

ECG

Normal sinus rhythm

Echocardiogram

Normal LV function

Assessment

A 38-year-old, African-American man in sickle cell crisis with probable acute chest syndrome, priapism, and constipation

QUESTIONS

Problem Identification

1.a. Create a list of the patient's drug therapy problems.

1.b. What signs, symptoms, and laboratory values are consistent with an acute sickle cell crisis in this patient?

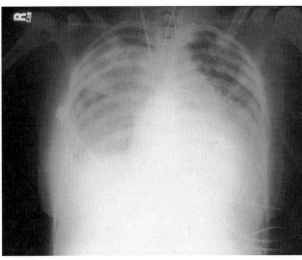

FIGURE 116-2. Lung radiograph of patient with acute chest syndrome secondary to sickle cell anemia. (*Photo courtesy of Kenneth I. Ataga, MD.*)

1.c. What signs, symptoms, and laboratory values support a diagnosis of acute chest syndrome in this patient?

1.d. What additional information is needed to satisfactorily assess this patient?

Desired Outcome

2. What are the goals of pharmacotherapy in this case?

Therapeutic Alternatives

3.a. What nondrug therapies might be useful for this patient?

3.b. What feasible pharmacotherapeutic alternatives are available for treatment of the patient's pain?

3.c. What feasible pharmacotherapeutic alternatives are available for treating opioid-induced constipation?

Optimal Plan

4. Outline a detailed therapeutic plan to treat all facets of this patient's acute sickle cell crisis, acute chest syndrome, priapism, and constipation. For all drug therapies, include the dosage form, dose, schedule, and duration of therapy.

Outcome Evaluation

5.a. What clinical and laboratory parameters are necessary to evaluate therapy for achievement of the desired therapeutic outcome and to detect or prevent adverse effects?

■ CLINICAL COURSE

The plans you recommended have been initiated, and on the fourth day of hospitalization the patient's pain is markedly improved, oxygen saturation improved to 98% on room air, he is afebrile, and his priapism has resolved. He has had two bowel movements but still feels his bowel habits have not yet returned to normal. He is only using two to three demands on his PCA per day and is asking to switch back to oral medication.

5.b. Considering this information, what changes (if any) in the pharmacotherapeutic plan are warranted while the patient is hospitalized?

5.c. What evidence exists to suggest that the patient is adherent with hydroxyurea therapy, and how should this therapy continue to be monitored?

Patient Education

6. What information should be provided to the patient to enhance compliance, ensure successful therapy, and minimize adverse effects?

■ SELF-STUDY ASSIGNMENTS

1. Determine the likelihood of the patient's offspring having sickle cell trait and/or disease if the father has:
   (a) Normal hemoglobin
   (b) Sickle cell trait
   (c) Sickle cell disease

2. Describe the complications associated with frequent crises in each organ system.

3. Discuss the differences between sickle cell anemia and β-thalassemia in terms of etiologies, laboratory abnormalities, and disease complications.

CLINICAL PEARL

Vaccination with pneumococcal conjugate 13-valent (PCV13) vaccine is necessary in addition to the 23-valent pneumococcal polysaccharide vaccine (PPSV23) for all adult sickle cell anemia patients with functional or anatomic asplenia if they have not received it previously. The PCV13 should be given at least 1 year after the last PPSV23 dose. For patients who have not received any pneumococcal vaccine, they should receive the PCV13 first, then the PPSV23 at least 8 weeks after receiving the PCV13, and a second dose 5 years after the first dose.

REFERENCES

1. Vichinsky EP, Neumayr LD, Earles AN, et al. Causes and outcomes of the acute chest syndrome in sickle cell disease. National Acute Chest Syndrome Study Group. N Engl J Med 2000;342:1855–1865.

2. Vichinsky EP, Styles LA, Colangelo LH, et al. Acute chest syndrome in sickle cell disease: clinical presentation and course. Cooperative Study of Sickle Cell Disease. Blood 1997;89:1787–1792.

3. Yawn BP, Buchanan GR, Afenyi-Annan AN, et al. Management of sickle cell disease: summary of the 2014 evidence-based report by expert panel members. JAMA 2014;312(10):1033–1048.

4. Morris CR, Singer ST, Walters MC. Clinical hemoglobinopathies: iron, lungs and new blood. Curr Opin Hematol 2006;13:407–418.

5. Bellet PS, Kalinyak KA, Shukla R, et al. Incentive spirometry to prevent acute pulmonary complications in sickle cell diseases. N Engl J Med 1995;333:699–703.

6. Demerol® (meperidine hydrochloride, USP) [Packet insert]. Bridgewater, NJ: Sanofi Aventis US, LLC; revised October 2011. http://www.accessdata.fda.gov/drugsatfda_docs/label/2011/005010s051lbl.pdf. Accessed Jan. 14, 2016.

7. Herndon CM, Jackson KC, Hallin PA. Management of opioid-induced gastrointestinal effects in patients receiving palliative care. Pharmacotherapy 2002;22:240–250.

8. Argoff CE, Brennan MJ, Camilleri M, et al. Consensus recommendations on initiating prescription therapies for opioid-induced constipation. Pain Medicine 2015;16:2324–2337.

9. Steinberg MH, Barton F, Castro O, et al. Effect of hydroxyurea on mortality and morbidity in adult sickle cell anemia: risks and benefits up to 9 years of treatment. JAMA 2003;289:1645–1651.

117

USING LABORATORY TESTS IN INFECTIOUS DISEASES

Chief of Staph . . . . Level III

Anthony J. Guarascio, PharmD, BCPS

Branden Nemecek, PharmD, BCPS

LEARNING OBJECTIVES

After completing this case study, the reader should be able to:

- Discuss the possible etiology of bacterial disease following a viral illness such as influenza.

- Discuss the use of rapid diagnostic testing methods that help differentiate coagulase-negative staphylococci from *Staphylococcus aureus*.

- Design a therapeutic plan to treat a bloodstream infection due to *Staphylococcus aureus* based on laboratory-based information.

- Evaluate culture and sensitivity results, and determine the clinical significance of the MIC for *S. aureus*.

- Recommend a plan for monitoring efficacy and adverse effects of antimicrobial therapy.

PATIENT PRESENTATION

▧ Chief Complaint

Patient's wife states of her husband, "Lately he has not been acting like himself. He has been very dizzy, tired and has not been eating or drinking well."

▧ HPI

David Covey is a 72-year-old man who came to the ED via ambulance. The patient's history is obtained from his wife. She describes a change in mental status, lethargy, and shortness of breath, along with a significant decrease in activity and nutritional intake. The symptoms started 3 days ago and have progressively worsened. Over the past 24 hours he has become very nauseated and developed a fever (39°C). She states that Mr Covey has not eaten anything over this time period. He was recently hospitalized (last week) for 4 days due to influenza A pneumonia confirmed by PCR.

▧ PMH

Diabetes mellitus
Resistant hypertension
Depression
Influenza pneumonia

▧ FH

Both parents are deceased (mother, aged 88, of PE; father, aged 71, of stroke). He is married without any children.

▧ SH

Retired steel mill worker and union chief, distant history of tobacco and alcohol use with no current use

▧ Meds

Metformin 1000 mg PO BID
Glyburide 5 mg PO daily
Spironolactone 25 mg PO daily
Lisinopril 40 mg PO Q HS
Amlodipine 10 mg PO daily
Paroxetine 10 mg PO daily

▧ All

Penicillin: hives when he was a child
Morphine: itching

▧ ROS

Patient's primary complaint is of nausea and dizziness but due to current status unable to review further

▧ Physical Examination

Gen

The patient is frail, disheveled, appearing in respiratory distress

VS

BP 108/58, P 108, RR 36, T 39°C; Wt 64.2 kg, Ht 68 in

Skin

Warm and diaphoretic

HEENT

PERRLA; EOM intact; dry mucous membranes, teeth clean and intact, pharynx negative

Neck/Lymph Nodes

No nodules, negative lymphadenopathy

Chest

Respiratory distress with marked effort and use of accessory muscles; generalized bilateral wheezing

CV

Tachycardic; normal S_1 and S_2; no heaves, thrills, or bruits

Abd

Soft, non-distended; non-tender, no splenomegaly

Genit/Rect

Not performed

MS/Ext

Deferred

Neuro

Decreased responses; delayed recognition; responds to painful stimuli

▌ Labs

Na 148 mEq/L	Hgb 10.6 g/dL	WBC 16.3×10^3/mm³
K 5.4 mEq/L	Hct 29.8%	Segs 70%
Cl 102 mEq/L	RBC 3.34×10^6/mm³	Bands 22%
CO_2 18 mEq/L	Plt 280×10^3/mm³	Lymphs 6%
BUN 68 mg/dL	MCV 86.1 μm³	Monos 2%
SCr 2.9 mg/dL	D-dimer 0.2 μg/mL	INR 1.2
Glu 58 mg/dL	Influenza A/B PCR: negative	Nares MRSA swab: positive

O_2 saturation 92%

▌ Urinalysis

Color, yellow; specific gravity, 1.170; pH 5; +1 protein; negative nitrites; negative LE; 15–20 RBC; few bacteria; 0–3/HPF WBC; moderate uric acid crystals

▌ Chest X-Ray

Concerning for patchy infiltrates with left lower lobe consolidation

▌ Electrocardiogram

Normal sinus rhythm with heart rate of 108 bpm, no axis deviation, no peaked T waves or T-wave inversion. No prior ECG for comparison

▌ Assessment

1. Respiratory distress with differential diagnosis pneumonia or pulmonary embolus
2. Acute kidney injury of unknown cause
3. Lab abnormalities (hyperkalemia, hypoglycemia)

▌ Plan

1. Collect two sets of blood cultures and a sputum specimen. Collect urine sample for urinalysis and culture.
2. Initiation of empiric antibiotics vancomycin and piperacillin/tazobactam per pharmacy to dose protocol.
3. Initiation of fluid resuscitation to address acute kidney injury, hypotension, hypoglycemia and hyperkalemia.

QUESTIONS

Problem Identification

1.a. Create a list of this patient's drug therapy problems.

1.b. What subjective and objective data indicate the presence of infection?

1.c. What indicates a possible urinary tract infection on urinalysis? Does Mr Covey's urinalysis represent the presence of an infection?

1.d. What are the criteria for SIRS and sepsis? Does Mr Covey meet these criteria?

1.e. Define acute kidney injury and how it may affect antimicrobial management.

TABLE 117-1	*S. aureus* Susceptibility Report
Antibiotic	**MIC/Interpretation**
Clindamycin	≤0.25/susceptible[a]
Erythromycin	≥8/resistant
Gentamicin	≤0.5/susceptible
Levofloxacin	0.25/susceptible
Oxacillin	≥4/resistant
Penicillin	≥0.5/resistant
Rifampin	≤0.5/susceptible
Trimethoprim/sulfamethoxazole	≤10/susceptible
Vancomycin	1/susceptible
Tetracycline	≤1/susceptible

[a]Positive for inducible clindamycin resistance.

Desired Outcome

2. What are the pharmacotherapy goals for Mr Covey's case?

Therapeutic Alternatives

3.a. Create a list of appropriate antibiotics to empirically treat Mr Covey's infection pending final culture and sensitivity results.

3.b. Identify appropriate initial fluid management for Mr Covey.

3.c. What pharmacologic therapies need to be held during this initial presentation?

▌ CLINICAL COURSE

In the ED, the patient responds well to IV fluids with normalization of potassium and improvement in blood pressure and blood glucose. Shortly after the patient arrived to the Medical floor, the microbiology lab calls the physician and reports that Mr Covey's Gram stain from both blood cultures reveal gram-positive cocci in clusters, and the Alere rapid immunochromatographic assay and culture colony PBP2a test has returned as presumptive positive for MRSA. Sputum culture also reveals preliminary results of gram-positive cocci in clusters. Final culture and susceptibility results are pending. The following day, blood and sputum culture and susceptibility results become available. Table 117-1 depicts the final culture susceptibility report that is identical for both sputum and blood isolates.

Optimal Plan

4.a. When should Mr Covey's blood cultures have been drawn in relation to antibiotic administration?

4.b. What is the clinical advantage of using a rapid identification test, such as rapid culture colony PBP2a test, to help determine the staphylococcal species?

4.c. What is the preferred antibiotic for this patient, including dose, route, frequency, and duration of therapy?

4.d. Develop a plan for monitoring for therapeutic drug monitoring and the occurrence of adverse drug events with the chosen antibiotic.

Outcome Evaluation

5.a. What effect does the MIC of the organism have on the current treatment plan?

5.b. When are serum vancomycin concentrations collected to determine the appropriateness of drug dosing? How often are serum vancomycin concentrations checked? What is the goal trough serum concentration in this patient?

5.c. Outline a follow-up plan for monitoring the efficacy of this therapeutic regimen.

5.d. Outline a follow-up plan for re-initiation of diabetes and anti-hypertensive therapies.

Patient Education

6. What patient counseling information should Mr Covey receive prior to discharge to address all medical conditions?

■ SELF-STUDY ASSIGNMENTS

1. Which organisms most frequently represent contaminants in blood cultures?

2. What is the role of rapid diagnostic testing in the treatment of bloodstream infections?

3. How do you utilize MRSA nasal swab surveillance results?

4. How would the therapeutic management of this patient change if kidney injury progressed to necessitate hemodialysis?

CLINICAL PEARL

The blood is a sterile body fluid; therefore, when a blood culture grows pathogenic bacteria, the source of the bacteria must always be investigated. The infectious source must be identified to assist in determining the appropriate antimicrobial selection and duration of therapy to increase the likelihood of clinical success.

REFERENCES

1. Sobel JD, Kaye D. Chap 74. Urinary tract infections. In: Bennett JE, Dolin R, Blaser MJ, eds. Mandell, Douglas, and Bennett's Principles and Practice of Infectious Diseases, 8th ed. Philadelphia, PA, Saunders Elsevier, 2014:886–913.

2. Gilbert JS, Weiner DE, Gipson DS, Perazella MA, Tonelli M, eds. National Kidney Foundation's Primer on Kidney Diseases. 6th ed. Philadelphia, PA Saunders Elsevier, 2014:294–303 and 337–346.

3. Metersky ML, Masterson RG, Lode H, File TM Jr, Babinchak T. Epidemiology, microbiology, and treatment considerations for bacterial pneumonia complicating influenza. Int J Infect Dis 2012;16(5):e321–e331.

4. Polenakovik HM, Pleiman CM. Ceftaroline for methicillin-resistant Staphylococcus aureus bacteraemia: case series and review of the literature. Int J Antimicrob Agents 2013;42(5):450–455.

5. Liu C, Bayer A, Cosgrove SE, et al. Clinical practice guidelines by the Infectious Diseases Society of America for the treatment of methicillin-resistant Staphylococcus aureus infections in adults and children. Clin Infect Dis 2011;52:1–38.

6. Trienski TL, Barrett HL, Pasquale TR, DiPersio JR, File TM Jr. Evaluation and use of a rapid Staphylococcus aureus assay by an antimicrobial stewardship program. Am J Health Syst Pharm 2013;70(21):1908–1912.

7. Goff DA, Jankowski C, Tenover FC. Using rapid diagnostic tests to optimize antimicrobial selection in antimicrobial stewardship programs. Pharmacotherapy 2012;32(8):677–687.

8. Rybak M, Lomaestro B, Rotschafer JC, et al. Therapeutic monitoring of vancomycin in adult patients: a consensus review of the American Society of Health-System Pharmacists, the Infectious Diseases Society of America, and the Society of Infectious Diseases Pharmacists. Am J Health Syst Pharm 2009;66:82–98.

9. CLSI. Performance Standards for Antimicrobial Susceptibility Testing; Twenty-Fifth Informational Supplement. CLSI Document M100-S25. Wayne, PA, Clinical and Laboratory Standards Institute, 2015.

10. Prybylski JP. Vancomycin trough concentration as a predictor of clinical outcomes in patients with Staphylococcus aureus bacteremia: A meta-analysis of observational studies. Pharmacotherapy 2015;35(10):889–898.

118

BACTERIAL MENINGITIS

This Is Spinal Tap............................. Level II

S. Travis King, PharmD, BCPS

LEARNING OBJECTIVES

After completing this case study, the reader should be able to:

- List risk factors and common presenting signs and symptoms of bacterial meningitis in infants and children.

- Differentiate common bacterial pathogens associated with meningitis in children of different ages.

- Recommend appropriate empiric and definitive antimicrobial and adjunctive therapy for bacterial meningitis.

- Identify appropriate monitoring parameters for antimicrobial therapy of bacterial meningitis.

PATIENT PRESENTATION

■ Chief Complaint

From mom: "Why is my baby so sleepy? And what is this purple rash?"

■ HPI

David St. Hubbins is a 2 yo, 13.6 kg male toddler who presented to the emergency department with his mother. Mom reports that she noticed him sleeping longer than normal since yesterday evening after returning from daycare, as well as this morning. She also reports that he had a poorer than normal appetite at dinner and breakfast. She also notes the rapid appearance of a purplish rash on his extremities, trunk, and back. At 08:00 she checked his temperature, reporting a temperature of 39.1°C. At this point, the mother reports that she called her sister who is a nurse, and was told to go straight to the emergency room. When aroused prior to transport, David was irritable and frequently crying. She indicates that during transport, David was in and out of sleep and did not respond well to normal stimuli. There was one episode of slight vomiting during transit.

■ PMH

David was born via an uncomplicated vaginal delivery at 39 weeks. Mother reports one episode of otitis media at 13 months of age, treated with amoxicillin.

■ FH

Mother is in good health; father has hypercholesterolemia; maternal grandparents both with metabolic syndrome; paternal grandfather in good health; maternal grandmother alive, history of breast cancer.

■ SH

Lives with mother and father. Father is a rock musician and mother is a teacher. David began attending daycare 3 months ago. Father is a smoker. No pets in the home.

Meds

None; immunizations up to date per the U.S. CDC Advisory Committee for Immunization Practices (ACIP)

All

NKDA

Review of Systems

Refer to HPI

Physical Examination

Gen

Lethargic toddler with generalized rash in mild-moderate distress

VS

SBP 75, HR 152, RR 48, T 39.4°C; Wt 13.6 kg, SatO$_2$ (RA): 98%

HEENT

PERRLA, tympanic membranes erythematous bilaterally

Chest

Lungs clear bilaterally

CV

Sinus tachycardia, regular rhythm, no murmurs, rubs, gallops

Abd

Soft, distended, (+) BS, (+) purpuric rash

Extremities

Capillary refill 4 seconds, extremities mottled and cool to the touch; (+) mildly blanching, purpuric rash is present; petechial lesions noted

Neuro

Listless; arousable to strong stimuli only, (–) Brudzinski's, (–) Kernig's, (+) Babinski

Labs

Na 135 mEq/L	Hgb 13.2 g/dL	pH 7.32
K 3.9 mEq/L	Hct 39.6%	PaO$_2$ 80 mm Hg
Cl 110 mEq/L	Plt 160 × 10³/mm³	PaCO$_2$ 40 mm Hg
CO$_2$ 14 mEq/L	WBC 25 × 10³/mm³	HCO$_3$ 15 mEq/L
SCr 0.9 mg/dL	Neutrophils 70%	Base excess 5.3 mEq/L
BUN 19 mg/dL	Bands 16%	Serum procalcitonin:
Glucose 130 mg/dL	Lymphocytes 10%	20.2 ng/mL
Ca 9.2 mg/dL	Monocytes 2%	
Mg 1.4 mEq/L	Eosinophils 1%	
PO$_4$ 4.2 mg/dL	Basophils 1%	
T. protein 6.6 g/dL		
Alb 4.1 g/dL		
Bili 0.7 mg/dL		
AST 86 IU/L		
ALT 20 IU/L		
ALP 285 IU/L		

CSF serology/urine antigen testing:

Haemophilus influenzae type B (–); *Streptococcus pneumoniae* (–); group B *Streptococcus* (–)

CSF analysis:

Color/appearance: straw/cloudy, glucose 38 mg/dL, protein 315 mg/dL, WBC 420/mm³ (2% lymphocytes, 2% monocytes, 96% neutrophils), RBC 500/mm³
CSF Gram stain: Gram-negative diplococci

Cultures

Blood, Urine, and CSF cultures: Pending

Chest X-Ray

No acute cardiopulmonary process noted

Assessment

1. Acute bacterial meningitis, suspected meningococcal

2. Hypotension/metabolic acidosis

QUESTIONS

Problem Identification

1.a. Create a list of the patient's drug-related problems.

1.b. What risk factors does this patient have for bacterial meningitis?

1.c. What organisms are most commonly associated with bacterial meningitis?

1.d. What information (signs, symptoms, laboratory values) indicates the presence or severity of meningitis in this patient?

Desired Outcome

2. What are the goals of pharmacotherapy in this situation?

Therapeutic Alternatives

3.a. What non-drug therapies might be useful for managing this patient?

3.b. What feasible pharmacotherapeutic alternatives are available for treatment of the disease or drug therapy problem?

Optimal Plan

4.a. What drug, dosage form, dose, schedule, and duration of therapy are best for this patient?

4.b. What alternatives would be appropriate if the initial therapy fails or cannot be used?

4.c. What adjunctive therapies should be given to this patient?

Outcome Evaluation

5.a. What clinical and laboratory parameters are necessary to evaluate the therapy for achievement of the desired therapeutic outcome and to detect or prevent adverse effects?

■ CLINICAL COURSE

The patient received fluids, supportive care and empiric antibiotics according to the hospital sepsis protocol. The patient was begun on vancomycin and ceftriaxone empirically. He also received dexamethasone (0.15 mg/kg every 6 hours starting with the first dose of antibiotics). Blood cultures returned positive for *N. meningitidis*. CSF cultures return positive for *N. meningitidis*. Urine cultures remain negative.

Susceptibility testing of *N. meningitidis* from CSF culture demonstrates the following profile:

penicillin MIC: 0.1 mcg/mL
ceftriaxone MIC: 0.06 mcg/mL
rifampin MIC: 0.25 mcg/mL
ciprofloxacin MIC: 0.03 mcg/mL

Repeat procalcitonin on day 3 of admission is 6.3 ng/mL

Repeat CBC at that time revealed: Hgb/Hct 13.5 g/dL/40.5%, Platelets $225 \times 10^3/mm^3$, and WBC $12 \times 10^3/mm^3$ (66% neutrophils, 32% lymphocytes, 1% basophils, 1% eosinophils).

Patient Education

6.a. What information should be provided to the patient to enhance compliance, ensure successful therapy, and minimize adverse effects?

Self-Study Assignments

1. Discuss the impact of vaccination on reducing the rates of meningitis and other invasive diseases in pediatric patients. What impact may be anticipated following the approval of the *N. meningitidis*, serotype B vaccine?

2. Detail the pharmacokinetic properties that influence the ability of antimicrobials to penetrate the blood-brain barrier.

3. Discuss the role of procalcitonin in the work-up of bacterial vs aseptic meningitis.

4. Discuss the management alternatives when treating meningitis caused by drug-resistant meningococcal and pneumococcal pathogens.

CLINICAL PEARL

The *N. meningitis*, serotype B vaccine may be administered in addition to the quadrivalent vaccine to patients between the ages of 16 and 23 years. If patients are deemed to be at risk for meningococcal disease (asplenia, complement deficiency, microbiology lab personnel), they should receive the serotype B vaccine.

REFERENCES

1. Tunkel AR, Hartman BJ, Kaplan SL, et al. Practice guidelines for the management of bacterial meningitis. Clin Infect Dis 2004;39:1267–1284.

2. Chavez-Bueno S, McCracken GH. Bacterial meningitis in children. Pediatr Clin North Am 2005;52:795–810.

3. Centers for Disease Control and Prevention. Prevention and Control of Meningococcal Disease Recommendations of the Advisory Committee on Immunization Practices (ACIP). MMWR 2005;54(No. RR-7).

4. Cohn A, MacNeil J. The Changing Epidemiology of Meningococcal Disease. Infect Dis Clin North Am 2015 Dec;29(4):667–677.

5. Brouwer MC, Tunkel AR, van de Beek D. Epidemiology, diagnosis, and antimicrobial treatment of acute bacterial meningitis. Clin Microbiol Rev 2010 Jul;23(3):467–492.

6. Bonadio W. Pediatric lumbar puncture and cerebrospinal fluid analysis. J Emerg Med. 2014 Jan;46(1):141–150.

7. Alkholi UM, Abd Al-Monem N, Abd El-Azim AA, Sultan MH. Serum procalcitonin in viral and bacterial meningitis. J Glob Infect Dis 2011 Jan;3(1):14–18.

8. Brouwer MC, McIntyre P, Prasad K, van de Beek D. Corticosteroids for acute bacterial meningitis. Cochrane Database Syst Rev 2015 Sep 12;9:CD004405.

9. Wall EC, Ajdukiewicz KM, Heyderman RS, Garner P. Osmotic therapies added to antibiotics for acute bacterial meningitis. Cochrane Database Syst Rev 2013 Mar 28;3:CD008806.

10. World Health Organization. Chapter 11: Antimicrobial Susceptibility Testing of Neisseria meningitidis, Haemophilus influenzae, and Streptococcus pneumoniae. In: Laboratory Methods for the Diagnosis of Meningitis Caused by Neisseria meningitidis, Streptococcus pneumoniae, and Haemophilus influenzae. 2009. Available: *http://www.cdc.gov/meningitis/lab-manual/*. Accessed March 30, 2016.

119

ACUTE BRONCHITIS

The Collegiate Cough .... Level II

Jessica Helmer Brady, PharmD, BCPS

LEARNING OBJECTIVES

After completing this case study, the reader should be able to:

- Identify signs and symptoms of acute bronchitis and their duration, and evaluate relevant laboratory values to rule out more serious illness such as pneumonia.

- Discuss why obtaining sputum cultures and Gram stains is not relevant in evaluation and treatment of patients with uncomplicated acute bronchitis.

- Discuss why antibiotic treatment is not indicated for uncomplicated acute bronchitis.

- Select nonpharmacologic and pharmacologic treatment alternatives for supportive care, incorporating data regarding efficacy.

PATIENT PRESENTATION

Chief Complaint

"I can't seem to stop coughing! It's keeping me and my roommate awake at night, not to mention totally disrupting my classes. And now my throat is also really sore. I even tried my roommate's asthma inhaler in hopes that my cough would stop, but it didn't. I just want an antibiotic to make this all go away!"

HPI

Allie Comeaux, a 21-year-old college student, is being seen at her university's Student Health Center for complaints of a productive, purulent cough and sore throat for the past 5 days. On questioning, Allie denies that she has had any fever, chills, or myalgias. She does express concern that a dorm mate was recently hospitalized with pneumonia. She admits to using her roommate's asthma inhaler, which she recalls was albuterol, with no relief. While her throat is still sore, she is most concerned with her disruptive cough. "My history professor even asked me to leave the class when I couldn't stop coughing!"

PMH

Mild acne × 5 years
Irregular menstrual cycle, ranging from 25 to 40 days in length
Current with age-appropriate vaccinations, with the exception of influenza and human papillomavirus

FH

Father, 51, has been diagnosed with hypertension and hyperlipidemia and has a distant history of alcohol abuse. Mother, 50, is menopausal. The patient also has two younger brothers, ages 16 and 18, with no health issues.

SH

Allie lives at University dorm with a suitemate. She smokes "socially" when out with friends but denies alcohol use due to her father's history of alcohol abuse. She also denies any illicit drug use. She is currently a junior kinesiology major and hopes to attend physical therapy school on completion of her degree. She is also on the University Dance line. Allie states that she is sexually active with her boyfriend of 8 months. They use condoms as a method of birth control, although inconsistently.

Meds

Acetaminophen 650 mg PO PRN headache or menstrual cramps
Benzoyl peroxide 2.5% cream topically daily PRN acne

All

Penicillin—"all-over body rash"

ROS

No fever, chills, myalgia, chest pain, or shortness of breath; no nausea, vomiting, or diarrhea

Physical Examination

Gen

Well-developed, thin female in NAD

VS

BP 104/68 mm Hg, P 64, RR 14, T 37°C; Wt 50 kg, Ht 5'6"

HEENT

PERRLA, conjunctivae clear, TMs intact. No epistaxis or nasal discharge. No sinus swelling or tenderness, and mucous membranes are moist. There are no oropharyngeal lesions.

Neck/Lymph Nodes

Supple without adenopathy or thyromegaly

Chest

(—) Rhonchi, rales, increased fremitus, wheezing, or egophony; negative bronchophony

CV

RRR without MRG

Abd

Soft, nontender, (+) BS

Genit/Rect

Deferred

MS/Ext

Pulses 2+ throughout

Neuro

A & O × 3; 2+ reflexes throughout, 5/5 strength; CN II–XII intact

Labs

Na 140 mEq/L	Hgb 14 g/dL	WBC 6 × 10³/mm³
K 4.5 mEq/L	Hct 38%	Segs 55%
Cl 102 mEq/L	RBC 5.0 × 10⁶/mm³	Bands 3%
HCO₃ 24 mEq/L	Plt 250 × 10³/mm³	Lymphs 33%
BUN 14 mg/dL		Monos 6%
SCr 0.7 mg/dL		Eos 2%
FPG 88 mg/dL		Basos 1%

Sputum Culture

No pathogens isolated

Assessment

1. Presumed acute bronchitis.

2. Sexual/reproductive health issues should be further explored and addressed.

3. (+) Smoking history, although patient states, "I only smoke when I'm out, so I can stop at any time."

QUESTIONS

Problem Identification

1.a. Create a list of the patient's drug therapy problems.

1.b. What information (signs, symptoms, laboratory values) indicates the presence or severity of acute bronchitis?

1.c. What additional information must be considered before deciding whether antimicrobial therapy is indicated?

Desired Outcome

2. What are the goals of pharmacotherapy in this case?

Therapeutic Alternatives

3.a. What nondrug therapies might be useful for this patient?

3.b. What feasible pharmacotherapeutic alternatives are available for treatment of uncomplicated acute bronchitis?

3.c. What are the most likely alternatives for smoking cessation?

3.d. What sexual/reproductive health considerations are applicable to this patient?

3.e. What psychosocial considerations are applicable to this patient?

Optimal Plan

4.a. What drugs, dosage form, dose, schedule, and duration of therapy are best to alleviate this patient's symptoms of acute bronchitis?

4.b. What medication and dosage should be recommended for this patient's smoking cessation plan?

Outcome Evaluation

5. What clinical and laboratory parameters are necessary to evaluate the therapy for achievement of the desired outcome and to detect or prevent adverse effects?

Patient Education

6. What information should be provided to the patient to enhance adherence, ensure successful therapy, and minimize adverse effects?

■ FOLLOW-UP QUESTION

1. What vaccinations should this patient receive?

■ SELF-STUDY ASSIGNMENTS

1. Outline a treatment plan for a patient with chronic bronchitis presenting with an acute exacerbation, and contrast how this treatment would differ from treatment for a patient with a new diagnosis of acute bronchitis.

2. Prepare a patient education pamphlet on acute bronchitis. Be sure to address why antibiotics are not usually first-line therapy for uncomplicated acute bronchitis.

3. Discuss the differences in presentation and treatment of uncomplicated acute bronchitis for a child versus an adult versus an elderly patient.

CLINICAL PEARL

Many patients who present with symptoms of acute bronchitis expect to receive an antibiotic. Therefore, time should be spent with the patient to explain what goes into the decision to not prescribe an antibiotic, and why excessive use of unnecessary antibiotics could harm the community at large.

REFERENCES

1. Braman SS. Chronic cough due to acute bronchitis: ACCP evidence-based clinical practice guidelines. Chest 2006;129:95S–103S.
2. Wenzel RP, Fowler AA. Acute bronchitis. N Engl J Med 2006;355:2125–2130.
3. Becker LA, Hom J, Villasis-Keever M, van der Wouden JC. Beta2-agonists for acute bronchitis. Cochrane Database Syst Rev 2011;(7):CD001726.
4. Albert RH. Diagnosis and treatment of acute bronchitis. Am Fam Physician 2010;82(11):1345–1350.
5. Gonzales R, Bartlett JG, Besser RE, et al. Principles of appropriate antibiotic use for treatment of uncomplicated acute bronchitis: background. Ann Intern Med 2001;134:521–529.
6. Phillips TG, Hickner J. Calling acute bronchitis a chest cold may improve patient satisfaction with appropriate antibiotic use. J Am Board Fam Pract 2005;18:459–463.
7. Brunton S, Carmichael BP, Colgan R, et al. Acute exacerbation of chronic bronchitis: a primary care consensus guideline. Am J Manag Care 2004;10:689–696.
8. Irwin RS, Baumann MH, Boulet L, et al. Diagnosis and management of cough executive summary: ACCP evidence-based clinical practice guidelines. Chest 2006;129:1S–23S.
9. Petrosky E, Bocchini JA, Hariri S, et al. Use of 9-valent Human Papillomavirus (HPV) vaccine: Updated HPV vaccination recommendations of the Advisory Committee on Immunization Practices. MMWR 2015;64(11):300–304.

120

COMMUNITY-ACQUIRED PNEUMONIA

The Coughing Conundrum . . . . Level II

Trent G. Towne, PharmD, BCPS, AQ-ID

Sharon M. Erdman, PharmD

LEARNING OBJECTIVES

After completing this case study, the reader should be able to:

- Recognize the common signs, symptoms, physical examination, laboratory, and radiographic findings in a patient with community-acquired pneumonia (CAP).

- Describe the most common causative pathogens of CAP, including their frequency of occurrence and susceptibility to frequently used antimicrobials.

- Discuss the risk stratification strategies that can be employed to determine whether a patient with CAP should be treated as an inpatient or outpatient.

- Provide recommendations for initial empiric antibiotic therapy for an inpatient or outpatient with CAP based on clinical presentation, severity of infection, age, allergies, and comorbidities.

- Define the goals of antimicrobial therapy for a patient with CAP, as well as the monitoring parameters that should be used to assess the response to therapy and the occurrence of adverse effects.

- Describe the clinical parameters that should be considered when changing a patient from IV to oral antimicrobial therapy in the treatment of CAP.

PATIENT PRESENTATION

■ Chief Complaint

"I have been short of breath and have been coughing up rust-colored phlegm for the past 3 days."

■ HPI

James Thompson is a 55-year-old African-American man with a 3-day history of worsening shortness of breath, subjective fevers, chills, right-sided chest pain, and a productive cough. The patient states that his initial symptom of shortness of breath began approximately 1 week ago after delivering mail on an extremely cold winter day. After several days of not feeling well, he went to an immediate care clinic and received a prescription for levofloxacin 750 mg orally once daily for 5 days, which he did not fill due to financial reasons. He has been taking acetaminophen and an over-the-counter cough and cold preparation, but feels that his symptoms are getting "much worse." The patient began experiencing right-sided pleuritic chest pain and a productive cough with rust-colored sputum over the past 3 days, and feels that he has been feverish with chills, although he did not take his temperature. On presentation to the ED, he is febrile and appears visibly short of breath.

PMH

Hypertension × 15 years
Type 2 diabetes mellitus × 10 years

SH

Lives with wife and four children
Employed as a mail carrier for the US Postal Service
Denies alcohol, tobacco, or intravenous drug use

Home Medications

Prescription

Patient states that he only sporadically takes his medications due to financial reasons
Lisinopril 10 mg orally once daily
Hydrochlorothiazide 25 mg orally once daily
Metformin 1000 mg orally twice daily

Over-the-Counter

Acetaminophen 650 mg orally every 6 hours as needed for pain
Guaifenesin/dextromethorphan (100 mg/10 mg/5 mL) two teaspoonfuls every 4 hours as needed for cough

All

Amoxicillin (rash—as a child). Patient has received cephalexin as an adult without problem.

ROS

Patient is a good historian. He has been experiencing shortness of breath, a productive cough with rust-colored sputum, subjective fevers, chills, and pleuritic chest pain that is "right in the middle of my chest." He denies any nausea, vomiting, constipation, or problems urinating.

Physical Examination

Gen

Patient is a well-developed, well-nourished, African-American man in moderate respiratory distress appearing somewhat anxious and uncomfortable.

VS

BP 155/85, P 127, RR 30, T 39.5°C; Wt 110 kg, Ht 5′11″

Skin

Warm to the touch; poor skin turgor

HEENT

PERRLA; EOMI; dry mucous membranes

Neck/Lymph Nodes

No JVD; full range of motion; no neck stiffness; no masses or thyromegaly; no cervical lymphadenopathy

Lungs/Thorax

Tachypneic, labored breathing; coarse rhonchi throughout right lung fields; decreased breath sounds in right middle and right lower lung fields

CV

Audible S_1 and S_2; tachycardic with regular rate and rhythm; no MRG

Abd

NTND; (+) bowel sounds

Genit/Rect

Deferred

Extremities

No CCE; 5/5 grip strength; 2+ pulses bilaterally

Neuro

A & O × 3; CN II–XII intact

Labs on Admission

Na 140 mEq/L	Hgb 12.1 g/dL	WBC 23.1 × 10³/mm³
K 4.3 mEq/L	Hct 35%	Neutrophils 67%
Cl 102 mEq/L	RBC 3.8 × 10⁶/mm³	Bands 15%
CO₂ 22 mEq/L	Plt 220 × 10³/mm³	Lymphs 12%
BUN 42 mg/dL	MCV 91 μm³	Monos 6%
SCr 1.4 mg/dL	MCHC 35 g/dL	
Glu 295 mg/dL		

ABG

pH 7.38; $PaCO_2$ 29; PaO_2 70 make HCO_3 25 mEq/L with 87% O_2 saturation on room air

Chest X-Ray

Right middle and right lower lobe consolidative airspace disease, likely pneumonia. Left lung is clear. Heart size is normal.

Chest CT Scan Without Contrast

No axillary, mediastinal, or hilar lymphadenopathy. The heart size is normal. There is consolidation of the right lower lobe and lateral segment of the middle lobe, with air bronchograms. No significant pleural effusions. The left lung is clear.

Sputum Gram Stain

>25 WBCs/hpf, <10 epithelial cells/hpf, many Gram (+) cocci in pairs

Sputum Culture

Pending

Blood Cultures × Two Sets

Pending

Other Lab Tests

Streptococcus pneumoniae urine antigen—Pending
Legionella pneumophila urine antigen—Pending

Assessment

Probable multilobar CAP involving the RML and RLL
Hypoxemia

QUESTIONS

Problem Identification

1.a. Create a list of the patient's drug therapy problems.

1.b. What clinical, laboratory, and radiographic findings are consistent with the diagnosis of CAP in this patient?

1.c. What are the common causative bacteria of CAP?

1.d. What clinical, laboratory, and physical examination findings should be considered when deciding on the site of care (inpatient or outpatient) for a patient with CAP?

Desired Outcome

2. What are the goals of pharmacotherapy in the treatment of CAP?

Therapeutic Alternatives

3. What feasible pharmacotherapeutic alternatives are available for treatment of CAP for both inpatients and outpatients?

Optimal Plan

4.a. What drug, dose, route of therapy, dosing schedule, and duration of treatment should be used in this patient?

■ CLINICAL COURSE

While in the ED, the patient was placed on 4 L NC of O₂, and his oxygen saturation improved to 98%. The patient was initiated on ceftriaxone 1 g IV daily and azithromycin 500 mg IV daily and admitted to the hospital. Over the next 48 hours, the patient's clinical status improved with decreasing fever, tachypnea, tachycardia, and shortness of breath. On hospital day 2, the *S. pneumoniae* urine antigen was positive, and the sputum culture demonstrated the growth of *S. pneumoniae*, resistant to erythromycin (MIC ≥1 mcg/mL), but susceptible to penicillin (MIC ≤2 mcg/mL), ceftriaxone (MIC ≤1 mcg/mL), levofloxacin (MIC ≤0.5 mcg/mL), and vancomycin (MIC ≤1 mcg/mL).

4.b. Given this new information, what changes in the antimicrobial therapy would you recommend?

4.c. What oral antibiotic would be suitable to complete the course of therapy for CAP in this patient? When is it appropriate to convert a patient from IV to oral therapy for the treatment of CAP?

Outcome Evaluation

5. What clinical and laboratory parameters should be monitored to ensure the desired therapeutic outcome, and to detect or prevent adverse effects?

Patient Education

6. By hospital day 4, the patient's clinical symptoms of pneumonia had almost completely resolved, and the patient was discharged home on oral antibiotics to complete a 7-day course of treatment. What information should be provided to the patient about his oral outpatient antibiotic therapy to enhance adherence, ensure successful therapy, and minimize adverse effects?

■ SELF-STUDY ASSIGNMENTS

1. Review the most recent practice guidelines for the treatment of CAP published by the Infectious Diseases Society of America (IDSA)/American Thoracic Society, and evaluate changes from the last published guidelines.

2. Review national, regional, and local patterns of *S. pneumoniae* susceptibility and compare the data with what is seen at your institution or clinic.

3. Describe the role of short-course (5-day) antibiotic therapy in the management of CAP.

CLINICAL PEARL

Influenza and pneumococcal vaccines for appropriate patient types are important components in the prevention of CAP as well as for reducing the morbidity and mortality associated with CAP.

REFERENCES

1. Mandell LA, Wunderink RG, Anzueto A, et al. Infectious Diseases Society of America/American Thoracic Society consensus guidelines on the management of community-acquired pneumonia in adults. Clin Infect Dis 2007;44(Suppl 2):S27–S72.
2. Prina E, Ranzani OT, Torres A. Community-acquired pneumonia. Lancet 2015;386:1097–108.
3. Infections of the lower respiratory tract. In: Tile, PM, ed. Bailey and Scott's Diagnostic Microbiology. 13th ed. St Louis, MO: Mosby Inc; 2014:878–891.
4. Segreti J, House HR, Siegel RE. Principles of antibiotic treatment of community-acquired pneumonia in the outpatient setting. Am J Med 2005;118(7A):21S–28S.
5. Bochud PY, Moser F, Erard P, et al. Community-acquired pneumonia: a prospective outpatient study. Medicine 2001;80(2):75–87.
6. File TM. Community-acquired pneumonia. Lancet 2003;362:1991–2001.
7. Fine MJ, Auble TE, Yealy DM, et al. A prediction rule to identify low-risk patients with community-acquired pneumonia. N Engl J Med 1997;336:243–250.
8. Lim WS, van der Eerden MM, Laing R, et al. Defining community-acquired pneumonia severity on presentation to hospital: an international derivation and validation study. Thorax 2003;58:377–382.
9. Pfaller MA, Farrell DL, Sader HS, Jones RN. AWARE Ceftaroline Surveillance Program (2008–2010): trends in resistance patterns among *Streptococcus pneumoniae*, *Haemophilus influenzae*, and *Moraxella catarrhalis* in the United States. Clin Infect Dis 2012;55(Suppl 3):S187–S193.
10. Fine MJ, Stone RA, Singer DE, et al. Process and outcomes of care for patients with community-acquired pneumonia: results from the Pneumonia Patients Outcomes Research Team (PORT) cohort study. Arch Intern Med 1999;159:970–980.

121

HOSPITAL-ACQUIRED PNEUMONIA

The HAPpening................................Level III

Kendra M. Damer, PharmD

LEARNING OBJECTIVES

After completing this case study, the reader should be able to:

- Recognize the signs and symptoms of hospital-acquired pneumonia (HAP).

- Identify the most common causative organisms associated with HAP, and recognize the impact of bacterial resistance on the etiology and treatment of HAP.

- Design an appropriate empiric antimicrobial therapy regimen for a patient with suspected HAP.

- Formulate a list of alternative antimicrobial therapy options for the treatment of HAP based on the most common causative organisms.

- Recommend a directed/targeted antimicrobial therapy regimen for a patient with HAP based on patient-specific data and final microbiology culture and susceptibility results.

PATIENT PRESENTATION

Chief Complaint

"My chest hurts, I can't catch my breath, and this cough is getting worse."

HPI

Justin Case is a 60-year-old man with a past medical history significant for MI who was admitted to the hospital 5 days ago to undergo a scheduled surgical procedure following a recent diagnosis of colorectal adenocarcinoma with metastatic lesions to the liver. The patient was taken to the OR on hospital day 2 and underwent an exploratory laparotomy, diverting ileostomy, and Hickman catheter placement in preparation for chemotherapy. Postoperatively, the patient was transferred to the progressive ICU for his recovery without complication. The patient had no new complaints until hospital day 5 when he complained of retrosternal crushing chest pain radiating to the left shoulder and left jaw, shortness of breath, and a worsening cough with sputum production. The patient was noted to be in respiratory distress with a RR of 43 breaths/min, HR 153 bpm, BP 162/103 mm Hg, and O_2 saturation of 87%. He was then transferred to the medical ICU and underwent endotracheal intubation due to worsening respiratory status. Cardiac markers were obtained, given the patient's symptoms and history of MI. Imaging and blood & sputum cultures were obtained after patient transfer.

PMH

CAD, S/P MI 3 years ago for which he did not undergo any surgical intervention

SH

Lives with his wife
Smokes one ppd × 40 years
Denies alcohol or illicit drug use

Meds

Patient states that he did not take any medications at home. Hospital medications include (ICU medication list):

Aspirin 325 mg PO × 1 dose, then 81 mg PO daily
Enoxaparin 70 mg subcutaneously every 12 hours
Esomeprazole 40 mg PO daily
Fentanyl 25 mcg/hour IV continuous infusion
Lorazepam 2 mg/hour IV continuous infusion
Metoprolol 25 mg PO every 12 hours
Nicotine patch 21 mg per day applied daily

All

NKDA

ROS

Patient is experiencing significant chest pain, shortness of breath, and a cough with sputum production. He denies nausea, vomiting, or difficulty urinating. He complains of mild abdominal pain near his ostomy and incision sites.

Physical Examination

Gen

WDWN Caucasian man, initially anxious, ill-appearing, and in moderate respiratory distress; now, S/P endotracheal intubation and in NAD

VS

BP 162/103 mm Hg, P 147 bpm, RR 42 breaths/min, T 38.5°C; Wt 70 kg, Ht 5′6″

Skin

Warm; no rash; no skin breakdown

HEENT

PERRLA; moist mucous membranes

Neck/Lymph Nodes

Supple; no lymphadenopathy

Lungs/Thorax

Scattered rhonchi with expiratory wheezing; diffuse bilateral crackles; decreased breath sounds in bilateral bases; right IJ Hickman catheter intact without erythema

CV

Tachycardic with regular rhythm; no MRG

Abd

Soft; mildly distended; hypoactive BS; large liver palpated in RUQ; ileostomy in RLQ is pink and functioning; surgical incision is C/D/I

Genit/Rect

Deferred

MS/Ext

1+ pitting edema; 2+ pulses bilaterally; good peripheral perfusion

Neuro

Prior to intubation, A & O × 3; CN II–XII intact; patient is now intubated and sedated

Labs

Lab Parameter	Admission	Hospital Day 5
Na (mEq/L)	130	141
K (mEq/L)	4.1	5.1
Cl (mEq/L)	92	110
CO_2 (mEq/L)	24	19
BUN (mg/dL)	22	34
SCr (mg/dL)	1	1.1
Glu (mg/dL)	113	148
Ca (mg/dL)	9.4	9.2
WBC (mm^{-3})	9.5×10^3	17×10^3
Neutros (%)	89	88
Bands (%)	0	5
Lymphs (%)	5	4
Monos (%)	6	3
Eos (%)	0	0
Hgb (g/dL)	11.9	12.4
Hct (%)	35	37
Plts (mm^{-3})	448×10^3	584×10^3

Cardiac Markers

CK 871 IU/L, troponin-I 1.23 ng/mL

ABG

pH 7.39; $PaCO_2$ 30; PaO_2 51 make HCO_3 25 mEq/L with 87% O_2 saturation on room air (pre-intubation)

pH 7.44; $PaCO_2$ 29; PaO_2 89 make HCO_3 23 mEq/L with 100% O_2 saturation on 40% inspired oxygen (post-intubation)

■ **Chest X-Ray**

New bilateral opacities are noted in the left upper lobe and right middle lobe; likely infectious process. Some increased alveolar infiltrates in the perihilar location and involving the lower lobes.

■ **Chest CT Scan with IV Contrast**

No evidence of pulmonary embolism. The heart size is normal. There are small mediastinal and axillary lymph nodes; none are pathologically enlarged. There are small bilateral pleural effusions with adjacent atelectasis. There are pleural-based airspace opacities within the left upper lobe and right middle lobe; this is most consistent with an acute infectious process.

■ **EKG**

Sinus tachycardia, low voltage QRS, septal infarct (age undetermined); ST- and T-wave abnormality; consider inferior ischemia. Inverted T waves noted in the inferior leads.

■ **Sputum Gram Stain**

Greater than 25 WBC/hpf, <10 epithelial cells/hpf, 1+ (few) Gram-positive cocci, 3+ (many) Gram-negative rods

■ **Sputum Culture**

Pending

■ **Blood Cultures × Two Sets**

Pending

■ **Assessment**

Presumed bilobar HAP involving the LUL and RML
NSTEMI

QUESTIONS

Problem Identification

1.a. Create a list of the patient's drug therapy problems.

1.b. What subjective and objective data are consistent with the diagnosis of HAP in this patient?

1.c. What are the most common causative organisms associated with HAP?

Desired Outcome

2. What are the goals of pharmacotherapy in the treatment of this patient's HAP?

Therapeutic Alternatives

3. What feasible pharmacotherapeutic alternatives are available for treatment of HAP?

Optimal Plan

4.a. What drug(s), dosage form, dose, dosing schedule, and duration of therapy represent(s) an appropriate empiric antimicrobial therapy for this patient?

4.b. What alternative antimicrobial therapy options exist in the event the initial therapy fails or is not tolerated by the patient?

■ CLINICAL COURSE

Following endotracheal intubation, the patient experienced improved oxygen saturation and a normalization of his respiratory

and heart rates. The patient was initiated on therapy for NSTEMI per cardiology. The patient was initiated on appropriate empiric antimicrobial therapy while awaiting the results of sputum and blood cultures. The blood and sputum cultures revealed *Klebsiella pneumoniae*. The organism's susceptibility profile is provided below. Over the next 72 hours, the patient's clinical status improved with decreased sputum production, oxygen requirement, temperature, and WBC count, and improvement in chest x-ray findings was also noted, resulting in extubation on hospital day 8. The patient was transferred to the progressive ICU for his continued recovery.

Antimicrobial Agent	MIC (mg/L)	Interpretation
Ampicillin	≥32	Resistant
Ampicillin/sulbactam	≥32	Resistant
Piperacillin/tazobactam	≤4	Susceptible
Cefazolin	32	Resistant
Ceftriaxone	≤1	Susceptible
Cefepime	≤1	Susceptible
Meropenem	≤0.25	Susceptible
Gentamicin	≤1	Susceptible
Tobramycin	≤1	Susceptible
Ciprofloxacin	≤0.25	Susceptible
Levofloxacin	≤0.12	Susceptible
Trimethoprim/sulfamethoxazole	≥320	Resistant

4.c. Based on the new data listed above, provide a recommendation for directed/targeted therapy for this patient's HAP.

Outcome Evaluation

5. What clinical and laboratory parameters are necessary to monitor for the achievement of the identified goals of therapy as well as to detect or prevent adverse effects associated with the antimicrobial therapy?

Patient Education

6. What information should be provided to the patient to enhance adherence, ensure successful therapy, and minimize adverse effects?

■ SELF-STUDY ASSIGNMENTS

1. Review national, regional, and local patterns of bacterial susceptibility for the most common causative organisms associated with HAP to determine appropriate empiric antimicrobial therapy choices for your geographic location.

2. Evaluate the literature to determine the most appropriate duration of therapy for HAP according to the causative microorganism.

3. Review the published literature to determine the role and utility of severity scoring (eg, acute physiologic assessment and chronic health evaluation II [APACHE II] and clinical pulmonary infection score [CPIS]) for the diagnosis, and/or treatment of HAP.

4. Given the patient's recent NSTEMI and PMH of MI, evaluate the literature to determine the most appropriate recommendations for the medical management of CAD both as an inpatient and on hospital discharge.

CLINICAL PEARL

Delays in initiation of appropriate empiric antimicrobial therapy have been associated with significant increases in hospital lengths of stay, health care costs, and mortality among patients with HAP.

REFERENCES

1. ATS/IDSA Therapeutics Work Group. Guidelines for the management of adults with hospital-acquired, ventilator-associated, and healthcare-associated pneumonia. Am J Respir Crit Care Med 2005;171:388–416.
2. Lancaster JW, Lawrence KP, Fong JJ, et al. Impact of an institution-specific hospital-acquired pneumonia protocol on the appropriateness of antibiotic therapy and patient outcomes. Pharmacotherapy 2008;28(7):852–862.
3. Gastermeier P, Sohr D, Geffers C, Ruden H, Vonberg RP, Welte T. Early and late-onset pneumonia: is this still a useful classification? Antimicrob Agents Chemother 2009;53(7):2714–2718.
4. Ferrer M, Liapikou A, Valendia M, et al. Validation of the American Thoracic Society–Infectious Diseases Society of America guidelines for hospital-acquired pneumonia in the intensive care unit. Clin Infect Dis 2010;50:945–952.
5. Niederman MS. Use of broad-spectrum antimicrobials for the treatment of pneumonia in seriously ill patients: maximizing clinical outcomes and minimizing selection of resistant organisms. Clin Infect Dis 2006;42:S72–S81.
6. Torres A, Ferrer M, Badia JR. Treatment guidelines and outcomes of hospital-acquired and ventilator-associated pneumonia. Clin Infect Dis 2010;51(Suppl 1):S48–S53.
7. Napolitano LM. Use of severity scoring and stratification factors in clinical trials of hospital-acquired and ventilator-associated pneumonia. Clin Infect Dis 2010;51(Suppl 1):S67–S80.
8. Liu C, Bayer A, Cosgrove SE, et al. Clinical practice guidelines by the Infectious Diseases Society of America for the treatment of methicillin resistant *Staphylococcus aureus* infections in adults and children. Clin Infect Dis 2011;52:1–38.
9. Corey GR, Kollef MH, Shorr AF, et al. Televancin for hospital-acquired pneumonia: clinical response and 28-day survival. Antimicrob Agents Chemother 2014;58(4)2030–2037.
10. Pugh R, Grant C, Cooke RPD, Dempsey G. Short-course versus prolonged-course antibiotic therapy for hospital-acquired pneumonia in critically ill adults. Cochrane Database Syst Rev 2015;Aug 24:8:CD007577.

122

OTITIS MEDIA

Up To My Ears with Ear Infections . . . . Level II

Rochelle Rubin, PharmD, BCPS

Lauren Camaione, PharmD

LEARNING OBJECTIVES

After completing this case study, the reader should be able to:

- Identify the signs and symptoms of acute otitis media (AOM).
- Identify risk factors associated with an increased incidence of AOM.
- Identify the pathogens most commonly causing AOM.
- Recommend an effective and economical treatment regimen including specific agent(s), route of administration, and dose(s) of antibiotics and analgesic medications.
- Recognize the role of delaying antibiotic therapy for AOM.
- Educate parents about recommended drug therapy using appropriate nontechnical terminology.

PATIENT PRESENTATION

Chief Complaint

Per patient's mom: "I've had it up to my ears with his ear infections!"

HPI

Seth Jacobs is a 16-month-old boy who is brought to his pediatrician by his distraught mother on a Monday morning in early March. Mom describes a 2-day history of tugging at his right ear and crying, and a 2-day history of decreased appetite, decreased playfulness, and difficulty sleeping. Mom states that his temperature last night was elevated by electronic axial thermometer (39.5°C), so she gave him 5 mL of ibuprofen every 12 hours × 2 doses. When Seth is asked if anything hurts, he does not respond. Mom requests all recommendations be written as prescriptions (even ibuprofen) for day care administration. She also notes that it is tax season and she needs Seth to be able to return to day care immediately so she can return to work as an accountant.

PMH

Former full-term, NSVD, 4-kg healthy infant at birth, breastfed for 6 months.

Immunizations are up-to-date, including four doses of 13-valent pneumococcal conjugate vaccination (Prevnar-13).

First episode of AOM at age 4 months treated with amoxicillin without adverse effects. Recurrent AOM × 3 over the past year; most recent episode 2 weeks ago treated with high-dose amoxicillin for 10 days without adverse effects.

Seth was seen approximately 1 month ago for persistent nonproductive cough of 5-day duration. A diagnosis of acute bronchiolitis was made and symptoms improved with ibuprofen treatment, fluids, and rest.

FH

Both parents in good health. Two siblings, 3 and 6 years old, in good health.

SH

Seth lives at home with his parents and two sisters. Both parents are employed and work out of the house. Seth and his 3-year-old sister attend day care. His elder sister attends elementary school. There is a pet dog in the home. Seth uses a pacifier regularly throughout the day. There is no smoking in the house.

Meds

Ibuprofen suspension 100 mg/5 mL, 100 mg (5 mL) Q 12 H × 2 doses in the last 24 hours

All

NKDA

ROS

Head: Otorrhea noted; ears tender to the touch

Respiratory: (per mom) denies wheezing. Has lingering, mild cough still present, no sputum production.

■ Physical Examination

Gen

WDWN Caucasian male, now crying

VS

BP 104/60, HR 130, RR 26, T 39.1°C; Wt 10 kg, Ht 30″

Skin

Warm and dry; no rashes

HEENT

Both TMs erythematous (with R > L); right TM with moderate bulging and limited mobility; copious cerumen and purulent fluid behind TM; otorrhea noted; left TM landmarks appear normal including the pars flaccida, the malleus, and the light reflex below the umbo. However, the right TM landmarks are difficult to visualize and the fluid is obstructing visualization of the umbo. Throat is erythematous; nares patent.

Neck/Lymph nodes

Supple; no lymphadenopathy

Chest

Mild crackles at bases bilaterally, improved since bronchiolitis visit 1 month ago

CV

RRR, no murmurs

Abd

Soft, nontender

Genit/Rect

Tanner stage I; rectal exam not performed

MS/Ext

No CCE; moves all extremities well; warm, pink, no rashes; normal range of motion

Neuro

Responsive to stimulation, DTR 2+ no clonus, CN intact

■ Labs

None

■ Assessment

Right ear AOM

QUESTIONS

Problem Identification

1.a. Create a drug therapy problem list for this patient.

1.b. What subjective and objective data support the diagnosis of AOM, and is the diagnosis certain or uncertain in this case?

1.c. How would you distinguish AOM from OME?

1.d. Which diagnosis does Seth have?

1.e. How is the severity of otitis media determined?

1.f. How severe is Seth's infection?

1.g. What risk factors for AOM are present in this child?

1.h. What organisms typically cause AOM?

Desired Outcome

2. What are the goals of pharmacotherapy for AOM in this child?

Therapeutic Alternatives

3.a. What pharmacotherapeutic alternatives are available for treatment of AOM in this patient?

3.b. Should this patient receive antibiotic therapy at this time, or should watchful waiting (observation) be the course of action? Defend your answer.

3.c. What measures are available to prevent AOM infections in children?

Optimal Plan

4.a. If antibiotics are indicated, which of the alternatives would you recommend to treat this child's AOM? Include the dose, schedule, duration of therapy, and rationale for your selection.

4.b. What other therapies would you recommend to treat this child's symptoms?

Outcome Evaluation

5. How should the therapy you recommended be monitored for efficacy and adverse effects?

Patient Education

6. How would you provide important information about this therapy to the child's mother?

■ SELF-STUDY ASSIGNMENTS

1. Describe a scenario in which it would be appropriate to use azithromycin to treat AOM.

CLINICAL PEARL

Streptococcus pneumoniae has been shown to cause 40–50% of childhood AOM cases. First-line treatment remains high-dose amoxicillin despite significant resistance because the high dose used is generally effective against susceptible, intermediate, and often resistant pneumococci and it is a low-cost, safe, acceptable tasting therapeutic option with a narrow microbiologic spectrum.

REFERENCES

1. Lieberthal AS, Carroll AE, Chonmaitree T, et al. Clinical practice guideline: Diagnosis and management of acute otitis media. Pediatrics 2013;131:e964–e999.

2. American Academy of Pediatrics, American Academy of Otolaryngology-Head and Neck Surgery, American Academy of Pediatrics Subcommittee on Otitis Media with Effusion. Otitis media with effusion. Pediatrics 2004;113:1412–1429.

3. Neto JFL, Hemb L, Silva DB. Systematic literature review of modifiable risk factors for recurrent otitis media in childhood. J Pediatr 2006;82:87–96.

4. Atkinson H, Sebastian W, Coatesworth AP. Acute Otitis Media. Postgrad Med 2015;127(4):386–390.

5. Bertin L, Pons G, d'Athis P, et al. A randomized, double-blind, multicentre controlled trial of ibuprofen versus acetaminophen and placebo for symptoms of acute otitis media in children. Fundam Clin Pharmacol 1996;10:387–392.

6. Centers for Disease Control and Prevention. Active Bacterial Core Surveillance Report, Emerging Infections Program Network, *Streptococcus pneumoniae*, 2010. Atlanta, GA, Centers for Disease Control and Prevention, 2012. Available at: *http://www.cdc.gov/abcs/reports-findings/survreports/spneu12.pdf*. Accessed March 30, 2016.

7. Venekamp RP, Sanders S, Glasziou PP, et al. Antibiotics for acute otitis media in children. Cochrane Database Syst Rev 2013;(1):CD000219.

8. Spiro DM, Tay KY, Arnold DH, Dziura JD, Baker MD, Shapiro ED. Wait-and-see prescription for the treatment of acute otitis media. JAMA 2006;196:1235–1241.

9. Centers for Disease Control and Prevention. Advisory committee on immunization practices (ACIP) recommended immunization schedules for persons aged 0 through 18 years and adults aged 19 years and older—Unitied States, 2013. MMWR 2013;62(Suppl 1):6–9.

10. Centers for Disease Control and Prevention (CDC). Licensure of a 13-valent pneumococcal conjugate vaccine (PCV13) and recommendations for use among children—Advisory Committee on Immunization Practices (ACIP), 2010. MMWR Morb Mortal Wkly Rep 2010;59(9):258–261.

123

RHINOSINUSITIS

Sick Sinus. . . . . Level II

Michael B. Kays, PharmD, FCCP

LEARNING OBJECTIVES

After completing this case study, the reader should be able to:

- Compare and contrast the clinical signs and symptoms of acute viral and bacterial rhinosinusitis in a given patient, noting the cardinal symptoms of acute rhinosinusitis.

- Differentiate viral from bacterial etiology in rhinosinusitis based on a patient's symptoms.

- Identify the most common pathogens that cause acute bacterial rhinosinusitis.

- Identify adult patients with a diagnosis of acute bacterial rhinosinusitis who may be candidates for observation without use of antibiotics.

- Formulate a treatment plan for a patient with acute bacterial rhinosinusitis based on duration of symptoms, severity of symptoms, and history of previous antibiotic use.

- Revise the treatment plan for a patient who fails the initially prescribed therapy.

PATIENT PRESENTATION

■ Chief Complaint

"I feel awful and congested, and my head hurts. I think my sinus infection is back."

■ HPI

Kyle Rhiner is a 49-year-old man who presents to his primary care physician with fever, purulent nasal discharge from the left naris, facial pain (L > R), nasal congestion, headache, and fatigue. He states that his symptoms began 8 days ago, but the symptoms initially improved over the first 4–5 days. However, the symptoms have become progressively worse over the last few days. He also complains of intense facial pressure when he bends forward to tie his shoes or to pick up something. He has noticed a decreased ability to smell and states that foods do not taste the same as before. He has experienced occasional episodes of nausea, dizziness, tremors, and palpitations for the last week and states that he has difficulty sleeping. He has been taking ibuprofen as needed and loratadine 5 mg/pseudoephedrine sulfate 120 mg every 12 hours but has received little relief from his symptoms. He denies vomiting, diarrhea, chills, diaphoresis, dyspnea, productive cough, or allergies. Mr Rhiner states that he was treated for a sinus infection about 3–4 weeks ago. When questioned further, he states that he presented to an urgent care clinic complaining of a runny nose, congestion, sneezing, cough, and a mild sore throat for 2–3 days. He was leaving the following day for a business trip and asked the physician for an antibiotic prescription. He told the physician that azithromycin has always worked for him so he was prescribed a Z-Pak. His symptoms slowly improved over several days, and he was symptom-free for a few days before his current symptoms began 8 days ago. He states that he only gets sick occasionally and has not had an infection in the last year prior to these episodes.

■ PMH

Sinus infection 3–4 weeks ago
Hypertension (well controlled with medication)
Hypercholesterolemia

■ FH

Father died of MI at 64 years of age.
Mother with hypertension and diabetes mellitus.

■ SH

Smokes cigars on occasion (one to two per week). Denies cigarette smoking and illicit drug use. Drinks socially (three to four beers and one bottle of red wine per week). He is divorced with two children (23-year-old son, 21-year-old daughter).

■ Meds

Lisinopril 20 mg PO daily
Hydrochlorothiazide 25 mg PO daily
Simvastatin 40 mg PO daily
Ibuprofen 200–400 mg PO as needed
Claritin-D 12 hours (loratadine 5 mg/pseudoephedrine sulfate 120 mg) PO Q 12 H

■ All

None

■ ROS

Patient with an 8-day history of fever, purulent nasal drainage, congestion, facial pain, headache, fatigue, hyposmia, and occasional nausea, dizziness, and palpitations. The symptoms improved initially but have progressively worsened over the last few days. In addition, the patient complains of insomnia, which may be contributing to the fatigue. He has hypertension and hypercholesterolemia, and he was treated for sinusitis approximately 3–4 weeks ago.

■ Physical Examination

Gen

Tired-looking, overweight white man in mild distress; appears uncomfortable

VS

BP 158/102, P 90, RR 16, T 39.3°C; Wt 118 kg, Ht 6′1″

Skin

Warm to touch; good skin turgor; no other abnormalities

HEENT

NC/AT; PERRLA; EOMI; funduscopic exam normal; injected conjunctivae; anicteric sclerae. Thick, purulent, yellow-green nasal discharge; mucosal hypertrophy (L > R) without evidence of nasal polyps. Facial pain over left maxillary and frontal sinuses. No oral lesions; no periorbital swelling. Tympanic membranes intact, non-erythematous, nonbulging. Throat erythematous.

Neck/Lymph Nodes

Supple, no JVD, mild lymphadenopathy

Lungs/Thorax

CTA; no crackles or wheezing

CV

Slightly tachycardic; normal S_1 and S_2, no MRG

Abd

Soft, nontender; bowel sounds present; no masses

Genit/Rect

Deferred

MS/Ext

No CCE

Neuro

A & O × 3; CN II–XII intact

■ **Labs**

None obtained

■ **Assessment**

Recurrent rhinosinusitis
Hypertension
Dizziness, tremors, palpitations

QUESTIONS

Problem Identification

1.a. Create a list of the patient's drug therapy problems.

1.b. What subjective and objective data support the diagnosis of acute bacterial rhinosinusitis versus viral rhinosinusitis?

1.c. What are the three cardinal symptoms of acute rhinosinusitis?

1.d. What diagnostic studies (cultures, radiographs, sinus CT, etc.), if any, should be obtained before recommending therapy?

1.e. Should the patient have been treated with an antibiotic for his initial presentation 3–4 weeks ago? Why or why not? If yes, what antibiotic should the patient have received?

Desired Outcome

2. What are the goals of pharmacotherapy for this patient?

Therapeutic Alternatives

3.a. What are the most likely causative bacterial pathogens in this patient?

3.b. Based on the patient's current symptoms, is he a candidate for watchful waiting (ie, observation without antibiotic therapy) as a therapeutic option in his treatment plan?

3.c. What antibiotics and dosage regimens are appropriate treatment options for the patient at this time?

3.d. What are the most likely reasons why this patient has an infection despite receiving previous antibiotic therapy?

Optimal Plan

4.a. Based on the patient's clinical presentation, what antibiotic would you recommend for therapy? Include drug name, dosage form, schedule, and duration of therapy.

4.b. What adjunctive measures can be employed to optimize the patient's medical therapy?

4.c. What alternatives, if any, would be appropriate if the patient fails to respond to the initial regimen?

Outcome Evaluation

5. What clinical parameters are necessary to evaluate the therapy for achievement of the desired therapeutic outcome and to detect or prevent adverse effects?

Patient Education

6. What information should be provided to the patient to ensure successful therapy, enhance adherence, and minimize adverse effects?

■ SELF-STUDY ASSIGNMENTS

1. Determine if a change in mucus color from clear to yellow or green is an indication of a bacterial infection or if it is the natural course of a viral infection.

2. If the patient had a penicillin allergy, review the likelihood of an allergic reaction if he had received a cephalosporin.

3. Review the pharmacokinetic and pharmacodynamic properties of antibacterial agents commonly used in the treatment of acute bacterial rhinosinusitis.

4. Review the most common mechanisms of bacterial resistance in pathogens frequently encountered in acute bacterial rhinosinusitis.

CLINICAL PEARL

The etiology of most cases of acute rhinosinusitis is viral; however, an antibiotic is prescribed in approximately 80% of cases. In patients with a clinical diagnosis of acute bacterial rhinosinusitis, the spontaneous resolution rate is 50–60%. This information is important to consider when evaluating antimicrobial efficacy from comparative clinical studies.

REFERENCES

1. Chow AW, Benninger MS, Brook I, et al. IDSA clinical practice guideline for acute bacterial rhinosinusitis in children and adults. Clin Infect Dis 2012;54:e72–e112.

2. Rosenfeld RM, Piccirillo JF, Chandrasekhar SS, et al. Clinical practice guideline (update): adult sinusitis. Otolaryngol Head Neck Surg 2015;152 (2 Suppl):S1–S39.

3. Rosenfeld RM, Andes D, Bhattacharyya N, et al. Clinical practice guidelines: adult sinusitis. Otolaryngol Head Neck Surg 2007;137(Suppl 3):S1–S31.

4. Benninger MS, Payne SC, Ferguson BJ, Hadley JA, Ahmad N. Endoscopically directed middle meatal cultures versus maxillary sinus taps in acute bacterial maxillary rhinosinusitis: a meta-analysis. Otolaryngol Head Neck Surg 2006;134:3–9.

5. Smith SS, Kern RC, Chandra RK, Tan BK, Evans CT. Variations in antibiotic prescribing of acute rhinosinusitis in United States ambulatory settings. Otolaryngol Head Neck Surg 2013;148:852–859.

6. Donnelly JP, Baddley JW, Wang HE. Antibiotic utilization for acute respiratory tract infections in U.S. emergency departments. Antimicrob Agents Chemother 2014;58:1451–1457.

7. Benninger M, Brook I, Farrell DJ. Disease severity in acute bacterial rhinosinusitis is greater in patients infected with *Streptococcus pneumoniae* than in those infected with *Haemophilus influenzae*. Otolaryngol Head Neck Surg 2006;135:523–528.

8. Karageorgopoulos DE, Giannopoulou KP, Grammatikos AP, Dimopoulos G, Falagas ME. Fluoroquinolones compared with β-lactam antibiotics for the treatment of acute bacterial sinusitis: a meta-analysis of randomized controlled trials. CMAJ 2008;178:845–854.

9. Jones RN, Sader HS, Mendes RE, Flamm RK. Update on antimicrobial susceptibility trends among *Streptococcus pneumoniae* in the United States: report of ceftaroline activity from the SENTRY Antimicrobial Surveillance Program (1998–2011). Diagn Microbiol Infect Dis 2013;75:107–109.

10. Flamm RK, Mendes RE, Hogan PA, Ross JE, Farrell DJ, Jones RN. In vitro activity of linezolid as assessed through the 2013 LEADER surveillance program. Diagn Microbiol Infect Dis 2015;81:283–289.

124

ACUTE PHARYNGITIS

A Serious Pain in the Neck . . . . Level I

Anthony J. Guarascio, PharmD, BCPS

Catherine Johnson, PhD, FNP, PNP

LEARNING OBJECTIVES

After completing this case study, the reader should be able to:

- Evaluate the need for antibiotic therapy in a patient with pharyngitis based on signs and symptoms as well as microbiological and immunological diagnostic studies.

- Identify the most common organisms responsible for causing pharyngitis.

- Select an appropriate pharmacologic regimen for a patient with acute pharyngitis, including route, frequency, and duration.

- List the suppurative and nonsuppurative complications of acute pharyngitis, as well as the prevalence of these complications, and the measures to prevent occurrence.

PATIENT PRESENTATION

■ Chief Complaint

"It hurts to swallow."

■ HPI

David Jacobs is a 5-year-old boy who presents to his pediatrician complaining of sore throat. His mother states he has had fever of 102°F on and off for the past 24 hours and was treated with acetaminophen. He has also been sleeping more than usual over the past 2 days. He has refused to eat anything solid since this time but has been drinking liquids. His mother states he does not have a cough, shortness of breath, or difficulty breathing. The patient mentions that both his stomach and head aches, but his mother states he has not vomited. Mother notes no recent illness in the family.

■ PMH

The patient has had prior cases of otitis media, his last over a year ago. Otherwise he is healthy. His mother states that he is up-to-date on all vaccinations.

■ FH

Noncontributory

■ SH

David lives with his parents and infant sister. He attends a local day care and preschool.

■ Meds

None

■ All

Amoxicillin: rash, hives

■ ROS

Negative except for complaints noted in the HPI

■ Physical Examination

Gen

WDWN 5-year-old male, clearly fatigued

VS

BP 104/70, P 92, RR 22, T 38.8°C, Wt 21 kg, Ht 45″

Skin

Pale, warm, faint scarlatiniform rash on arms and trunk

HEENT

PERRLA; tonsils erythematous with associated white exudates; uvula edematous; soft palate with notable petechiae, TM normal

Neck/Lymph Nodes

Multiple enlarged anterior cervical lymph nodes, greater than 2 cm in size

Lungs/Thorax

CTA bilaterally, (–) shortness of breath, (–) cough

CV

RRR, normal S_1 and S_2

Abd

Soft, nontender, nondistended, (+) BS

Genit/Rect

Deferred

Neuro

CN I–XII intact

▧ Labs

RADT: negative
Throat culture: results pending

▧ Assessment

A 5-year-old male presents to the pediatrician with suspected group A β-hemolytic streptococcus (GABHS) pharyngitis.

QUESTIONS

Problem Identification

1.a. What are the signs and symptoms in this patient that are indicative of possible GABHS infection in comparison with symptoms of viral pharyngitis?

1.b. What diagnostic tool(s) may be used to facilitate a diagnosis? Describe differences in implementation and sensitivity/specificity between testing methods and how these differences influence clinical interpretation.

1.c. When can throat culture results be expected to return? Based on clinical interpretation of DJ's signs and symptoms, what is the expected result of this culture?

Desired Outcome

2. List the goals of therapy for both treatment and the prevention of clinical and pharmacologic complications.

Therapeutic Alternatives

3.a. What nonpharmacologic therapies are available for treatment of GABHS acute pharyngitis?

3.b. What are the pharmacologic options for GABHS acute pharyngitis?

Optimal Plan

4.a. Assuming DJ's throat culture returns positive for GABHS, what is the preferred treatment for DJ's acute pharyngitis? Include dose, route, frequency, and duration.

4.b. Which option would be most appropriate if DJ had not reported an amoxicillin allergy?

Outcome Evaluation

5.a. What should be monitored to evaluate successful therapy and/or development of adverse effects?

5.b. What would be the appropriate management strategy if DJ's infection did not resolve?

Patient Education

6. What information should be shared with DJ and his parents regarding his clinical condition as well as his drug therapy?

■ SELF-STUDY ASSIGNMENTS

1. Create a table that lists the preferred and alternative therapeutic options for GABHS pharyngitis and includes the following comparative data:
   - Drug
   - Dose
   - Frequency
   - Duration
   - Available dosage forms
   - Adverse effects
   - Cost

2. Prepare a one-page paper that describes the incidence, risk factors, signs/symptoms, and onset of scarlet fever, rheumatic fever, and poststreptococcal glomerulonephritis.

CLINICAL PEARL

While early initiation of antibiotic therapy can reduce the duration of GABHS symptoms, withholding antibiotics until laboratory confirmation of GABHS bacterial disease in the majority of clinical circumstances can reduce the potential for inappropriate antibiotic therapy while still preventing the spread of GABHS to others.

Acknowledgment

This case is based on the case written by John L. Lock, PharmD, BCPS, AQ-ID, for the 9th edition of the Casebook.

REFERENCES

1. Gerber MA, Baltimore RS, Eaton CB, et al. Prevention of rheumatic fever and diagnosis and treatment of acute streptococcal pharyngitis. Circulation 2009;119:1541–1551.
2. Shulman ST, Bisno AL, Clegg HW, et al. Practice guidelines for the diagnosis and management of group A streptococcal pharyngitis: 2012 update by the Infectious Diseases Society of America. Clin Infect Dis 2012;55:1279–1282.
3. Wessels MR. Streptococcal pharyngitis. N Engl J Med 2011;364:648–655.
4. Tanz RR, Gerber MA, Kabat W, Rippe J, Seshadri R, Shulman ST. Performance of a rapid antigen-detection test and throat culture in community pediatric offices: implications for management of pharyngitis. Pediatrics 2009;123:437–444.
5. McIsaac WJ, Kellner JD, Aufricht P, Vanjaka A, Low DE. Empirical validation of guidelines for the management of pharyngitis in children and adults. JAMA 2004;291:1587–1595.
6. Center for Medicare and Medicaid Services. 2014 Clinical Quality Measures (CQMs): Pediatric Recommended Core Measures. *https://www.cms.gov/Regulations-and-Guidance/Legislation/EHRIncentivePrograms/Downloads/2014_CQM_PrediatricRecommended_CoreSetTable.pdf.* Accessed March 30, 2016.
7. Tanz RR, Shulman ST, Shortridge VD, et al. Community-based surveillance in the United States of macrolide-resistant pediatric pharyngeal group A streptococci during 3 respiratory disease seasons. Clin Infect Dis 2004;39:1794–1801.
8. Centers for Disease Control and Prevention. Is It Strep Throat? *http://www.cdc.gov/Features/strepthroat/.* Accessed March 30, 2016.

125

INFLUENZA

Run Over by the Flu .... Level II

Margarita V. Divall, PharmD, MEd, BCPS

LEARNING OBJECTIVES

After completing this case study, the reader should be able to:

- Recognize the clinical presentation of influenza.

- Discuss influenza-related complications.

- Develop a patient-specific treatment plan for influenza.

- Identify appropriate target populations for vaccination against influenza.

- Compare and contrast available options for preventing influenza.

- Discuss strategies to control influenza outbreaks.

PATIENT PRESENTATION

■ Chief Complaint

"I feel like a truck ran over me. Every muscle and bone hurts, and I am burning up."

■ HPI

Vladimir Kharitonov is a 67-year-old Russian man who presents in mid-December to an urgent care clinic with complaints of 1-day history of fever, up to 39°C (102.2°F), muscle and bone aches, feeling tired, and headache. He has not had anything to eat in the past 12 hours due to loss of appetite and has not taken his glyburide this morning. He has been in his usual state of health previously and reports that some of his coworkers have been sick with the "flu." He decided to come to the clinic in hopes that an antibiotic can allow him to recover sooner since his son is getting married next weekend. He missed his regular physical appointment 1 month ago because he was "too busy."

■ PMH

Type 2 DM for 14 years
Hyperlipidemia
HTN

■ FH

Father and sister with type 2 DM

■ SH

Lives at home with his wife; works full time; quit smoking 10 years ago, but smokes occasionally when really stressed or in a social setting; drinks alcohol in a social setting—mostly vodka

■ Meds

Aspirin 81 mg PO daily
Hydrochlorothiazide 25 mg PO daily
Glyburide 5 mg PO every morning
Metformin 1 g PO twice daily
Lantus 35 units SC at bedtime
Lipitor 10 mg PO daily
Centrum Silver one tablet PO daily

■ All

NKDA

■ ROS

Complains of severe fatigue, body aches, alternating between being too cold and sweating, sore throat, nonproductive cough, and a headache. He denies nasal congestion, nausea, vomiting, or diarrhea.

■ Physical Examination

Gen

WDWN overweight man in NAD

VS

BP 150/90 (patient reports similar readings at home), P 95, RR 18, T 38.5°C; Wt 95.5 kg, Ht 5'10"

Skin

Warm and moist secondary to diaphoresis, no lesions

HEENT

PERRLA; EOMI; TMs intact; wears dentures; mild pharyngeal erythema with no exudates

Neck/Lymph Nodes

Neck is supple and without adenopathy; no JVD

Lungs/Thorax

CTA; no crackles or wheezing

CV

RRR; normal S_1, S_2; no murmurs

Abd

Soft, slightly obese; NT/ND; normal BS

Genit/Rect

Not performed

MS/Ext

Muscle strength and tone 4–5/5; no CCE

Neuro

A & O × 3; CN II–XII intact; decreased sensation to light touch of the lower extremities (both feet)

■ Labs

Na 138 mEq/L	Hgb 13.2 g/dL	WBC 10 × 10³/mm³	Fasting lipid profile
K 3.8 mEq/L	Hct 41%	Neutros 50%	T. chol 177 mg/dL
Cl 98 mEq/L	Plt 275 × 10³/mm³	Bands 4%	LDL 110 mg/dL
CO_2 24 mEq/L		Eos 0%	HDL 35 mg/dL
BUN 26 mg/dL		Lymphs 39%	Trig 160 mg/dL
SCr 1.3 mg/dL		Monos 7%	
Glu 135 mg/dL			
A1C 7.1%			

■ **Diagnostic Tests**

QuickVue rapid influenza test—positive

■ **Assessment**

A 67-year-old man with diabetes, HTN, and hyperlipidemia presents with influenza.

QUESTIONS

Problem Identification

1.a. Create a list of patient's drug therapy problems.

1.b. What information (signs, symptoms, and laboratory values) indicates the presence of influenza?

1.c. What diagnostic tests are available to confirm and differentiate among the different types and subtypes of influenza? Should laboratory testing be performed in all patients presenting with flu-like illness?

1.d. What influenza-related complications is this patient at risk for developing?

Desired Outcome

2. What are the goals of pharmacotherapy in this case?

Therapeutic Alternatives

3.a. List available options for treating influenza in this patient. Include the drug name, dose, dosage form, route, frequency, and treatment duration. Are these options affected by the type of influenza that this patient experiences and/or time since onset of illness?

3.b. What other therapies are available to help this patient with his symptoms?

3.c. Should all patients with confirmed influenza receive treatment with antiviral medications?

Optimal Plan

4.a. Provide your individualized treatment recommendations for treating this patient's influenza, including symptom management.

4.b. Outline your plans for managing each of the patient's other drug therapy problems.

Outcome Evaluation

5. What clinical and laboratory parameters are necessary to evaluate the therapy for achievement of the desired therapeutic outcome and detect or prevent adverse effects?

Patient Education

6. What information should be provided to the patient to enhance adherence, ensure successful therapy, and minimize adverse effects?

■ CLINICAL COURSE

In October of the following year, Mr Kharitonov presents for his routine physical exam. He has been doing very well. His diabetes, hypertension, and hyperlipidemia are well controlled.

■ FOLLOW-UP QUESTIONS

1. What indications does this patient have for administration of the seasonal influenza vaccine?

2. If the vaccine is desirable, what is the optimal time frame for this patient to receive vaccination(s)?

3. What are all available options for vaccination against seasonal influenza?

4. Provide your individualized recommendations for protecting this patient against influenza virus infections.

■ CLINICAL COURSE: ALTERNATIVE THERAPY

As Mr Kharitonov is leaving, he thanks you and promises to follow your recommendations. He states that he is worried about making anyone else sick, because of his son's upcoming wedding. "My cousins back in Russia keep telling me they use elderberry syrup to keep from getting sick during flu season. Could that help keep my wife from getting this flu?" See Section 19 in this Casebook for information regarding the use of elderberry for influenza treatment and prevention.

■ SELF-STUDY ASSIGNMENTS

1. Prepare an educational pamphlet on influenza prevention and treatment directed at both patients and general practice physicians. Be sure to include recommendations for controlling influenza outbreaks.

2. Investigate the role of pharmacists as immunization providers.

3. Investigate the threat of human infection with avian influenza viruses. Are currently available influenza prevention strategies effective against avian flu?

CLINICAL PEARL

Development of antibodies takes approximately 2 weeks after influenza vaccination in adults, during which time they remain at high risk for influenza infection. If the immunization occurs during an influenza outbreak, chemoprophylaxis with antiviral agents can be administered for 2 weeks immediately after vaccination to minimize the risk of infection. The live attenuated influenza vaccine (LAIV) can cause a false-positive result for up to 7 days on a rapid influenza diagnostic test since these tests cannot differentiate between live attenuated and wild-type influenza viruses.

REFERENCES

1. Harper SA, Bradley JS, Englund JA, et al. Seasonal influenza in adults and children—diagnosis, treatment, chemoprophylaxis and institutional outbreak management: clinical practice guidelines of the Infectious Diseases Society of America for seasonal influenza in adults and children. Clin Infect Dis 2009;48:1003–1032.

2. Fiore AE, Fry A, Shay D, et al. Antiviral agents for the treatment and chemoprophylaxis of influenza—recommendations of the Advisory Committee on Immunization Practices (ACIP). MMWR Recomm Rep 2011;60(1):1–24.

3. United States Centers for Disease Control and Prevention. Guidance for clinicians on the use of rapid influenza diagnostic tests. Available at: *http://www.cdc.gov/flu/professionals/diagnosis/clinician_guidance_ridt.htm*. Accessed March 30, 2016.

4. United States Centers for Disease Control and Prevention. FDA-cleared RT-PCR assays and other molecular assays for influenza viruses. Available at: *http://www.cdc.gov/flu/pdf/professionals/diagnosis/table1-molecular-assays.pdf*. Accessed March 30, 2016.

5. Center for Disease Control and Prevention. Influenza antiviral medications: summary for clinicians. Available at: *http://www.cdc.gov/flu/professionals/antivirals/*. Accessed March 30, 2016.

6. Louie JK, Yang S, Acosta M, et al. Treatment with neuraminidase inhibitors for critically ill patients with influenza A (H1N1)pdm09. Clin Infect Dis 2012;55(9):1198–1204.

7. Prevention and control of influenza with vaccines: recommendations of the Advisory Committee on Immunization Practices—United States, 2015–2016 influenza season. MMWR Morb Mortal Wkly Rep 2015;64(30):818–825.

8. James PA, Oparil S, Carter BL. 2014 evidence-based guidelines for the management of high blood pressure in adults: report from the panel members appointed to the Eighth Joint National Committee (JNC 8). JAMA 2014;311(5):507–520.

9. Stone NJ, Robinson JG, Lichtenstein AH, et al. 2013 ACC/AHA Guideline on the Treatment of Blood Cholesterol to Reduce Atherosclerotic Cardiovascular Risk in Adults: A Report of the American College of Cardiology/American Heart Association Task Force on Practice Guidelines. Circulation 2014;129(25 Suppl 2):S1–S45.

10. Black S, Nicolay U, Del Giudice G, Rappuoli R. Influence of Statins on Influenza Vaccine Response in Elderly Individuals. J Infect Dis 2015;213(8):1224–1228.

126

SKIN AND SOFT TISSUE INFECTION

A Pain in the Butt.............................. Level II

Jarrett R. Amsden, PharmD, BCPS

LEARNING OBJECTIVES

After completing this case study, the reader should be able to:

- Evaluate the signs and symptoms of skin and soft tissue infections (SSTIs).

- Recommend appropriate empiric nonpharmacologic and pharmacologic treatment options for patients presenting with SSTIs.

- Differentiate between the definition and clinical manifestations of mild, moderate and severe SSTI.

- Compare and contrast the clinical characteristics and presentation of a purulent vs nonpurulent SSTI.

- Design an antimicrobial treatment regimen for a purulent and nonpurulent SSTIs that are either: mild, moderate or severe.

- Develop a list of alternative therapeutic options for the treatment of purulent and nonpurulent SSTIs that are either: mild, moderate or severe.

- Identify treatment modalities for decolonizing a patient with recurrent purulent SSTIs.

PATIENT PRESENTATION

■ Chief Complaint

"I have a boil on my butt, and I cannot sit down for class."

■ HPI

Jimmie Chipwood is a 19-year-old college student who presents to the ED with a new-onset "boil" on his right buttock. He noticed some pain and irritation in the right buttock area over the past week, but thought it was due to having slid into second base during a baseball game. The pain gradually increased over the next few days, and he went to the student health center, where they cleaned the wound and gave him a prescription for clindamycin 300 mg QID for 7 days. They recommended he try to keep the area covered until the antibiotic began to work. Today, Jimmie returned to the student health center for further evaluation and was referred to the ED for further care for his continued SSTI. At the ED, Jimmie says the area on his buttock is worse, and he cannot sit down for class. He reports only partial adherence to the clindamycin regimen, because he often forgets to take it and says it makes him nauseous.

■ PMH

Right gluteal skins and soft tissue infection, diagnosed approximately 1 week ago (Rx for clindamycin was given, but the patient reports nonadherence).

■ Surgical History

2010—appendectomy
2012—repair of left ACL

■ SH

Denies any alcohol or illicit drug use.

■ Meds

Clindamycin 300 mg PO QID × 7 days (prescribed at student health center visit 1 week ago; patient did not complete full course).

■ All

Penicillin (hives as a child)

■ Immunizations

Up-to-date per student health center records

■ ROS

Negative except for complaints noted in HPI

■ Physical Examination

Gen

WDWN Caucasian male in no acute distress, but with noticeable pain when he walks and tries to sit

VS

BP 129/74, P 96, RR 16, T 37.5°C; Wt 77.5 kg, Ht 6′0″

Skin

Right gluteal area: red, erythematous, warm, and tender to touch; localized fluid collection that appears fluctuant, consistent with a carbuncle and surrounding erythema

HEENT

PERRLA; EOMI, oropharynx clear

Neck/Lymph Nodes

Supple, no lymphadenopathy

Lungs/Thorax

CTA, no rales or wheezing

CV

RRR, no MRG

Abd

Soft, NT/ND; (+) BS

Genit/Rect

Large 2 cm × 4 cm red swollen area over the right buttock, with a localized fluid collection and surrounding erythema

MS/Ext

Upper extremities: WNL
Lower extremities: could not be adequately assessed due to patient's inability to sit; 2+ pulses bilaterally

Neuro

A & O × 3

■ Labs

Na 138 mEq/L	Hgb 15.5 g/dL	WBC 11.3 × 10³/mm³
K 3.2 mEq/L	Hct 44%	Neutros 89%
Cl 98 mEq/L	Plt 279 × 10³/mm³	Lymphs 10%
CO_2 23 mEq/L		Monos 1%
BUN 33 mg/dL		
SCr 0.9 mg/dL		
Glu 95 mg/dL		
Ca 9.4 mg/dL		

■ Urine Drug Screen

(–) Alcohol, (–) marijuana, (–) cocaine and other substances

■ Assessment

Progressive right gluteal SSTI with focal area of fluctuance/fluid

QUESTIONS

Problem Identification

1.a. Classify this patient's SSTI as purulent or nonpurulent and either: mild, moderate or severe.

1.b. What subjective and objective clinical data are consistent with the diagnosis of purulent SSTI?

1.c. What are the most common causative organisms of a purulent vs nonpurulent SSTI?

Desired Outcome

2.a. What are the goals of nonpharmacologic management of this patient's SSTI?

2.b. What are the goals of pharmacotherapy for the treatment of this patient's SSTI?

Therapeutic Alternatives

3.a. Create a list of nonpharmacologic treatment or supportive options for this patient in the treatment of SSTI.

3.b. What feasible oral antimicrobial options are available for the treatment of purulent and nonpurulent SSTIs?

Optimal Plan

4.a. What is the most appropriate treatment course for this patient (pharmacologic vs nonpharmacologic)?

4.b. What antimicrobial agent (or agents), dosage form, dose, schedule, and duration of therapy are best for this patient, if any?

■ CLINICAL COURSE

The patient was treated in the ED with I&D alone and was given wound care instructions. The fluid was not sent for culture and sensitivity. He returns to the ED 8 days later with a recurrent boil in the same right buttock area. On physical exam, the patient is found to have a new area of fluid collection (1 cm × 3 cm) and surrounding erythema. An MRI of the gluteal area was negative for deep tissue involvement and extension to other adjacent areas. Two sets of blood cultures were drawn and are pending, and a second I&D of the area was performed. The patient did have his nares and groin area swabbed for MRSA detection, but the results are pending. The patient has reported mild fevers without chills, but he has not taken his temperature at home. His current temperature is 37.7°C and all other vital signs are stable. Given the current information, the ED physician does not think Jimmie needs to be admitted.

Microbiology

Blood cultures × 2 sets: pending
Culture of abscess fluid from right buttock: pending
Nares swab: pending
Groin swab: pending

Imaging Studies

Negative for deep tissue involvement; localized area of inflammation and fluid consistent with an abscess.

Optimal Plan (continued)

4.c. Was I&D alone an appropriate management strategy for the initial presentation of this patient case?

4.d. Based on the above information, the patient has failed oral clindamycin (arguably) and an initial I&D. Does this patient need antibiotic therapy in addition to the second I&D and if so, what antimicrobial regimen would you now recommend for this patient? (Please specify dose, schedule, and duration of therapy.)

4.e. What are some nonpharmacologic (focus on hygiene or environmental) measures (outside of proper local/wound care) you could recommend for Jimmie to use at home/school/in the locker room?

4.f. What decolonization measures could be considered for Jimmie, if his nares and/or groin culture(s) is/are positive for MRSA? (Please discuss the relative options for both, if you would treat them differently.)

Outcome Evaluation

5. What clinical and laboratory parameters are necessary to evaluate the therapy for its effectiveness in treating this patient's SSTI?

Patient Education

6. What information should be provided to the patient to ensure successful therapy?

■ SELF-STUDY ASSIGNMENTS

1. Compare and contrast the therapeutic alternatives for the treatment of mild, moderate and severe SSTIs with purulence vs SSTIs without purulence.

2. Prepare a table that differentiates the presentation, signs, and symptoms of the patient in this case with those of a patient presenting with erysipelas, diabetic foot infection, as well as necrotizing fasciitis and also the organisms involved in each infection, respectively.

CLINICAL PEARL

Necrotizing fasciitis is a severe, progressing form of cellulitis that affects the subcutaneous tissues and moves along the superficial fascia. The infection may encompass all the tissues from the skin to the muscle. The most commonly implicated organisms are *Streptococcus pyogenes* or *Clostridium perfringens*, however in patients with exposures to fresh water *Aeromonas hydrophila* should be suspected and for those with exposures to salt water *Vibrio vulnificus* should be considered. The empiric treatment is doxycycline plus ciprofloxacin or doxycycline plus ceftazidime for *A. hydrophila* and *V. vulnificus*, respectively.[1]

REFERENCES

1. Stevens DL, Bisno AL, Chambers HF, et al. Practice guidelines for the diagnosis and management of skin and soft tissue infections: 2014 Update by the Infectious Diseases Society of America. Clin Infect Dis 2014;59:e10–52.

2. Stevens DL, Bisno AL, Chambers HF, et al. Practice guidelines for the diagnosis and management of skin and soft-tissue infections. Clin Infect Dis 2005;41:1373–1406.

3. Liu C, Bayer A, Cosgrove SE, et al. Clinical practice guidelines by the Infectious Diseases Society of America for the treatment of methicillin-resistant *Staphylococcus aureus* infections in adults and children. Clin Infect Dis 2011;52:1–38.

4. Stryjewski ME, Chambers HF. Skin and soft-tissue infections caused by community-acquired methicillin-resistant *Staphylococcus aureus*. Clin Infect Dis 2008;46:S368–S377.

5. Stein GE, Throckmorton JK, Scharmen AE, et al. Tissue penetration and antimicrobial activity of standard- and high-dose trimethoprim/sulfamethoxazole and linezolid in patients with diabetic foot infection. J Antimicrob Chemother 2013;68:2852–2858.

6. Ruhe JJ, Smith N, Bradsher RW, et al. Community-onset methicillin-resistant *Staphylococcus aureus* skin and soft-tissue infections: impact of antimicrobial therapy on outcome. Clin Infect Dis 2007;44:777–784.

7. Rajendran PM, Young D, Maurer T, et al. Randomized, double-blind, placebo-controlled trial of cephalexin for treatment of uncomplicated skin abscesses in a population at risk for community-acquired methicillin-resistant *Staphylococcus aureus* infection. Antimicrob Agent Chemother 2007;51:4044–4048.

8. Miller LG, Diep BA. Colonization, fomites, and virulence: rethinking the pathogenesis of community-associated methicillin-resistant *Staphylococcus aureus* infection. Clin Infect Dis 2008;46:752–760.

9. Barrett TW, Moran GJ. Update on emerging infections: news from the Centers for Disease Control and Prevention. Methicillin-resistant *Staphylococcus aureus* infections among competitive sports participants—Colorado, Indiana, Pennsylvania, and Los Angeles County, 2000–2003. Ann Emerg Med 2004;43:41–45.

10. McConeghy KW, Mikolich DJ, LaPlante KL. Agents for the decolonization of methicillin-resistant *Staphylococcus aureus*. Pharmacotherapy 2009;29:263–280.

127

DIABETIC FOOT INFECTION

Let's Nail That Infection . . . . Level II

Renee-Claude Mercier, PharmD, BCPS-AQ ID, PhC, FCCP

Paulina Deming, PharmD, PhC

LEARNING OBJECTIVES

After completing this case study, the reader should be able to:

- Recognize the signs and symptoms of diabetic foot infections and identify the risk factors and the most likely pathogens associated with these infections.

- Recommend appropriate antimicrobial regimens for diabetic foot infections, including for patients with drug allergies or renal insufficiency.

- Recommend appropriate home IV therapy and proper counseling to patients.

- Outline monitoring parameters for achievement of the desired pharmacotherapeutic outcomes and prevention of adverse effects.

- Counsel diabetic patients about adequate blood glucose control as part of an overall plan for good foot health.

PATIENT PRESENTATION

■ Chief Complaint

As per the Spanish interpreter: "He had an ingrown toe nail that became infected several weeks ago, and now the whole foot is swollen."

■ HPI

Jesus Chavez is a 67-year-old Hispanic man, Spanish-speaking only, who presents to the ED complaining of a sore and swollen foot. Three weeks ago he noticed that his right great toe became swollen and red due to an ingrown toenail. The patient tried to fix the nail with scissors and tweezers, but the swelling got worse, and thick, foul-smelling drainage became noticeable approximately 2 weeks ago. The patient was visiting family in Mexico at the time and now has just returned home to New Mexico. History is per translation by a hospital interpreter. The patient is accompanied by his wife who also only speaks Spanish.

Primary care physician is Dr Martinez at First Choice Clinic in Albuquerque.

■ PMH

Type 2 DM × 18 years
Hospitalized 2 months ago for HHS
Left second toe amputation 1 year ago secondary to diabetic foot infection
Hyperlipidemia
Hypertension
Chronic renal insufficiency

FH

Father is deceased (56-year-old) secondary to MI, type 2 DM, HTN
Mother is deceased secondary to breast cancer (41-year-old)
One daughter, alive and well, 42-year-old

SH

The patient lives with his wife in Albuquerque, New Mexico. He denies tobacco and illicit drug use; however, he admits to a long history of drinking four to five beers per day. He admits to nonadherence with his medications and glucometer.

Meds

Lantus SoloStar 40 units once daily
Humalog KwikPen 12 units with each meal
Metformin 1,000 mg PO twice daily
Aspirin 81 mg PO once daily
Lisinopril 20 mg PO once daily
Atorvastatin 40 mg PO daily

All

Sulfa—severe rash.

ROS

Negative except as noted in the HPI

Physical Examination

Gen

Patient is a thin Hispanic man who appears very concerned about losing his foot.

VS

BP 126/79, P 92, RR 20, T 38.4°C; Wt 60 kg, Ht 5′10″

Skin

Warm, coarse, and very dry

HEENT

PERRLA; EOMI; funduscopic exam is normal with absence of hemorrhages or exudates. TMs are clouded bilaterally but with no erythema or bulging. Oropharynx shows poor dentition but is otherwise unremarkable.

Neck/Lymph Nodes

Neck is supple; normal thyroid; no JVD; no lymphadenopathy

Chest

CTA

Heart

RRR, normal S_1 and S_2

Abd

Distended, (+) BS, no guarding, no hepatosplenomegaly or masses felt

Ext

2+ edema with markedly diminished sensation of the right foot. Significant swelling and induration extend from first metatarsal to midfoot (4 cm × 5 cm) consistent with cellulitis. Purulent foul-smelling drainage expressed from great toe wound. Wound probe 2 cm deep. Pedal pulses present but diminished. Normal range of motion. Poor nail care with some fungus and overgrown toenails.

Neuro

A & O × 3; CN II–XII intact. Motor system intact (overall muscle strength 4–5/5). Sensory system exam showed a decreased sensation to light touch of the lower extremities (both feet); intact upper body sensation.

Labs

Na 136 mEq/L	Hgb 14.1 g/dL
K 3.6 mEq/L	Hct 42.3%
Cl 98 mEq/L	Plt 390 × 10³/mm³
CO_2 24 mEq/L	WBC 17.3 × 10³/mm³
BUN 30 mg/dL	PMNs 78%
SCr 2.4 mg/dL	Lymphs 17%
Glu 323 mg/dL	Monos 5%
A1C 11.8%	
ESR 73 mm/h	

X-Ray

Right foot: There is soft tissue swelling from first metatarsal to midfoot consistent with cellulitis. No fluid collection noted. No evidence of adjacent periosteal reactions or erosions to suggest radiographic evidence of osteomyelitis. No definite subcutaneous air is evident. Presence of vascular calcifications.

Assessment

Diabetic foot infection with significant cellulitis in a patient with poorly controlled diabetes mellitus.

Clinical Course

On the day of admission, the patient went to surgery for I&D. Blood and tissue specimens were sent for culture and sensitivity testing.

QUESTIONS

Problem Identification

1.a. Create a list of the patient's drug therapy problems.

1.b. What signs, symptoms, or laboratory values indicate the presence of an infection?

1.c. What risk factors for infection does the patient have?

1.d. What organisms are most likely involved in this infection?

Desired Outcome

2. What are the therapeutic goals for this patient?

Therapeutic Alternatives

3.a. What nondrug therapies might be useful for this patient?

3.b. What feasible pharmacotherapeutic alternatives are available for the empiric treatment of diabetic foot infection?

3.c. What economic and social considerations are applicable to this patient?

Optimal Plan

4. Outline a drug regimen that would provide optimal initial empiric therapy for the infection.

Outcome Evaluation

5.a. What clinical and laboratory parameters are necessary to evaluate your therapy for achievement of the desired therapeutic outcomes and monitoring for adverse effects?

■ CLINICAL COURSE

Mr Chavez received the empiric therapy you recommended until the tissue cultures were reported positive for *Bacteroides fragilis* and *Staphylococcus aureus*, and reported sensitive to vancomycin, linezolid, quinupristin/dalfopristin, and daptomycin and resistant to oxacillin (and other β-lactams), tetracycline, erythromycin, clindamycin, and sulfamethoxazole/trimethoprim. Susceptibilities are not available for *B. fragilis*. The blood cultures were all found to have no growth. The patient remained hospitalized for an additional 10 days and received a more directed antimicrobial regimen and multiple surgical debridements of the wound. The cellulitis slowly improved over this time, and multiple x-rays did not suggest osteomyelitis. He was then discharged to complete his antimicrobial regimen on an outpatient basis. Over the next 2 weeks, he received wound care at home and showed significant but slow progress in healing of the wound.

5.b. What therapeutic alternatives are available for treating this patient after results of cultures are known to contain MRSA and *B. fragilis*?

5.c. Design an optimal drug treatment plan for treating the mixed infection while he remains hospitalized.

5.d. Design an optimal pharmacotherapeutic plan for completion of his treatment after he is discharged from the hospital.

Patient Education

6. What information should be provided to the patient to enhance adherence, ensure successful therapy, and minimize adverse effects with IV vancomycin and oral metronidazole?

■ SELF-STUDY ASSIGNMENTS

1. Review in more detail different therapeutic options available for home IV therapy, including the antimicrobial agents suitable for use, types of IV lines available, and contraindications to home IV therapy.

2. Outline the patient counseling you would provide for successful home IV therapy.

3. Describe how you would educate this diabetic patient about proper foot care to prevent further skin or tissue breakdown.

CLINICAL PEARL

Treatment of diabetic foot infections with antimicrobial agents alone is often inadequate; local wound care (incision, drainage, debridement, and amputation), good glycemic control, and immobilization of the limb are often required.

REFERENCES

1. Lipsky BA, Berendt AR, Cornia PB, et al. 2012 Infectious Diseases Society of America clinical practice guideline for the diagnosis and treatment of diabetic foot infections. Clin Infect Dis 2012;54:132–173.

2. Levin ME. Management of the diabetic foot: preventing amputation. South Med J 2002;95:10–20.

3. Echániz-Aviles G, Velazquez-Meza ME, Vazquez-Larios Mdel R, Soto-Noguerón A, Hernández-Dueñas AM. Diabetic foot infection caused by community-associated methicillin-resistant *Staphylococcus aureus* (USA300). J Diabetes 2015 Nov;7(6):891–892.

4. Lipsky BA, Cannon CM, Ramani A, et al. Ceftaroline fosamil for treatment of diabetic foot infections: the CAPTURE study experience. Diabetes Metab Res Rev 2015;31(4):395–401.

5. Lipsky BA, Tabak YP, Johannes RS, Vo L, Hyde L, Weigelt JA. Skin and soft tissue infections in hospitalised patients with diabetes: culture isolates and risk factors associated with mortality, length of stay and cost. Diabetologia 2010;53:914–923.

6. Liu C, Bayer A, Cosgrove SE, et al. Clinical Practice Guidelines by the Infectious Diseases Society of America for the Treatment of Methicillin-Resistant Staphylococcus aureus infections in Adults and Children. Clin Infect Dis 2011;52:1–38.

7. Martí-Carvajal AJ, Gluud C, Nicola S, et al. Growth factors for treating diabetic foot ulcers. Cochrane Database Syst Rev 2015 Oct 28;10:1–144.

8. Guillamet CV, Kollef MH. How to stratify patients at risk for resistant bugs in skin and soft tissue infections? Curr Opin Infect Dis 2016;29(2):116–123.

9. Weigelt J, Itani K, Stevens D, Lau W, Dryden M, Knirsch C. Linezolid versus vancomycin in the treatment of complicated skin and soft tissue infections. Antimicrob Agents Chemother 2005;46:2260–2266.

10. Nicolau DP, Stein GE. Therapeutic options for diabetic foot infections: a review with an emphasis on tissue penetration characteristics. J Am Podiatr Med Assoc 2010;100:52–63.

128

INFECTIVE ENDOCARDITIS

Toxic Choices. . . . . Level II

Kristen L. Bunnell, PharmD, BCPS

Manjunath (Amit) P. Pai, PharmD

Keith A. Rodvold, PharmD, FCCP, FIDSA

LEARNING OBJECTIVES

After completing this case study, the reader should be able to:

• Identify major and minor diagnostic criteria for infective endocarditis.

• Select an appropriate empiric antibiotic regimen for presumed infective endocarditis.

• Design a pharmacotherapy regimen for endocarditis that takes into account patient-specific factors such as medication allergies, comorbidities, social history, and financial status.

• Recognize severe adverse reactions experienced by a patient receiving therapy for infective endocarditis and revise the therapeutic plan.

• Establish monitoring parameters for a selected drug therapy in the treatment of a patient with infective endocarditis.

PATIENT PRESENTATION

■ Chief Complaint

"I thought I'd feel a lot better after this surgery."

■ HPI

Bob Williams is a 66-year-old man who presents for a follow-up appointment six months after aortic valve replacement surgery for severe aortic stenosis. He reports that he's been compliant with his cardiac rehabilitation and has been taking all of his prescribed medications. However, he still feels weak and has experiencing fevers (temperatures not taken) over the last two weeks.

■ PMH

Aortic stenosis, s/p AVR with bioprosthetic valve (diagnosed 2 years ago, surgery 6 months ago)
Hypertension (diagnosed 10 years ago)
Diabetes, Type 2 (diagnosed 2 years ago)

■ FH

Father: hypertension, died of myocardial infarction at age 76

■ SH

Previous tobacco 1/2 ppd quit 8 years ago; no illicit drugs or EtOH

■ Meds

Lisinopril 10 mg PO daily
Amlodipine 10 mg PO daily
Rivaroxaban 20 mg PO daily
Metformin 1,000 mg PO twice daily

■ All

NKDA

■ ROS

Noncontributory except for complaints noted in HPI

■ Physical Examination

Gen

Patient is a Caucasian man in no apparent distress, alert and oriented

VS

BP 152/92, P 90, RR 22, T 38.9°C; Wt 92 kg, Ht 6′0″

Skin/Nails

No evidence of rash, lesions, or petechiae

HEENT

PERRLA, EOMI, anicteric sclerae, no Roth spots, normal oral mucosa and palate

Neck/Lymph Nodes

No lymphadenopathy, JVD, or thyromegaly

Lungs

Clear to auscultation; no wheezing, rales, or rhonchi

CV

RRR, normal S_1 and S_2, S_3 present, III/VI holosystolic murmur

Abd

Nontender, nondistended

Genit/Rect

Normal; guaiac-negative stool

Ext

Reflexes bilaterally 5/5 UE, 4/5 LE; no edema

Neuro

Nonfocal; alert and oriented × 3; negative asterixis

■ Labs

Na 136 mEq/L	Hgb 12.2 g/dL	WBC 13.3 × 10³/mm³
K 4.1 mEq/L	Hct 32.6%	Neutros 78%
Cl 102 mEq/L	Plt 220 × 10³/mm³	Bands 8%
CO_2 25 mEq/L	RDW 14.2%	Lymphs 12%
BUN 15 mg/dL	MCV 81.1 mm³	Monos 2%
SCr 0.8 mg/dL	MCH 26.3 pg/cell	Alb 2.1 g/dL
Glu 98 mg/dL	MCHC 34 g/dL	INR 1.0
ESR 140 mm/h		

■ ECG

Nonspecific T-wave changes

■ Chest X-Ray

Normal heart size. Lungs well expanded without opacities or infiltrates

■ Two-Dimensional Echocardiogram (Transthoracic)

Vegetations not visualized on heart valves

■ Transesophageal Echocardiogram

A six-millimeter vegetation is noted on the aortic valve with mild aortic regurgitation. Mild dehiscence of prosthetic valve is noted. No perivalvular abscess noted. (See Fig. 128-1 for location of heart valves and other cardiac structures.)

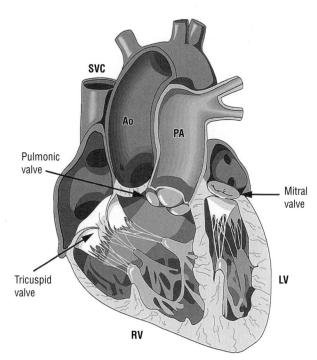

FIGURE 128-1. Diagram illustrating the location of the tricuspid, pulmonic, and mitral valves. Ao, aorta; LV, left ventricle; PA, pulmonary artery; RV, right ventricle; SVC, superior vena cava.

Blood Cultures

Two out of two sets are positive for *Staphylococcus aureus* (09:30 from left antecubital, 09:37 from right hand)

Assessment

A 66-year-old male with an aortic bioprosthetic valve replacement with several weeks of fever, positive blood cultures for *S. aureus*, and documented endocardial vegetation

QUESTIONS

Problem Identification

1.a. Create a list of the patient's drug therapy problems.

1.b. What major and minor diagnostic criteria indicate the presence of endocarditis in this patient?

1.c. What risk factors does this patient have for developing endocarditis?

1.d. Based on this patient's risk factors and location of the vegetation, does this patient have right- or left-sided endocarditis, and what is the prognostic relevance of left-sided versus right-sided endocarditis?

1.e. What are the most common microorganisms that cause infective endocarditis after cardiothoracic surgery?

Desired Outcome

2. What are the goals of pharmacotherapy for infective endocarditis?

Therapeutic Alternatives

3.a. What is an appropriate empiric regimen for Mr Williams? Include the drug names, doses, and dosage forms in your answer.

3.b. Describe alternative pharmacologic as well as non-pharmacologic approaches to the treatment of methicillin-resistant *S. aureus* endocarditis.

■ CLINICAL COURSE (PART 1)

Mr Williams is initiated on vancomycin, gentamicin, and rifampin. Susceptibility testing subsequently showed *Staphylococcus aureus* to be resistant to oxacillin, but sensitive to vancomycin (MIC = 2 mcg/mL), trimethoprim–sulfamethoxazole (MIC ≤ 20 mcg/mL), gentamicin (MIC ≤ 0.5 mcg/mL), linezolid (MIC = 1 mcg/mL), and daptomycin (MIC 0.5 mcg/mL). Cardiac surgery evaluated the patient and determined that because of the extent of valve dehiscence, surgery is indicated to repair the valve.

Optimal Plan

4.a. Because MRSA has been definitively identified as the infecting pathogen, outline a detailed pharmacotherapy plan that includes monitoring parameters, therapeutic goals, and durations of therapy for each agent.

4.b. On day 3 of therapy, a gentamicin trough of 0.6 mcg/mL and a peak of 3.1 mcg/mL are obtained around the 4th dose. Serum creatinine is 0.92 mg/mL. How should the regimen be adjusted?

■ CLINICAL COURSE (PART 2)

On post-operative day #4 from valve repair and debridement, Mr Williams' blood cultures return with gram stain positive for gram positive cocci in clusters. Blood cultures positive for MRSA with the same susceptibility pattern have now been identified from 2/2 sets on hospital day #1, and #3, #5, and #6. The most recent vancomycin trough obtained before the 6th dose was 19 mcg/mL, and the most recent gentamicin trough was 2.4 mcg/mL. Repeat labs are as follows:

Na 137 mEq/L   K 4.8 mEq/L   Cl 102 mEq/L
CO_2 20 mEq/L   BUN 31 mg/dL   SCr 1.4 mg/dL
Glu 110 mg/dL

4.c. Describe factors that may have led to therapeutic failure in this clinical scenario.

4.d. How can the antimicrobial regimen be modified based upon suspected clinical vancomycin failure and potential adverse drug reactions? Describe an alternative agent, dose schedule, and monitoring parameters.

Outcome Evaluation

5. What clinical and laboratory parameters are necessary to evaluate achievement of desired therapeutic outcomes and detect or prevent adverse effects?

■ CLINICAL COURSE (PART 3)

Mr Williams is started on daptomycin and his MRSA bacteremia clears on Day 8 of therapy. His serum creatinine decreased over 7 days and stabilized to 0.76 mg/dL, with appropriate adjustments made to his daptomycin interval. The patient is transferred to a skilled nursing facility on Day 16 for completion of antimicrobial therapy.

Patient Education

6. Prior to the patient being discharged from the nursing facility, what information should you relay to Mr Williams regarding his outpatient care and follow-up?

■ SELF-STUDY ASSIGNMENTS

1. Evaluate the clinical literature that assesses the risk of nephrotoxicity associated with higher doses of vancomycin (≥4 g per day) and targeted vancomycin concentrations.

2. Compare and contrast the potential safety concerns with the use of linezolid, daptomycin, ceftaroline, or telavancin to treat MRSA-related infections for a greater than 14-day duration of therapy.

3. Analyze the clinical literature reporting the clinical outcomes of patients who receive high-dose (≥8 mg/kg) daptomycin for treatment of *S. aureus* infections.

4. What is the role for combination antibacterial therapy in the treatment of *S. aureus* endocarditis? Consider what agents might be used, the evidence, and increased risks or benefits with combination therapy.

5. What is the role of long-term oral antibacterial therapy for bacterial suppression in cases of recurrent infective endocarditis when surgery is not a viable option?

CLINICAL PEARL

Prosthetic valve endocarditis occurs with a yearly incidence of 0.8–3.6%, and *S. aureus* is the most frequent causative pathogen. This challenging clinical scenario requires the use of combination therapy with potentially toxic agents including aminoglycosides and rifampin. Treatment failures associated with vancomycin are possible, but the ideal agent or combination of agents to use for prosthetic valve MRSA endocarditis after vancomycin failure is unknown.

REFERENCES

1. Whitlock RP, Sun JC, Fremes SE, Rubens FD, Teoh KH. Antithrombotic and thrombolytic therapy for valvular disease. Antithrombotic therapy and prevention of thrombosis, 9th ed: American College of Chest Physicians evidence-based clinical practice guidelines. CHEST 2012;141(2 Suppl):e576S–e600S.
2. Nishimura RA, Otto CM, Bonow RO, et al. 2014 AHA/ACC guideline for the management of patients with valvular heart disease. *J Am Coll Cardiol* 2014;63(22):e57–185.
3. Baddour LM, Wilson WR, Bayer AS, et al. Infective endocarditis in adults: diagnosis, antimicrobial therapy, and management of complications. A scientific statement for healthcare professionals from The American Heart Association. *Circulation* 2015;132:1435–1486.
4. Cahill TJ, Prendergast BD. Infective endocarditis. *Lancet* 2016 Feb 27;387(10021):882–893.
5. Liu C, Bayer A, Cosgrove SE, et al. Clinical practice guidelines by the Infectious Diseases Society of America for the treatment of methicillin-resistant *Staphylococcus aureus* infections in adults and children. *Clin Infect Dis* 2011;52:1–38.
6. McConeghy KW, Bleasdale SC, Rodvold KA. The empirical combination of vancomycin and a beta-lactam for staphylococcal bacteremia. *Clin Infect Dis* 2013;57:1760–1765.
7. Kullar R, Casapao AM, Davis SL, et al. A multicenter evaluation of the effectiveness and safety of high-dose daptomycin for the treatment of infective endocarditis. *J Antimicrob Chemother* 2013;68:2921–2926.
8. Sakoulas G, Moise PA, Casapao AM, et al. Antimicrobial salvage therapy for persistent Staphylococcal bacteremia using daptomycin plus ceftaroline. *Clin Ther* 2014;36(10):1317–1333.
9. Miro JM, Garcia-de-la-Maria C, Amero Y, et al. Addition of gentamicin or rifampin does not enhance the effectiveness of daptomycin in treatment of experimental endocarditis due to methicillin-resistant *Staphylococcus aureus*. *Antimicrob Agents Chemother* 2009;53(10):4172–4127.
10. Tong SYC, Davis JS, Eichenberger E, Holland TL, Fowler VG. *Staphylococcus aureus* infections: epidemiology, pathophysiology, clinical manifestations, and management. *Clin Microbiol Rev* 2014;28(3):603–661.

129

TUBERCULOSIS

Close Encounters . . . . Level II

Sharon M. Erdman, PharmD

Kendra M. Damer, PharmD

LEARNING OBJECTIVES

After completing this case study, the reader should be able to:

- Recognize the typical signs and symptoms of active pulmonary tuberculosis.

- Design a therapeutic regimen for the treatment of a patient with newly diagnosed active pulmonary tuberculosis based on patient-specific history and physical characteristics, history of present illness, subjective and objective findings, and desired clinical response.

- Develop a monitoring plan for a patient receiving treatment for active pulmonary tuberculosis to ensure efficacy and prevent/minimize toxicity.

- Provide patient education on the proper administration of drug therapy for active pulmonary tuberculosis including directions for use, the administration of therapy in relation to meals, the importance of adherence, and potential side effects of the medications.

- Recognize potential drug interactions that may occur with agents used in the treatment of active pulmonary tuberculosis.

PATIENT PRESENTATION

▓ Chief Complaint

"I have been coughing up blood for the past 3 days."

▓ HPI

Jose Rodriguez is a 35-year-old Hispanic man who presents to the ED at the county hospital in Indianapolis, Indiana, with a 3- to 4-week history of a productive cough, which was originally productive of yellow sputum but is now accompanied by the presence of blood in the sputum for the past 3 days. Along with the cough, the patient also complains of subjective fevers, chills, night sweats, dyspnea, fatigue, and an unintentional 20-lb weight loss over the past several weeks.

▓ PMH

None

▓ FH

Mother has DM and HTN.
Father died of MI 6 months ago.

▓ SH

The patient moved to the United States from Mexico 4 years ago but has not recently traveled.

Patient has a 10-pack-year history of smoking but quit several weeks ago when the current illness started. The patient denies illicit drug use, but does report drinking alcohol on weekends.

Patient is a laborer and is currently working for cash on a new home construction project in close contact with other workers. Several of his coworkers have recently moved to the United States from Mexico and have similar respiratory symptoms. The patient does not have any medical insurance.

Patient is homeless and stays at homeless shelters or friends' houses as needed.

▓ Meds

OTC antitussives, which have not provided any relief

▓ All

No known drug allergies

▓ ROS

Patient complains of a productive cough with hemoptysis for the past few days. He also complains of shortness of breath that worsens with exertion, subjective fevers, chills, night sweats, fatigue, and a 20-lb weight loss over the past several weeks.

Physical Examination

Gen

Somewhat thin-appearing Hispanic male in mild respiratory distress

VS

BP 131/70, P 100, RR 24, T 38.8°C, 93% O_2 saturation on room air; Wt 65 kg, Ht 5′9″

Skin

No lesions

HEENT

PERRLA, EOMI, no scleral icterus

Neck

Supple

Chest

Rhonchi and dullness to percussion in RUL

CV

Slightly tachycardic, no MRG

Abd

Soft NTND; (+) bowel sounds; no hepatosplenomegaly

Ext

No CCE, pulses 2+ throughout; full ROM

Neuro

A & O × 3; CN II–XII intact; reflexes 2+, sensory and motor levels intact

Labs

Na 143 mEq/L	Hgb 11.6 g/dL	WBC 12.3 × 10³/mm³	Bili 0.6 mg/dL
K 3.7 mEq/L	Hct 34.8%	Neutros 74%	Alk phos 120 IU/L
Cl 106 mEq/L	RBC 3.8 × 10⁶/mm³	Bands 8%	ALT 45 IU/L
CO₂ 22 mEq/L	Plt 269 × 10³/mm³	Lymphs 10%	AST 34 IU/L
BUN 21 mg/dL	MCV 92 μm³	Monos 8%	
SCr 0.9 mg/dL	MCHC 33 g/dL		
Glu 101 mg/dL			

Tuberculin Skin Test result: Pending
Interferon Gamma Release Assay: Pending
Sputum AFB smear: Numerous AFB (Fig. 129-1)
Sputum AFB culture: Pending
HIV antibody test (ELISA and Western blot): Pending

Radiology

CXR: RUL cavitary lesion with surrounding consolidation/air space disease (Fig. 129-2)

Chest CT: Focal airspace disease with tree-in-bud pattern in the RUL, including a cavitary lesion measuring 3.5 cm × 3.5 cm. Right hilar lymphadenopathy with scattered mediastinal lymphadenopathy. There is no pleural effusion or pneumothorax. Findings are consistent with active tuberculosis infection.

Assessment

Active pulmonary tuberculosis

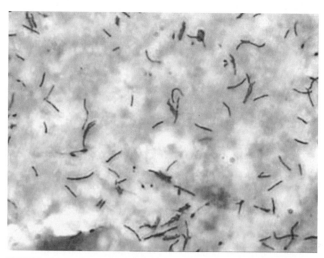

FIGURE 129-1. AFB smear. AFB (*shown as thin rods*) are tubercle bacilli.

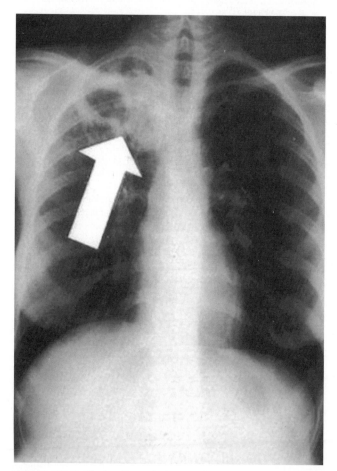

FIGURE 129-2. Chest radiograph. *Arrow* points to cavitation in patient's upper right lobe.

QUESTIONS

Problem Identification

1.a. What clinical, laboratory, and radiographic findings are consistent with the diagnosis of active pulmonary TB in this patient?

1.b. What factors place this patient at increased risk for acquiring TB?

Desired Outcome

2. What are the therapeutic goals in the treatment of active pulmonary tuberculosis?

Therapeutic Alternatives

3.a. What nonpharmacologic therapies should be considered in the management of a patient with active pulmonary tuberculosis?

3.b. What are the general principles of therapy in the management of active pulmonary tuberculosis?

3.c. What pharmacologic therapies and dosing strategies are available for the treatment of active pulmonary tuberculosis?

Optimal Plan

4.a. What specific drug regimen should be used for the treatment of this patient's active pulmonary tuberculosis, including the drugs, dosage forms, doses, schedule for administration, and duration of therapy? Include regimens that employ weekly, twice-weekly, or thrice-weekly administration of antituberculosis medications.

4.b. What economic and social considerations are applicable to this patient?

4.c. How should other close contacts of the patient be evaluated and treated?

Outcome Evaluation

5. What clinical and laboratory parameters should be monitored throughout the course of therapy to evaluate the effectiveness of therapy as well as to detect or prevent the development of adverse effects?

Patient Education

6. What information should be provided to the patient to ensure successful therapy, enhance adherence, minimize adverse effects, and avoid drug interactions?

■ CLINICAL COURSE

The patient was admitted to the hospital and placed into respiratory isolation in a negative-pressure hospital room. Because the initial sputum sample demonstrated the presence of numerous AFB, the patient was started on the antituberculosis therapy you recommended while waiting for the results of culture and susceptibility tests. On hospital day 2, his Tuberculin Skin Test (TST) was measured as 20 mm, the Interferon Gamma Release Assay (IGRA) was positive, and his HIV test result was negative. The patient tolerated the four-drug antituberculosis regimen during the initial weeks of therapy, and subsequent sputum AFB smears became negative 2 weeks after the initiation of therapy. The sputum AFB culture eventually grew *Mycobacterium tuberculosis*, which was susceptible to isoniazid, rifampin, pyrazinamide, ethambutol, and streptomycin. During the third week of antituberculosis therapy, an increase in the patient's AST (140 IU/L) and ALT (120 IU/L) was noted, although the patient appeared asymptomatic. The total bilirubin and alkaline phosphatase remained within normal limits. Follow-up mycobacterial sputum cultures obtained after 2 months of antituberculosis therapy were negative.

■ FOLLOW-UP QUESTIONS

1. How should the results of the susceptibility report of this patient's *M. tuberculosis* isolate influence his drug therapy?

2. How should the increase in AST and ALT in this patient be managed? What changes should be made to the current antituberculosis regimen and/or monitoring plan?

3. How should a patient with AST and ALT elevations greater than five times the upper limit of normal be managed?

■ SELF-STUDY ASSIGNMENTS

1. Review the differences (eg, methodology, turnaround time, advantages, disadvantages, cost) between the TST and IGRAs in the diagnosis of active pulmonary and latent tuberculosis. Discuss the populations or scenarios where the IGRA may be preferred over the TST.

2. Review the safety and efficacy of rifapentine in the management of active pulmonary tuberculosis and latent tuberculosis.

3. Perform a literature search to determine the national and regional rates of isoniazid resistance in clinical isolates of *M. tuberculosis*. How do these rates compare with those reported in other areas of the world where tuberculosis is endemic?

4. Review the management strategies of active pulmonary tuberculosis in an HIV-infected patient on antiretroviral therapy, with special attention to potential drug interactions between first-line antituberculosis agents and the non-nucleoside reverse transcriptase inhibitors or protease inhibitors.

CLINICAL PEARL

The treatment of tuberculosis in patients with HIV infection is often modified based on the many drug interactions that can occur among the rifamycins and antiretroviral agents.

REFERENCES

1. Sia IG, Wieland ML. Current concepts in the management of tuberculosis. Mayo Clin Proceed 2011;86(4):348–361.

2. American Thoracic Society, Centers for Disease Control and Prevention, Infectious Diseases Society of America. Treatment of tuberculosis. Am J Respir Crit Care Med 2003;167:603–662.

3. Zumla A, Raviglione M, Hafner R, Fordham von Reyn C. Tuberculosis. N Engl J Med 2013;368:745–755.

4. American Thoracic Society, Centers for Disease Control and Prevention, Infectious Diseases Society of America. Controlling tuberculosis in the United States. Am J Respir Crit Care Med 2005;172:1169–1227.

5. American Thoracic Society. Targeted tuberculin testing and treatment of latent tuberculosis infection. Am J Respir Crit Care Med 2000;161:S221–S247.

6. CDC. Reported Tuberculosis in the United States, 2014. Atlanta, GA, U.S. Department of Health and Human Services, CDC, October 2015.

7. Munsiff SS, Kambili C, Ahuja SD. Rifapentine for the treatment of pulmonary tuberculosis. Clin Infect Dis 2006;43:1468–1475.

8. O'Grady J, Mauerer M, Mwaba P, et al. New and improved diagnostics for detection of drug-resistant pulmonary tuberculosis. Curr Opin Pulm Med 2011;17(3):134–141.

9. Chang KC, Leung CC, Yew WW, Chan SL, Tam CM. Dosing schedules of 6-month regimens and relapse for pulmonary tuberculosis. Am J Respir Crit Care Med 2006;174:1153–1158.

10. Saukkonen JJ, Cohn DL, Jasmer RM, et al. An official ATS statement: hepatotoxicity of antituberculosis therapy. Am J Respir Crit Care Med 2006;174:935–952.

130

CLOSTRIDIUM DIFFICILE INFECTION

C. Diff-icult to Treat . . . . Level II

Michael J. Gonyeau, BS, PharmD, FCCP, BCPS

LEARNING OBJECTIVES

After completing this case study, the reader should be able to:

- Identify signs and symptoms of Clostridium difficile infection (CDI).

- Discuss CDI complications.

- Evaluate treatment options and develop an optimal patient-specific treatment plan for initial and recurrent CDI including drug, dose, frequency, route of administration, and duration of therapy.

- Develop a pertinent monitoring plan for a CDI regimen from a therapeutic and toxic standpoint.

- Discuss novel agents/treatment approaches being developed for CDI treatment.

PATIENT PRESENTATION

■ Chief Complaint

"I have been having to go to the bathroom a lot more frequently, and my stomach hurts a lot."

■ HPI

John Quinn, a 73-year-old man, is transferred to your medical team from the MICU after being admitted for urosepsis and hypotension requiring pressor support. Over the past 2 days, he has been complaining of frequent foul-smelling stools. One week prior to being transferred to your team, he was admitted to the hospital complaining of urinary frequency and urgency for 3 days, nausea, vomiting, and left-sided flank pain, as well as lightheadedness and dizziness. In the ED, the patient was noted to be hypotensive (BP 92/63 mm Hg) and tachycardic (HR 112–124), with an elevated lactate level and leukocytosis. He was transferred to the MICU for pressor support and started on an empiric regimen of ceftriaxone 2 g IV daily, levofloxacin 750 mg IV daily, and vancomycin 1 g IV Q 12 H for diagnosed urosepsis. Urine (×2) and blood (×3) cultures were subsequently found to be growing *E. coli* and enteric gram-negative rods, respectively, and antibiotic coverage was narrowed to ceftriaxone 2 g IV daily on day 5. The patient's blood pressure was stabilized, and he was transferred to the internal medicine service on day 7 of hospitalization. He is now complaining of new-onset diarrhea and abdominal pain, as described above.

■ PMH

Type 2 DM
Hyperlipidemia
HTN
s/p MI 2003

■ SH

Lives at home alone, lifetime smoker (half pack per day for 54 years), drinks alcohol socially

■ Medications

Metoprolol XL 100 mg PO once daily
Amlodipine 5 mg PO once daily
Pravastatin 20 mg PO once daily
Omeprazole 20 mg PO once daily
Metformin 500 mg PO twice daily

■ All

NKDA

■ Physical Examination

Gen

Patient is overweight and complains of abdominal discomfort.

VS

BP 139/85, P 98, RR 20, T 38.8°C; Ht 5'8", Wt 87.2 kg

Skin

Warm and moist secondary to diaphoresis, no lesions

HEENT

PERRLA; EOMI; TMs intact; clear oropharynx, moist oral mucosa

Neck/Lymph Nodes

Neck is supple and without adenopathy; no JVD

Lungs/Thorax

CTA

CV

RRR; normal S_1, S_2; no murmurs

Abd

Abdomen is soft and nondistended, diffusely tender to palpation. Slight rebound and guarding. Positive bowel sounds.

Genit/Rect

Not performed

MS/Ext

Muscle strength and tone 5/5 in upper and lower; no C/C/E

Neuro

A & O × 3; CN II–XII intact

■ Labs

Na 138 mEq/L	Hgb 16.1 g/dL	WBC 16.9 ×	T. chol 205 mg/dL
K 3.5 mEq/L	Hct 49.8%	10^3/mm³	LDL 137 mg/dL
Cl 102 mEq/L	Plt 375 × 10³/mm³	Neutros 50%	HDL 29 mg/dL
CO_2 22 mEq/L	A1C 7.9%	Bands 9%	Trig 197 mg/dL
BUN 36 mg/dL		Eos 0%	
SCr 1.8 mg/dL		Lymphs 34%	
(baseline		Monos 7%	
0.9 mg/dL)			
Glu 181 mg/dL			
Alb 1.9 mg/dL			

CXR

Clear

EKG

NSR, unchanged from previous

Clostridium difficile toxin EIA test

A/B toxin assay positive

Fecal leukocytes

Not performed

Assessment

A 73-year-old man presents with frequent, foul-smelling stools for 2 days with recent history of having received broad-spectrum antibiotics and currently receiving ceftriaxone for urosepsis (day 9); *C. difficile* toxin positive.

QUESTIONS

Problem Identification

1.a. Create a list of the patient's drug therapy problems.

1.b. How common is CDI in hospitalized patients?

1.c. What risk factors for CDI are present in this patient?

1.d. What information (signs, symptoms, laboratory values) indicates the presence of CDI?

1.e. Which antibiotics are most likely to cause CDI?

Desired Outcome

2. What are the goals of pharmacotherapy in this case?

Therapeutic Alternatives

3.a. What nonpharmacologic strategies would be prudent to implement in this patient?

3.b. List available options for treating CDI in this patient. Include the drug name, dose, dosage form, route, frequency, and treatment duration.

■ CLINICAL COURSE

Metronidazole 500 mg PO every 8 hours was initiated. Two days after starting metronidazole, the patient continued to have frequent foul-smelling stools, diffuse cramping and abdominal pain, and mild fever. A subsequent *C. difficile* toxin EIA test remained positive. At that time, metronidazole was changed to 500 mg PO every 6 hours and cholestyramine 2 g PO every 8 hours was initiated.

Optimal Plan

4.a. Your medical team wants to start the patient on loperamide 2 mg PO after each bowel movement. Do you agree with this course of action? Why or why not?

4.b. Was the initial therapy appropriate in this case? Why or why not?

4.c. Outline your plans for managing each of the patient's other drug therapy problems.

Outcome Evaluation

5. What clinical and laboratory parameters are necessary to evaluate the therapy for achievement of the desired therapeutic outcome and detect or prevent adverse effects?

Patient Education

6. What information should be provided to the patient to enhance adherence, ensure successful therapy, and minimize adverse effects?

■ FOLLOW-UP QUESTIONS

1. What if our patient does not respond to initial therapy?

2. What if our patient develops similar signs and symptoms 3 weeks after successful CDI treatment?

■ SELF-STUDY ASSIGNMENTS

1. Evaluate the relationship of PPI use and CDI recurrence and develop a plan to assess patient need for PPI use on discharge.

2. Conduct a literature search and develop a policy regarding infection control procedures to reduce the risk of CDI.

3. Assess the potential use of probiotics as an adjunct in the treatment, as well as prevention of recurrent CDI.

4. Conduct a literature search to assess the potential role of fecal microbiota transplant in the treatment of recurrent CDI.

CLINICAL PEARL

CDIs are an increasing concern in hospitalized patients due to increased incidence of highly toxigenic and treatment-resistant strains. There are a number of additional antibiotics or antiprotozoal agents under investigation for treatment of CDI including nitazoxanide, tinidazole, ramoplanin, fusidic acid, and bacitracin (although rapidly developing resistance limits a number of these options). Clinical effectiveness of some of these agents looks promising, but their place in therapy is still to be determined.

REFERENCES

1. Surawicz CM, Brandt LJ, Binion DG, et al. Guidelines for diagnosis, treatment, and prevention of *Clostridium difficile* infections. Am J Gastroenterol 2013;108(4):478–479.

2. Cohen SH, Gerding DN, Johnson S, et al. Clinical practice guidelines for *Clostridium difficile* infection in adults: 2010 update by the Society for Healthcare Epidemiology of America (SHEA) and the Infectious Diseases Society of America (IDSA). Infect Control Hosp Epidemiol 2010;31:431–455.

3. Pepin J, Saheb N, Coulombe MA, et al. Emergence of fluoroquinolones as the predominant risk factor for Clostridium difficile-associated diarrhea: a cohort study during an epidemic in Quebec. Clin Infect Dis 2005;41:1254–1260.

4. Bagdasarian N, Rao K, Malani PN. Diagnosis and treatment of Clostridium difficile in adults: a systematic review. JAMA 2015;313:398.

5. Debast SB, Bauer MP, Kuijper EJ. European Society of Clinical Microbiology and Infectious Diseases: update of the treatment guidance document for Clostridium difficile infection. Clin Microbiol Infect 2014;20(Suppl 2):1–26.

6. McFarland LV. Meta-analysis of probiotics for the prevention of antibiotic associated diarrhea and the treatment of Clostridium difficile disease. Am J Gastroenterol 2006;101:812–822.

7. Johnson S, Louie TJ, Gerding DN, et al. Vancomycin, metronidazole, or tolevamer for Clostridium difficile infection: results from two multinational, randomized, controlled trials. Clin Infect Dis 2014;59:345.

8. Rokas KE, Johnson JW, Beardsley JR, et al. The Addition of Intravenous Metronidazole to Oral Vancomycin is Associated with improved mortality in critically ill patients with Clostridium difficile infection. Clin Infect Dis 2015;61:934.

131

INTRA-ABDOMINAL INFECTION

Like Mother, Like Son . . . . Level II

Paulina Deming, PharmD, PhC

Renee-Claude Mercier, PharmD, BCPS, PhC

LEARNING OBJECTIVES

After completing this case study, the reader should be able to:

- Recognize the clinical manifestations of bacterial peritonitis.

- Identify the normal microflora found in the various segments of the GI tract.

- List the goals of antimicrobial therapy for bacterial peritonitis.

- Recommend appropriate empiric and definitive antibiotic therapy for spontaneous bacterial peritonitis (also known as primary bacterial peritonitis).

- Monitor antibiotic therapy for safety and efficacy.

- Recommend secondary prophylaxis for spontaneous bacterial peritonitis.

- Establish a long-term plan for the patient regarding alcohol abuse and hepatitis C, including monitoring parameters and counseling.

PATIENT PRESENTATION

■ Chief Complaint

"My belly hurts so bad I can barely move."

■ HPI

John Chavez is a 47-year-old Hispanic man who was brought to the ED by his wife. She stated that he has been suffering from nausea, vomiting, and severe abdominal pain for the last 2–3 days. His intake of food and fluids has been minimal over the past several days.

■ PMH

Cirrhosis, diagnosed 2014 with onset of ascites
GERD
Cholecystectomy 15 years ago
Chronic hepatitis C virus infection, diagnosed 2014

■ FH

Mother was alcoholic; died 10 years ago in car accident. Father's history unknown.

■ SH

Retired construction worker; EtOH abuse with 10–12 cans of beer per day × 25 years, sober for 6 months; however, recently did binge drink after an argument with his wife; denies use of tobacco or illicit drugs; poor adherence to medications and dietary restrictions

■ Meds

Spironolactone 100 mg PO once daily
Omeprazole 20 mg PO once daily
Maalox 30 mL PO QID PRN

■ All

NKDA

■ ROS

As noted in the HPI. Denies any hematemesis or melena.

■ Physical Examination

Gen

Thin man who appears older than his stated age, disoriented, and in severe pain

VS

BP 154/82, P 102, RR 32, T 38.2°C; current Wt 92 kg, (IBW 68 kg)

Skin

Jaundiced, warm, coarse, and very dry. Spider angiomata present on chest, back and arms.

HEENT

Yellow sclera; PERRLA; Oropharynges show poor dentition but are otherwise unremarkable

Neck/Lymph Nodes

Supple; normal size thyroid; no JVD or palpable lymph nodes

Chest

Lungs are CTA; shallow and frequent breathing

Heart

Tachycardia, normal S_1 and S_2 with no S_3 or S_4

Abd

Distended; pain on pressure or movements; pain is sharp and diffuse throughout abdomen; (+) guarding. (+) HSM. Decreased bowel sounds.

Genit/Rect

Prostate normal size; guaiac (–) stool

Ext

No clubbing or cyanosis; bilateral pitting pedal edema 1+

Neuro

Oriented to place; lethargic and apathetic, slumped posture, slowed movements

■ Labs

Na 142 mEq/L	Hgb 13.1 g/dL	AST 190 IU/L
K 3.9 mEq/L	Hct 40.6%	ALT 220 IU/L
Cl 96 mEq/L	Plt 65 × 10³/mm³	Alk phos 350 IU/L
CO_2 20 mEq/L	WBC 12.25 × 10³/mm³	T. bili 2.2 mg/dL
BUN 44 mg/dL	Neutros 73%	D. bili 1.8 mg/dL
SCr 1.2 mg/dL	Bands 9%	Albumin 2.8 g/dL
Glu 101 mg/dL	Lymphs 13%	INR 1.34
	Monos 5%	

▪ Abdominal US

Nodular liver consistent with cirrhosis; ascites; splenomegaly

▪ Blood Cultures

Pending × 2

▪ Paracentesis

Ascitic fluid: leukocytes 720/mm^3, protein 2.8 g/dL, albumin 1.1 g/dL, pH 7.28, lactate 30 mg/dL. Gram stain: numerous PMNs, no organisms.

▪ Assessment

Spontaneous bacterial peritonitis (SBP)

▪ CLINICAL COURSE

Because of the patient's history of cirrhosis and use of diuretics, recent low intake of fluids, and the high BUN-to-creatinine ratio, the patient was thought to be dehydrated and was given 1 L/h of 0.9% NaCl IV in the ED. His breathing became progressively worse, and he had to be intubated and transferred to the intensive care unit.

QUESTIONS

Problem Identification

1.a. Create a list of the patient's drug therapy problems.

1.b. What signs, symptoms, and laboratory values indicate the presence of SBP?

1.c. What risk factors for infection are present in this patient?

1.d. Which organisms are the most likely cause of this infection?

Desired Outcome

2. What are the therapeutic goals for this patient?

Therapeutic Alternatives

3.a. What nondrug therapies might be useful for this patient?

3.b. What feasible pharmacotherapeutic alternatives are available for the treatment of SBP?

Optimal Plan

4.a. Given this patient's condition, which drug regimens would provide optimal therapy for the infection?

4.b. In addition to antimicrobial therapy, what other drug-related interventions are required for this patient?

4.c. Which antimicrobial therapies should be avoided to prevent exacerbating kidney failure in this patient?

4.d. What pharmacotherapeutic therapies should be used for prevention of recurrent SBP?

Outcome Evaluation

5. What clinical and laboratory parameters are necessary to evaluate the therapy for achievement of the desired therapeutic outcome and to detect or prevent adverse effects?

Patient Education

6. What information should be provided to the patient to enhance adherence, ensure successful therapy, and minimize adverse effects?

▪ CLINICAL COURSE

After 48 hours of IV antibiotics, Mr Chavez was extubated. The blood cultures were reported positive for *Klebsiella pneumoniae*, resistant to ampicillin and ampicillin/sulbactam, and sensitive to aztreonam, ceftriaxone, levofloxacin, gentamicin, and piperacillin/tazobactam. The ascitic fluid culture grew *K. pneumoniae* as well. He received cefotaxime 2 g IV Q 8 H for a total of 10 days. After 3 days of antimicrobial treatment, repeat blood cultures were negative. He rapidly improved, and on discharge his mental status had returned to baseline.

▪ SELF-STUDY ASSIGNMENTS

1. Develop a table that illustrates the primary differences (clinical manifestations, pathogens involved, diagnosis methods, and treatment) between primary and secondary bacterial peritonitis.

2. Describe risk factors, modes of transmission, diagnostic methods, prognosis, and therapeutic options associated with hepatitis C.

3. Develop a table that compares the pharmacotherapeutic options for patients to assist in reducing alcohol cravings and consumption.

CLINICAL PEARL

Bacteremia is present in up to 75% of patients with primary peritonitis caused by aerobic bacteria but is rarely found in those with peritonitis caused by anaerobes. Ascitic fluid cultures are often negative and a diagnosis of SBP is frequently made based on ascitic fluid PMN counts and the patient's clinical presentation.

Patients with hepatitis C virus infections may not be diagnosed with HCV for many years until complications of liver disease, such as SBP, manifest. Hepatitis C is curable and successful viral eradication can prevent the development of cirrhosis, end-stage liver disease, and hepatocellular carcinoma.

REFERENCES

1. Garcia-Tsao G, Lim J, Veterans Affairs Hepatitis C Resource Center Program. Management and treatment of patients with cirrhosis and portal hypertension: recommendations from the department of Veterans Affairs Hepatitis C Resource Center Program and the National Hepatitis C Program. Am J Gastroenterol 2009;104:1802–1829.

2. Angeli P, Gines P, Wong F, et al. Diagnosis and management of acute kidney injury in patients with cirrhosis: revised consensus recommendations of the International Club of Ascites. Gut 2015;64:531–537.

3. Runyon BA, McHutchison JG, Antillon MR, Akriviadis EA, Montano AA. Short-course versus long-course antibiotic treatment of spontaneous bacterial peritonitis: a randomized controlled study of 100 patients. Gastroenterology 1991;100:1737–1742.

4. Runyon BA. American Association for the Study of Liver Diseases (AASLD) Practice Guideline: Management of adult patients with ascites due to cirrhosis: update 2012. Hepatology 2009;49:2087–2107.

5. Felisart J, Rimola A, Arroyo V, et al. Cefotaxime is more effective than is ampicillin–tobramycin in cirrhotics with severe infections. Hepatology 1985;5:457–462.

6. Such J, Runyon BA. Spontaneous bacterial peritonitis. Clin Infect Dis 1998;27:669–676.

7. Sigal SH, Stanca CM, Fernandez J, Arroyo V, Navasa M. Restricted use of albumin for spontaneous bacterial peritonitis. Gut 2007;56:597–599.

132

LOWER URINARY TRACT INFECTION

Where Is the Bathroom? . . . . Level I

Sharon M. Erdman, PharmD

Melissa Badowski, PharmD, BCPS, AAHIVP

Keith A. Rodvold, PharmD, FCCP, FIDSA

LEARNING OBJECTIVES

After completing this case study, the reader should be able to:

- Recognize the common signs and symptoms of acute uncomplicated cystitis/urinary tract infections (UTI) in females.

- Design a therapeutic regimen for the treatment of acute uncomplicated cystitis after consideration of symptoms, medical history, allergies, objective findings, and desired clinical response.

- Describe parameters that should be monitored during the treatment of acute uncomplicated cystitis to ensure efficacy and minimize toxicity.

- Provide patient education on the proper administration of antibiotic therapy for acute uncomplicated cystitis including directions for use, the administration of therapy in relation to meals, the importance of medication adherence (including the need to complete the entire prescribed course), proper storage, and potential side effects of the medication.

PATIENT PRESENTATION

■ Chief Complaint

"It burns when I urinate. I am urinating all the time."

■ HPI

Sarah Ramsey is a 26-year-old woman who presents to a family practice clinic in Seattle with complaints of dysuria, urinary frequency and urgency, and suprapubic tenderness for the past 2 days.

■ PMH

Patient has been diagnosed with three UTIs over the past 8 months based on symptoms, each treated with oral TMP–SMX

■ FH

Mother has DM; remainder of FH is noncontributory

■ SH

Denies smoking but admits to occasional marijuana use and social EtOH use. Patient has been sexually active with one partner for the past 9 months and typically uses spermicide-coated condoms for contraception.

■ Meds

None

■ All

No known allergies

■ ROS

Patient reports urethral pain and burning with urination, as well as mild suprapubic tenderness. Patient denies systemic symptoms such as fever, chills, vomiting, or back pain, and does not report any urethral or vaginal discharge. Upon further questioning, the patient notes that the UTIs started soon after she met her boyfriend, and she does not always completely empty her bladder after sexual intercourse.

■ Physical Examination

Gen

Cooperative woman in no acute distress

VS

BP 110/60, P 68, RR 16, T 36.8°C; Wt 57 kg, Ht 5'5"

Skin

No skin lesions

HEENT

PERRLA; EOMI; TMs intact

Neck/Lymph Nodes

Supple without lymphadenopathy

Chest

CTA

CV

RRR, no MRG

Back

No CVA tenderness

Abd

Soft; (+) bowel sounds; no organomegaly or tenderness

Pelvic

No vaginal discharge or lesions; LMP 2 weeks ago; mild suprapubic tenderness

Ext

Pulses 2+ throughout; full ROM

Neuro

A & O × 3; CN II–XII intact; reflexes 2+; sensory and motor levels intact

■ Labs

Urinalysis

Yellow, cloudy; pH 5.0; WBC 50 cells/hpf; RBC 1–5 cells/hpf; protein neg; trace blood; glucose (–); leukocyte esterase (+); nitrite positive; many bacteria (Fig. 132-1)

Urine Culture

Not performed

■ Assessment

Acute uncomplicated cystitis (Fig. 132-2)

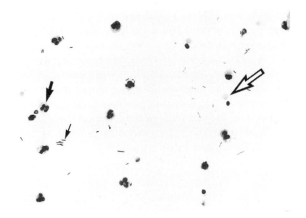

FIGURE 132-1. Urine sediment with neutrophils (*solid arrow*), bacteria (*small arrow*), and occasional red blood cells (*open arrow*) (Wright–Giemsa × 1650). (*Photo courtesy of Lydia C. Contis, MD.*)

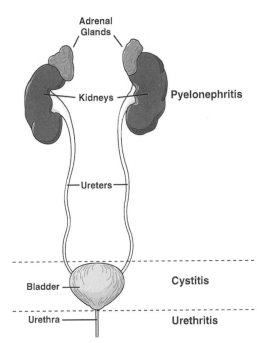

FIGURE 132-2. Anatomy and associated infections of the urinary tract.

QUESTIONS

Problem Identification

1.a. What clinical and laboratory findings are consistent with the diagnosis of acute uncomplicated cystitis in this patient?

1.b. How is the clinical presentation and diagnostic approach to acute uncomplicated cystitis different from that of urethritis (caused by *Chlamydia trachomatis*, *Neisseria gonorrhoeae*, or herpes simplex virus) or vaginitis (caused by *Candida* or *Trichomonas* species)?

1.c. Should urine cultures be obtained in patients with acute uncomplicated cystitis?

1.d. What are the most common causative pathogens of acute uncomplicated cystitis in females including their frequency of causing infection?

1.e. What are the risk factors for the development of urinary tract infections and, specifically, acute uncomplicated cystitis?

Desired Outcome

2. What are the therapeutic goals in the treatment of acute uncomplicated cystitis?

Therapeutic Alternatives

3.a. What are important antibiotic characteristics that should be considered in the treatment of acute uncomplicated cystitis?

3.b. What nonpharmacologic therapies may be useful in preventing acute uncomplicated cystitis?

3.c. What pharmacotherapeutic alternatives are available for empiric first- and second-line treatment of acute uncomplicated cystitis?

Optimal Plan

4.a. What drug, dosage form, dose, schedule, and duration of therapy are best for the treatment of this patient's acute uncomplicated cystitis?

4.b. What long-term treatment strategies could be employed for this patient with recurrent acute uncomplicated cystitis?

4.c. How should this patient be managed if she presents with continuing symptoms of a UTI 3 days after finishing the antibiotic treatment originally prescribed?

Outcome Evaluation

5. What clinical and laboratory parameters should be monitored to evaluate the efficacy of therapy and to detect or prevent adverse effects?

Patient Education

6. What information should be provided to the patient to enhance adherence, ensure successful therapy, and minimize adverse effects?

■ SELF-STUDY ASSIGNMENTS

1. Review the safety and efficacy of single-dose, 3-, 5-, and 7-day antimicrobial therapy for the treatment of acute uncomplicated cystitis.

2. Perform a literature search to obtain current data on the national and regional rates of resistance of outpatient urinary tract isolates of *Escherichia coli* to TMP–SMX and fluoroquinolone antibiotics. How do these rates compare with those reported at your institution, your clinic, or your geographic area?

3. If this patient were pregnant, what antibiotics would be appropriate for treatment?

4. Differentiate between reinfection and relapse infection.

CLINICAL PEARL

UTIs occur rarely in young males, unless there is an underlying structural abnormality or instrumentation of the urinary tract.

REFERENCES

1. Gupta K, Hooton TM, Naber KG, et al. International clinical practice guidelines for the treatment of acute uncomplicated cystitis and pyelonephritis in women: a 2010 update by the Infectious Diseases Society of America and the European Society for Microbiology and Infectious Diseases. Clin Infect Dis 2011;52:e103–e120.

2. Hooton TM. Clinical practice. Uncomplicated urinary tract infection. N Engl J Med 2012;366:1028–1037.

3. Dielubanza EJ, Schaeffer AJ. Urinary tract infections in women. Med Clin North Am 2011;95:27–41.

4. Grigoryan L, Trautner BW, Gupta K. Diagnosis and management of urinary tract infections in the outpatient setting. JAMA 2014;312(16):1677–1684.

5. Etienne M, Lefebvre E, Frebourg N, et al. Antibiotic treatment of acute uncomplicated cystitis based on rapid urine test and local epidemiology: lessons from a primary care series, BMC Infectious Diseases 2014;14:137–144.

6. Guay DR. Cranberry and urinary tract infections. Drugs 2009;69:775–807.

7. Oplinger M, Andrews CO. Nitrofurantoin contraindication in patients with a creatinine clearance below 60 mL/min: looking for the evidence. Ann Pharmacother 2013;47:106–111.

8. Singh N, Gandhi S, McArthur E, et al. Kidney function and the use of nitrofurantoin to treat urinary tract infections in older women. CMAJ 2015;187:648–656.

9. Sanchez GV, Master RN, Karlowsky JA, Bordon JM. *In vitro* antimicrobial resistance of urinary *Escherichia coli* isolates among US outpatients from 2000 to 2010. Antimicrob Agents Chemother 2012;56:2181–2183.

10. Gupta K. Emerging antibiotic resistance in urinary tract pathogens. Infect Dis Clin North Am 2003;17:243–259.

133

PYELONEPHRITIS

Resistant Rod . . . . Level II

Elizabeth A. Coyle, PharmD, FCCM, BCPS

LEARNING OBJECTIVES

After completing this case study, the reader should be able to:

- Differentiate the signs, symptoms, and laboratory findings associated with pyelonephritis from those seen in lower urinary tract infections.

- Recommend appropriate empiric antimicrobial and symptomatic pharmacotherapy for a patient with suspected pyelonephritis.

- Make appropriate adjustments in pharmacotherapy based on patient response and culture results, recognizing the prevalence of *Escherichia coli* and the risk of resistance.

- Design a monitoring plan for a patient with pyelonephritis that allows objective assessment of the response to therapy.

PATIENT PRESENTATION

■ Chief Complaint

"I am freezing and my back is killing me."

■ HPI

Isabella Toms is a 22-year-old college student with type 1 diabetes, who presents to the ER complaining that she has had pain in her right flank region over the last 24 hours, as well as pain in her abdomen.

She complains of some nausea and reports that she woke up this morning with severe stomach and back pain, but has not vomited. The patient states she has not eaten for 24 hours, but has been able to drink water and non–diet soda, and has continued to keep her insulin pump on, but has not given any additional regular insulin. The patient reports she recently started treatment for a urinary tract infection about 2 days ago with trimethoprim/sulfamethoxazole. She states that she has been feeling feverish and has the chills. She reports no substernal chest pain, shortness of breath, cough, or sputum production. She denies any diarrhea or rash.

■ PMH

Type 1 diabetes, diagnosed at age 11; has an insulin pump

■ FH

Mother and father are in their 40s and healthy; one sister with asthma, and an older brother with Crohn disease

■ SH

Nonsmoker, no IVDA, drinks alcohol socially. Single, but has a steady boyfriend and is sexually active. Currently is a first-year law student at the local university.

■ Meds

Ortho-Novum 7/7/7 one tablet daily
Insulin pump; regular insulin basal rate of 28 units per day
Regular insulin 2 units with breakfast, lunch, and supper
Trimethoprim/sulfamethoxazole one double strength tablet twice daily for 3 days (she has completed 2 days of therapy)

■ All

Penicillin (develops an itchy rash)

■ ROS

She has a history of UTIs and has had two UTIs in the past year, the most recent 2 days ago

■ Physical Examination

Gen

Conscious, alert, and oriented young Caucasian woman in mild distress

VS

BP 112/68, P 65, RR 16, T 39.0°C, O_2 sat 98% room air; Wt 63 kg (IBW 61.1 kg), Ht 5'7"

Skin

No tenting; dry skin; no signs of redness or rash

HEENT

EOMI; funduscopic examination WNL; pharynx clear and dry

Neck

Supple, no JVD

Chest

CTA

CV

RRR

TABLE 133-1	Laboratory Tests and Urinalyses on Days 1–3 of Hospitalization		
Parameter (Units)	Day 1	Day 2	Day 3
Serum chemistry			
Na (mEq/L)	141	139	141
K (mEq/L)	3.9	4.0	4.1
Cl (mEq/L)	99	101	102
CO_2 (mEq/L)	27	28	28
BUN (mg/dL)	19	14	12
SCr (mg/dL)	1.1	1.0	1.0
Glucose (mg/dL)	65	92	89
Hematology			
Hgb (g/dL)	13.9	13.8	13.6
Hct (%)	40.6	40.3	40.5
Plt (×10³/mm³)	275	276	276
WBC (×10³/mm³)	26.3	20.4	12.5
PMN/B/L/M (%)	80/13/7/0	85/10/5/0	86/6/7/1
Urinalysis			
Appearance	Hazy		
Color	Amber		
pH	5.0		
Specific gravity	1.017		
Blood	2+		
Ketones	Negative		
Leukocyte esterase	3+		
Nitrites	2+		
Urine protein, qualitative	Trace		
Urine glucose, qualitative	Trace		
WBC/hpf	487		
RBC/hpf	102		
Bacteria	Many		
WBC casts	2+		

B, bands; L, lymphocytes; M, monocytes; PMN, polymorphonuclear leukocytes.

Abd

Soft with suprapubic tenderness to deep palpation; no rebound or guarding; active bowel sounds. There is no hepatosplenomegaly or masses.

Back

No paraspinal or spinal tenderness

Genit/Rect

Normal female genitalia; no abnormal vaginal discharge; normal sphincter tone; last menstrual period 1 week ago

Ext

No CCE; pulses 2+ bilaterally

Neuro

A & O × 3; CN II–XII intact; sensory and perception intact

■ Labs and UA on Admission

See Table 133-1

■ Chest X-Ray

No infiltrates, no consolidation seen

■ CT Abdomen with Contrast

Findings: Liver, gallbladder, pancreas, spleen, and adrenals are unremarkable. No evidence of ascites or focal areas of fluid collection. The left kidney is unremarkable. A hypoattenuating lesion is seen involving the right kidney from mid- to lower pole.

Impression: Hypoattenuating lesion in right kidney consistent with pyelonephritis; correlate with clinical picture.

■ Abdominal Ultrasound

Findings: There is a hypoechoic region within the lateral cortex of the right kidney, which does not display through transmission.

Impression: Focal cortical thickening with decreased echogenicity involving the mid right renal cortex, similar to the recent CT scan, most likely representing focal pyelonephritis. No renal abscess identified. No hydronephrosis.

■ Urine Gram Stain

Many gram-negative rods.

■ Blood Culture

Many gram-negative rods.

■ Vaginal Swab

Negative

■ Assessment

Pyelonephritis
Bacteremia
Type 1 diabetes

QUESTIONS

Problem Identification

1.a. Create a list of the patient's drug therapy problems.

1.b. What information (signs, symptoms, laboratory tests) indicates the presence and severity of pyelonephritis in this patient?

1.c. List any potential contributing factors that may have predisposed this patient to developing pyelonephritis.

1.d. What additional information is needed to fully assess the patient?

Desired Outcome

2. What are the goals of pharmacotherapy in this patient?

Therapeutic Alternatives

3.a. What nondrug therapies might be useful for this patient?

3.b. What organisms are commonly associated with pyelonephritis?

3.c. How often is antimicrobial resistance to *E. coli* seen in the community?

3.d. What feasible pharmacotherapeutic alternatives are available for the empiric treatment of pyelonephritis?

Optimal Plan

4. Outline an antimicrobial regimen that will provide appropriate empiric therapy for pyelonephritis in this patient.

Outcome Evaluation

5.a. What clinical and laboratory parameters are necessary to evaluate the antibiotic therapy for achievement of the desired therapeutic outcomes and to detect or prevent adverse effects?

■ CLINICAL COURSE

The patient was started on the empiric antimicrobial regimen you recommended. She required acetaminophen Q 6 H for pain. Her fevers subsided with the initiation of acetaminophen and

TABLE 133-2	Culture Results of Urine and Blood Samples Taken on Day 1 and Reported on Day 3

Urine culture
Result: >100,000 cfu/mL *Escherichia coli*

Antibiotic	Kirby–Bauer Interpretation
Ampicillin/sulbactam	Intermediate
Ampicillin	Resistant
Cefazolin	Intermediate
Cefuroxime	Sensitive
Ceftriaxone	Sensitive
Levofloxacin	Sensitive
Piperacillin/tazobactam	Sensitive
Tobramycin	Sensitive
TMP/SMX	Resistant

Day 1 blood cultures × 2 sets
Result: Many *E. coli*

Antibiotic	Kirby–Bauer Interpretation
Ampicillin/sulbactam	Intermediate
Ampicillin	Resistant
Cefazolin	Intermediate
Cefuroxime	Sensitive
Ceftriaxone	Sensitive
Levofloxacin	Sensitive
Piperacillin/tazobactam	Sensitive
Tobramycin	Sensitive
TMP/SMX	Resistant

Vaginal swab
No growth × 3 days
Day 2 blood cultures
Results: No growth to date
Day 3 blood cultures
Results: No growth to date

antibiotics. On day 3 of hospitalization, she was much improved and was ready for discharge. Laboratory tests for days 2 and 3 are included in Table 133-1. Culture results from admission were finalized on day 3 (late in the day) and are shown in Table 133-2.

Outcome Evaluation (continued)

5.b. What recommendations, if any, do you have for changes in the initial drug regimen?

Patient Education

6. What information should be provided to the patient on discharge to enhance adherence, ensure successful therapy, and minimize adverse effects?

■ SELF-STUDY ASSIGNMENTS

1. Develop a protocol for switching patients from IV to oral therapy when treating pyelonephritis.

2. Perform a literature search to find clinical trials comparing drug therapy in pyelonephritis, and compare inclusion criteria, drug regimens, outcomes, and costs of therapy.

3. Develop a clinical pathway that could be used for the management of suspected pyelonephritis.

CLINICAL PEARL

Pyelonephritis can be managed with many different drugs; choose drugs that are bactericidal and cleared in the active form by the kidney. Drugs suitable for once-daily therapy help to reduce treatment costs.

REFERENCES

1. Filiatrault L, McKay RM, Patrick DM, et al. Antibiotic resistance in isolates recovered from women with community-acquired urinary tract infections presenting to tertiary care emergency department. CJEM 2012;14(5):295–305.

2. Gupta K, Hooton TM, Naber KG, et al. International clinical practice guidelines for the treatment of acute uncomplicated cystitis and pyelonephritis in women: a 2010 update by the Infectious Diseases Society of America and the European Society for Microbiology and Infectious Diseases. Clin Infect Dis 2011;52(5):e103–e120.

3. Colgan R, Williams M. Diagnosis and treatment of acute pyelonephritis in women. Am Fam Physician 2011;84(5):519–526.

4. Eliakim-Raz N, Yahar D, Paul M, Leibovici L. Duration of antibiotic treatment for acute pyelonephritis and septic urinary tract infection–7 days versus longer treatment: systemic review and meta-analysis of randomized controlled trials. J Antimcrob Chemother 2013;68:2183–2191.

5. Peterson J, Kaul S, Khashab M, Fisher AC, Kahn JB. A double-blind, randomized comparison of levofloxacin 750 mg once-daily for five days with ciprofloxacin 400/500 mg twice-daily for 10 days for the treatment of complicated urinary tract infections and acute pyelonephritis. Urology 2008;71(1):17–22.

6. Abbo LM, Hooten TM. Antimicrobial Stewardship and Urinary Tract Infections. Antibiotics 2014;3:174–192.

7. Wagenlehner F, Umeh O, Steenbergen J, Yuan G, Darouiche RO. Ceftolozane-tazobactam compared with levofloxacin in the treatment of complicated urinary-tract infections, including pyelonephritis: a randomized, double-blind, phase 3 trial (ASPECT-cUTI). The Lancet 2015;385:1949–1956.

8. Zasowski EJ, Rybak JM, Rybak MJ. The β-lactams Strike Back: Cetazidime–Avibactam. Pharmacotherapy 2015;35(8):755–770.

134

PELVIC INFLAMMATORY DISEASE AND OTHER SEXUALLY TRANSMITTED INFECTIONS

Frankie and Jenny Were Lovers . . . . Level II

Neha Sheth Pandit, PharmD, AAHIVP, BCPS

Christopher Roberson, MS, AGNP-BC, ACRN

LEARNING OBJECTIVES

After completing this case study, the reader should be able to:

• Identify relevant information from patient history, physical examination, and laboratory data suggestive of the diagnosis of a sexually transmitted infection (STI).

• List major complications of STIs and appropriate strategies for prevention and/or treatment.

- Discuss other health issues that may be present in patients referred for treatment of STIs, including immunization needs and risk reduction.

- Provide appropriate treatment plans for patients with STIs, including drug(s), dosage form, doses, route of administration, frequency, duration, and monitoring.

- Compare and contrast criteria and options for ambulatory and inpatient treatment of women with pelvic inflammatory disease (PID).

- Recognize opportunities and provide appropriate recommendations for immunizations, including human papillomavirus (HPV) vaccine.

- Develop patient counseling strategies regarding drug treatment and possible adverse effects.

PATIENT PRESENTATION 1

■ Chief Complaint

"My lady and I don't feel good."

■ HPI

Frankie Mason is a 20-year-old man who presents to a health clinic with complaints of 5 days of painful urination and increasing amounts of discolored urethral discharge. Today, he noted four painful blisters on the penis. He is single, heterosexual, sexually active with two to three concurrent partners, and admits to unprotected sex "at least once" in the past 2 weeks. He does not know the sexual histories of his current or past sexual partners or their sexual partners and he admits to over 15 lifetime sexual partners. He denies oral or rectal intercourse.

■ PMH

History of genital herpes 2 years ago. He has not undergone testing for HIV. He has been immunized against hepatitis B but has not been immunized against HPV as "it's only for women." He is unaware of hepatitis A or C as infectious diseases, asking "Do you get that from sex or restaurant food?" No active medical problems.

■ FH

Noncontributory

■ SH

Denies IV drug and cigarette use; has two to four beers "on weekends"; may be unreliable in keeping follow-up appointments because he states, "I don't like doctors."

■ Meds

None

■ All

Ciprofloxacin ("makes me dizzy")

■ ROS

Occasional headaches; denies stomach pain, constipation, vision problems, night sweats, weight loss, or fatigue

■ Physical Examination

Gen

Patient is a well-developed male in NAD, very talkative

VS

BP 104/80, HR 72, RR 12, T 37.6°C; Wt 78 kg

Skin

No rashes or other lesions seen

HEENT

No erythema of pharynx or oral ulcers

Neck/Lymph Nodes

No lymphadenopathy; neck supple

Chest

Normal breath sounds; good air entry

CV

RRR; no murmurs

Abd

No tenderness or rebound; no HSM

Genit/Rect

Tanner stage V; testes descended, nontender, without erythema. Thick yellow urethral discharge; four small erupting vesicles on penile tip and glans; negative rectal examination; no scrotal tenderness or swelling. No genital growths visualized.

MS/Ext

No inguinal or other lymphadenopathy; no lesions or rashes; muscle strength and tone normal

Neuro

CN II–XII intact; DTRs 2+ bilaterally and symmetric

■ Urethral Smear

15 WBC/hpf; Gram stain (+) for intracellular gram-negative diplococci

■ Other Tests

A urine specimen was sent for NAAT for gonococcus and *Chlamydia*

■ Assessment

1. Urethritis caused by gonococcal infections, r/o chlamydial coinfection

2. Recurrent genital herpes

PATIENT PRESENTATION 2

■ Chief Complaint

"I have bad stomach pain."

■ HPI

Jenny Klein is a 20-year-old female sexual partner of Frankie who reports a 1 day history of increasingly severe dysuria, lower abdominal pain, and vaginal discharge. She is sexually active with "only Frankie," has no previous history of urinary or genital infections, and denies IV drug use. She is unaware of Frankie's multiple sexual partners. Her last menses started 10 days ago and last intercourse was 7 days ago without the use of a condom. She noted the vaginal discharge yesterday, which she describes as thick and yellow. She denies oral or rectal intercourse. She admits to three lifetime sexual partners.

■ PMH

No previous pregnancies and current negative pregnancy test. She has received a complete hepatitis B series. She has not been immunized against hepatitis A and has not received the HPV vaccine series, because her mother did not consent to the vaccine. She believes she is "low risk" for HPV.

■ FH

HTN in maternal grandmother

■ SH

Denies nicotine or recreational drug use; occasional 1–2 glasses of wine; does not use hormonal or other contraception; reports occasional use of condoms; no routine medical care

■ Meds

None

■ All

NKDA

■ ROS

Occasional painful menses self-treated with brand name menstrual treatment (Pamprin or Midol—she does not recall exactly)

■ Physical Examination

Gen

Well-developed woman in moderate-to-severe abdominal discomfort

VS

BP 110/76, HR 100, RR 16, T 39.2°C; Wt 62 kg

Skin

No rashes seen

HEENT

No erythema of pharynx or oral ulcers

Neck/Lymph Nodes

No lymphadenopathy; neck supple

Chest

Normal breath sounds; good air entry; breasts Tanner stage V

CV

Regular rate and rhythm; no murmurs

Abd

Guarding of right and mid–lower quadrants with palpation

Genit/Rect

Pubic hair Tanner stage V; vulva with no ulcers, erythema, or excoriations. Vaginal area with large amount of thick yellow-white discharge. Cervix shows erythema and extensive yellow-white discharge; no masses on bimanual examination; cervical motion

tenderness; adnexal tenderness and fullness on right. No genital growths visualized.

■ Vaginal Saline Wet Preparation and KOH

Examination of vaginal discharge: Increased WBCs (too numerous to count), pH 5.0, no yeast or hyphae seen; "whiff" test positive with KOH preparation; many clue cells present.

MS/Ext

No adenopathy, lesions, or rashes; no arthritis or tenosynovitis

Neuro

CN II–XII intact, DTRs 2+ and symmetric bilaterally

■ Labs

Na 138 mEq/L	Hgb 12.2 g/dL	WBC 12.75 × 10³/mm³
K 4.2 mEq/L	Hct 37%	Neutros 66%
Cl 102 mEq/L	Plt 250 × 10³/mm³	Bands 12%
BUN 22 mg/dL	SCr 0.9 mg/dL	Lymphs 10%
Glu 106 mg/dL		Monos 12%

■ Urine Dipstick

Small leukocytes, nitrites neg; protein 100 mg/dL; otherwise unremarkable

■ Other Tests

Vaginal specimen sent for NAAT for gonococcus and *Chlamydia*

■ Assessment

PID (infection of the upper genital tract and cervicitis)
Bacterial vaginosis

QUESTIONS

Problem Identification

1.a. For each patient, create a list of drug therapy problems.

1.b. What information indicates the presence or severity of each STD in each patient?

1.c. Should any additional tests be performed in these patients?

1.d. What complications of infection can be reduced or avoided with appropriate therapy for each patient?

Desired Outcome

2. State the goals of treatment for each patient.

Therapeutic Alternatives

3. What therapeutic options are available for treatment of each patient?

Optimal Plan

4.a. What treatment regimen (drug, dosage form, dose, route of administration, frequency, and duration) is appropriate for these patients?

4.b. What alternatives would be appropriate if the initial therapy cannot be used?

Outcome Evaluation

5.a. What clinical and laboratory parameters are necessary to evaluate the therapy for achievement of the desired outcome and to detect or prevent adverse effects?

■ CLINICAL COURSE

One day later, *Chlamydia* and gonorrhea NAAT-positive test results received on samples from both patients.

Outcome Evaluation (continued)

5.b. What changes, if any, in antibacterial therapy are required?

Patient Education

6. What information should be provided to Frankie and Jenny to enhance adherence, ensure success of therapy, and minimize adverse effects?

■ SELF-STUDY ASSIGNMENTS

1. Review the legal status of expedited partner therapy (EPT) in your area of practice. Discuss the ethical implications of this practice (see *www.cdc.gov/std/ept*).

2. Survey 10 local community pharmacists to assess their knowledge of EPT. Would they dispense the ordered medications?

3. Review nonprescription brand name products for management of dysmenorrhea and accompanying pain for ingredients, effectiveness, and cost. Develop recommendations for the most cost-effective therapy.

4. Review the current pre-exposure prophylaxis (PrEP) guidelines for HIV to see if either patient would be a good candidate for prophylaxis medication. If so, develop recommendations for PrEP with an appropriate monitoring plan.

CLINICAL PEARLS

1. Although partner notification and treatment may be enhanced through "EPT" strategies, misconceptions regarding legality and ethics of this practice limit implementation of this public health initiative.

2. Advertised brand name nonprescription products for menstrual problems are almost always an expensive choice when compared with single-agent alternatives. Most "brands" offer multiple formulations so it is often difficult to know the exact ingredients used by a patient.

3. Health care providers should view a diagnosis of STI as an immunization opportunity to enhance care of the individual while furthering public health initiatives for disease prevention.

Acknowledgment

This case is based on the case written by Denise L. Howrie, PharmD, and Pamela J. Murray, MD, MHP, for the 9th edition of the Casebook.

REFERENCES

1. Workowski KA, Bolan GA. Sexually transmitted diseases treatment guidelines, 2015. MMWR Recomm Rep 2015;64(RR-03):1–137.
2. Papp JR, Schachter J, Gaydos CA, Van Der Pol B. Recommendations for the laboratory-based detection of *chlamydia trachomatis* and *neisseria gonorrhoeae*–2014. MMWR Recomm Rep 2014;63:1–24.
3. Lyss SB, Kamb ML, Peterman TA, et al. Chlamydia trachomatis among patients infected with and treated for Neisseria gonorrhoeae in sexually transmitted disease clinics in the United States. Ann Intern Med 2003;139:178–185.
4. Trent M. Pelvic inflammatory disease. Pediatr Rev 2013;34:163–171.
5. Brunham RC, Gottlieb SL, Paavonen J. Pelvic inflammatory disease. N Engl J Med 2015;372:2039–2048.
6. Llata E, Bernstein KT, Kerani RP, et al. Management of pelvic inflammatory disease in selected US sexually transmitted disease clinics: Sexually transmitted disease surveillance network, January 2010-December 2011. Sex Transm Dis 2015;42:429–433.
7. Centers for Disease Control and Prevention. Guidance on the Use of Expedited Partner Therapy in the Treatment of Gonorrhea. Available at: *http://www.cdc.gov/std/ept/GC-Guidance.htm*. Accessed March 25, 2016.
8. Centers for Disease Control and Prevention. Expedited Partner Therapy in the Management of Sexually Transmitted Diseases. Atlanta, GA, US Department of Health and Human Services, 2006. *http://www.cdc.gov/std/treatment/eptfinalreport2006.pdf*. Accessed March 25, 2016.
9. Gift TL, Kissiner P, Mohammed H, Leichliter JS, Hogben M, Golden MR. The cost and cost-effectiveness of expedited partner therapy compared with standard partner referral for the treatment of chlamydia or gonorrhea. Sex Transm Dis 2011;38:1067–1073.
10. Petrosky E, Bocchini JA, Hariri S, et al. Use of 9-valent human papillomavirus (HPV) vaccine: Updated HPV vaccination recommendations of the Advisory Committee on immunization practices. MMWR 2015;64:300–304.

135

SYPHILIS

Here Today … Gone Tomorrow? . . . . Level I

John S. Esterly, PharmD, BCPS, AQ-ID

Marc H. Scheetz, PharmD, MSc, BCPS, AQ-ID

LEARNING OBJECTIVES

After completing this case study, the reader should be able to:

- Discuss the diagnosis of syphilis and differentiate among the temporal stages of the disease.

- Develop a pharmacotherapeutic treatment plan individualized for the patient's stage of syphilis.

- Recommend alternate treatment regimens when the primary therapeutic option is contraindicated.

- Describe appropriate monitoring, follow-up, and counseling of patients with a syphilitic infection to ensure success of treatment.

PATIENT PRESENTATION

■ Chief Complaint

"This rash started 3–4 days ago on my back and stomach. My whole left side has been hurting, and I've also been feeling weaker than usual lately."

■ HPI

John Rutherford, a 27-year-old man with a past medical history of HIV on HAART, presents with left upper quadrant/left back/left side pain and a diffuse rash. He states the rash started 3–4 days ago, and is mostly on his chest, abdomen, and arms. He also has seven macules on his scalp. The rash is nonpainful and nonpruritic, except on his scalp where he has developed a few scabs from itching; no drainage from any lesions is noted. He also has been having some chest pain that is worse with breathing. He notes nausea, though no vomiting, and reports ongoing nonbloody diarrhea for months. He presents to the ED primarily because of pain in his upper left back that radiates around his left side. His urine is very dark, brownish-red; however, he has no dysuria. The patient also states he has felt weaker than usual for the past few days.

PMH

Hepatitis B, now immune
HIV diagnosed 6 months ago, on HAART

FH

Both parents with hypertension, still living

SH

Unemployed
Tobacco 1.5 ppd since early teens
Social alcohol usage (average four drinks per week)
Occasional methamphetamine use—both smoked and injected (with clean needles)
Previous MSM Hx (four partners in last 6 months) with inconsistent use of condoms

Meds

Tenofovir/emtricitabine 300/200 mg PO once daily
Raltegravir 400 mg PO BID
Acetaminophen–hydrocodone 325/5 mg PO Q 6 H PRN

All

Codeine

ROS

Constitutional: reports weakness and malaise; denies fever
Eyes: denies vision changes
Ears, nose, and throat: denies sore throat, rhinorrhea, or sinus pressure
Lymphatic: denies lymph node swelling
Respiratory: denies shortness of breath, dyspnea on exertion, or cough
Cardiovascular: reports some chest pain on inspiration
Gastrointestinal: reports intermittent nausea, no vomiting, and consistent diarrhea
Neurologic: denies neuropathy symptoms
Musculoskeletal: reports arthralgias and myalgias
Skin: rash on scalp, abdomen, arms, and legs present
Pain: reports persistent abdominal and left side pain

Physical Examination

Gen

Awake and alert, NAD. Appropriate. Oriented to person, place, and year.

VS

T 98.4°F, BP 114/70, HR 92, RR 16, O_2 sat 98; Ht 61 in, Wt 59 kg

Skin

Numerous palpable, blanchable macules mostly ~5 mm with one area of confluence on the left lower abdomen. Macules present on both arms, chest, and back. Four to five scabs with surrounding erythema on scalp.

HEENT

Moist mucous membranes, neck supple. No cervical, postauricular, or supraclavicular lymphadenopathy. No obvious oral lesions. Mild icterus.

Neck/Lymph Nodes

Supple; no lymphadenopathy, bruits, JVD, or thyromegaly

Chest

CTA bilaterally. No crackles or wheezes.

CV

RRR; S_1, S_2; no m/r/g

Abd

Soft, nondistended. Diffuse tenderness with minimal localization to the RUQ and more prominent on the epigastrium, LUQ, and back. (+) BS. No rebound or guarding.

Extremities

Warm, well perfused, no edema. 2+ DP and PT pulses

GU

Rash extending to penis; no other lesions present. Moderate inguinal lymphadenopathy.

Rectal

Scar from recently healed ulcer noted

Musculoskeletal

No joint swelling, or effusions

Neuro

CN II–XII grossly intact. No dysmetria. Strength 5/5 on all four extremities.

Labs

Na 138 mEq/L	WBC 9.3 × 10³/mm³
K 3.9 mEq/L	Plt 391 × 10³/mm³
Cl 96 mEq/L	ALT 66 IU/L
CO₂ 28 mEq/L	AST 95 IU/L
BUN 7 mg/dL	Alk phos 1271 IU/L
SCr 0.7 mg/dL	T. bili 5.0 mg/dL
Glu 100 mg/dL	CD4 460 cells/mm³
Hgb 12.3 g/dL	HIV viral load <48 copies/mL
Hct 36.9%	

Other

RPR: Titers positive at 1:256.
FTA-ABS: Positive.
Hepatitis B: HBsAb positive, HBsAg negative.
Hepatitis C: RNA negative.

CT abdomen and pelvis: Mild hepatosplenomegaly with minimal intrahepatic biliary ductal dilatation and prominence of the common duct. There are multiple tortuous perirectal vessels that may represent varices secondary to portal hypertension. Proctitis is present with innumerable reactive perirectal and pelvic lymph nodes.

■ **Assessment**

1. The patient is a 27-year-old man with a history of HIV and newly diagnosed syphilis that appears to be in a secondary stage based on signs, symptoms, and report of sexual history.

2. This patient may be at higher risk for disease progression, specifically neurosyphilis, due to HIV coinfection.

QUESTIONS

Problem Identification

1.a. Which populations are most at risk for syphilis?

1.b. What information (signs, symptoms, laboratory values) indicates the presence or stage of syphilis?

1.c. What laboratory tests are used in the diagnosis of syphilis, and how should they be interpreted?

Desired Outcome

2. What are the goals of pharmacotherapy in this case?

Therapeutic Alternatives

3.a. What pharmacotherapeutic alternatives are available for this patient?

3.b. What nondrug measures should be implemented in this case?

Optimal Plan

4. What is the recommended treatment (drug, dose, and duration) for this patient?

Outcome Evaluation

5. What clinical and laboratory parameters are necessary to evaluate the therapy for achievement of the desired therapeutic outcome and to detect or prevent adverse effects?

Patient Education

6.a. What information should be provided to the patient to enhance adherence, ensure successful therapy, and minimize adverse effects?

6.b. What information should be provided to the patient to prevent a future sexually transmitted disease?

■ SELF-STUDY ASSIGNMENTS

1. Describe the differences in syphilis presentation in relation to disease progression.

2. Discuss the tests or procedures that should be used to diagnose and monitor the progression/regression of syphilis over time.

3. Identify potential confounding factors that may impact test results in HIV-infected patients.

CLINICAL PEARL

Patients undergoing penicillin therapy for syphilis will frequently experience the Jarisch–Herxheimer reaction within the first 24 hours of treatment. This is an inflammatory response to the breakdown of spirochetes and subsequent release of endotoxins. Usually manifesting as fever, chills, myalgias, arthralgias, and headache, it is generally self-limiting and may be treated with analgesics and antipyretics as needed.

REFERENCES

1. Centers for Disease Control and Prevention. Sexually Transmitted Disease Surveillance, 2013. Atlanta, U.S. Department of Health and Human Services, December 2014. Available at: *http://www.cdc.gov/std/stats13/syphilis.htm.* Accessed November 11, 2015.

2. Centers for Disease Control and Prevention. Sexually transmitted diseases treatment guidelines, 2015. MMWR Morb Mortal Wkly Rep 2015;64(RR-3):34–50. Available at: *www.cdc.gov.* Accessed Novemeber 12, 2015.

3. Tramont EC. *Treponema pallidum* (syphilis). In: Mandell GL, Bennett JE, Dolin R, eds. Principles and Practice of Infectious Diseases, 7th ed. Philadelphia, Churchill Livingstone, 2010:3035–3053.

4. Panel on Opportunistic Infections in HIV-infected Adults and Adoloescents. Guidelines for the prevention and treatment of opportunistic infections in HIV-infected adults and adolescents: recommendations from CDC, the National Institutes of Health, and the HIV Medicine Association of the Infectious Diseases Society of America. Available at: *http://aidsinfo.nih.gov/contentfiles/lvguidelines/adult_oi.pdf.* Accessed November 12, 2015.

5. Bai ZG, Wang B, Yang K, et al. Azithromycin versus penicillin G benzathine for early syphilis. Cochrane Database Syst Rev 2012;6:CD007270.

6. Warwick Z, Dean G, Fisher M. Should syphilis be treated differently in HIV-positive and HIV-negative individuals? Treatment outcomes at a university hospital, Brighton, UK. Int J STD AIDS 2009;20(4):229–230.

7. See S, Scott EK, Levin MW. Penicillin-induced Jarisch-Herxheimer Reaction. Ann Pharmacother 2005;39(12):2128–2130.

136

GENITAL HERPES, GONOCOCCAL, AND CHLAMYDIAL INFECTIONS

Triple Threat . . . . Level II

Suellyn J. Sorensen, PharmD, BCPS, FASHP

LEARNING OBJECTIVES

After completing this case study, the reader should be able to:

* Identify subjective and objective data consistent with genital herpes, gonorrhea, and chlamydia.

* Recommend appropriate therapies for the treatment of genital herpes, gonorrhea, and chlamydia.

* Provide effective and comprehensive counseling for patients with genital herpes, gonorrhea, and chlamydia.

* Identify drug interactions of clinical significance and provide recommendations for managing them.

PATIENT PRESENTATION

■ **Chief Complaint**

"I have painful sores in my genital area, and I have terrible headaches and muscle aches."

HPI

Megan Thompson is a 19-year-old nulligravida woman who presents to the county health STD clinic for evaluation of genital lesions that have been present for 3 days. She has also noticed a white nonodorous vaginal discharge that has lasted 14 days. She admits to anal and vaginal intercourse with two regular partners in the last 60 days. It has been 5 days since her last sexual encounter.

PMH

Recurrent UTIs; most recent 3 months ago
Vaginal candidiasis; most recent 6 months ago
Gonorrhea 5 years ago
Trichomonas vaginalis 2 years ago

FH

Mother with type 2 DM; father died at age 50 of an acute MI

SH

Lives with her boyfriend and works at a local grocery store. She admits to occasional use of alcohol and marijuana.

Meds

Ethinyl estradiol and norethindrone (Junel) 21 1/20 one tablet PO daily
Multivitamin with iron one tablet PO daily
Ibuprofen 200 mg PO PRN
Ciprofloxacin 250 mg PO once daily

All

Penicillin (hives and tongue swelling)

ROS

(–) Cough, night sweats, weight loss, dysuria, or urinary frequency; (+) diarrhea and anorectal pain; LMP 6 weeks ago

Physical Examination

Gen

Thin, young woman in NAD

VS

BP 136/71 mm Hg, P 78 bpm, RR 17, T 37.8°C; Wt 51 kg, Ht 5′5″

Skin

Dry, no lesions, normal color and temperature

HEENT

PERRLA, EOMI without nystagmus

Neck

Supple; no adenopathy, JVD, or thyromegaly.

Chest

Air entry equal; no crepitations or wheezing

CV

RRR, normal S_1 and S_2; no S_3 or S_4; no murmurs or rubs

Abd

Soft, mild tenderness to palpation in RLQ, (+) bowel sounds, no HSM

Genit/Rect

Tender inguinal adenopathy. External exam clear for nits and lice, several extensive shallow small painful vesicular lesions over vulva and labia, swollen and red. Vagina red, rugated, moderate amounts of creamy white discharge. Cervix pink, covered with above discharge, nontender, ~3 cm. Corpus nontender, no palpable masses. Adnexa with no palpable masses or tenderness. Rectum with no external lesions; (+) diffuse inflammation and friability internally, no masses.

Ext

Peripheral pulses 2+ bilaterally, DTRs 2+, no joint swelling or tenderness

Neuro

Alert and oriented, CN II–XII intact

Labs

Na 135 mEq/L	Hgb 12.9 g/dL	WBC 6.3×10^3/mm³	RPR nonreactive
K 4.0 mEq/L	Hct 37.3%	PMNs 64%	Preg test: hCG
Cl 102 mEq/L	Plt 255×10^3/mm³	Bands 2%	pending
CO_2 27 mEq/L		Eos 1%	HIV serology:
BUN 11 mg/dL		Lymphs 24%	ELISA pending
SCr 0.9 mg/dL		Monos 9%	
Glu 72 mg/dL			

Other

Vaginal discharge: Whiff test (–); pH <4.5; wet mount *Trichomonas* (–), clue cells (–), yeast (+)

Clinical Course

The following results were reported 2 days later:

Vulval swab DFA monoclonal stain: HSV-2 isolated
Vaginal and rectal swab gonorrhea NAAT (PCR): *Neisseria gonorrhoeae* (+)
Vaginal and rectal swab chlamydia NAAT (PCR): *Chlamydia trachomatis* (+)

Assessment

A 19-year-old woman who may be pregnant and has primary genital HSV-2 infection, vaginal candidiasis, and gonococcal and chlamydial infections of the vagina, cervix, and rectum.

QUESTIONS

Problem Identification

1.a. Create a list of the patient's drug therapy problems.

1.b. What subjective and objective clinical data are consistent with a primary genital herpes infection?

1.c. Could any of the patient's problems have been caused by drug therapy?

Desired Outcome

2. What are the goals of pharmacotherapy in this case?

Therapeutic Alternatives

3.a. What nondrug therapies might be useful for this patient?

3.b. What feasible pharmacotherapeutic alternatives are available for treatment of genital herpes, chlamydia, and gonorrhea?

Optimal Plan

4.a. What drug, dosage form, dose, schedule, and duration of therapy are best for treating this patient's genital herpes, chlamydial, and gonococcal infections?

4.b. If an NAAT (also called PCR) test was negative for chlamydia but positive for gonorrhea, would treatment for chlamydia still be warranted?

Outcome Evaluation

5. What clinical and laboratory parameters are necessary to evaluate the therapy for achievement of the desired therapeutic outcome and to detect or prevent adverse effects?

Patient Education

6. What information should be provided to the patient to enhance adherence, ensure successful therapy, and minimize adverse effects?

■ FOLLOW-UP QUESTIONS

1. Six months later, Megan calls the STD clinic complaining of genital lesions that look and feel the same as the lesions she had 6 months earlier when seen and treated in the clinic. Should this episode of recurrent genital herpes be treated? If so, what therapies would be appropriate?

2. Is daily suppressive therapy indicated because she had a recurrent episode?

3. When is herpes treatment indicated for sexual partners?

4. When is chlamydia and gonorrhea treatment indicated for sexual partners?

5. What additional pharmacotherapeutic interventions should be made to address the drug therapy problems that were identified in question 1.a.?

■ SELF-STUDY ASSIGNMENTS

1. Determine whether there is a role for vaccines in the future management of herpes simplex disease.

2. Recommend alternative agents for the treatment of acyclovir-resistant herpes.

3. Explain the relationship between herpes simplex and HIV infections. Is there a role for herpes simplex virus–suppressive therapy in preventing HIV transmission?

4. Describe herpes simplex complications that may require hospitalization, and recommend an appropriate treatment regimen.

CLINICAL PEARL

Most genital herpes infections are transmitted by persons who have asymptomatic viral shedding and are unaware that they have the infection. Systemic antiviral drugs control the signs and symptoms of genital herpes infection, but they do not eradicate latent virus.

REFERENCES

1. Centers for Disease Control and Prevention. 2015 STD treatment guidelines. MMWR Morb Mortal Wkly Rep. 2015;64(RR-135). Available at: *http://www.cdc.gov/mmwr/pdf/rr/rr6403.pdf.* Accessed March 30, 2016.

2. Valtrex caplets package insert. Research Triangle Park, NC, GlaxoSmithKline, January 2013.

3. Comparative drug prices. Available at: *www.rxpricequotes.com.* Accessed March 30, 2016.

4. Famvir tablets package insert. East Hanover, NJ, Novartis Pharmaceuticals Corporation, April 2013.

5. Centers for Disease Control and Prevention. Update to CDC's sexually transmitted diseases treatment guidelines, 2010: oral cephalosporins no longer recommended treatment for gonococcal infections. MMWR Morb Mortal Wkly Rep 2012;61(31):590–594. Available at: *http://www.cdc.gov/mmwr/preview/mmwrhtml/mm6131a3.htm?s_cid=mm6131a3_w.* Accessed March 30,2016.

6. Corey L, Wald A, Patel R, et al. Once daily valacyclovir to reduce the risk of transmission of genital herpes. N Engl J Med 2004;350:11–20.

7. Centers for Disease Control and Prevention. Expedited Partner Therapy in the Management of Sexually Transmitted Diseases. Atlanta, GA, US Department of Health and Human Services, 2006. Available at: *http://www.cdc.gov/std/treatment/EPTFinalReport2006.pdf.* Accessed March 30, 2016.

8. Centers for Disease Control and Prevention. Guidance on the Use of Expedited Partner Therapy in the Treatment of Gonorrhea. Atlanta, GA, US Department of Health and Human Services, November 2012. Available at: *http://www.cdc.gov/std/treatment/EPTFinalReport2006.pdf.* Accessed March 30, 2016.

137

OSTEOMYELITIS AND SEPTIC ARTHRITIS

I Must Be Getting Old . . . . Level II

R. Brigg Turner, PharmD, BCPS

Jacqueline Schwartz, PharmD

LEARNING OBJECTIVES

After completing this case study, the reader should be able to:

- Describe the most common presenting signs and symptoms of osteomyelitis and septic arthritis.

- Recommend an antimicrobial treatment plan with empiric and definitive therapy for osteomyelitis and septic arthritis.

- Develop alternative treatment approaches for osteomyelitis and septic arthritis when the preferred regimen cannot be used.

- Create monitoring parameters to evaluate the efficacy and toxicity of antimicrobial therapy for osteomyelitis and septic arthritis.

- Provide patient education on the proper administration of home infusion antibiotics for osteomyelitis and septic arthritis.

PATIENT PRESENTATION

■ Chief Complaint

"Back spasms."

HPI

Richard Frost is a 52-year-old male with a history of chronic back pain who presents with a 1-week history of back spasms localized in the thoracic region. He was doing relatively well until 1 week ago when he went bowling and also did some maintenance around his house, whereupon his back felt tight. There is radiation of pain to his upper right leg with movement. He had a similar episode three months ago that resolved after approximately 2 days with no treatment. He reports this episode to be more severe. He denies nausea, vomiting, fevers, chills, chest pain, shortness of breath, and bowel or bladder incontinence. He reports decreased oral intake over the past week due to pain and general malaise.

PMH

Patient reports chronic back pain starting approximately 10 years ago. He does not routinely seek medical care and does not report any chronic conditions.

FH

Noncontributory

SH

He has smoked one pack of cigarettes per day for the past 20 years. He admits to IV heroin use for the past 3–4 years.

Meds

Acetaminophen and ibuprofen as needed for back pain; he has increased use of these medications over the past week

All

No known allergies

ROS

No positive findings with regard to head, eyes, ears, nose, throat; cardiorespiratory systems; or recent illness. Skin lesion noted as discussed below. No other significant trauma.

Physical Examination

Gen

He does not appear to be in any acute distress

VS

BP 152/109, P 84 bpm, RR 18, T 36.4°C; 96% SpO$_2$ on room air, Ht 5'8", Wt 90 kg

Skin

Open left lateral leg ulcer 4 × 2 in in size with foul-smelling, purulent drainage. Patient reports this ulcer to be a result of burning his leg on a motorcycle approximately 1 year previously. He has not previously sought medical care for this condition.

HEENT

Pupils equal/round, reactive to light, conjunctiva clear. Poor dentition noted.

Neck/Lymph nodes

No lymphadenopathy

Lungs/Thorax

Clear to auscultation bilaterally, no wheezing, rhonchi, or rales

CV

Regular rate and rhythm; no appreciable murmurs, gallops, or rubs

Abd

Soft, nontender, nondistended; bowel sounds present

Genit/Rect:

Genitalia normal

MS/Ext

Decreased dorsiflexion on the left foot, which he states is chronic. He has reproducible pain in the thoracic spine.

Neurologic

Cranial nerves II-XII are intact

Psychiatric

Oriented to person, place, and time. Mood and affect are appropriate.

Labs

Na 130 mEq/L	Hgb 13.7 g/dL
K 4.0 mEq/L	Hct 41.1%
Cl 95 mEq/L	Plt 341 × 10^3/mm^3
CO$_2$ 23 mEq/L	WBC 22.7 × 10^3/mm^3
BUN 34 mg/dL	Neutros 71%
SCr 0.87 mg/dL	Bands 17%
Glu 120 mg/dL	Lymphs 3%
Ca 9.4 mg/dL	Monos 9%
ESR 73 mm/hour	
CRP 84.2 mg/L	

CT scan

CT scan of abdomen and pelvis are unremarkable. Thoracic spine shows degenerative disk diseases from T1-T5.

MRI

MRI shows T2-T3 osteomyelitis and paravertebral abscess

Blood cultures x two sets

Pending

Other

HCV Ab positive; HIV non-reactive

Assessment

1. Paravertebral abscess and osteomyelitis in the presence of chronic back pain. Soft-tissue infection on the left lateral leg.

2. Hyponatremia likely secondary to volume depletion related to decreased oral intake over the past week.

3. Chronic tobacco smoker.

4. Infection with hepatitis C virus.

QUESTIONS

Problem Identification

1.a. Create a list of the patient's drug therapy problems.

1.b. What information (signs, symptoms, and laboratory values) indicates the presence or severity of osteomyelitis?

1.c. What are the common sources of infection for osteomyelitis? What are possible sources of infection for this patient's osteomyelitis?

TABLE 137-1	Blood Culture Susceptibilities of *Staphylococcus Aureus:* Final Report
Cefazolin	Susceptible
Clindamycin	Susceptible
Oxacillin	Susceptible
Trimethoprim/sulfamethoxazole	Susceptible
Vancomycin	Susceptible, MIC = 0.5 mg/L

Desired Outcome

2. What are the goals of pharmacotherapy in this case?

Therapeutic Alternatives

3.a. What are the most likely causative pathogens in this patient?

3.b. What pharmacotherapeutic options are available for the empiric treatment of osteomyelitis?

Optimal Plan

4.a. What empiric drug, dosage form, dose, and schedule are best for this patient?

■ CLINICAL COURSE

The patient was taken to interventional radiology and a culture from CT-guided aspiration of his paravertebral abscess was obtained. Blood cultures were drawn and the patient was treated initially with empiric vancomycin plus cefepime. After two days, paravertebral abscess culture and blood cultures (2 out of 4) revealed methicillin-susceptible *Staphylococcus aureus* with susceptibilities reported in the **Table 137-1**. A transthoracic echocardiogram found an ejection fraction of approximately 65%, trace aortic and mitral regurgitation, and no evidence of vegetation or perivalvular abscess. The patient has improvement of symptoms, he is clinically stable, and the physician determines discharge is appropriate and orders placement of a peripherally inserted central catheter.

Optimal Plan (continued)

4.b. What definitive drug, dosage form, dose, schedule, and duration of therapy are best for this patient?

Outcome Evaluation

5. What clinical and laboratory parameters are necessary to evaluate the therapy for achievement of the desired therapeutic outcome and to detect or prevent adverse effects?

Patient Education

6. What information should be provided to the patient and patient's caregiver to enhance adherence, ensure successful therapy, and minimize adverse effects?

■ SELF-STUDY ASSIGNMENTS

1. Devise alternative IV and oral treatment regimens in the event that the patient could not tolerate the antibiotic initially used.

2. Describe differences in signs, symptoms, laboratory values, and treatment options if this patient were diagnosed with septic arthritis of a joint instead of osteomyelitis.

3. Devise short and long term pain management for patients with osteomyelitis and substance abuser disorders.

4. Discuss the considerations that need to be made when sending a patient home with a peripherally inserted central catheter.

CLINICAL PEARL

Staphylococcus aureus bacteremia is a serious condition requiring specialized care. Consultation with infectious diseases specialists results in better patient care and outcomes. All patients should have a thorough physical exam performed to identify metastatic foci including an echocardiogram to detect vegetation, intracardiac abscess, or valvular perforation to aid in the diagnosis of infective endocarditis.

REFERENCES

1. Berbari EF, Kanj SS, Kowalski TJ, et al. 2015 Infectious Disease Society of America (IDSA) clinical practice guidelines for the diagnosis and treatment of native vertebral osteomyelitis in adults. Clin Infect Dis 2015;61:e26–46.

2. McHenry M, Easley K, Locker G. Vertebral osteomyelitis: long-term outcome for 253 patients from 7 Cleveland-area hospitals. Clin Infect Dis 2002;34:1342–1350.

3. Weissman S, Parker R, Siddiqui W, Dykema S, Horvath J. Vertebral osteomyelitis: retrospective review of 11 years experience. Scan J Infect Dis 2014;46:193–199.

4. Lipsky B, Berendt A, Cornia P, et al. 2012 Infectious Disease Society of America clinical practice guidelines for the diagnosis and treatment of diabetic foot infections. Clin Infect Dis 2012;54:e132–173.

5. Liu C, Bayer A, Cosgrove S, et al. Clinical practice guidelines by the Infectious Disease Society of America for the treatment of methicillin-resistant Staphylococcus aureus infections in adults and children. Clin Infect Dis 2011;52:e18–e55.

6. Butalia S, Palda VA, Sargeant RJ, Detsky AS, Mourad O. Does this patient with diabetes have osteomyelitis of the lower extremity? JAMA 2008;299:806–813.

7. Stevens DL, Bisno AL, Chambers HF, et al. Practice guidelines for the diagnosis and management of skin and soft tissue infections: 2014 update by the Infectious Diseases Society of America. Clin Infect Dis 2014;59:e10–e52.

8. Zimmerli W. Clinical practice. Vertebral osteomyelitis. N Engl J Med 2010;362:1022–1029.

9. Babouee Flury B, Elzi L, Kolbe M, et al. Is switching to an oral regimen safe after 2 weeks of intravenous treatment for primary bacterial vertebral osteomyelitis? BMC Infect Dis 2014;14:226.

10. Tice AD, Rehm SJ, Dalovisio JR, et al. Practice guidelines for outpatient parenteral antimicrobial therapy. IDSA guidelines. Clin Infect Dis 2004;38(12):1651–1672.

138

SEPSIS

Time Is of the Essence . . . . Level III

Trisha N. Branan, PharmD, BCCCP

Christopher M. Bland, PharmD, BCPS, FIDSA

LEARNING OBJECTIVES

After completing this case study, the reader should be able to:

• Compare and contrast the different syndromes related to sepsis (systemic inflammatory response syndrome, sepsis, severe sepsis, septic shock).

- State patient variables used to diagnose sepsis.
- Identify the initial treatment goals for patients after the diagnosis of sepsis.
- Formulate a comprehensive treatment plan for the initial management of patients with sepsis.
- Recommend appropriate supportive care therapies for patients with sepsis.

PATIENT PRESENTATION

■ Chief Complaint

The patient presents from her nursing home with altered mental status and lethargy that has progressively worsened over the last 24 hours.

■ HPI

Ruth Carter is an 80-year-old Caucasian female who resides in a nursing home with a past medical history that includes hypertension, dementia, chronic kidney disease, depression, and GERD. She was discharged last week from another hospital after being treated for 5 days for a urinary tract infection. Patient did well through the first two days after discharge, but has become increasingly lethargic and drowsy in the last 24 hours. Patient is barely responsive at the time of assessment. Patient has had no reports of fever, nausea, vomiting, or pain.

■ PMH

HTN
Dementia
CKD, stage II
Depression
GERD

■ PSH

Non-contributory

■ FH

No HTN, DM, CAD, cancer, or vascular disease

■ SH

Lives in a nursing home due to dementia
No tobacco, alcohol, or illicit drug use

■ Medications PTA

Clonidine 0.2 mg/24 H transdermal patch every week
Acetaminophen 500 mg PO Q 6 H as needed for pain/fever
Lorazepam 0.5 mg PO QHS
Hydralazine 50 mg PO TID
Omeprazole 20 mg PO QAM
Rivastigmine 4.6 mg/24 H transdermal patch Q HS
Levofloxacin 500 mg PO Q 24 H for 3 days (received 5 days of inpatient therapy; completed total course 2 days ago)

■ Allergies

NKDA

■ Review of Systems

Unable to obtain due to patient's mental status

■ Physical Exam

Gen

Unresponsive, thin appearing female in acute distress

Vital Signs

BP 86/42 mm Hg, P 118–142 bpm, RR 14–35 bpm, T 35.6°C; SpO$_2$: 94% on 8 L NC, Ht 5′3″, Wt 50.8 kg

Skin

Skin is warm, dry and pink, intact with no rashes or lesions

HEENT

Normocephalic, no scleral icterus, no sinus tenderness
Neck/Lymph Nodes: Supple, non-tender, no carotid bruits, no JVD, no lymphadenopathy

Lungs

Decreased air entry in the bases, otherwise clear, tachypnea

CV

Tachycardia, regular rhythm, no murmur, gallop, or edema

Abdomen

Soft, NT/ND, normal bowel sounds, no masses

Musculoskeletal

Normal range of motion and strength, no tenderness or swelling

Neuro

Responsive to painful stimuli at this time, unable to assess further

■ Labs

Na 135 mEq/L	Mg 2.2 mg/dL	WBC 19.3 × 10³/mm³	pH 7.15
K 4.4 mEq/L	Phos 3.1 mg/dL	PMNs 72%	PaCO$_2$ 28 mm Hg
Cl 105 mEq/L	Alb 2.3 g/dL	Bands 18%	PaO$_2$ 165 mm Hg
CO$_2$ 12 mEq/L	Alk Phos 55 IU/L	Lymphs 5%	HCO$_3$ 9.8 mEq/L
BUN 42 mg/dL	T. bili 0.4 mg/dL	Monos 5%	Lactate 6.3 mmol/L
SCr 2.3 mg/dL	AST 15 IU/L	Hgb 12.2 g/dL	
Glu 195 mg/dL	ALT 10 IU/L	Hct 38%	
Ca 7.2 mg/dL		Plt 205 × 10³/mm³	

Urinalysis

Color: Yellow
Appearance: Cloudy
WBC 12/hpf
RBC 5/hpf
Leukocyte esterase: Positive
Nitrite: Positive
Epithelial cells: 3–5/hpf
pH 5
Bacteria 15/hpf

■ Other

EKG: sinus tachycardia (HR 122), QRS 98/QT-QT$_c$ 358/425.

■ Clinical Course

After several hours in the ED, Ms Carter's blood pressure failed to improve despite receiving 2 liters of normal saline. Her mental status did not improve and her urinary output has been approximately 50 mL over last 3 hours (via foley catheter). She was intubated and placed on mechanical ventilation secondary to respiratory failure and concern for airway protection due to her mental status. The intensivist is called to evaluate the patient. The intravenous medications she received in the ED included:

Normal saline 2 liters
Etomidate 20 mg
Succinylcholine 75 mg
Midazolam 2 mg
Norepinephrine 15 mcg/min
Ceftriaxone 2 gm × 1 dose

■ Assessment

An 80-year-old-female is admitted to the ICU with concerns of septic shock, respiratory failure, and acute kidney injury secondary to a UTI.

QUESTIONS

Problem Identification

1.a. Create a list of this patient's drug therapy and disease state problems.

1.b. What information (signs, symptoms, laboratory values) indicates the presence or severity of the problem or disease?

Desired Outcome

2. What are the goals of patient care in this case?

Therapeutic Alternatives

3.a. What interventions and/or therapies should be accomplished as soon as severe sepsis or septic shock is suspected or diagnosed in a patient?

3.b. What type of fluid therapy should be recommended for resuscitation of septic patients?

3.c. When should a vasopressor agent be considered in the treatment of sepsis-induced hypotension and which agents are appropriate?

3.d. When should you consider inotropic agents in this patient's therapy, and which agents are appropriate?

3.e. What is the role of corticosteroid therapy in septic shock?

3.f. What additional supportive care issues should be implemented for all severe sepsis or septic shock patients?

3.g. What ethical considerations are applicable to this patient?

Optimal Plan

4. Ms Carter has been admitted to the ICU with acute respiratory failure requiring mechanical ventilation, septic shock, and acute kidney injury secondary to a urinary tract infection. Design an optimal septic shock pharmacotherapy treatment plan for Ms Carter.

Outcome Evaluation

5. What clinical and laboratory parameters are necessary to evaluate the therapy for achievement of the desired therapeutic outcome and to detect or prevent an adverse effect?

Patient Education

6. What information should be provided to the patient's family to enhance compliance, ensure successful therapy, and minimize adverse effects?

■ SELF-STUDY ASSIGNMENTS

1. Compare and contrast the available literature supporting the use of regular insulin infusions to achieve glycemic control in patients with sepsis focusing on target blood glucose values.

2. Compare and contrast available literature discussing the use of corticosteroids in severe sepsis focusing on dosing, administration, and diagnosis of sepsis-induced adrenal insufficiency.

CLINICAL PEARL

Antibiograms are an important tool in antimicrobial selection in sepsis syndromes. Patients can present with sepsis from a variety of settings such as the community, nursing home, or in-hospital settings. By knowing the typical resistance patterns of the most common pathogens within a given setting, the most likely beneficial empiric regimen can be selected to ensure coverage of the infecting pathogen.

REFERENCES

1. Dellinger RP, Levy MM, Rhodes A, et al. Surviving sepsis campaign: International guidelines for management of severe sepsis and septic shock: 2012. Crit Care Med 2013;41(2):580–637.

2. Rivers E, Nguyen B, Havstad S, et al. Early goal-directed therapy in the treatment of severe sepsis and septic shock. N Engl J Med 2001;345:1368–1377.

3. Yealy D, Kellum J, Huang D, et al. The ProCESS Investigators. A randomized trial of protocol-based care for early septic shock. N Engl J Med 2014;370:1683–1693.

4. Peake S, Delaney A, Bailey M, et al. Goal-directed resuscitation for patients with early septic shock. N Engl J Med 2014;371:1496–1506.

5. Mouncey P, Osborn T, Power S, et al. Trial of early, goal-directed resuscitation for septic shock. N Engl J Med 2015;372:1301–1311.

6. Yunos N, Bellomo R, Hegarty C, et al. Association between a chloride-liberal vs chloride-restrictive intravenous fluid administration strategy and kidney injury in critically ill adults. JAMA 2012;308(15):1566–1572.

7. Myburgh JA, Finger S, Bellomo R, et al. CHEST investigators; Australian and New Zealand Intensive Care Society Clinical Trials Group. Hydroxyethyl starch or saline for fluid resuscitation in intensive care. N Engl J Med 2012;367:1901–1911.

8. Sprung CL, Annane D, Keh D, et al. Hydrocortisone therapy for patients with septic shock. N Engl J Med 2008;358:111–124.

9. Finfer S, Chittock DR, Su SY, et al; NICE-SUGAR Study Investigators. Intensive versus conventional glucose control in critically ill patients. N Engl J Med 2009;360:1346–1349.

10. Gupta K, Hooton T, Naber K, et al. International clinical practice guidelines for the treatment of acute uncomplicated cystitis and pyelonephritis in women: a 2010 update by the Infectious Diseases Society of America and the European Society for Microbiology and Infectious Diseases. Clin Infect Dis 2011;52(5):e103–120.

139

DERMATOPHYTOSIS

Toeing the Line.................................Level I

Scott J. Bergman, PharmD, BCPS (AQ-ID)

Natalie R. Schwarber, PharmD

LEARNING OBJECTIVES

After completing this case study, the reader should be able to:

- Recognize the signs and symptoms of a dermatophyte infection.

- Evaluate the risk factors for developing a dermatophyte infection.

- Recommend an appropriate treatment plan for a dermatophyte infection.

- Explain the best way for the patient to use a selected antifungal product.

PATIENT PRESENTATION

Chief Complaint

"My feet itch."

HPI

Dave Harvester is a 41-year-old man who presents to the local pharmacy because of recent itching in the area of his feet. He is an assistant manager at a local retail store who plays basketball at the YMCA for exercise three times a week. He sweats profusely during games and always showers before going home. He has not changed laundry detergent recently, but he admits that he does not always wash his athletic clothes between workouts. He says his feet have always smelled bad, but he first started to notice the burning and itching about 6 weeks ago. He started applying some deodorizing spray to his feet a week ago, but thus far it has only made a slight improvement in itching. Now his groin is starting to itch as well.

PMH

Appendectomy 20 years ago
GERD diagnosed 5 years ago
Type 2 diabetes mellitus diagnosed 1 year ago
High cholesterol diagnosed 1 year ago

SH

Recent sexual activity (within past month)
Denies tobacco use
Drinks beer on weekends and after games or practice

Meds

Pantoprazole 40 mg daily
Simvastatin 20 mg daily
Metformin 500 mg twice daily
Men's multivitamin daily

All

Penicillin (rash as a baby)

ROS

Denies fever and chills. Fatigued, only after basketball practice. Reports frequent trauma to feet while playing in games. Complains of itching between his toes and groin area.

Physical Examination (Limited)

Gen

An obese, but healthy-looking man wearing sandals, shorts, and a T-shirt

VS

BP 118/78 mm Hg, P 60 bpm, RR 18; Wt 105 kg, Ht 5'11"

Skin

Visible regions are soft and moist

Abd

Fat rolls can be seen around his belly

Genit/Rect

Not directly examined, but patient reports pruritus and burning of skin around groin, not on penis or scrotum. Redness can be seen on the medial aspects of the upper thighs.

MS/Ext

Foul-smelling, dry, scaling feet with white flaking between toes. Toenails on both feet appear to have yellow-brown discoloration. The nails of some of the toes are thicker than the rest, particularly on the right foot.

Labs

None available, but patient states his cholesterol and blood sugars are "good."

Assessment of Current Problems

1. Athlete's foot (tinea pedis)

2. Jock itch (tinea cruris)

3. Possible onychomycosis

4. Unsanitary foot and body hygiene

QUESTIONS

Problem Identification

1.a. What are this patient's drug therapy problems?

1.b. What information leads you to this conclusion?

1.c. What risk factors does the patient have for these conditions?

1.d. What pathogen is most likely to cause these infections?

1.e. What tests could be done at a physician's office to confirm diagnosis of these conditions?

Desired Outcome

2. What are the goals of treatment in this case?

Therapeutic Alternatives

3.a. What nonpharmacologic measures should be recommended to this patient?

3.b. What pharmacologic treatments can be sold to this patient without a prescription for these conditions? Include drug, formulation, route of administration, and duration.

3.c. What additional pharmacologic treatments for these conditions could be used if a prescription is obtained from the patient's physician? Include drug, formulation, and route of administration.

■ CLINICAL COURSE

You recommend an OTC product and see the patient in your pharmacy 2 months later. He tells you that his itching has stopped, but his toenails have grown thick and crusty. They are also darker yellow than before. He has an appointment with his physician next week.

Optimal Plan

4.a. What treatment option would you recommend for this patient's onychomycosis and why? Include drug, dosage form, strength, frequency, and duration of therapy.

4.b. If this treatment fails to work or is not tolerated, what alternatives exist?

Outcome Evaluation

5.a. How would you determine whether your treatment succeeded?

5.b. What side effects can occur with oral and topical antifungal treatments, and how should you monitor for the occurrence of such side effects?

Patient Education

6. What would you say to the patient (in layman's terms) when counseling on how to treat his condition with the selected antifungal product? Include how to take the medication and what to expect from it in terms of efficacy and possible side effects.

■ FOLLOW-UP QUESTIONS

1. What is "pulse" therapy for superficial fungal infections, and what are its advantages and disadvantages?

2. What are the differences between appropriate treatment of onychomycosis and tinea pedis?

3. If itraconazole had been prescribed for this patient, what could be some possible reasons for lack of efficacy?

■ SELF-STUDY ASSIGNMENTS

1. Explain the situations where it is necessary to refer a patient to a physician for the treatment of tinea infections and when oral therapy is preferred over topical agents.

2. Compare and contrast the mechanisms of action for the azole and allylamine antifungals.

3. Review the rates and precipitating factors of oral terbinafine- and oral itraconazole-associated hepatotoxicity.

Over 70% of the population will experience a mycotic infection of the skin, hair, or nail at some point in their lifetime.

REFERENCES

1. Gupta AK, Cooper EA. Update in antifungal therapy of dermatophytosis. Mycopathologia 2008;166:353–367.
2. Westerberg DP, Voyack MJ. Onychomycosis: current trends in diagnosis and treatment. Am Fam Physician 2013(Dec 1);88(11):762–770.
3. Ely JW, Rosenfeld S, Seabury Stone M. Diagnosis and management of tinea infections. Am Fam Physician 2014(Nov 15);90(10):702–710.
4. Andrews MD, Burns M. Common tinea infections in children. Am Fam Physician 2008;77(10):1415–1420.
5. Khanna D, Bharti S. Luliconazole for the treatment of fungal infections: an evidence-based review. Core Evid 2014;9:113–124.
6. Tavaborole topical solution (Kerydin) for onychomycosis. Med Lett Drugs 2015(Mar 2);27(1463):35.
7. Lipner SR, Scher RK. Efinaconazole in the treatmet of onychomycosis. Infect Drug Resist 2015;8:163–172.
8. Gupta AK, Simpson FC. Medical devices for the treatment of onychomycosis. Dermatol Ther 2012;25(6):574–581.

140

BACTERIAL VAGINOSIS

Competition Among Bacteria.................Level I

Charles D. Ponte, BS, PharmD, BC-ADM, BCPS, CDE, CPE, FAADE, FAPhA, FASHP, FCCP, FNAP

LEARNING OBJECTIVES

After completing this case study, the reader should be able to:

- Identify predisposing factors associated with bacterial vaginosis.
- List the common clinical and diagnostic findings associated with bacterial vaginosis.
- Develop a therapeutic plan for the management of bacterial vaginosis.
- Describe the role of the pharmacist in the overall management of infectious vaginitis.

PATIENT PRESENTATION

■ Chief Complaint

"I think I might have a yeast infection."

■ HPI

Judy Heyman is a 30-year-old female graduate student who comes to the Family Practice Center for an acute visit. She states that

1 month ago she was seen at an urgent care center for severe facial pain and headache. She was diagnosed with an acute sinus infection and given a prescription for a 2-week course of doxycycline (100 mg PO BID). During treatment, she developed a vaginal yeast infection. She self-treated it with a nonprescription antifungal cream that alleviated her symptoms. She states that she completed her course of doxycycline despite some mild diarrhea attributed to the drug. Presently, she complains of some mild vaginal discomfort (worse with intercourse) and a "fishy" vaginal odor. Her last period was approximately 5 weeks ago. She admits to inconsistent use of a diaphragm and foam for contraception.

▨ PMH

Venereal warts—2011
GERD

▨ FH

Noncontributory

▨ SH

Is a graduate student in the College of Business and Economics. Has multiple sexual partners (including women); male partners rarely use condoms. Has smoked one pack of cigarettes per day since age 16. Alcohol use consists of a glass of wine nightly and occasional beer. Smokes an occasional marijuana joint.

▨ Meds

Prilosec 20 mg PO Q HS
Multivitamin one PO daily
Calcium supplement with vitamin D one PO daily

▨ All

Cats → itchy eyes and sneezing; house dust → watery eyes, sneezing; penicillin → hive-like pruritic rash, some tightness in her chest; topical clindamycin → facial rash when used to treat acne 15 years ago.

▨ ROS

Noncontributory except that she has noticed a small amount of thin, white mucus on her underclothing and her period is approximately 7 days late

▨ Physical Examination

Limited because of acute visit for specific gynecologic complaint

Gen

Patient is a healthy-appearing 30-year-old woman in NAD

VS

BP 130/75 mm Hg, P 90 bpm, RR 16, T 37.4°C; Wt 51.5 kg, Ht 5'3"

Genit/Rect

External genitalia WNL; no discharge expressed from the urethra, vagina with a small amount of thin white mucus; positive "whiff" test; pH 5.0. Cervix—not completely visualized; appears clear with a small amount of mucoid discharge from the os. Uterus is slightly enlarged, nontender, retroflexed, no cervical motion tenderness. Adnexa without tenderness or masses.

▨ Labs

Microscopic examination of vaginal secretions: 20–25 WBC/hpf; 10–15 clue cells/hpf; 0 lactobacilli/hpf; 15–20 squamous epithelial cells/hpf
Serum pregnancy test—negative

▨ Assessment

Vaginal candidiasis—resolved
Bacterial vaginosis

QUESTIONS

Problem Identification

1.a. Create a list of the patient's drug therapy problems.

1.b. What clinical or laboratory information indicates the presence of bacterial vaginosis (Table 140-1)?

1.c. What is the pathophysiologic basis for the development of bacterial vaginosis?

1.d. Could the patient's problem have been caused by drug therapy?

Desired Outcome

2. What are the goals of pharmacotherapy in this case?

Therapeutic Alternatives

3.a. What feasible pharmacotherapeutic alternatives are available for the treatment of bacterial vaginosis?

3.b. What economic, psychosocial, and ethical considerations are applicable to this patient?

Optimal Plan

4.a. What drug, dosage form, dose, schedule, and duration of therapy are best for this patient?

TABLE 140-1	Characteristics of Different Types of Vaginitis			
Characteristic	Candida	Bacterial	Trichomonas	Chemical
Pruritus	++	+/–	+/–	++
Erythema	+	+/–	+/–	+
Abnormal discharge	+	+	+/–	–
Viscosity	Thick	Thin	Thick/thin	–
Color	White	Gray	White, yellow, green–gray	–
Odor	None	Foul, "fishy"	Malodorous	–
Description	Curdlike	Homogeneous	Frothy	–
pH	3.8–5.0	>4.5	5.0–7.5	–
Diagnostic tests	Potassium hydroxide preparation shows long, threadlike fibers of mycelia microscopically	(+) Whiff test, clue cells	Pear–shaped protozoa, cervical "strawberry" spots	–

4.b. What alternatives would be appropriate if the initial therapy fails or cannot be used?

Outcome Evaluation

5. What clinical and laboratory parameters are necessary to evaluate the therapy for achievement of the desired therapeutic outcome and to detect or prevent adverse effects?

Patient Education

6. What information should be provided to the patient to enhance adherence, ensure successful therapy, and minimize adverse effects?

■ CLINICAL COURSE

After completion of the treatment you recommended, the patient returns to the clinic in 10 days for follow-up. She voices no complaints except that she has been experiencing some vaginal itching, dysuria, and continued painful intercourse. Physical examination reveals a thick, whitish material adherent to the vaginal mucosa. The vulva appears erythematous with excoriations on the labia majora. Microscopic analysis of vaginal secretions revealed hyphae and budding yeast. No white cells are noted. Vaginal pH is normal. The patient is diagnosed with vaginal candidiasis.

■ FOLLOW-UP QUESTIONS

1. What is the most likely cause of this patient's vaginal candidiasis?

2. What other issues should be addressed with the patient during this follow-up visit?

3. What is the role of the pharmacist in the management of patients with infectious vaginitis?

■ SELF-STUDY ASSIGNMENTS

1. Discuss the management of a patient who fails a specific course of treatment for bacterial vaginosis.

2. Discuss the pros and cons of screening asymptomatic pregnant women for the presence of bacterial vaginosis.

3. Describe the best therapeutic approach for a woman diagnosed with bacterial vaginosis who is breastfeeding her infant.

4. Discuss the role of sexual transmission in the pathogenesis of bacterial vaginosis.

CLINICAL PEARL

Patients should be counseled that oral metronidazole may cause a mild disulfiram (Antabuse)-like reaction if alcohol is consumed during therapy. Symptoms may include flushing, GI distress, sweating, thirst, and blurred vision. Advise patients to abstain from alcoholic beverages during therapy and for 72 hours following its completion.

REFERENCES

1. Biggs WS, Williams RM. Common gynecologic infections. Prim Care 2009;36:33–51.

2. Allsworth JE, Peipert JF. Severity of bacterial vaginosis and the risk of sexually transmitted infection. Am J Obstet Gynecol 2011;113:e1–e6.

3. Nyirjesy P. Vulvovaginal candidiasis and bacterial vaginosis. Infect Dis Clin North Am 2008;22:637–652.

4. McCormack WM. Bacterial vaginosis. In: Mandell GL, Bennett JE, Dolin R, eds. Mandell, Douglas, and Bennett's: Principles and Practice of Infectious Diseases, Vol 1, 7th ed. Philadelphia, PA, Elsevier, 2009:1502–1504.

5. Centers for Disease Control and Prevention. Diseases characterized by vaginal discharge. Sexually transmitted diseases treatment guidelines, 2015. MMWR Morb Mortal Wkly Rep 20105;6459(RR-123):1–14009. Available at: www.cdc.gov/std/tg2015/default.htm. www.cdc.gov. Accessed Jan 21, 2016.

6. Sobel JD. What's new in bacterial vaginosis and trichomoniasis? Infect Dis Clin North Am 2005;19:387–406.

7. Swidsinski A, Mendling W, Loening-Baucke V, et al. An adherent *Gardnerella vaginalis* biofilm persists on the vaginal epithelium after standard therapy with oral metronidazole. Am J Obstet Gynecol 2008;198:e1–e6.

8. Petrova MI, Lievens E, Malik S, Imholz N, Lebeer S. Lactobacillus species as biomarkers and agents that can promote various aspects of vaginal health. Front Physiol 2015;6:81.

9. Nygren P. Evidence on the benefits and harms of screening and treating pregnant women who are asymptomatic for bacterial vaginosis: an update review for the U.S. Preventive Services Task Force. Ann Intern Med 2008;148:220–233.

10. Lamont RF, Nhan-Chang Cl, Sobel JD, et al. Treatment of abnormal vaginal flora in early pregnancy with clindamycin for the prevention of spontaneous pre-term birth: a systematic review and metaanalysis. Am J Obstet Gynecol 2011;205:177–190.

141

CANDIDA VAGINITIS

It's Back..Level I

Rebecca M. T. Law, BS Pharm, PharmD

LEARNING OBJECTIVES

After completing this case study, the reader should be able to:

- Distinguish *Candida* vaginitis (vulvovaginal candidiasis, VVC) from other types of vaginitis.

- Know when to refer a patient with symptoms of vaginitis to a physician for further evaluation and treatment.

- Choose an appropriate treatment regimen for the patient with VVC.

- Choose appropriate alternatives for the patient with recurrent VVC, while considering issues relating to non-*albicans* VVC.

- Educate patients with vaginitis about proper use of pharmacotherapeutic treatments and nonpharmacologic management strategies.

PATIENT PRESENTATION

■ Chief Complaint

"I'm having the same problem I had 2 weeks ago, and my doctor is away until next Monday. Can you give me some more of these suppositories?"

▓ HPI

Sophie Kim is a 32-year-old woman who presents to your pharmacy with the above complaint. Upon further questioning, you find that she was diagnosed 3 weeks ago by her physician as having another vaginal *Candida* infection. She was prescribed nystatin suppositories 100,000 units intravaginally for 14 nights, which was the same as what she had been prescribed for her previous episode of vaginal candidiasis 2 months earlier. She stated that she had finished the prescription 1 week ago and had felt better then. However, 3 days ago she began to notice mild vaginal itching again. She thought it was her new control-top panty hose and stopped wearing them, but the itching got worse and became fairly severe with a burning sensation. There was also a white, dry, curd-like vaginal discharge that was nonodorous. This seemed to be identical to what she had experienced 3 weeks ago. Her physician is away until next week, and she wondered if the pharmacy can give her some more suppositories.

▓ PMH

Diabetes type 1 since age 11. Her blood glucose is well controlled, and her physician is keeping a close eye due to her pregnancy.

Recurrent leg ulcers and foot infections for which she has been prescribed antibiotics on a frequent basis. Currently, there are no ulcers or infections, and she is not on antibiotics.

Last month, she began using tights (with an adjustable waist) to help prevent varicose veins.

▓ SH

Nonsmoker; drinks alcohol in moderate amounts (one to two drinks maximum) at social functions. She is married and is 7.5 months pregnant.

▓ Meds

Insulin glargine 15 units SC Q AM for past year
Insulin lispro 6 units SC 15 minutes prior to breakfast, 8 units 15 minutes prior to lunch, and 10 units 15 minutes prior to dinner, for past 4 months
Materna 1 PO Q AM

▓ All

NKDA

▓ ROS

Not performed

▓ Physical Examination

VS

BP 120/78 mm Hg; Wt 70 kg, Ht 5'5"

Note: No further assessments performed

▓ Labs

Not available

QUESTIONS

Problem Identification

1.a. What signs and symptoms indicate the presence and severity of vulvovaginal candidiasis (VVC, *Candida* vaginitis) (Table 141-1)?

1.b. What predisposing factors for VVC might exist in this patient?

1.c. How common is VVC?

Desired Outcome

2. What are the goals of therapy for this patient?

Therapeutic Alternatives

3. What pharmacotherapeutic alternatives are available for the treatment of VVC?

Optimal Plan

4. Design a pharmacotherapeutic plan for this patient.

Outcome Evaluation

5. What parameters should be monitored to assess the efficacy of the treatment and to detect adverse effects?

Patient Education

6. What information should the patient receive about her treatment?

■ CLINICAL COURSE

The recommended treatment was successful. Two months later, Sophie had another episode of VVC, which was again successfully treated. She delivered a healthy 7-lb baby boy born at term.

TABLE 141-1	Characteristics of Different Types of Vaginitis			
Characteristic	**Candida**	**Bacterial**	**Trichomonas**	**Chemical**
Pruritus	++	+/−	+/−	++
Erythema	+	+/−	+/−	+
Abnormal discharge	+	+	+/−	−
Viscosity	Thick	Thin	Thick/thin	−
Color	White	Gray	White, yellow, green–gray	−
Odor	None	Foul, "fishy"	Malodorous	−
Description	Curdlike	Homogeneous	Frothy	−
pH	3.8–5.0	>4.5	5–7.5	−
Diagnostic tests	Potassium hydroxide prep. shows long, thread–like fibers of mycelia microscopically	+ Whiff test, clue cells	Pear–shaped protozoa, cervical "strawberry" spots	−

For some discussion of above conditions and diagnostic considerations see: Diseases characterized by vaginal discharge: vulvovaginal candidiasis. CDC 2015 sexually transmitted diseases treatment guidelines, . Available at: *http://www.cdc.gov/std/tg2015/candidiasis.htm* and Section 4: Management and treatment of specific syndromes: vaginal discharge (bacterial vaginosis, vulvovaginal candidiasis, trichomoniasis). Canadian Guidelines on Sexually Transmitted Infections, 2010. . Ottawa, ON, Public Health Agency of Canada. Available at: *http://www.phac–aspc.gc.ca/std–mts/sti–its/cgsti–ldcits/section–4–8–eng.php*

A month after that, she had another episode of VVC, and she is now nursing.

■ FOLLOW-UP QUESTION

1. What is the most appropriate course of action for management of this patient's recurrent VVC?

■ SELF-STUDY ASSIGNMENTS

1. Obtain information on tests used to diagnose different types of vaginitis.

2. Compare the retail cost of nonprescription vaginitis treatments in your area.

3. Outline your plans for communicating your treatment recommendations to the patient's physician.

CLINICAL PEARL

Patients with symptoms suggestive of bacterial vaginosis or sexually transmitted infection (fever, abdominal or back pain, foul-smelling discharge) should be referred to a physician for further evaluation and treatment.

REFERENCES

1. Centers for Disease Control and Prevention (CDC), Workowski KA, Bolan GA. Diseases characterized by vaginal discharge: vulvovaginal candidiasis. 2015 Sexually transmitted diseases treatment guidelines. Available at: *http://www.cdc.gov/std/tg2015/candidiasis.htm*. Accessed March 25, 2016.

2. Public Health Agency of Canada (PHAC). Section 4: Management and treatment of specific syndromes: vaginal discharge (bacterial vaginosis, vulvovaginal candidiasis, trichomoniasis). In: Canadian Guidelines on Sexually Transmitted Infections—January 2010. Ottawa, ON, Public Health Agency of Canada. Available at: *http://www.phac-aspc.gc.ca/std-mts/sti-its/cgsti-ldcits/section-4-8-eng.php*. Accessed March 25, 2016.

3. Young G, Jewell D. Topical treatment for vaginal candidiasis (thrush) in pregnancy. Cochrane Database Syst Rev. 2001;(4):CD000225. Abstract available at: *http://onlinelibrary.wiley.com/doi/10.1002/14651858.CD000225/abstract*. Accessed on March 25, 2016.

4. Sobel JD, Chaim W, Nagappan V, Leaman D. Treatment of vaginitis caused by *Candida glabrata*: use of topical boric acid and flucytosine. Am J Obstet Gynecol 2003;189:1297–1300.

5. Wooltorton E. Drug advisory: the interaction between warfarin and vaginal miconazole. CMAJ 2001;165(7):938. Available at: *http://www.cmaj.ca/content/165/7/938.3.full*. Accessed March 25, 2016.

6. Sanchez JM, Moya G. Fluconazole teratogenicity. Prenat Diagn 1998;18:862–863.

7. Jick SS. Pregnancy outcomes after maternal exposure to fluconazole. Pharmacotherapy 1999;19:221–222.

8. Falagas ME, Betsi GI, Athanasiou S. Probiotics for prevention of recurrent vulvovaginal candidiasis: a review. J Antimicrob Chemother 2006;58:266–272.

9. Hilton E, Isenberg HD, Alperstein P, France K, Borenstein MT. Ingestion of yogurt containing Lactobacillus acidophilus as prophylaxis for *Candidal* vaginitis. Ann Intern Med 1992;116:353–357.

10. Ray D, Goswami R, Banerjee U, et al. Prevalence of *Candida glabrata* and its response to boric acid vaginal suppositories in comparison with oral fluconazole in patients with diabetes and vulvovaginal candidiasis. Diabetes Care 2007;30:312–317.

142

INVASIVE FUNGAL INFECTIONS

The Brewer's Yeast . . . . Level II

Douglas Slain, PharmD, BCPS, FCCP, FASHP

LEARNING OBJECTIVES

After completing this case study, the reader should be able to:

- Construct a prudent empiric antifungal regimen for a patient with candidemia.

- Determine situations to use echinocandins for invasive *Candida* infections.

- Discuss how the identification of non-albicans *Candida* species can influence antifungal selection.

PATIENT PRESENTATION

■ Chief Complaint

"I am burning up and feel like I have the flu."

■ HPI

August Hops is a 50-year-old man who has been experiencing fever and chills and has not been feeling well over the past 4 days. He was admitted to our hospital yesterday. He was at home receiving home therapy with daptomycin 700 mg IV once daily (day 12 of a 14-day course) via PICC line for MRSA bacteremia, which he developed after having an appendectomy at an outside community hospital about a month ago. During that hospitalization, he also received a course of piperacillin–tazobactam for his appendicitis. His postoperative stay was complicated by a surgical site infection and MRSA bacteremia. He had his catheter removed at that time and was started on vancomycin, until he developed a rash and possible neutropenia. He was then switched to (and eventually sent home on) daptomycin. Prior to being discharged from the outside hospital, Mr Hops also received 7 days of fluconazole 200 mg PO daily for a urine sample from a Foley catheter that grew 100,000 colonies/mL of *C. glabrata*. He never grew *Candida* from any other site.

A set of blood cultures was drawn on this admission to our hospital and is showing no growth at 24 hours. His surgical site does not look infected. His PICC line was removed, and blood and urine cultures were drawn. Piperacillin–tazobactam was added to the daptomycin empirically on admission.

■ PMH

GERD
Hyperlipidemia
HTN
Chronic knee pain (bilateral)

◼ PSH

S/P hernia repair
S/P appendectomy 1 month ago

◼ FH

Father died of CHF, mother still alive with no major medical problems

◼ SH

He is the brewmaster at the local brewery. Married, has four adult children. Denies smoking or excessive ethanol use.

◼ Home Meds

Omeprazole 40 mg PO once daily
Simvastatin 40 mg PO once daily
Metoprolol XL 50 mg PO once daily
Ibuprofen 600 mg PO TID PRN

◼ All

Vancomycin—reaction: neutropenia and rash.

◼ Physical Examination

Gen

Patient is a 50-year-old Caucasian man who is resting somewhat comfortably in bed. Weight: 125 kg; height: 5′11″.

VS

BP 130/85 mm Hg, P 70 bpm, RR 20, T 38.5°C, O_2 sat 97

Skin

Mildly clammy, no Janeway lesions or Osler's nodes

HEENT

PERRLA, EOMI, nares patent

Neck/Lymph Nodes

Neck supple; no lymphadenopathy

Lungs/Thorax

CTA

Heart

EKG: Regular rate and rhythm. No murmurs.

Abd

Bowel sounds faint, mildly distended. Has not had BM for 2 days.

GU

Grossly normal, UA pending

MS/Ext

No abnormalities

◼ Neuro

Intact

◼ Labs

Na 137 mEq/L	Hgb 12.9 g/dL	WBC 13.4 × 10³/mm³	AST 35 IU/L
K 4.3 mEq/L	Hct 40%	PMNs 70%	ALT 30 IU/L
Cl 99 mEq/L	Plt 332 × 10³/mm³	Bands 10%	Alk phos
CO_2 27 mEq/L	CK 56 IU/L	Lymphs 14%	140 IU/L
BUN 7 mg/dL		Monos 5%	T. bili 1.1 mg/dL
SCr 0.8 mg/dL		Eos 1%	
Glu 98 mg/dL		Lipase 92 IU/L	
Mg 2.2 mg/dL		Amylase 112 IU/L	

◼ Chest X-Ray

No infiltrates

◼ Assessment

1. Infection? (New source vs nonresponding MRSA bacteremia.)
2. Constipation.

◼ Plan

1. Infection:
   - ✓ Continue daptomycin 700 mg IV daily and piperacillin–tazobactam 3.375 mg IV Q 8 H.
   - ✓ Order an abdominal CT.
   - ✓ Draw blood cultures.
   - ✓ Order a TEE.
2. Constipation:
   - ✓ Senna/docusate tablet PO now and daily PRN
   - ✓ Docusate sodium capsule 100 mg PO daily

◼ CLINICAL COURSE

TEE shows no signs of vegetation. CT of abdomen showed no signs of intra-abdominal infection. Despite two more days of continued daptomycin therapy, the patient continues to be febrile with leukocytosis, but WBC is slightly improved.

Culture and sensitivity data are now available:

- *Blood cultures* positive at 72 hours (drawn on admission):
  - ✓ PICC line catheter: Rare budding yeast and rare coagulase-negative staphylococci
  - ✓ Left peripheral: Rare budding yeast

The lab states that it appears to be germ tube negative. The team added fluconazole dosed as an 800 mg IV loading dose, then 400 mg IV daily and discontinued piperacillin–tazobactam. They also ordered a funduscopic eye exam to check the patient for *Candida* endophthalmitis.

QUESTIONS

Problem Identification

1.a. Create a list of the patient's drug therapy problems.

1.b. What information (signs, symptoms, and laboratory values) indicates the presence or severity of each of the drug therapy problems?

Desired Outcome

2. What are the goals of pharmacotherapy for this patient's drug therapy problems?

Therapeutic Alternatives

3.a. What nondrug therapies might be useful for this patient?

3.b. What feasible pharmacotherapeutic alternatives are available for treating this infection?

Optimal Plan

4. What drug, dosage form, dose, schedule, and duration are best for this patient?

Outcome Evaluation

5. What clinical and laboratory parameters are necessary to evaluate the therapy for achievement of the desired therapeutic outcome and to detect or prevent adverse effects?

Patient Education

6. What information should be provided to the patient and/or the patient's caregiver to enhance adherence, ensure successful therapy, and minimize adverse effects?

■ FOLLOW-UP QUESTIONS

1. What risk factors does Mr Hops have for developing candidemia?

2. What duration of antifungal therapy should be prescribed for Mr Hops?

■ SELF-STUDY ASSIGNMENTS

1. Explain how use of T2-Polymerase chain reaction or MALDI-TOF technology in the microbiology laboratory can affect antifungal drug usage.

2. Explain how this patient's therapy would be different if he developed *Candida* endophthalmitis.

3. Research available literature to determine whether any antifungal agents have displayed useful activity against *Candida* in biofilm.

CLINICAL PEARL

Despite the general enhanced in vitro *Candida* activity of voriconazole over fluconazole, therapy with voriconazole may be affected by azole-class resistance mechanisms.

REFERENCES

1. Parkins MD, Sabuda DM, Elsayed S, Laupland KB. Adequacy of empirical antifungal therapy and effect on outcome among patients with invasive *Candida* species infections. J Antimicrob Chemother 2007;60:613–618.

2. Pappas PG, Kauffman CA, Andes D, et al. Clinical practice guidelines for the management of candidiasis: 2016 update by the Infectious Diseases Society of America. Clin Infect Dis 2016 Feb 15;62(4):e1–e50.

3. Gubbins PO, Heldenbrand S. Clinically relevant drug interactions of current antifungal agents. Mycoses 2010;53:95–113.

4. Souza MN, Ortiz SO, Mello MM, et al. Comparison between four usual methods of identification of Candida species. Rev Inst Med Trop Sao Paulo 2015;57:281–287.

5. Cauda R. Candidemia in patients with an inserted medical device. Drugs 2009;69(Suppl 1):33–38.

6. Chen SC, Sorrell TC. Antifungal agents. Med J Aust 2007;187:404–409.

7. Andes DR, Safdar N, Baddley JW, et al. Impact of Treatment Strategy on Outcomes in Patients with Candidemia and Other Forms of Invasive Candidiasis: A Patient-Level Quantitative Review of Randomized Trials. Clin Infect Dis 2012;54:1110–1122.

8. Cleary JD, Schwartz M, Rogers PD, de Mestral J, Chapman SW. Effects of amphotericin B and caspofungin on histamine expression. Pharmacotherapy 2003;23:966–973.

143

INFECTIONS IN IMMUNOCOMPROMISED PATIENTS

Making a Rash Decision . . . . Level II

Aaron Cumpston, PharmD, BCOP

Douglas Slain, PharmD, BCPS, FCCP, FASHP

LEARNING OBJECTIVES

After completing this case study, the reader should be able to:

• Construct a prudent empiric antibiotic regimen for a febrile neutropenic patient.

• Determine appropriate situations to use vancomycin in empiric antimicrobial regimens for the treatment of febrile neutropenic episodes.

• Describe situations in which antibiotic monotherapy versus combination therapy would be warranted in the empiric treatment of febrile neutropenia.

PATIENT PRESENTATION

■ Chief Complaint

"I have a fever and chills."

■ HPI

Scarlet Hives is a 60-year-old woman with a history of IgG kappa multiple myeloma who is undergoing an autologous hematopoietic cell transplant. Her stem cells were collected by peripheral blood collection, which were mobilized with cyclophosphamide and filgrastim. During collection she developed a vesicular rash involving her left lower abdominal quadrant, which was documented by PCR analysis to be herpes zoster. This was treated with valacyclovir. Her preparative regimen for transplant was high-dose melphalan, followed by stem cell rescue with her peripheral blood stem cells. Eight days after stem cell infusion, she spiked a fever of 38.6°C (101.5°F). She now also complains of chills and nausea.

PMH

IgG kappa multiple myeloma
GERD
HTN
Hyperlipidemia
CAD
Peripheral neuropathy
Type 2 DM
Chronic back pain

Surgical History

Hysterectomy—17 years ago

FH

Mother died of CAD at early age; father died at age 67 from lung cancer; has one sister and one brother, both living and well.

SH

High school cafeteria manager of 22 years, now retired. She is married and lives with her husband. She has three children. Denies smoking or ethanol use.

Home Meds

Esomeprazole 40 mg PO once daily
Atorvastatin 80 mg PO once daily
Fentanyl patch 75 mcg Q 48 H
Neurontin 800 mg PO TID
Lisinopril 5 mg PO once daily
Metoprolol 75 mg PO BID
Multivitamin PO once daily
Oxycodone IR 15 mg Q 6 H PRN pain
Pioglitazone 15 mg PO once daily
Promethazine 25 mg PO Q 6 H PRN nausea
Valacyclovir 500 mg PO once daily, after previously completing 1,000 mg TID × 7 days for treatment course
Fluconazole 400 mg PO once daily
Levofloxacin 500 mg PO once daily
Filgrastim 480 mcg subcutaneously daily

All

Ceftazidime—bad rash

ROS

(+) Fever/chills, (+) nausea; denies vomiting, cough, diarrhea

Physical Examination

Gen

Patient is a 60-year-old Caucasian woman who appears alert and oriented

VS

BP 115/83 mm Hg, P 115 bpm, RR 16, T 38.6°C; O_2 sat 98%; Wt 191 lb, Ht 5'1"

Skin

Warm and dry. No erythema or induration around port on left chest. Resolving herpes zoster rash on abdomen; lesions are crusted and healing.

HEENT

PERRLA, EOMI, (–) tonsillar erythema, (–) rhinorrhea, (–) mucositis

Neck/Lymph Nodes

Neck supple; no lymphadenopathy

Lungs/Thorax

Normal; no wheezes, crackles, or rhonchi

Heart

Tachycardic but regular rhythm; no murmurs, rubs, or gallops

Abd

Soft, NT, (+) bowel sounds

Genit/Rect

Deferred

MS/Ext

No deformity, mild weakness, no peripheral edema

Neuro

A & O × 3; CN II–XII grossly intact

Labs

Na 135 mEq/L	WBC 0.2×10^3/mm³	AST 16 IU/L
K 3.6 mEq/L	PMNs 14%	ALT 15 IU/L
Cl 95 mEq/L	Bands 5%	Alk phos 38 IU/L
CO_2 21 mEq/L	Lymphs 81%	LDH 187 IU/L
BUN 16 mg/dL	Hgb 8.9 g/dL	T. bili 0.6 mg/dL
SCr 1.0 mg/dL	Hct 25.3%	
Glu 149 mg/dL	RBC 2.6×10^6/mm³	
Ca 8.0 mg/dL	Plt 21×10^3/mm³	

UA

Pending

Blood Cultures

PICC line: Pending
Peripheral: Pending

Chest X-Ray

Interval presence of a 2.2-cm oval-shaped density projecting at the level of the retrocardiac aspect of the medial left lung base

CT Scan with IV Contrast

Normal, no evidence of pulmonary nodule that was a concern on chest x-ray

Assessment

1. Multiple myeloma s/p autologous stem cell transplant
2. Neutropenic fever
3. Concern for possible pneumonia, ruled out by CT scan

Plan

1. Begin empiric antimicrobials:

   Piperacillin–tazobactam 4.5 g IV Q 8 H (infused over 30 minutes)

2. Discontinue prophylactic levofloxacin.

3. Monitor for rash due to history of ceftazidime allergy.

4. Monitor renal function and hydrate with IV fluids due to IV contrast with CT scan.

5. Continue home medications.

QUESTIONS

Problem Identification

1.a. Create a list of the patient's drug therapy problems.

1.b. What information (signs, symptoms, and laboratory values) indicates the presence or severity of each of the drug therapy problems?

Desired Outcome

2. What are the goals of pharmacotherapy in this patient's case?

Therapeutic Alternatives

3.a. What nondrug therapies might be useful for this patient?

3.b. What feasible pharmacotherapeutic alternatives are available for treating this febrile episode?

Optimal Plan

4. What drug(s), dosage form(s), dose(s), schedule, and duration of therapy are best for the empiric treatment of this febrile episode in this patient?

Outcome Evaluation

5. What clinical and laboratory parameters are necessary to evaluate the therapy for achievement of the desired therapeutic outcome and to detect or prevent adverse effects?

Patient Education

6. What information should be provided to the patient to enhance adherence, ensure successful therapy, and minimize adverse effects?

■ CLINICAL COURSE

On day 2 of admission, the patient is still febrile and the following laboratory results are reported: SCr 2.1 mg/dL, Hgb 8.4 g/dL, Hct 22.8%, and platelets $9 \times 10^3/mm^3$. The WBC is $0.2 \times 10^3/mm^3$.

BP 120/75, P 100, RR 18, T 38.3°C, O_2 sat 98% RA

Urine and blood cultures (PICC line and peripheral): No growth at 24 hours

The team continued to monitor the patient as planned. She started developing a systemic erythematous rash. On day 3, her piperacillin–tazobactam was changed to imipenem–cilastatin due to the presumed drug rash. Her rash continued to worsen while taking imipenem. On day 5 (WBC = $0.3 \times 10^3/mm^3$) of the admission, caspofungin was added for empiric coverage of persistent fevers. On day 6, her WBC was $0.6 \times 10^3/mm^3$ with an ANC of $0.520 \times 10^3/mm^3$. At this time, her blood cultures (from the PICC line) became positive for gram-positive cocci in pairs and chains. The team added vancomycin 1500 mg Q 24 H and stopped the imipenem–cilastatin since the rash was still worsening and the patient was no longer neutropenic. The PICC line was removed, and caspofungin was also discontinued the next day. The final

identification of the organism in the blood was reported on day 8 as *Enterococcus faecalis*, sensitive to ampicillin and vancomycin. The patient became afebrile after initiation of vancomycin. Her creatinine had normalized by this time, she was no longer neutropenic, and her rash was starting to resolve. She was discharged to complete a 2-week course of vancomycin. All subsequent blood and urine cultures were negative for microbial growth.

■ FOLLOW-UP QUESTIONS

1. What other antibiotic therapies could have been used for the treatment of Mrs Hives's bacteremia?

2. What is the possibility of cross-reactivity between ceftazidime and aztreonam?

3. When should vancomycin be considered as an initial empiric agent in febrile neutropenic patients?

■ SELF-STUDY ASSIGNMENTS

1. Review the criteria for classification of febrile neutropenic patients as either "low" or "high" risk. What types of neutropenic patients would be considered "low risk" and might benefit from oral antibiotic regimens?

2. Construct a treatment algorithm for neutropenic patients with bloodstream infections caused by vancomycin-resistant *Enterococcus faecium* (VRE). The algorithm should include decisions based on renal function and drug contraindications.

CLINICAL PEARL

Bacterial infections in neutropenic patients have evolved from the historical isolation of gram-negative pathogens to the most common bacteria isolated currently being gram-positive organisms. This is especially true when fluoroquinolone prophylaxis is used.

REFERENCES

1. Freifeld AG, Bow EJ, Sepkowitz KA, et al. Clinical practice guideline for the use of antimicrobial agents in neutropenic patients with cancer: 2010 update by the Infectious Diseases Society of America. Clin Infect Dis 2011;52:e56–e93.

2. Mermel LA, Farr BM, Sherertz RJ, et al. Guidelines for the management of intravascular catheter-related infections. Clin Infect Dis 2009;49:1–45.

3. National Comprehensive Cancer Network (NCCN) Clinical Practice Guidelines in Oncology (v2.2015). Prevention and treatment of cancer-related infections. Available at: *http://www.nccn.org/professionals/physician_gls/PDF/infections.pdf*. Accessed January 18, 2016.

4. Tomblyn M, Chiller T, Einsele H, et al. Guidelines for preventing infectious complications among hematopoietic cell transplantation recipients: a global perspective. Biol Blood Marrow Transplant 2009;15:1143–1238.

5. Paul M, Soares-Weiser K, Leibovici L. Beta lactam monotherapy versus beta lactam-aminoglycoside combination therapy for fever with neutropenia: systematic review and meta-analysis. BMJ 2003;326:1111–1119.

6. Gilbert DN, Chambers HF, Eliopoulos GM, Saag MS, eds. The Sanford Guide to Antimicrobial Therapy 2015. 45th Edition. Antimicrobial Therapy, Inc, Sperryville, VA, 2012.

7. Frumin J, Gallagher JC. Allergic cross-sensitivity between penicillin, carbapenem, and monobactam antibiotics: what are the chances? Ann Pharmacother 2009;43:304–315.

144

ANTIMICROBIAL PROPHYLAXIS FOR SURGERY

In Life, Preparation Is Everything . . . . Level II

Curtis L. Smith, PharmD, BCPS

LEARNING OBJECTIVES

After completing this case study, the reader should be able to:

- Recommend appropriate antimicrobial prophylaxis for a given surgical procedure.

- Discuss the timing of antimicrobial prophylaxis for surgery, including doses prior to surgery and dosing after surgery.

- Describe the controversy regarding mechanical bowel preparation prior to colorectal surgery.

- Identify the pros and cons to using oral antimicrobial decontamination prior to colorectal surgery.

- Evaluate the need for perioperative β-blocker therapy in a specific surgical patient.

PATIENT PRESENTATION

■ Chief Complaint

"I have colon cancer and I'm here for surgery."

■ HPI

Edward Adler is a 72-year-old man who was recently diagnosed with anemia and generalized weakness. The workup for anemia included a colonoscopy, which showed a malignant neoplasm of the proximal ascending colon. The neoplasm was identified, and the biopsy revealed moderately-differentiated adenocarcinoma. The patient denies any current abdominal pain or change in bowel habits, but reports a 20-lb weight loss over the past several months. He is eating but has less of an appetite than normal.

■ PMH

Positive for HTN, CAD, TIA, and chronic rhinitis; also mild osteoarthritis, for which he has required no regularly scheduled medications in the past. History of gastritis and anemia.

■ PSH

Tonsillectomy, left inguinal hernia repair, colonoscopy with biopsy.

■ SH

Positive for smoking history of one half of a pack daily; quit 20 years ago.

■ Meds

Atenolol 100 mg PO daily
Hydrochlorothiazide 12.5 mg PO daily
Atorvastatin 40 mg PO daily
Sertraline 100 mg PO daily
Omeprazole 20 mg PO daily
Aspirin 81 mg PO daily
Triamcinolone nasal spray, two sprays in the morning
Ferrous sulfate 325 mg PO TID
Multivitamin one PO once daily

■ All

None

■ ROS

Cardiopulmonary: Denies chest pain, shortness of breath, or wheezing.
Gastrointestinal: Denies history of hepatitis, ulcers, or jaundice.
Genitourinary: He has no history of hematuria or renal calculi.
Musculoskeletal: Positive for arthritis of both wrists and hands.
Psychiatric: Positive for some depression.

■ Physical Examination

Gen

He has the appearance of a normally developed white man who appears his stated age. He is alert, awake, and in no obvious distress.

VS

BP 132/86 mm Hg, P 68 bpm, RR 11, T 37.1°C; Wt 69 kg, Ht 172.7 cm

Skin

Warm and dry. Multiple seborrheic dermatomes over the abdomen and chest.

HEENT

Face reveals no asymmetry. Pupils are equal. Eyes have no icterus or exophthalmus, extraocular muscles intact. He is wearing corrective lenses.

Neck/Lymph Nodes

No adenopathy or thyromegaly. There is no jugular venous distention.

Lungs/Thorax

Clear to auscultation

CV

Regular rate and rhythm without murmurs

Abd

The patient has a faint, left inguinal scar from prior left inguinal hernia repair. The abdomen is without palpable masses, splenomegaly, or hepatomegaly. No tenderness noted.

Genit/Rect

Not examined

MS/Ext

No scoliosis. He has normal lordotic and kyphotic components to the vertebral curvature. No paravertebral tenderness or spasm. Leg lengths and shoulder heights are grossly equal. He was examined in the sitting and supine positions. Extremities: no gross deformities, rashes, or ecchymoses. 2+ pulses in all four extremities.

Neuro

No gross motor or sensory deficits or hyperreflexia. Good grip strength bilaterally.

◼ Labs

Na 132 mEq/L	Hgb 9.9 g/dL	WBC $6.0 \times 10^3/mm^3$
K 4.1 mEq/L	Hct 30.2%	PMNs 70%
Cl 97 mEq/L	RBC $4.06 \times 10^6/mm^3$	Bands 0%
CO_2 26 mEq/L	Plt $324 \times 10^3/mm^3$	Eos 5%
BUN 14 mg/dL	MCV 74 μm³	Lymphs 13%
SCr 0.9 mg/dL	MCHC 32.8 g/dL	Monos 12%
Glu 93 mg/dL		
Alb 3.9 g/dL		

◼ Assessment

1. Adenocarcinoma of the proximal ascending colon
2. Right hemicolectomy planned

QUESTIONS

Problem Identification

1.a. Based on the planned surgical procedure, what is the risk for a surgical wound infection in this patient postoperatively?

1.b. List all of the patient's drug-related problems, including potential postoperative problems.

Desired Outcome

2. What are the goals of antimicrobial pharmacotherapy for prevention of a surgical wound infection?

Therapeutic Alternatives

3.a. Discuss the pharmacologic options available for this patient to prevent a surgical wound infection. When would you dose antimicrobials related to the surgical procedure, and how long would you continue antibiotics after the procedure?

3.b. Will a mechanical bowel preparation prior to surgery benefit this patient?

3.c. What are the potential advantages and disadvantages associated with giving oral antibiotics prior to a colorectal surgical procedure?

Optimal Plan

4.a. What would you recommend for antimicrobial prophylaxis prior to this surgical procedure?

4.b. Will this patient require additional antimicrobial dosing during the procedure? How long would you continue antibiotics following the procedure?

4.c. Should this patient receive perioperative β-blocker therapy?

Outcome Evaluation

5. What clinical parameters should be monitored to assess the development of a surgical wound infection?

Patient Education

6. What information should be provided to this patient regarding the risk of surgical wound infections and the use of antibiotics to prevent this risk?

◼ SELF-STUDY ASSIGNMENTS

1. Construct a chart listing surgical procedures requiring preoperative antimicrobial prophylaxis and the recommended agent(s) to use.

2. Perform a literature search and assess the current information regarding the use of oral antibiotics prior to colorectal surgery.

3. Perform a literature search and assess the current information regarding using perioperative β-blockers (based on both patient characteristics and surgical procedure).

CLINICAL PEARL

Patients who receive antibiotics for surgical prophylaxis within 3 hours after the surgical incision have a three times higher risk of surgical wound infection compared to patients who receive antibiotics within 2 hours before the incision.

REFERENCES

1. Edwards JR, Peterson KD, Mu Y, et al. National Healthcare Safety Network (NHSN) report: data summary for 2006 through 2008, issued December 2009. Am J Infect Control 2009;37(10):783–805.
2. Hawn MT, Richman JS, Vick CC, et al. Timing of surgical antibiotic prophylaxis and the risk of surgical site infection. JAMA Surg. 2013 Jul;148(7):649–657.
3. Fleisher LA, Fleischmann KE, Auerbach AD, et al. 2014 ACC/AHA guideline on perioperative cardiovascular evaluation and management of patients undergoing noncardiac surgery: a report of the American College of Cardiology/American Heart Association Task Force on Practice Guidelines. Circulation. 2014 Dec 9;130(24):e278–333.
4. Deveraux PJ, Mirkobrada M, Sessler DI, et al. Aspirin in patients undergoing noncardiac surgery. N Engl J Med 2014;370:1484–1503.
5. Gould MK, Garcia DA, Wren SM, et al. American College of Chest Physicians. Prevention of VTE in nonorthopedic surgical patients: antithrombotic therapy and prevention of thrombosis, 9th ed. American College of Chest Physicians Evidence-Based Clinical Practice Guidelines. Chest 2012;141(2 Suppl):e227S–e277S.
6. Bratzler DW, Dellinger EP, Olsen KM, et al. Clinical practice guidelines for antimicrobial prophylaxis in surgery. Am J Health Syst Pharm 2013;70:195–283.
7. Classen DC, Evans RS, Pestotnik SL, Horn SD, Menlove RL, Burke JP. The timing of prophylactic administration of antibiotics and the risk of surgical-wound infection. N Engl J Med 1992;326:281–286.
8. Scher KS. Studies on the duration of antibiotic administration for surgical prophylaxis. Am Surg 1997;63:59–62.
9. Nelson RL, Gladman E, Barbateskovic M. Antimicrobial prophylaxis for colorectal surgery. Cochrane Database Syst Rev 2014 May 9;5:CD001181.
10. Dahabreh IJ, Steele DW, Shah N, Trikalinos TA. Oral Mechanical Bowel Preparation for Colorectal Surgery: Systematic Review and Meta-Analysis. Dis Colon Rectum 2015 Jul;58(7):698–707.

145

PEDIATRIC IMMUNIZATION

Back to School. . . . . Level II

Jean-Venable "Kelly" R. Goode, PharmD, BCPS, FAPhA, FCCP

LEARNING OBJECTIVES

After completing this case study, the reader should be able to:

- Develop a plan for administering any needed vaccines, when given a patient's age, immunization history, and medical history.

- Describe appropriate use of pediatric vaccines.

- Educate a child's parents on the risks associated with pediatric vaccines and ways to minimize adverse effects.

- Recognize inappropriate reasons for deferring immunization.

PATIENT PRESENTATION

■ Chief Complaint

"My daughter is here for the 'Back to School' program."

■ HPI

Allison Showalter is a 4-year-old girl who is generally healthy. She presents today (August 30, 2015) to the pharmacy with her mother for evaluation and to receive any needed immunizations. Allison will be entering junior kindergarten in the fall, and she needs to have an updated immunization record.

■ PMH

Some prenatal care, delivered at 42 weeks' gestation via uncomplicated vaginal delivery; birth weight 7 lb, 4 oz. Mother states that her child has had a couple of ear infections and three or four "colds," no other illnesses.

■ FH

Mother is 4 months pregnant

■ SH

Lives with mother, age 30, and father, age 32. No siblings. Mother works part-time. Father works as an electrician.

■ Meds

Amoxicillin suspension 540 mg PO Q 8 H
No recent OTC medication use

■ All

NKDA

■ ROS

Negative

■ Physical Examination

Gen

Alert, happy, appropriately developed 4-year-old child in NAD. Wt 18 kg (75th percentile), height 40 in (50th percentile).

VS

BP 105/65 mm Hg, P 110 bpm, RR 28, T 36.7°C (axillary)

HEENT

AF open, flat; PERRL; funduscopic exam not performed; ears slightly red; normal looking TMs, landmarks visualized, no effusion present; nose clear; throat normal

Lungs

Clear bilaterally

CV

RRR, no murmurs

Abd

Soft, nontender, no masses or organomegaly; normal bowel sounds

Genit/Rect

Normal external genitalia; rectal exam deferred, no fissures noted

Ext

Normal

Neuro

Alert; normal DTRs bilaterally

■ Labs

See Table 145-1. Immunization Record Card
No other labs obtained

■ Assessment

Normal-appearing child, in need of immunizations

TABLE 145-1 Immunization Record Card

Immunization Record Card
Name: Allison Showalter:

Vaccine	Dose/Route/Site	Date	Health Professional	VIS
Hepatitis B	0.5 mL IM thigh	3/15/2011	Colter, RN	Hep B
Pediarix (DTaP, Hep B, IPV)	0.5 mL IM thigh	5/20/2011	Edwards, RN	DTaP, Hep B, IPV
PCV-13	0.5 mL IM thigh	5/20/2011	Edwards, RN	PCV
Hib (HibTITER)	0.5 mL IM thigh	5/20/2011	Edwards, RN	Hib
Pediarix	0.5 mL IM thigh	7/29/2011	Edwards, RN	DTaP, Hep B, IPV
PCV-13	0.5 mL IM thigh	7/29/2011	Edwards, RN	PCV
Hib (HibTITER)	0.5 mL IM thigh	7/29/2011	Edwards, RN	Hib
Pediarix	0.5 mL IM thigh	9/30/2011	Jones, RN	DTaP, Hep B, IPV
PCV-13	0.5 mL IM thigh	9/30/2011	Jones, RN	PCV
Hib (HibTITER)	0.5 mL IM thigh	9/30/2011	Jones, RN	Hib
Hib (HibTITER)	0.5 mL IM thigh	4/1/2012	Edwards, RN	Hib
PCV-13	0.5 mL IM thigh	4/1/2012	Edwards, RN	PCV

QUESTIONS

Problem Identification

1. Create a list of the patient's immunization-related problems including any contraindications or precautions for vaccination.

Desired Outcome

2.a. What immediate goals are reasonable in this case?

2.b. What long-term goals are appropriate for comprehensive management of this patient?

Therapeutic Alternatives

3.a. How do health care providers determine which vaccines an infant or child needs?

3.b. What is the proper immunization administration technique for children, including location and needle size?

3.c. What vaccines should be administered to this child today, including dose, route, and any alternatives?

Optimal Plan

4.a. What immunization schedule should be followed for this patient today?

4.b. In addition to immunizations received today, what should be the plan for providing additional immunizations and when should they be administered?

Outcome Evaluation

5. How should the response to the immunization plan be assessed?

Patient Education

6. What important information about vaccination needs to be explained to this child's mother?

■ FOLLOW-UP QUESTIONS

1. The next year, the mother brings the child to a pediatric influenza immunization clinic. The mother mentions that the child was diagnosed with diabetes about 3 months ago. The child's immunization record reveals influenza vaccine 0.5 mL × 1 dose last fall. What is your recommendation for influenza vaccine for this child?

2. What other immunizations are indicated for this child who now has a chronic condition, diabetes mellitus?

■ SELF-STUDY ASSIGNMENTS

1. Search the internet for the immunization laws and allowed exemptions in your state. What vaccines are required for child-care and school entry?

2. Review the most current immunization recommendations for persons aged 0–6 years, and provide a summary of how your recommendations for this case would be different if a 6-month-old patient in need of immunizations came into your clinic today.

3. Search the internet for immunization-related websites about vaccine-associated adverse effects; compare and contrast these sites, and evaluate them against reliable websites for vaccine information.

CLINICAL PEARL

All states have immunization laws, but there are differences in the requirements and types of exemptions allowed. Vaccine requirements for school entry help ensure that most people are protected through immunization. Pharmacists should advocate for parents and caregivers to have their children immunized on time to protect them against vaccine-preventable diseases.

REFERENCES

1. Centers for Disease Control and Prevention. Advisory Committee on Immunization Practices (ACIP). Recommended immunization schedules for persons aged 0–18 years—United States, 2015. MMWR 2015;64(04):93–94 (updated annually at: http://www.cdc.gov/vaccines/schedules/hcp/child-adolescent.html). Accessed March 25, 2016.

2. American Academy of Pediatrics. Active and passive immunization. In: Red Book—Report of the Committee on Infectious Diseases. Pickering LK, ed., 30th ed. Elk Grove Village, IL, American Academy of Pediatrics, 2015:1–101.

3. Chen RT, Clark TA, Halperin SA. The yin and yang of paracetamol and paediatric immunizations. Lancet 2009;374:1305–1306.

4. Centers for Disease Control and Prevention. General recommendations on immunization. Recommendations of the Advisory Committee on Immunization Practices (ACIP). MMWR 2011;60(RR-2):1–60.

5. Centers for Disease Control and Prevention. Licensure of a Diphtheria and Tetanus Toxoids and Acellular Pertussis Adsorbed and Inactivated Poliovirus Vaccine and Guidance for Use as a Booster Dose. MMWR 2015;64(34):948–949.

6. Marin M, Broder KR, Temte JL, et al. Use of combination measles, mumps, rubella, and varicella vaccine. Recommendations of the Advisory Committee on Immunization Practices (ACIP). MMWR 2010;59(RR-3):1–12.

7. Centers for Disease Control and Prevention. Prevention and control of influenza with vaccines: Recommendations of the Advisory Committee on Immunization Practices, United States, 2015–16 Influenza Season. MMWR 2015;64(30)818–825.

8. Centers for Disease Prevention and Control. Prevention of pneumococcal disease among infants and children—use of 13-valent pneumococcal conjugate vaccine and 23-valent pneumococcal polysaccharide vaccine. MMWR 2010;59(RR-11):1–18.

146

ADULT IMMUNIZATION

Immunizations: Not Just Kid Stuff . . . . Level II

Jean-Venable "Kelly" R. Goode, PharmD, BCPS, FAPhA, FCCP

LEARNING OBJECTIVES

After completing this case study, the reader should be able to:

• Develop a plan for administering any needed vaccines when given a patient's age, immunization history, and medical history.

• Recognize appropriate precautions and contraindications for vaccination, including inappropriate reasons for deferring vaccination.

- Explain appropriate administration of vaccines, including timing and spacing of both inactive and live attenuated vaccines.

- Recognize the differences in vaccines for young adults currently in use in the United States.

PATIENT PRESENTATION

■ Chief Complaint

"I'm here to get my new prescription filled."

■ HPI

Sandra Williams is a 23-year-old woman who presents to your pharmacy in January with a new prescription for prednisone 40 mg PO BID for 10 days. She has had a moderate asthma exacerbation. She just started her new job as an elementary school teacher. She is a new patient to your pharmacy. She inquires about your "One less" signs which refers to a national HPV vaccination campaign.

■ PMH

Moderate persistent asthma
Chickenpox at age 5 per patient
Splenectomy secondary to car accident 3 months ago

■ FH

One sister—healthy
Mother—healthy
Father with type 2 diabetes

■ SH

Does not smoke
Drinks alcohol socially

■ Meds

Albuterol MDI two inhalations PRN
Pulmicort DPI two inhalations once daily

■ All

NKDA

■ Immunization Record

No vaccines since kindergarten except:

- Meningococcal vaccine before she started her freshman year in college

- One dose of hepatitis B vaccine before she started her freshman year in college

- MMR vaccine before she started her freshman year in college, Td 10 years ago at her adolescent well check-up

■ ROS

WDWN African-American woman in NAD

■ VS

BP 120/72 mm Hg (left arm, large cuff, seated), P 76 bpm; Wt 54 kg, Ht 5′5″

■ Physical Examination

Deferred

■ Assessment

A 23-year-old woman recently treated for a moderate asthma exacerbation. She is in need of immunizations today.

QUESTIONS

Problem Identification

1.a. Create a list of the patient's immunization-related problems, including any contraindications or precautions for vaccination.

1.b. Create a list of this patient's drug-related problems.

Desired Outcome

2.a. What immediate immunization goals are reasonable in this case?

2.b. Provide the rationale for administering each of the recommended vaccines to this patient.

2.c. What long-term goals are appropriate for comprehensive management of this patient?

Therapeutic Alternatives

3. Identify the therapeutic alternatives for addressing this patient's immunization needs.

Optimal Plan

4. What immunization schedule should be followed for this patient today, including dose and route of administration and the plan for providing additional immunizations?

Outcome Evaluation

5. How should the response to the immunization plan be assessed?

Patient Education

6. What important information about vaccination needs to be explained to this patient?

■ FOLLOW-UP QUESTIONS

1. What screening questions should a patient be asked prior to administering any vaccinations?

2. What must be documented after a health care practitioner administers a vaccination?

■ SELF-STUDY ASSIGNMENTS

1. Review the most current immunization recommendations for adults, and provide a summary of how your recommendations for this case would be different if this person were 65 years of age.

2. Develop a list of diseases and medications indicating that a patient may be a candidate for immunization.

3. Research the laws in your state to verify which vaccines pharmacists may administer. Also, explore how to implement an immunization service in your practice.

4. Review the guidelines for vaccination of pregnant women.

5. Search the internet for immunization-related websites about vaccine-associated adverse effects; compare and contrast these sites, and evaluate them against reliable websites for vaccine information.

CLINICAL PEARL

Delays in vaccination put patients at risk of vaccine-preventable diseases. However, there is no need to restart an immunization series if the interval between doses is longer than that recommended in the routine schedule. Instead of starting over, merely count the doses administered (provided that they were given at an acceptable minimum interval) and complete the series.

REFERENCES

1. Centers for Disease Control and Prevention. Advisory Committee on Immunization Practices. Recommended adult immunization schedule for immunization schedules for adults aged 19 years and older—United States, 2015. MMWR 2015;64(4):91–92. (Updated annually at *http://www.cdc.gov/vaccines/schedules/hcp/adult.html*). Accessed March 25, 2016.

2. Centers for Disease Control and Prevention. Use of 13-valent pneumococcal conjugate vaccine and 23-valent pneumococcal polysaccharide vaccine for adults with immunocompromising conditions: recommendations of the Advisory Committee on Immunization Practices (ACIP). MMWR 2012;61(40):816–819.

3. Centers for Disease Control and Prevention. Prevention and control of meningococcal disease: recommendations of the Advisory Committee on Immunization Practices (ACIP). MMWR 2013;62(RR02):1–22.

4. Centers for Disease Control and Prevention. Updated recommendations for prevention of invasive pneumococcal disease among adults using the 23-valent pneumococcal. MMWR 2010;59(34):1102–1106.

5. Kobayashi M, Bennett NM, Gierke R, et al. Intervals between PCV13 and PPSV23 vaccines: recommendations of the Advisory Committee on Immunization Practices (ACIP). MMWR 2015;64(34):944–947.

6. Centers for Disease Control and Prevention. Human papillomavirus vaccine: recommendations of the Advisory Committee on Immunization Practices (ACIP). MMWR 2014;63(RR05):1–30.

7. Centers for Disease Control and Prevention. Updated recommendations for the use of tetanus toxoid, reduced diphtheria acellular pertussis (Tdap) vaccine from the Advisory Committee on Immunization Practices, 2010. MMWR 2011;60(01):13–15.

8. Centers for Disease Control and Prevention. Prevention and control of *Haemophilus influenza* Type B Disease: recommendations of the Advisory Committee on Immunization Practices (ACIP). MMWR 2014;63(RR01);1–14.

9. Centers for Disease Control and Prevention. Prevention and control of influenza with vaccines: Recommendations of the Advisory Committee on Immunization Practices, United States, 2015–16 Influenza Season. MMWR 2015;64(30)818–825.

10. Petrosky E, Bocchini JA, Hariri S, et al. Use of 9-Valent Human Papillomavirus (HPV) Vaccine: Updated HPV Vaccination Recommendations of the Advisory Committee on Immunization Practices MMWR 2015;64(11);300–304.

147

HIV INFECTION

The Antiretroviral-Naive Patient................. Level II

Rodrigo M. Burgos, PharmD, AAHIVE

Sarah M. Michienzi, PharmD

LEARNING OBJECTIVES

After completing this case study, the reader should be able to:

- Describe when antiretroviral therapy should be initiated in patients with HIV infection, and determine the desired outcome of such therapy.

- Recommend appropriate first-line antiretroviral therapies for the antiretroviral-naive person.

- Provide patient education on the proper dose, administration, and adverse effects of antiretroviral agents.

PATIENT PRESENTATION

▓ Chief Complaint

"I am here for regular care. It hurts to swallow."

▓ HPI

Jenny Baird is a 34-year-old woman diagnosed with HIV infection 2 years ago during a routine exam. At the time of diagnosis, the patient was asymptomatic. She is currently antiretroviral therapy (ART) naïve, and since her diagnosis, she has been following up regularly every 4 months. However, up to this point, she has not been ready to commit to ART. Today she returns for a follow-up visit and reports painful and difficult swallowing over the past 2–3 weeks.

▓ PMH

HIV infection, diagnosed 2 years ago; risk factor heterosexual contact
Bronchitis
Asthma
GERD

▓ FH

Noncontributory

▓ SH

History of crack cocaine use, last use 1 month ago
Smokes marijuana once per month, mainly as an appetite enhancer
Tobacco 0.5 ppd
EtOH, one to two drinks on weekends
Unemployed, lives with partner
Sexually active with stable partner, 100% condom use as sole method of contraception; partner is HIV (–) and is aware of her HIV status

▓ Medications

Multivitamin with minerals PO once daily
Tums PRN heartburn
Albuterol HFA MDI, two puffs Q 6 H PRN SOB

▓ All

TMP/SMX (rash)

▓ ROS

Difficulty and pain on swallowing

▓ Physical Examination

Gen

Thin, well-developed black female in NAD, alert and oriented × 3

VS

BP 110/64 mm Hg, P 80 bpm, RR 18, T 35.9°C; Wt 58 kg, Ht 5′5″

Skin

Anicteric, has large tattoo on back, no other skin lesions noted

HEENT

(+) Oral lesions and white plaques, sinuses nontender, PERRLA, ears and nose clear

Neck

Supple, no thyromegaly, R neck lymph node 0.7 cm in diameter

Chest

Lungs clear

CV

S_1, S_2 without S_3, S_4, or murmur

Abd

(+) BS, soft, nontender, without HSM
(+) Bilateral inguinal lymph nodes 0.5 cm in diameter

GU

The pelvic exam reveals normal external genitalia. The vaginal vault is within normal limits. Perineum and perianal regions are free of grossly visible lesions. Guaiac (–) stools.

Ext

No wasting, no CCE

Neuro

No focal deficits

■ Labs

See **Table 147-1**

■ Assessment

A 34-year-old woman with HIV infection, ART-naïve, shows steady decline in CD4 cell count and rising levels of HIV viremia since her initial diagnosis 2 years ago, presenting with painful swallowing and white plaques on posterior pharynx, and mouth consistent with esophageal and oropharyngeal candidiasis.

QUESTIONS

Problem Identification

1.a. What information (signs, symptoms, and laboratory values) indicates the severity of HIV disease?

1.b. Is prophylactic therapy for any associated opportunistic pathogen indicated in this patient? Why or why not?

1.c. What is your recommendation regarding antiretroviral therapy for this patient?

Desired Outcome

2. What are the goals of pharmacotherapy in this case?

Therapeutic Alternatives

3.a. What therapeutic options are available for treating this antiretroviral-naive patient?

3.b. What economic, psychosocial, racial, and ethical considerations are applicable to this patient?

3.c. How would you evaluate patient readiness for antiretroviral treatment initiation?

TABLE 147-1 Laboratory Values for the Previous Visit and for Subsequent Visits

Parameter (Units)	2 Years Ago	This Visit	6 Weeks Later	12 Weeks Later
Weight (kg)	65	58	57	60
Hematology:				
Hgb (g/dL)	10.9	11.1	12.2	12.9
Hct (%)	32.9	33.6	36.5	37.3
Plt (x10³/mm³)	234	287	298	311
WBC (x10³/mm³)	7.1	5.7	6.9	7.1
Lymphs (%)	47.3	45.5	44.9	47.3
Monos (%)	6.4	6.6	6.1	6.4
Eos (%)	3.5	0.9	2.0	3.5
Basos (%)	0.3	0.2	0.4	0.3
Neutros (%)	42.5	46.8	46.6	42.5
ANC (x10³/mm³)	3.0	2.7	3.2	3.0
Chemistry:				
BUN (mg/dL)	5	10	9	7
SCr (mg/dL)	0.8	0.9	0.9	0.8
T. bili (mg/dL)	0.5	1.6	0.6	–
Alb (g/dL)	3.3	3.8	3.4	–
AST (IU/L)	17	19	18	–
ALT (IU/L)	12	13	14	–
Fasting glucose	115	93	92	
Fasting lipid profile:				
T. chol	–	162	164	–
Triglycerides	–	53	92	–
LDL	–	45	112	–
Surrogate markers:				
CD4 (%)	38	25	–	17
CD4 (cells/mm³)	689	477	–	529
CD8 (%)	48	48	–	59
HIV RNA (RT-PCR)[a] (copies/mL)	25,000	155,000	154	20
Antiviral resistance test (genotypic resistance test)	L63P	–	–	–
Hepatitis virus serologies:				
HBV Ab	Negative	–	–	–
HBV core Ab total	Negative	–	–	–
HBV Ag	Negative	–	–	–
HCV Ab	Negative	–	–	–
HAV Ab	Positive	–	–	–
Other tests:				
Human chorionic gonadotropin (hCG)	Negative	Negative		

[a]Reverse transcriptase polymerase chain reaction assay.

Optimal Plan

4.a. Propose an antiretroviral regimen for this woman. Indicate the drug name, dosage form, dose, schedule, and duration of therapy for the regimen you choose.

4.b. Design an antiretroviral regimen that would be appropriate if the patient informs you that she would like to consider becoming pregnant once her HIV infection is under control.

4.c. Recommend an antiretroviral regimen that would be appropriate if this patient has a history of chronic kidney disease, not requiring hemodialysis.

4.d. Discuss the role of HIV resistance testing in designing an initial regimen for the antiretroviral treatment-naive patient.

Outcome Evaluation

5. What clinical and laboratory parameters are necessary to evaluate the clinical efficacy and toxicity of the antiretroviral regimen

selected? Specify frequency with which you will monitor these parameters. Indicate therapeutic goal.

Patient Education

6.a. What important information would you provide to this patient about her therapy?

6.b. Explain in nontechnical terms the surrogate markers and their use in monitoring HIV disease.

6.c. Identify potential barriers to medication adherence, and discuss potential strategies to overcome these barriers and maximize treatment adherence.

■ CLINICAL COURSE

The provider and patient accepted your treatment recommendations. The patient returns to the clinic for follow-up 6 and 12 weeks after treatment initiation. She reports nausea from her medications that resolved after several days of therapy. Her treatment flow sheet is as follows:

Parameter	6 Weeks Later	12 Weeks Later
HIV RNA (RT-PCR) (copies/mL)	154	<20
CD4-lymphocyte count (cells/mm³)	NA	529
Symptoms of HIV infection	Asymptomatic	Asymptomatic
Adverse events reported	Mild nausea, no vomiting	None
Concomitant medications	Oral contraceptive daily	Oral contraceptive daily
	MVI with minerals daily	MVI with minerals daily
	Dapsone 100 mg daily	Dapsone 100 mg daily
	Albuterol INH PRN	Albuterol INH PRN
	Tums PRN	Tums PRN

■ FOLLOW-UP QUESTIONS

1. Provide an assessment of the antiretroviral regimen efficacy at each follow-up visit.

2. Identify potential problems with her concomitant medications and discuss alternatives.

■ SELF-STUDY ASSIGNMENTS

1. Review the current literature regarding recommended therapy for the antiretroviral-naive and treatment-experienced individuals. What is the recommended first-line therapy, and what are the indications to change to alternative therapy? What is known about therapy of HIV and survival?

2. Review the current literature regarding the development of HIV resistance to antiretroviral agents and strategies for the prevention and management of resistance.

CLINICAL PEARL

Updated guidelines recommend that ART be initiated in all HIV-infected patients, regardless of CD4 count. This recommendation is based on two randomized controlled trials, START

and TEMPRANO, which revealed greater clinical benefit when antiretroviral therapy is started early, as well an effort to prevent transmission. In addition to potency and efficacy factors, clinicians must take into account a wide range of individual factors, including comorbid conditions, transmitted resistant virus, adherence, potential adverse events, drug–drug or drug–food interactions, and consequences of virologic failure for the particular regimen selected. Clinicians should always individualize therapeutic choices based on available data and unique patient factors.

REFERENCES

1. Centers for Disease Control and Prevention. Revised surveillance case definitions for HIV infection among adults, adolescents, and children aged <18 months and for HIV infection and AIDS among children aged 18 months to <13 years—United States, 2008. MMWR 2008;57(RR-10):1–8.

2. Centers for Disease Control and Prevention. Appendix A: AIDS-defining conditions. MMWR 2008;57(RR-10):9.

3. Panel on opportunistic infections in HIV-infected adults and adolescents. Guidelines for prevention and treatment of opportunistic infections in HIV-infected Adults and Adolescents: recommendations from the Centers for Disease Control (CDC) and Prevention, the National Institutes of Health (NIH), and the HIV Medical Association of the Infectious Diseases Society of America. November 4, 2015. Available at: *https://aidsinfo.nih.gov/guidelines/html/4/adult-and-adolescent-oi-prevention-and-treatment-guidelines/0*. Accessed April 19, 2016.

4. Guidelines for the use of antiretroviral agents in HIV-infected adults and adolescents. Department of Health and Human Services (DHHS) Panel on Antiretroviral Guidelines for Adults and Adolescents, April 8, 2015. Available at: *https://aidsinfo.nih.gov/guidelines/html/1/adult-and-adolescent-treatment-guidelines/0*. Accessed April 19, 2016.

5. Guideline on when to start antiretroviral therapy and on pre-exposure prophylaxis for HIV. World Health Organization, September 2015. Available at: *http://apps.who.int/iris/bitstream/10665/186275/1/9789241509565_eng.pdf?ua=1*. Accessed April 19, 2016.

6. Gunthard HF, Aberg JA, Eron JJ, et al. Antiretroviral treatment of adult HIV infection: 2014 recommendations of the International Antiviral Society–USA Panel. JAMA 2014;312(4):410–425.

7. Recommendations for use of antiretroviral drugs in pregnancy HIV-1-infected women for maternal health and interventions to reduce perinatal HIV transmission in the United States. Department of Health and Human Services (DHHS) Panel on Antiretroviral Guidelines for Adults and Adolescents, August 16, 2015. Available at: *https://aidsinfo.nih.gov/guidelines/html/3/perinatal-guidelines/224*. Accessed April 19, 2016.

8. Paterson DL, Swindells S, Mohr J, et al. Adherence to protease inhibitor therapy and outcomes in patients with HIV infection. Ann Intern Med 2000;133:21–30.

9. Novak RM, Chen L, MacArthur RD, et al. Prevalence of antiretroviral drug resistance mutations in chronically HIV-infected, treatment-naive patients: implications for routine resistance screening before initiation of antiretroviral therapy. Clin Infect Dis 2005;40:468–474.

10. Little SJ, Holte S, Routy JP, et al. Antiretroviral-drug resistance among patients recently infected with HIV. N Engl J Med 2002;347:385–394.

148

BREAST CANCER

An Opportunity Lost..........................Level II

Neelam K. Patel, PharmD, BCOP

Bonnie Lin Boster, PharmD, BCOP

LEARNING OBJECTIVES

After completing this case study, the reader should be able to:

- Design a pharmacotherapeutic plan for treatment of locally advanced breast cancer.

- Develop an appropriate monitoring plan for patients receiving adjuvant hormonal therapy for treatment of breast cancer.

- Describe appropriate follow-up for patients after definitive treatment of breast cancer.

- Provide patient education on the proper dosing, administration, and adverse effects of letrozole and palbociclib.

- Compare and contrast the goals of treatment for locally advanced breast cancer versus metastatic breast cancer.

PATIENT PRESENTATION

■ Chief Complaint

"I have a lump in my breast."

■ HPI

Rosalita Garza is a 61-year-old woman presenting for evaluation of a new mass in her left breast. She first noticed a palpable breast mass on self-examination approximately 14 months ago but was unable to have this further investigated due to loss of health insurance. The patient describes the mass as intermittently painful. A mammogram was performed prior to her current visit, which was suspicious for malignancy.

■ PMH

Musculoskeletal injury in 2012. Fell from a chair while at work and suffered injuries to her cervical spine. She has required bone grafting from her right hip to her cervical spine. She is taking multiple medications for pain control.

Depression (diagnosed 7 years ago).

■ FH

Sister diagnosed with breast cancer at age 60, now 5 years postsurgery. The patient was unable to recall any further details. No other significant cancer history is noted.

■ SH

Lives with and acts as primary caretaker for her mother, who has dementia. Denies alcohol use and is a nonsmoker. Has a 35-year-old daughter who also lives with her.

■ Endocrine History

Menarche age 13; menopause age 55; first child age 26; $G_1P_1A_0$. Last Pap smear at age 40. Took Premarin as HRT for 5 years after the onset of menopause.

■ Meds

Protonix 40 mg PO once daily

Zoloft 50 mg PO once daily

Ambien CR 12.5 mg PO at bedtime PRN sleep

Neurontin 300 mg PO TID

Hydrocodone/acetaminophen 5 mg/300 mg, one to two tablets PO Q 6 H PRN pain

■ All

NKDA

■ ROS

Negative except for complaints noted above

■ Physical Examination

Gen

WDWN 61-year-old Hispanic female. Awake, alert, in NAD.

VS

BP 127/71 mm Hg, P 89 bpm, RR 16, T 36.7°C; Wt 137 lb, Ht 5'1″

HEENT

NC/AT; PERRLA; EOMI; ear, nose, and throat are clear

Neck/Lymph Nodes

Supple. No lymphadenopathy, thyromegaly, or masses. No supraclavicular or infraclavicular adenopathy.

Lungs

CTA and percussion

Breasts

Left: Notable for a 2.5-cm mass at the 6 o'clock position, approximately 3 cm from the nipple margin, not fixated to skin; no nipple

retraction or discharge is visualized; the mass is not tender to palpation; 1.5-cm, nontender, palpable mass in the axilla noted. *Right:* Without mass or lymphadenopathy.

CV

RRR; no murmurs, rubs, or gallops

Abd

Soft, NT/ND, normoactive bowel sounds. No appreciable hepatosplenomegaly.

Spine

Slight tenderness to percussion

Ext

No CCE

Neuro

No deficits noted

■ Labs

Na 142 mEq/L	Hgb 12.9 g/dL	WBC $8.7 \times 10^3/mm^3$	AST 36 IU/L
K 3.7 mEq/L	Hct 37.6%	Neutros 55%	ALT 17 IU/L
Cl 102 mEq/L	RBC $4.13 \times 10^6/mm^3$	Lymphs 35%	LDH 488 IU/L
CO_2 26 mEq/L	Plt $410 \times 10^3/mm^3$	Monos 8%	T. bili 0.2 mg/dL
BUN 9 mg/dL	PT 11.9 sec	Eos 2%	CA 27.29
SCr 0.7 mg/dL	INR 1.09		36.2 units/mL
Glu 83 mg/dL	aPTT 30.1 sec		

■ Chest X-Ray

Lungs are clear

■ Other

Diagnostic bilateral mammogram (Fig. 148-1):

1. American College of Radiology Category V, highly suspicious for malignancy in the left breast. There is a high-density, irregular mass measuring 2.2 cm with indistinct margins seen in the left breast lower hemisphere at 6 o'clock located 3 cm from the nipple.

2. In the right breast, no dominant mass, distortion, or suspicious calcifications are identified.

Unilateral ultrasound left breast and left axilla with biopsy:

1. An ill-defined, hypoechoic mass is noted in the 5:00–6:00 region. This measures approximately 2.5 cm × 2.3 cm × 1.5 cm and is located 3 cm from the nipple. A core biopsy of this mass was performed.

2. Suspicious lymph nodes are noted in the axilla. The largest node measures 1.8 cm × 1.8 cm × 1.4 cm. FNA of this lymph node was performed. In the infraclavicular region, a few hypoechoic lymph nodes were also seen and were located in the lateral aspect. The largest node measured 0.8 cm × 0.8 cm × 0.8 cm. FNA of this infraclavicular lymph node was performed. No suspicious internal mammary or supraclavicular lymph nodes were seen.

Core needle biopsy of left breast mass:

Left breast, 6 o'clock: infiltrating ductal carcinoma, modified Black's nuclear grade II (moderately differentiated), ER 95%, PR 95%, HER2 overexpression 2+, HER2 FISH negative (no amplification), and Ki-67 30% (moderate)

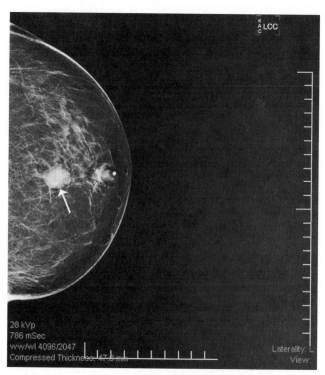

FIGURE 148-1. Mammogram of left breast. *Arrow* indicates area of abnormality highly suspicious for malignancy.

FNA of left axillary and infraclavicular lymph nodes:

1. Left axillary lymph node: metastatic adenocarcinoma consistent with breast primary

2. Left infraclavicular lymph node: metastatic adenocarcinoma consistent with breast primary

Bone scan:

1. No definite evidence of osseous metastases

2. Abnormality in cervical spine consistent with previous history of bone grafting

CT Abdomen:

No lesions suggestive of metastases.

CT chest:

No evidence of metastases.

■ Assessment:

Ms Garza is a 61-year-old woman who has newly diagnosed breast cancer.

QUESTIONS

Problem Identification

1.a. Create a list of potential drug therapy problems in the patient's medication regimen.

1.b. Given this clinical information, what is this patient's clinical stage of breast cancer?

Desired Outcome

2.a. What is the primary goal for cancer treatment in this patient?

2.b. What is the prognosis for this patient based on tumor size and nodal status?

2.c. In addition to the stage of disease, what other factors are important for determining the prognosis for breast cancer?

Therapeutic Alternatives

3. List the treatment modalities available for this patient's breast cancer, and discuss their advantages and disadvantages.

Optimal Plan

4. Design an appropriate plan for treating this patient's breast cancer, focusing on pharmacologic and nonpharmacologic measures. If the plan includes chemotherapy, identify a specific regimen, and provide your rationale for selecting it.

Outcome Evaluation

5.a. What parameters should be monitored to evaluate the efficacy and adverse effects of the therapy you recommended?

■ CLINICAL COURSE

The patient tolerated your treatment plan well. Twelve months after its completion, the patient returns to clinic complaining of lower back pain for the past 3–4 weeks. She has been taking hydrocodone/acetaminophen more regularly, "about two or three pills per day." This is a significant change since previously she reported not taking any. The patient is restaged with a bone scan, chest x-ray, abdominal CT, chest CT, and laboratory tests. Bone scan reveals metastases to the lumbar spine without spinal cord compression. Chest x-ray is negative. Abdominal CT shows a solitary liver metastasis. Chest CT is negative for metastases. LFTs are within normal limits. Ca 27.29 is 100.7 units/mL. Biopsy of the liver lesion confirms recurrence of ER-positive, PR-positive, HER2-negative breast cancer. The physician concludes that this patient's breast cancer is now metastatic to the bone and liver. The previous therapy is discontinued, and the patient is started on palbociclib and letrozole. The patient's updated information is below.

Labs

Na 140 mEq/L	Hgb 12.5 g/dL	WBC 6.7×10^3/mm³	AST 40 IU/L
K 3.9 mEq/L	Hct 36.4%	Neutros 64%	ALT 24 IU/L
Cl 103 mEq/L	RBC 4.1×10^6/mm³	Lymphs 30%	LDH 502 IU/L
CO₂ 28 mEq/L	Plt 356×10^3/mm³	Monos 3%	T. bili 0.5 mg/dL
BUN 11 mg/dL		Eos 3%	CA 27.29
SCr 0.65 mg/dL			100.7 units/mL
Glu 92 mg/dL			

Meds

Cardizem CD 180 mg PO once daily

Protonix 40 mg PO once daily

Zoloft 50 mg PO once daily

Ambien CR 12.5 mg PO at bedtime PRN sleep

Hydrocodone/acetaminophen 5 mg/300 mg, one to two tablets PO Q 6 H PRN pain

Outcome Evaluation (continued)

5.b. What is this patient's current clinical stage of breast cancer, and what is the primary goal for cancer treatment for this patient now?

5.c. Based on the patient's current medication list, create a list of potential drug therapy problems as she begins a new therapy for cancer.

5.d. Since the patient has developed bone metastases, what other medication should be added to her treatment plan? At what dose and schedule?

Patient Education

6. What information should be provided to the patient regarding her new chemotherapy for breast cancer?

■ SELF-STUDY ASSIGNMENTS

1. Perform a literature search to obtain recent information regarding clinical trials utilizing trastuzumab and pertuzumab in patients with HER2 overexpressing breast cancer.

2. Perform a literature search to obtain recent information regarding clinical trials using aromatase inhibitors (anastrozole, letrozole, or exemestane) in patients with early stage hormone receptor-positive breast cancer.

3. Develop a treatment plan for a patient presenting to the emergency center with febrile neutropenia after administration of chemotherapy.

4. Provide educational information regarding genetic testing for a patient with a family history of breast cancer.

CLINICAL PEARL

Even though metastatic breast cancer is usually considered to be incurable, some patients can live for a relatively long time with hormonal therapy (if hormone receptor-positive) and palliative chemotherapy. These therapies are administered to increase the patient's quality of life and prolong disease progression, and are typically used in a sequential manner until they are no longer effective, or side effects preclude their use. Although the average life span after diagnosis of metastatic disease is a few years, some patients can live a decade or more with the disease.

REFERENCES

1. Edge SB, Byrd DR, Compton CC, Fritz AG, Greene FL, Trotti A, eds. AJCC Cancer Staging Manual, 7th ed. New York, Springer, 2010.

2. Peto R, Davies D, Godwin J, et al. Comparisons between different polychemotherapy regimens for early breast cancer: meta-analyses of long-term outcome among 100,000 women in 123 randomised trials. Lancet 2012;379(9814):432–444.

3. De Laurentiis M, Cancello G, D'Agostino D, et al. Taxane-based combinations as adjuvant chemotherapy of early breast cancer: a meta-analysis of randomized trials. J Clin Oncol 2008;26:44–53.

4. Early Breast Cancer Trialists' Collaborative Group (EBCTCG). Aromatase inhibitors versus tamoxifen in early breast cancer: patient-level meta-analysis of the randomized trials. Lancet 2015;386(10001):1341–1352.

5. Davies C, Pan H, Godwin J, et al. Long-term effects of continuing adjuvant tamoxifen to 10 years versus stopping at 5 years after diagnosis of oestrogen receptor-positive breast cancer: ATLAS, a randomised trial. Lancet 2013;381:805–816.

6. Francis PA, Regan MM, Fleming GF, et al. Adjuvant ovarian suppression in premenopausal breast cancer. N Engl J Med 2015;372:436–446.

7. Khatcheressian JL, Hurley P, Bantug E, et al. Breast cancer follow-up and management after primary treatment: American Society of Clinical Oncology clinical practice guideline update. J Clin Oncol 2013;31(7):961–965.

8. NCCN Clinical Practice Guidelines in Oncology (NCCN Guidelines®) for Breast Cancer V.3.2015 © National Comprehensive Cancer Network, Inc 2015. All rights reserved. Accessed [September 14, 2015].

9. Van Poznak CH, Temin S, Yee GC, et al. American Society of Clinical Oncology executive summary of the clinical practice guideline update on the role of bone-modifying agents in metastatic breast cancer. J Clin Oncol 2011;29:1221–1227.

10. Ibrance® [package insert]. New York, NY: Pfizer Laboratories, Inc; 2015.

149

NON-SMALL CELL LUNG CANCER

It Takes Your Breath Away . . . . Level II

Julianna V. F. Roddy, PharmD, BCOP

Michelle L. Rockey, PharmD, BCOP

LEARNING OBJECTIVES

After completing this case study, the reader should be able to:

- Recognize the most common symptoms of non-small cell lung cancer (NSCLC).

- Identify potential complications associated with NSCLC.

- Design a treatment plan for patients with NSCLC.

- Recommend potential second-line chemotherapy agents and regimens for treating refractory and metastatic NSCLC.

- Design a pharmacotherapeutic plan for the treatment of hypercalcemia.

- Describe appropriate treatment strategies for brain metastases in NSCLC.

- Monitor carboplatin and paclitaxel therapy.

- Educate patients on the anticipated side effects of carboplatin, paclitaxel, radiation, nivolumab, and erlotinib therapy.

PATIENT PRESENTATION

■ Chief Complaint

"I have been coughing up blood."

■ HPI

This 66-year-old woman presents to her PCP with complaints of a dry, nonproductive cough for 2.5 months, dyspnea on exertion, and hemoptysis for 1 week.

■ PMH

Dyslipidemia
HTN
Anemia of unknown etiology × 1 year
Type 2 DM
PPD (−)

■ FH

Father died of colorectal cancer at age 68.
Aunt died of breast cancer at age 70.

■ SH

Married, lives with son and daughter; 30 pack-year cigarette smoking history (approximately 1 ppd × 30 years); occasional ETOH use; no known recent exposure to TB

■ Meds

Folic acid 1 mg PO daily
Ferrous sulfate 325 mg PO TID
Simvastatin 20 mg PO daily
Metformin 500 mg PO BID
Pantoprazole 40 mg PO daily

■ All

Penicillin (rash)
Sulfa (rash)

■ ROS

(+) For pulmonary symptoms as noted in HPI; no headaches, dizziness, or blurred vision

■ Physical Examination

Gen

Mildly overweight Caucasian woman in slight distress. ECOG performance status of 1.

VS

BP 169/100 mm Hg, P 90 bpm, RR 30, T 37.2°C; Wt 82 kg, Ht 5′6″

Skin

Patches of dry skin; no lesions

HEENT

PERRLA; EOMI; fundi benign; TMs intact

Neck/Lymph Nodes

No lymphadenopathy; neck supple

Lungs

Wheezing in RUL; remainder of lung fields clear

Heart

RRR; slight systolic murmur on left lateral side; normal S_1, S_2

Abd

Soft, nontender; no splenomegaly or hepatomegaly

Genit/Rect

Normal female genitalia; guaiac (−) stool

Neuro

A & O × 3; sensory and motor intact, 5/5 upper, 4/5 lower; CN II–XII intact; (−) Babinski

■ Labs

Na 138 mEq/L	Hgb 10.7 g/dL	Ca 9.7 mg/dL
K 3.6 mEq/L	Hct 34.6%	Mg 2.0 mg/dL
Cl 101 mEq/L	Plt 255 × 10³/mm³	
CO_2 23 mEq/L	WBC 9.9 × 10³/mm³	
BUN 11 mg/dL		
SCr 1.1 mg/dL		
Glu 182 mg/dL		

■ Chest X-Ray

PA and lateral views reveal a possible mass in right upper lobe (Fig. 149-1).

■ Assessment

A 66-year-old woman with new-onset hemoptysis is admitted for workup of a possible lung mass.

She has anemia and a history of dyslipidemia, DM type 2, and HTN.

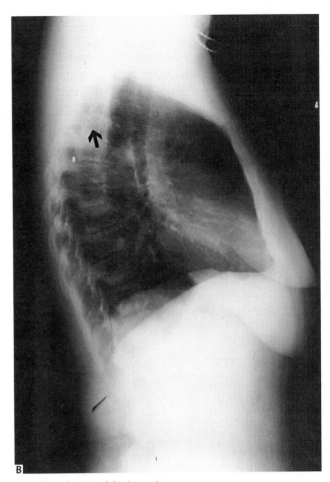

FIGURE 149-1. Chest x-ray with PA *(A)* and lateral *(B)* views showing a possible mass in the right upper lobe *(arrows)*.

■ Clinical Course

The patient was further evaluated for lung cancer on an outpatient basis. A bronchoscopy (with biopsy) was performed that identified squamous cell carcinoma. The chest CT scan revealed a 3-cm × 2-cm right lung mass (Fig. 149-2). A mediastinoscopy was performed to determine the resectability of the tumor. The mediastinoscopy and biopsy revealed unresectable stage IIIB NSCLC with metastases to the contralateral mediastinal nodes. A brain MRI was negative for disease. EGFR status was positive by IHC (non-sensitizing), and EML4-ALK and ROS1 gene rearrangement were negative. PFTs included FEV_1 1.49 L and FVC 1.9 L. An echocardiogram showed mild LVH with an LVEF of 55%. Patient has an EGOG performance status of 1.

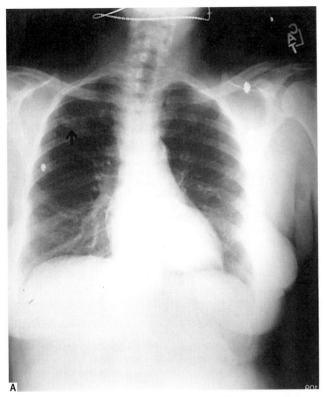

FIGURE 149-2. CT scan of the chest revealing a 2.5-cm × 2-cm right lung mass *(arrow)*.

QUESTIONS

Problem Identification

1.a. Identify the patient's drug therapy problems.

1.b. What signs, symptoms, and other information indicate the presence of NSCLC in this patient?

Desired Outcome

2. What is the goal for treatment of NSCLC in this patient? What is the likelihood of achieving this goal?

Therapeutic Alternatives

3.a. What chemotherapeutic regimens may be considered for NSCLC?

3.b. What nondrug therapies may be used for NSCLC?

Optimal Plan

4.a. Design a specific chemotherapeutic regimen to treat this patient, and explain why you chose this regimen.

4.b. What additional measures should be taken to ensure the tolerability of the regimen and to prevent adverse effects?

4.c. What additional laboratory and clinical information is needed before administration of the chemotherapy?

4.d. Calculate the patient's BSA, creatinine clearance, and the amount of each drug to be administered based on the regimen chosen.

4.e. Would the treatment plan for this patient change if she had presented initially with stage IV NSCLC or was not a radiation candidate with Stage IIIB NSCLC? If so, what would the treatment be?

Outcome Evaluation

5. What clinical and laboratory parameters are necessary to evaluate the therapy for achievement of the desired therapeutic outcome and the occurrence of adverse effects?

Patient Education

6. What information should be provided to the patient to optimize therapy and minimize adverse effects?

■ CLINICAL COURSE (PART 1)

The patient's subsequent courses were further complicated by the occurrence of DVT, weight loss, neutropenic fever, anemia, nausea/vomiting, and infections. At one point, the patient presented with a serum calcium level of 11.3 mg/dL and an albumin of 1.2 g/dL, with symptoms of weakness, confusion, nausea, and vomiting.

Follow-Up Questions

1. Calculate the patient's corrected calcium level and provide an interpretation of that value.

2. What treatment modalities may be used to correct hypercalcemia?

■ CLINICAL COURSE (PART 2)

A repeat chest CT before cycle 3 of carboplatin/paclitaxel showed an increase in the size of the initial lesion, and a PET-CT demonstrated a 2 × 2 cm suspicious lesion in the liver. Patient's performance status remains an ECOG of 1. The physician changed her therapy to gemcitabine/vinorelbine. After 2 cycles, a repeat PET-CT showed an increase in size of the liver lesion.

Follow-Up Questions

3. What treatment options are available for the patient at this time?

4. Design a specific chemotherapeutic regimen to treat this patient.

■ CLINICAL COURSE (PART 3)

Seven weeks after beginning the new chemotherapy regimen, the patient presents to the ED with complaints of headache and mental status changes as per the patient's husband and caregiver. An MRI of the head reveals multiple lesions, most likely brain metastases.

Follow-Up Questions

5. Briefly discuss options (drug and nondrug) to treat brain metastases.

6. What is the role of anticonvulsant agents in the setting of brain metastases?

■ SELF-STUDY ASSIGNMENTS

1. Review clinically important drug interactions for cancer patients started on phenytoin. Include appropriate monitoring parameters. Extend your review beyond the medications this patient is currently receiving.

2. The oncologist has decided to place this patient on erlotinib. Design a patient education session for this drug therapy.

CLINICAL PEARL

Approximately 85–90% of lung cancers are attributable to cigarette smoking. Smoking cessation is the only proven method to decrease the risk of lung cancer. Low-dose computed tomography (CT) in select high-risk smokers and former smokers decreases the mortality rate in lung cancer.

REFERENCES

1. National Comprehensive Cancer Network Clinical Practice Guidelines in Oncology. Non-small cell lung cancer, version 7, 2015. Available at: *www.nccn.org/professionals/physician_gls/PDF/nscl.pdf*. Accessed Oct. 5, 2015.

2. Belani CP, Choy H, Bonomi P, et al. Combined chemotherapy regimens of paclitaxel and carboplatin for locally advanced non-small-cell lung cancer: a randomized phase II locally advanced multi-modality protocol. J Clin Oncol 2005;23:5883–5891.

3. Fournel P, Robinet G, Thomas P, et al. Randomized phase III trial of sequential chemoradiotherapy compared with concurrent chemoradiotherapy in locally advanced non-small-cell lung cancer: Groupe Lyon-Saint-Etienne d'Oncologie Thoracique-Groupe Francis de Pneumo-Cancerologie NPC 95-01 study. J Clin Oncol 2005;23:5910–5917.

4. Hesketh PJ, Bohlke K, Lyman GH, et al. Antiemetics. American Society of Clinical Oncology Focused Guideline Update. J Clin Oncol 2015;33:1–8.

5. Rizzo DJ, Brouwers M, Hurley P, et al. American Society of Clinical Oncology/American Society of Hematology clinical practice guideline update on the use of epoetin and darbepoetin in adult patients with cancer. J Clin Oncol 2010;28:4996–5010.

6. Sandler A, Gray R, Perry M, et al. Paclitaxel–carboplatin alone or with bevacizumab for non-small-cell lung cancer. N Engl J Med 2006;355:2542–2550.

7. Rizvi NA, Mazieres J, Planchard D, et al. Activity and safety of nivolumab, an anti-PD-1 immune checkpoint inhibitor, for patients with advanced, refractory squamous non-small-cell lung cancer (CheckMate 063): a phase 2, single-arm trial. Lancet Oncol 2015;16:257–265.

8. Garon EB, Ciuleanu T, Arrieta O, et al. Ramucirumab plus docetaxel versus placebo plus docetaxel for second-line treatment of stage IV non-small-cell lung cancer after disease progression on platinum-based therapy (REVEL): a multicentre, double-blind, randomised phase 3 trial. Lancet 2014;384:665–673.

9. Weiss GJ, Langer C, Rosell R, et al. Elderly patients benefit from second-line cytotoxic chemotherapy: a subset analysis of a randomized phase III trial of pemetrexed compared with docetaxel in patients with previously treated advanced non-small-cell lung cancer. J Clin Oncol 2006;24:4405–4411.

10. Shepherd FA, Pereira JR, Ciuleanu T, et al. Erlotinib in previously treated non-small-cell lung cancer. N Engl J Med 2005;353:123–132.

150

COLON CANCER

Drug Therapy by Design . . . . Level II

Lisa E. Davis, PharmD, FCCP, BCPS, BCOP

LEARNING OBJECTIVES

After completing this case study, the reader should be able to:

- Identify common symptoms associated with colon cancer at presentation and with disease progression.

- Describe the treatment goals associated with early and advanced stages of colon cancer.

- Design an appropriate chemotherapy regimen for colon cancer based on patient-specific data.

- Formulate a monitoring plan for a patient receiving a prescribed chemotherapy regimen for colon cancer based on patient-specific information.

- Recommend alterations in a drug therapy plan for a patient with colon cancer based on patient-specific information.

- Use pharmacogenetic test results to design an appropriate drug therapy plan for a patient with colorectal cancer.

- Educate patients on the anticipated side effects of irinotecan, capecitabine, fluorouracil, oxaliplatin, bevacizumab, ziv-aflibercept, ramucirumab, regorafenib, cetuximab, panitumumab, and trifluorothymidine/tipiracil hydrochloride.

PATIENT PRESENTATION

Chief Complaint

"The pain below my right ribs is getting worse. Also, I'm having more numbness, cramping, and burning sensations in my hands and feet, especially when I'm working a lot. I don't think I can tolerate it much longer."

HPI

Peter Robinson is a 56-year-old man who presents with worsening pain in his hands and feet and increasing RUQ pain. He was diagnosed with stage IV colon cancer 11 months ago after presenting with abdominal pain, bloating and distention, a history of intermittent BRBPR, and no BM within the prior 4 days. He presented to the ED where a barium enema revealed an "apple core" lesion in his descending colon that was suggestive of malignancy (Fig. 150-1). An FDG-PET/CT scan showed a complete bowel obstruction and several areas of focal intense uptake in the liver, consistent with metastases. His preoperative CEA was 5.6 ng/mL. He subsequently underwent a laparotomy with a left hemicolectomy and lymphadenectomy. The pathology revealed a moderately differentiated adenocarcinoma with extension through the bowel wall to the serosal surface. The tumor was *KRAS* and *NRAS* gene wild-type. Ten of 13 lymph nodes were positive for tumor. Biopsy of a liver lesion confirmed hepatic metastases. A CT scan of the chest showed no evidence of lung metastases. Seven weeks later, chemotherapy

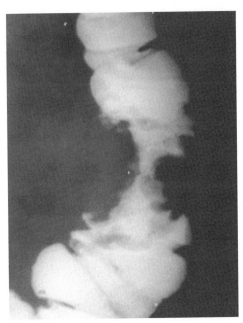

FIGURE 150-1. Annular, constricting adenocarcinoma of the descending colon. This radiographic appearance is referred to as an "apple-core" lesion and is always highly suggestive of malignancy. *(Reprinted with permission from Mayer RJ. Gastrointestinal tract cancer. In: Fauci AS, Kasper DL, Longo DL, et al., eds. Harrison's Principles of Internal Medicine, 17th ed. New York, McGraw-Hill Education, 2008:577.)*

was initiated with capecitabine, oxaliplatin (CapeOx), and bevacizumab. Except for occasional nausea, he generally tolerated the chemotherapy well. However, over the past 2 months he has been experiencing worsening redness and pain on the palms of his hands with numbness and tingling in his fingers and toes. Six days ago he received his 19th cycle of chemotherapy. *UGT1A1* testing showed that he was homozygous for the *UGT1A1*28* allele.

PMH

Type 2 diabetes mellitus × 9 years
Hypertriglyceridemia × 5 years

FH

The patient is the oldest of three brothers; both siblings are alive and well. He has been married for 26 years and has one daughter who is 20 years old. Both his mother and father are in good health. His paternal grandfather died in his 60s from colon cancer, and his mother died in her 60s from ovarian cancer; he is aware of no other family history of malignancy.

SH

Self-employed as a graphic designer. He smoked cigarettes, one pack per day, since age 19 but quit 10 years ago. He does not drink alcohol and has never tried illicit drugs.

Meds

Morphine sustained-release 60 mg PO twice daily
Bisacodyl 5 mg PO daily as needed
Metformin 750 mg PO once daily
Fenofibrate 120 mg PO once daily

All

NKDA

■ ROS

The patient reports diffuse abdominal pain that is continuous with a "grabbing, gnawing" sensation and painful redness and swelling on the palms of his hands. He rates the abdominal pain severity as 5–6 out of 10. The numbness, tingling, cramping, and burning sensations in his hands and feet have worsened in frequency and severity over the past 2 months and have not responded well to morphine. He rates the severity of the tingling and burning pain as 6/10. He denies fever, headaches, shortness of breath, cough, nausea, vomiting, or diarrhea. He reports no lesions in his mouth or difficulty swallowing. He has been having fewer bowel movements (about one every 3–4 days), but there is no pain or blood with passage of stool. He denies polyuria, polydipsia, and burning on urination. He has not noticed any bleeding or excessive bruising.

■ Physical Examination

Gen

Patient is a slightly overweight Caucasian man who appears fatigued.

VS

BP 164/93 mm Hg, P 79 bpm, RR 22, T 35.6°C; Wt 87 kg, Ht 5′9″

Skin

Redness and swelling of the palms of both hands and soles of feet

HEENT

PERRLA; EOMI; funduscopic exam without retinopathy; pale conjunctiva; no scleral icterus; moist mucous membranes; no lesions in oral cavity

Neck/Lymph Nodes

Supple neck; no lymphadenopathy

Lungs/Thorax

Symmetric chest expansion with respiratory effort; clear to A & P; regular breath sounds

CV

Normal heart sounds; regular rate and rhythm; no MRG

Abd

Well-healed scar on left upper abdomen; diffuse abdominal tenderness to palpation; no rebound tenderness; decreased bowel sounds

Genit/Rect

Prostate normal size; no masses palpated; stool heme negative

MS/Ext

Full ROM in all four extremities

Neuro

A & O × 3; cranial nerves II–XII grossly intact; reduced DTRs bilaterally; reduced feet sensitivity to light touch and pinprick bilaterally in stocking-glove distribution; vibration sensation reduced in distal legs

■ Labs

Na 137 mEq/L	Hgb 9.6 g/dL	WBC $8.1 \times 10^3/mm^3$	AST 52 IU/L
K 4.4 mEq/L	Hct 29%	Neutros 40%	ALT 45 IU/L
Cl 98 mEq/L	Plt $252 \times 10^3/mm^3$	Bands 3%	Alk phos 109 IU/L
CO_2 26 mEq/L	MCV 87 μm³	Eos 4%	LDH 370 IU/L
BUN 17 mg/dL	MCHC 33 g/dL	Lymphs 45%	T. bili 1.2 mg/dL
SCr 1.0 mg/dL		Monos 8%	T. chol 199 mg/dL
Glu 117 mg/dL			CEA 7.9 ng/mL
Ca 8.7 mg/dL			
Phos 3.4 mg/dL			
Mg 2.3 mg/dL			

■ Urinalysis

1+ glucose, (–) ketones, 1+ protein, (–) leukocyte esterase and nitrites; (–) RBC; 2–3 WBC/hpf

■ Abdominal CT

Multiple liver metastases, increased approximately 30% in diameter compared to prior scan; multiple new lesions present in both lobes of the liver

■ Chest CT

No evidence of pulmonary metastases

■ Assessment

Unresectable stage IV colon cancer, with disease progression on CapeOx plus bevacizumab chemotherapy

QUESTIONS

Problem Identification

1.a. Identify all of the patient's drug therapy problems.

1.b. What clinical, laboratory, and other information is consistent with colon cancer?

Desired Outcome

2. What are the goals of pharmacotherapy for this patient?

Therapeutic Alternatives

3.a. What chemotherapeutic options are appropriate for this patient?

3.b. What treatment modifications are appropriate to address escalating oxaliplatin-induced neuropathy?

Optimal Plan

4.a. What drugs, dosage forms, treatment schedule, and duration of therapy are best for treating this patient's colon cancer?

4.b. What additional drug treatment interventions should be considered for this patient?

Outcome Evaluation

5.a. How is the response to the treatment regimen for the colon cancer assessed?

5.b. What acute adverse effects are anticipated with the chemotherapy regimen, and what parameters should be monitored?

5.c. What pharmacologic measures can be instituted to prevent or manage the acute toxicities associated with the chemotherapy regimen?

5.d. What are the potential late-onset toxicities of the chemotherapy regimen, and how can they be detected and prevented?

Patient Education

6. What information should you provide to the patient to enhance adherence, ensure successful therapy, and minimize adverse effects?

■ CLINICAL COURSE (PART 1)

His hypertension resolved after two cycles of the chemotherapy regimen you recommended, and his neuropathic symptoms diminished over time and with drug therapy. He received PRBC transfusions when his hemoglobin dropped below 9 g/dL. His sustained-release morphine dose was increased to 120 mg PO Q 12 H, and immediate-release morphine sulfate 30 mg PO Q 4 H PRN pain was started. A scheduled regimen of docusate sodium 100 mg orally plus two senna tablets daily maintained a regular pattern of bowel movements. After seven more cycles of chemotherapy, he presented with worsening abdominal pain, fatigue, and new-onset dyspnea. An abdominal CT scan showed the liver lesions increased in size, and a chest CT showed multiple bilateral pulmonary nodules consistent with pulmonary metastases. His ALT and AST increased to five times the upper limit of normal.

Follow-Up Question

1. What treatment options would be appropriate to consider at this time?

Additional Case Questions

1. What is the role of *UGT1A1* genotyping in the treatment of colon cancer?
2. What is the role of *KRAS* and *NRAS* tumor gene testing in the treatment of colon cancer?
3. How should a patient who develops a thrombotic event during bevacizumab therapy be managed?

■ CLINICAL COURSE (PART 2)

The patient expressed interest in receiving further treatment for his colon cancer. After considering limited treatment options with his oncologist, he agreed to participate in a clinical trial. His analgesic therapy was modified, and his pain control was acceptable. His metastatic lesions remained stable (by clinical symptoms and CT scans) for 2 months.

■ SELF-STUDY ASSIGNMENTS

1. Develop an algorithm for treatment of colon cancer chemotherapy-induced diarrhea.
2. Develop patient-specific education materials regarding management of cutaneous toxicities of agents used in colon cancer treatment.

CLINICAL PEARL

There is no available test, including presence of tumor tissue epidermal growth factor receptor expression, that predicts response to cetuximab or panitumumab. However, tumors can be tested for the presence of *KRAS* and *NRAS* mutations that are predictive of lack of response to these agents. Patients with tumors that are *KRAS* or *NRAS* mutant are not appropriate candidates for treatment regimens that contain cetuximab or panitumumab. *BRAF* mutation testing can also be performed. *BRAF* mutations are generally present in *KRAS* and *NRAS* wild-type tumors. Tumors with *BRAF* mutations are unlikely to respond to an anti-EGFR antibody.

REFERENCES

1. Fakih MG. Metastatic colorectal cancer: current state and future directions. J Clin Oncol 2015;33:1809–1824.
2. Bennouna J, Sastre J, Arnold D, et al. Continuation of bevacizumab after first progression in metastatic colorectal cancer (ML18147): a randomised phase 3 trial. Lancet Oncol 2013;14:29–37.
3. Van Cutsem E, Tabernero J, Lakomy R, et al. Addition of aflibercept to fluorouracil, leucovorin, and irinotecan improves survival in a phase III randomized trial in patients with metastatic colorectal cancer previously treated with an oxaliplatin-based regimen. J Clin Oncol 2012;30:3499–3506.
4. Tabernero J, Yoshino T, Cohn AL, et al. Ramucirumab versus placebo in combination with second-line FOLFIRI in patients with metastatic colorectal carcinoma that progressed during or after first-line therapy with bevacizumab, oxaliplatin, and a fluoropyrimidine (RAISE): a randomised, double-blind, multicentre, phase 3 study. Lancet Oncol 2015;16:499–508.
5. Peeters M, Price TJ, Cervantes A, et al. Randomized phase III study of panitumumab with fluorouracil, leucovorin, and irinotecan (FOLFIRI) compared with FOLFIRI alone as second-line treatment in patients with metastatic colorectal cancer. J Clin Oncol 2010;28:4706–4713.
6. Sobrero AF, Maurel J, Fehrenbacher L, et al. EPIC: phase III trial of cetuximab plus irinotecan after fluoropyrimidine and oxaliplatin failure in patients with metastatic colorectal cancer. J Clin Oncol 2008;26:2311–2319.
7. Seymour MT, Brown SR, Middleton G, et al. Panitumumab and irinotecan versus irinotecan alone for patients with KRAS wild-type, fluorouracil-resistant advanced colorectal cancer (PICCOLO): a prospectively stratified randomised trial. Lancet Oncol 2013;14:749–759.
8. Fuchs CS, Moore MR, Harker G, et al. Phase III comparison of two irinotecan dosing regimens in second-line therapy of metastatic colorectal cancer. J Clin Oncol 2003;21:807–814.
9. Berry SR, Cosby R, Asmis T, et al. Continuous versus intermittent chemotherapy strategies in metastatic colorectal cancer: a systematic review and meta-analysis. Ann Oncol 2015;26:477–485.
10. Bidard FC, Tournigand C, André T, et al. Efficacy of FOLFIRI-3 (irinotecan D1, D3 combined with LV5-FU) or other irinotecan-based regimens in oxaliplatin-pretreated metastatic colorectal cancer in the GERCOR OPTIMOX1 study. Ann Oncol 2009;20:1042–1047.

151

PROSTATE CANCER

Missed Opportunity . . . . Level II

Diana Hey Cauley, PharmD, BCOP

LEARNING OBJECTIVES

After completing this case study, the reader should be able to:

- Describe typical symptoms associated with prostate cancer at initial diagnosis and at disease progression.
- Describe the standard initial treatment options for androgen-dependent metastatic prostate cancer.
- Recommend a pharmacotherapeutic plan for patients with castration-resistant metastatic prostate cancer.
- Counsel patients regarding the toxicities associated with the pharmacologic agents used in prostate cancer treatment.

PATIENT PRESENTATION

Chief Complaint

"I have blood in my urine, I'm using the bathroom all the time, and my shoulder is really hurting."

HPI

Paul Williams is a 73-year-old African-American man who usually has yearly physicals and PSA checks by his local physician. The levels have always been in the range of 4–6 ng/mL. He did not go in for his yearly physical last year, and he now presents with painless gross hematuria, shoulder pain, and a PSA level of 35.7 ng/mL. He has had increased urinary symptoms for the past 5 months.

PMH

Hypercholesterolemia
CHF
Diverticulitis
Severe GERD
Depression

FH

Father, lung cancer diagnosed age 71, died age 73; mother, breast cancer, died at age 93. He has a paternal aunt and paternal grandmother who both were diagnosed with unspecified malignancies.

SH

Retired highway maintenance employee. Christian by faith, Protestant by denomination. He has an associate degree. He drinks on average one six-pack of beer per day. He smoked 10 cigarettes a day for 21 years; stopped smoking at age 42. He is married with two children. He is an only child.

Meds

Valsartan 160 mg PO daily
Carvedilol 3.125 mg PO twice daily
Aspirin 81 mg PO daily
Furosemide 40 mg PO daily
Potassium chloride 10 mEq PO daily
Allopurinol 300 mg PO daily
Tamsulosin 0.4 mg, two capsules PO daily
Fluoxetine 20 mg PO daily
Atorvastatin 40 mg PO at bedtime
Ibuprofen 400 mg PO four times daily PRN pain
Esomeprazole 40 mg PO BID

All

None

ROS

He reports significant fatigue and severe pain in right shoulder. No fever, chills, or sweats. No epistaxis or dysphagia. Reports no chest pain, shortness of breath, dyspnea, or cough. No nausea, vomiting, diarrhea, or constipation. He reports dysuria × 5 months with dribbling, nocturia eight times per night, hesitancy, and incomplete voiding. He has recurring hematuria. He denies memory loss, diplopia, or neuropathy; he has had no falls recently. He reports a 15- to 20-year history of tinnitus.

Physical Examination

Gen

This is a pleasant, elderly gentleman who appears to be in moderate discomfort. Pain is 7 over 10 multifocally. ECOG performance status 1+.

VS

BP 136/61 mm Hg, P 80 bpm, RR 20, T 36.9°C; Wt 91.5 kg, Ht 5′6″

Skin

Warm and dry; no lesions or rashes

HEENT

Sclerae are anicteric. PERRLA; EOMI. Tympanic membranes are within normal limits bilaterally.

Neck/Lymph Nodes

No cervical or supraclavicular adenopathy

Lungs/Thorax

Lungs are clear in all fields. Respirations are even and unlabored.

CV

Normal rate and rhythm; S_1, S_2 normal; no murmurs, gallops, or rubs

Abd

There is a large midline abdominal hernia that does not appear incarcerated. No hepatosplenomegaly.

Genit/Rect

Patient is circumcised with a normal phallus. There are bilaterally descended testicles. No inguinal hernia on examination. Prostate is markedly enlarged and is asymmetric on the right. Texture is firm, but no discrete nodule palpated. Normal rectal tone.

MS/Ext

He has significant pain to touch on the superior aspect of the right shoulder; there is also pain on range of motion. There is tenderness in lumbar area. 1+ ankle and pedal edema is present. Pedal pulses are 2+ bilaterally.

Neuro

CN II–XII grossly normal. Cerebellar function remains intact.

Labs

Na 139 mEq/L	Hgb 9.5 g/dL	WBC 7.2 × 10³/mm³	Total bilirubin 0.2 mg/dL
K 4.0 mEq/L	Hct 27.1%	Neutros 70.3%	
Cl 107 mEq/L	RBC 3.6 × 10⁶/mm³	Baso 0.2%	ALT <12 IU/L
CO₂ 24 mEq/L	Plt 215 × 10³/mm³	Eos 2.3%	AST 20 IU/L
BUN 21 mg/dL	MCV 75 μm³	Lymphs 16.6%	LDH 742 IU/L
SCr 0.9 mg/dL	MCHC 35.1 g/dL	Monos 10.6%	Alk phos 912 IU/L
Glu 114 mg/dL		PSA 35.7 ng/mL	Albumin 4 g/dL
		Testosterone 276 ng/dL	Calcium 8.7 mg/dL

Bone Scan

Skeletal metastases involving the skull and right shoulder

Cystoscopy and Bladder Neck Biopsy

High-grade carcinoma consistent with prostatic adenocarcinoma, Gleason score 8 (4 + 4), extensively involving the bladder neck biopsy tissue

Perineal Prostate Biopsy

Prostatic adenocarcinoma, Gleason score 9 (4 + 5), positive perineural invasion

CT Abdomen

No significant retroperitoneal adenopathy. Multiple small, external iliac lymph nodes are present, predominantly on the left. Small, deep inguinal lymph nodes are also present.

Urinalysis

Clear; negative for glucose, ketones, leukocyte esterase, nitrites, and protein; trace hemoglobin; rare bacteria

Assessment

A 73-year-old man with newly diagnosed T4N1M1b prostate cancer presenting with painless gross hematuria, increased urinary symptoms, and elevated PSA of 35.7 ng/mL. Patient has metastatic androgen-dependent/hormone-sensitive disease and is here for consideration of initial treatment options.

QUESTIONS

Problem Identification

1.a. Identify the patient's primary drug therapy problem.

1.b. What information (signs, symptoms, laboratory values, and other information) indicates the presence and extent of his metastatic prostate cancer?

Desired Outcome

2. Considering this patient's disease stage and history, what are the goals of pharmacotherapy?

Therapeutic Alternatives

3.a. What nondrug therapies might be useful for this patient?

3.b. What feasible pharmacotherapeutic alternatives are available for the treatment of the metastatic hormone-dependent prostate cancer?

Optimal Plan

4.a. What drug, dosage form, dose, schedule, and duration of therapy are best for this patient?

4.b. What alternative would be appropriate if the initial therapy cannot be used?

Outcome Evaluation

5. What clinical and laboratory parameters are necessary to evaluate the therapy for achievement of the desired therapeutic outcome and to detect or prevent adverse effects?

Patient Education

6. What information should be provided to the patient to enhance adherence, ensure successful therapy, and minimize adverse effects?

CLINICAL COURSE

Mr Williams has been compliant with his treatment plan. The physician also started IV zoledronic acid for the metastatic bone disease and an oral calcium/vitamin D supplement. His testosterone has been castrate since therapy was begun 20 months ago. His pain has been better controlled with these interventions. The PSA 3 months ago was mildly elevated at 0.6 ng/mL, whereas it had been undetectable previously. His PSA has now increased to 38.5 ng/mL, and his testosterone level is 22 ng/mL. He is complaining of increased pain in his pelvis and more bone pain in his ribs and back over the past 2 months. He is still able to participate in church social activities and play golf on the weekends. A CT of the pelvis shows a new soft tissue mass on the posterolateral aspect of the urinary bladder on the right side and multiple new blastic lesions in the pelvis and spine. His bone scan shows numerous new intense foci in the skull, scapulae, spine, and femurs.

Follow-Up Questions

1. What pharmacotherapeutic options are available to the patient for his progressive, castrate-recurrent metastatic prostate cancer?

2. What therapeutic options are available for managing this patient's pain?

SELF-STUDY ASSIGNMENTS

1. Locate information resources that are available to prostate cancer patients and their families.

2. Provide the rationale for intermittent LHRH hormone ablation for locally advanced and metastatic prostate cancer patients.

3. Define the role of secondary hormonal agents (eg, ketoconazole, estrogens) for metastatic disease relapse.

4. Describe the clinical rationale for starting an antiandrogen 1–2 weeks before giving the first dose of an LHRH agonist.

5. Define the role of bisphosphonates in men with prostate cancer.

CLINICAL PEARL

Androgen deprivation therapy is continued when a metastatic prostate cancer patient progresses from an androgen-dependent to a castration-resistant state.

REFERENCES

1. REDBOOK Online [Internet Database]. Greenwood Village, Colo, Thomson Reuters (Healthcare) Inc. Updated periodically.

2. Klotz L, Boccon-Gibod L, Shore N, et al. The efficacy and safety of degarelix: a 12-month, comparative, randomized, open-label, parallel-group phase III study in patients with prostate cancer. BJU Int 2008;102:1531–1538.

3. NCCN Clinical Practice Guidelines in Oncology, V1.2015 Prostate Cancer. Available at: *http://www.nccn.org/professionals/physician_gls/pdf/prostate.pdf*. Accessed Oct. 27, 2015.

4. Sooriakumaran P, Khaksar SJ, Shah J. Management of prostate cancer. Part 2: localized and locally advanced disease. Expert Rev Anticancer Ther 2006;6:595–603.

5. Shah J, Khaksar SJ, Sooriakumaran P. Management of prostate cancer. Part 3: metastatic disease. Expert Rev Anticancer Ther 2006;6:813–821.

6. Kantoff PW, Higano CS, Shore ND, et al. Sipuleucel-T immunotherapy for castration-resistant prostate cancer. N Engl J Med 2010;363:411–422.

7. Beer TM, Armstrong AJ, Rathkopf DE, et al. Enzalutamide in metastatic prostate cancer before chemotherapy. N Engl J Med 2014;371:424–433.

8. Ryan CJ, Smith MR, de Bono JS, et al. Abiraterone in metastatic prostate cancer without previous chemotherapy. N Engl J Med 2013;368;138–148.

9. Parker C, Nilsson S, Heinrich D, et al. Alpha emitter radium-223 and survival in metastatic prostate cancer. N Engl J Med 2013;369:213–223.

10. Tannock IF, de Wit R, Berry WR, et al. Docetaxel plus prednisone or mitoxantrone plus prednisone for advanced prostate cancer. N Engl J Med 2004;351:1502–1512.

11. Petrylak DP, Tangen CM, Hussain MH, et al. Docetaxel and estramustine compared with mitoxantrone and prednisone for refractory prostate cancer. N Engl J Med 2004;351:1513–1520.

12. Tannock IF, Osoba D, Stockler MR, et al. Chemotherapy with mitoxantrone plus prednisone or prednisone alone for symptomatic hormone-resistant prostate cancer: a Canadian randomized trial with palliative end points. J Clin Oncol 1996;14:1756–1764.

13. Fizazi K, Carducci M, Smith M, et al. Denosumab versus zoledronic acid for treatment of bone metastases in men with castration-resistant prostate cancer: a randomised, double-blind study. Lancet 2011;377:813–822.

14. NCCN Clinical Practice Guidelines in Oncology, V2.2015. Adult cancer pain. Available at: *http://www.nccn.org/professionals/physician_gls/pdf/pain.pdf.* Accessed Nov. 13, 2015.

152

NON-HODGKIN LYMPHOMA

Striking Out Cancer........................... Level II

Keith A. Hecht, PharmD, BCOP

LEARNING OBJECTIVES

After completing this case study, the reader should be able to:

- Identify and describe the components of the staging workup and the corresponding staging and classification systems for non-Hodgkin lymphoma (NHL).

- Describe the pharmacotherapeutic treatment of choice and the alternatives available for treating NHL.

- Identify acute and chronic toxicities associated with the drugs used to treat NHL and the measures used to prevent or treat these toxicities.

- Identify monitoring parameters for response and toxicity in patients with NHL.

- Provide detailed patient education for the chemotherapeutic regimen.

PATIENT PRESENTATION

■ Chief Complaint

"What's the next step for my lymphoma?"

■ HPI

Homer Bunting is a 58-year-old man who presents to his oncologist's office for recommendations about treatment of a newly diagnosed diffuse, large B-cell lymphoma. He had been in relatively good health other than his long-standing hypertension and chronic heart failure. He initially presented to the ED 2 weeks ago with new onset of shortness of breath and fevers up to 100.8°F (38.2°C). He was then hospitalized for further evaluation and treatment. At that time, he stated that he had lost weight over the past few months. Physical examination findings were significant for decreased breath sounds (worse on the left side than the right) and enlarged, painless supraclavicular lymph nodes on the left side. The largest palpable lymph node measured approximately 2 cm in diameter. Splenomegaly was also noted. Chest x-ray revealed a large heterogeneous mass at the apex of the left lung also involving the mediastinum. Given the patient's lengthy smoking history, he was presumed to have lung cancer. CT-guided biopsy of the mass was performed. Pathology revealed cells consistent with lymphoma, but definitive diagnosis could not be made. An excisional biopsy of the enlarged supraclavicular lymph node was performed. Pathology showed diffuse large non-Hodgkin B-cell lymphoma. The oncologist on call was consulted, and it was recommended for him to follow up as an outpatient for further evaluation and treatment recommendations.

■ PMH

HTN × 10 years
Hypercholesterolemia × 5 years
NYHA Class II HF × 8 years

■ FH

The patient is the oldest of seven children (four brothers and two sisters), all alive and well. He has two children, both in good health. Family history of terminal prostate cancer in his father (died at age 63). No other history of malignancy that he is aware of.

■ SH

The patient is employed as an usher at a professional baseball park. He previously smoked 1–2 ppd for 32 years. He quit when he was diagnosed with HF, and he complains about the fans who smoke in the section of the ballpark where he works. He drinks one to two beers nightly when working. Diet is mostly ballpark food, heavy on the hot dogs, and bratwursts. He states that he does not eat many vegetables, unless popcorn counts. He has been married for 34 years. His wife is with him today in the clinic.

■ ROS

The patient reports continuing fever, typically ranging from 100.2 to 101°F (37.9–38.3°C) and cough with occasional hemoptysis. In addition, he describes an unexplained weight loss of approximately 25 lb over the past 3 months. He denies headaches, changes in vision, or fainting episodes. He reports no lesions in his mouth, difficulty swallowing, or nosebleeds. He states that he occasionally has some dyspnea on exertion, but he is able to carry out activities of daily living without limitations. He denies orthopnea, tachycardia, or swelling in the extremities. He also denies burning on urination, frequency, dribbling, or blood in the urine. He has not noticed any additional bleeding or bruising. He has not received any prior transfusions.

■ Meds

Lisinopril 20 mg PO once daily
Furosemide 20 mg PO once daily
Simvastatin 20 mg PO at bedtime
Esomeprazole 20 mg PO once daily
Temazepam 30 mg PO at bedtime as needed
Epoetin alfa 40,000 units subQ once weekly

■ All

Penicillin—rash

Physical Examination

Gen

Patient is a thin white man in no apparent distress

VS

BP 145/100 mm Hg, P 95 bpm, RR 14, T 37.9°C; Wt 72 kg, Ht 5′9″

Skin

No rashes or moles noted

HEENT

PERRLA; TMs clear; no masses in the tonsils, palate, or floor of the mouth; no stomatitis. Several missing teeth, but no gingival inflammation is noted.

Neck

Supple; no masses; no JVD; small scar from excisional biopsy of supraclavicular lymph node noted

Chest

Decreased breath sounds bilaterally, more on the left than the right; no wheezes or crackles

CV

RRR; no MRG

Abd

Soft, NT/ND. Spleen palpable just below the left costal margin. No hepatomegaly. Bowel sounds normoactive.

Genit/Rect

Normal male genitalia

Ext

Without edema, warm to the touch; pulses 2+ bilaterally

Neuro

Symmetric cranial nerve function. Symmetric facial muscle movement, and the tongue is midline. The palate is symmetric. Balance and coordination of the upper extremities are intact, with no evidence of tremor. There is symmetric coordination of rapidly alternating movements. Motor strength in the upper and lower extremities is normal and symmetric.

Lymph Node Survey

The lymph node survey is negative for any palpable peripheral nodes in the preauricular, postauricular, cervical, supraclavicular, infraclavicular, or axillary areas. No palpable inguinal nodes present. Small scar noted from excisional biopsy of left supraclavicular node.

Labs

Na 132 mEq/L	Hgb 10.3 g/dL	AST 29 IU/L	Phos 4.0 mg/dL
K 4.6 mEq/L	Hct 30%	ALT 27 IU/L	Uric acid 5.6 mg/dL
Cl 97 mEq/L	Plt 338 × 10³/mm³	Alk phos 75 IU/L	PT 12.2 sec
CO₂ 26 mEq/L	WBC 9.9 × 10³/mm³	LDH 623 IU/L	aPTT 21.7 sec
BUN 20 mg/dL	Neutros 70%	T. bili 0.6 mg/dL	
SCr 0.7 mg/dL	Bands 2%	T. prot 6.3 g/dL	
Glu 112 mg/dL	Lymphs 18%	Alb 3.7 g/dL	
	Monos 9%		
	Eos 1%		

CT Chest

Large lobular heterogeneous mass within the left chest and mediastinum that extends from the level of the left lung and apex of the diaphragm

Chest X-Ray

Large heterogeneous mass at the apex of the left lung also involving the mediastinum

Tumor Pathology

Diffuse large cell lymphoma, B-cell type; CD20+, CD45+, CD3−

Initial Assessment

Diffuse large cell lymphoma. Further staging will include bilateral BM biopsies, PET scan, HIV test, CT of the abdomen, and a baseline cardiac assessment in light of the patient's long-standing history of HTN.

Clinical Course

Bone marrow biopsies are negative for lymphoma. PET scanning revealed multiple foci of increased FDG uptake; increased uptake noted in the spleen, mediastinum, and left-side supraclavicular lymph nodes. The HIV test is negative. CT of the abdomen shows large heterogeneous soft tissue mass within the left upper quadrant that may be contiguous with previously noted left chest mass. The mass extends inferiomedially to the tail of the pancreas. There is an additional 4-cm low-density mass near the head of the pancreas. The spleen is enlarged. MUGA scan reveals an LVEF of 45%.

Assessment

Diffuse large B-cell lymphoma, stage III; IPI score of 2

QUESTIONS

Problem Identification

1.a. Identify all of the drug therapy problems of this patient.

1.b. What clinical and other information is consistent with the diagnosis of NHL?

1.c. Explain what system of staging was used and how his stage of disease was determined.

1.d. What laboratory and clinical features does this patient have that may affect his prognosis? How is the IPI determined?

Desired Outcome

2. What are the goals of therapy in this case?

Therapeutic Alternatives

3. What chemotherapy regimens are available for treatment of his NHL?

Optimal Plan

4.a. What drug, dosage form, schedule, and duration of therapy are best for treating this patient's NHL?

4.b. What other interventions should be made to maintain control of the patient's other concurrent diseases?

4.c. What nondrug therapies might be useful for this patient?

Outcome Evaluation

5.a. How is the response to the treatment regimen for the NHL assessed?

5.b. What acute adverse effects are associated with the chemotherapy regimen, and what parameters should be monitored?

5.c. What pharmacologic measures should be instituted to treat or prevent the acute toxicities associated with the chemotherapy regimen?

5.d. What are potential late complications of the chemotherapy regimen, and how can they be detected and prevented?

Patient Education

6. What information would you provide to the patient about the agents used to treat the NHL?

■ CLINICAL COURSE (PART 1)

The patient tolerated the first few cycles of chemotherapy well, with only some minimal nausea and vomiting. His antihypertensive medication was modified, increasing the lisinopril to 40 mg daily and maintaining the furosemide 20 mg daily, achieving average systolic BPs in the 120s and average diastolic BPs in the 70s. His fasting lipid panel was checked and was found to be within his goals. One week after completing the fourth cycle of chemotherapy, he presented to the ED with fever (temperature at presentation was 101.3°F [38.5°C]), cough, dyspnea, pain on inspiration, and fatigue. Laboratory evaluation showed an ANC of $0.352 \times 10^3/mm^3$. He was admitted to the hospital for evaluation and treatment of suspected neutropenic fever with pneumonia. Blood and sputum cultures were negative. The patient was treated with broad-spectrum antibiotics and became afebrile after 3 days. He was discharged from the hospital after the neutropenia resolved, completing a 14-day course of inpatient IV antibiotics. Imaging studies were performed while he was in the hospital to evaluate his lymphoma. PET and CT scans showed that he achieved a complete response.

Follow-Up Question

1. What measures should be taken to prevent neutropenic fever in subsequent courses of chemotherapy?

■ CLINICAL COURSE (PART 2)

The patient completed his planned course of chemotherapy without further event. Eighteen months later, the patient returns to the oncologist office after being diagnosed with relapsed lymphoma during a hospital admission for worsening dyspnea.

■ SELF-STUDY ASSIGNMENTS

1. What is the role of stem cell transplant in the treatment of aggressive NHL?

2. What therapeutic options are available for the treatment of relapsed diffuse large B-cell lymphomas?

3. If the patient had a history of Hepatitis B what diagnostic tests would be indicated? What antiviral therapy, if any, should be considered in patients with a history of hepatitis B who are receiving chemo-immunotherapy for treatment of diffuse large B-cell lymphoma?

CLINICAL PEARL

The role of CNS prophylaxis in the treatment of aggressive NHL, such as diffuse large B-cell lymphoma, is controversial. Features associated with an increased risk of relapse in the brain include initial presentation in paranasal sinus or testicular involvement and an elevated LDH combined with more than one site of extranodal involvement. Therapeutic options for CNS prophylaxis include intrathecal or high-dose IV methotrexate.

REFERENCES

1. Cheson BD, Fisher RI, Barrington SF, et al. Recommendations for initial evaluation, staging, and response assessment of Hodgkin and non-Hodgkin lymphoma: The Lugano classification. J Clin Oncol 2014;32:3059–3067.

2. Zhou Z, Sehn LH, Rademaker AW, et al. An enhanced International Prognostic Index (NCCN-IPI) for patients with diffuse large B-cell lymphoma treated in the rituximab era. Blood 2014;123:837–842.

3. Fisher RI, Gaynor ER, Dahlberg S, et al. Comparison of a standard regimen (CHOP) with three intensive chemotherapy regimens for advanced non-Hodgkin's lymphoma. N Engl J Med 1993;328:1002–1006.

4. Coiffier B, Thieblemont C, Van Den Neste E, et al. Long-term outcome of patients in the LNH-98.5 trial, the first randomized study comparing rituximab-CHOP to standard CHOP chemotherapy in DLBCL patients: a study by the Groupe d'Etudes des Lymphomes de l'Adulte. Blood 2010;116:2040–2045.

5. Basser RL, Green MD. Strategies for prevention of anthracycline cardiotoxicity. Cancer Treat Rev 1993;19:57–77.

6. Procrit [Package Insert]. Horsham, Pennsylvania, Janssen Products LP, 2013.

7. Smith TJ, Bohlke K, Lyman GH, et al. Recommendations for the use of WBC growth factors: American Society of Clinical Oncology clinical practice guideline update. J Clin Oncol 2015;33:3199–3212.

8. Hesketh PJ, Bohlke K, Lyman GH, et al. Antiemetics: American Society of Clinical Oncology focused guideline update. J Clin Oncol 2015;64:3635–3640.

9. Ganz WI, Sridhar KS, Ganz SS, et al. Review of tests for monitoring doxorubicin-induced cardiomyopathy. Oncology 1996;53:461–470.

10. Flowers CR, Seidenfeld J, Bow EJ, et al. Antimicrobial prophylaxis and outpatient management of fever and neutropenia in adults treated for malignancy: American Society of Clinical Oncology clinical practice guideline. J Clin Oncol 2013;31(6):794–810.

153

HODGKIN LYMPHOMA

The Firefighter . . . . Level I

Cindy L. O'Bryant, PharmD, BCOP

Ashley Glode, PharmD, BCOP

LEARNING OBJECTIVES

After completing this case study, the reader should be able to:

- Recognize the signs and symptoms commonly associated with Hodgkin lymphoma (HL).

- Discuss the pharmacotherapeutic treatment of choice and the alternatives available for treating HL.

- Identify acute and chronic toxicities associated with the medications used to treat HL and the measures used to prevent, treat, and monitor these toxicities.

- Determine monitoring parameters for response and toxicity in patients with HL.
- Formulate appropriate educational information to provide to a patient receiving chemotherapy treatment for HL.

PATIENT PRESENTATION

■ Chief Complaint

"I have been having night sweats, fever, and have been a lot more tired lately. I also have a growth on my chest that has gotten bigger over the past few weeks."

■ HPI

Mike McCaffrey is a 27-year-old man who presents with a 1-month history of night sweats, fever, fatigue, and a 9-kg weight loss. He was previously working in finance but desired a career change and has been training for his interview and physical fitness test to join the local fire station. He served as a volunteer firefighter in college and missed that line of work. He denies any shortness of breath, and first attributed his fatigue to increased exercise. His wife also noticed a mass on his chest that has gotten progressively larger over the past 2 weeks. He initially associated the mass with an "elbow to the chest" he received during a recreation league basketball game. An ultrasound of the mediastinum showed a lymph node that measured approximately 11 cm. On physical exam, enlarged supraclavicular lymph nodes were noted on both the right and left. As a result, an excisional lymph node biopsy was performed that demonstrated classical HL, nodular sclerosing (NS) subtype.

■ PMH

None

■ FH

The patient's parents and one sibling (brother, also a firefighter) are all in good health. Paternal grandfather died of colon cancer.

■ SH

Worked in finance, now training to join the local fire squadron. Drinks socially, about 2 beers per week. He has never smoked. He does not use illicit drugs. The patient is married and wishes to start a family.

■ Meds

Ibuprofen 400 mg PO Q 4–6 H PRN pain/fever

■ All

NKDA

■ ROS

(+) For fevers, night sweats, fatigue and weight loss of approximately 9 kg over the past month.

(–) For vision changes, headaches, shortness of breath, chest pain, nausea, vomiting, diarrhea, constipation, or urinary symptoms. Denies feeling depressed or having loss of pleasure with activities. His performance status is 1 on the ECOG scale.

■ Physical Examination

Gen

The patient is a healthy-appearing man in no apparent distress

VS

BP 128/72 mm Hg, P 62 bpm, RR 16, T 37.6°C; Wt 87 kg, Ht 5′11″

Skin

Soft, diffusely enlarged soft tissue swelling in the middle of the upper chest just below the neck; no erythema or warmth; no rashes

HEENT

PERRL; EOMI; TMs intact

Lymph Nodes

Supraclavicular lymph nodes are enlarged on both the right and left. The mediastinal mass is palpable. No other lymph nodes are palpable bilaterally.

Chest

Respirations with normal rhythm; clear to auscultation

CV

RRR; no JVD, murmurs, or gallops

Abd

Soft and nontender with no masses; bowel sounds are normoactive

Genit/Rect

Normal male genitalia; stool is guaiac (–)

MS/Ext

Without edema

Neuro

A & O × 3; CN II–XII intact; remainder of exam is nonfocal

■ Labs

Na 137 mEq/L	Hgb 13.1 g/dL	AST 19 IU/L	PT 12.9 sec
K 4.1 mEq/L	Hct 39.3%	ALT 22 IU/L	aPTT 27.1 sec
Cl 103 mEq/L	Plt 310 × 10³/mm³	Alk phos 74 IU/L	Phos 3.1 mg/dL
CO_2 24 mEq/L	WBC 10.9 × 10³/mm³	LDH 372 IU/L	Magnesium
BUN 14 mg/dL	Neutros 80.5%	T. bili 0.4 mg/dL	1.2 mEq/L
SCr 0.7 mg/dL	Lymphs 13.2%	T. prot 7.7 g/dL	Uric acid 7.5 mg/dL
Glu 82 mg/dL	Monos 5.4%	Alb 3.2 g/dL	ESR 63 mm/h
	Eos 0.9%		

■ Ultrasound

There are singular, enlarged abnormal lymph nodes in the right and left supraclavicular regions. The largest node on the right measures 2.1 cm × 1.4 cm × 1.8 cm and on the left 1.7 cm × 0.9 cm × 1.1 cm. The large mediastinal node is 10.7 cm × 6.4 cm × 8.7 cm. The nodes contain solid echogenic material and have increased vascular flow.

■ Tumor Pathology

Identification of Reed–Sternberg cells classifying this as HL, NS type (see Fig. 153-1). Immunohistochemistry: CD15+, CD30+, CD20–, CD45–.

■ PET/Helical CT Scan

Enlarged nodes demonstrating hypermetabolic activity are noted in the bilateral supraclavicular chains. There is involvement of the superior middle mediastinum showing bulky disease and hilar nodal chains within the chest. The bilateral lungs and myocardium

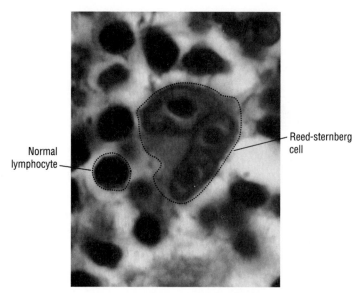

Normal lymphocyte

Reed-sternberg cell

FIGURE 153-1. Reed–Sternberg cell (center) surrounded by normal lymphocytes. *(Source: National Cancer Institute.)*

are negative for disease. Normal physiologic liver, GI, and urinary activity are noted. Diffuse increased uptake within the bone marrow; it is unclear whether this is lymphoma or hyperplasia.

■ Bone Marrow Biopsy

Bilateral biopsies are negative for HL.

■ Assessment

Classical HL, nodular sclerosis subtype, early stage IIB, unfavorable with bulky disease.

QUESTIONS

Problem Identification

1.a. What clinical and other information is consistent with the diagnosis of HL?

1.b. Explain what system of staging was used and how his stage of disease was determined.

Desired Outcome

2. What are the goals of therapy in this case?

Therapeutic Alternatives

3. What treatment options are available for managing this patient's HL?

Optimal Plan

4.a. What drug regimen, dose, schedule, and duration of chemotherapy are best for treating this patient's HL?

4.b. Are additional treatment modalities other than chemotherapy indicated for treating this patient's HL?

Outcome Evaluation

5.a. What clinical and laboratory parameters are necessary to evaluate the therapy for achievement of the desired therapeutic outcome for treatment of HL?

5.b. What acute adverse effects are associated with the chemotherapy regimen?

5.c. What clinical or laboratory parameters are necessary to detect and prevent acute and long-term adverse events commonly associated with treatment of HL?

Patient Education

6. What information should be provided to the patient to enhance compliance, ensure successful therapy, and minimize adverse effects for treatment of HL?

■ CLINICAL COURSE

The patient's treatment was administered in the outpatient setting. He received day 1 of his first cycle of chemotherapy and experienced acute nausea and vomiting. Five days after his first treatment he experienced mild mucositis and mild constipation. The patient was instructed to maintain good oral hygiene, use a soft toothbrush, and avoid alcohol and spicy or acidic foods. He was started on a mouthwash (diphenhydramine, lidocaine, and aluminum/magnesium hydroxide) with instructions to swish and spit four times a day. He was educated to maintain good hydration, a high-fiber diet and to start docusate sodium 50 mg orally once daily for constipation. He successfully received cycles 2 through 4 of chemotherapy in the outpatient clinic without incident. After completing 4 cycles he was restaged with a PET/CT scan to assess his response to chemotherapy. Restaging showed the patient had a complete response with a Deauville score of 2, and he received 2 more cycles of chemotherapy followed by involved-site radiation. On subsequent follow-up, the patient is in remission.

Follow-Up Question

1. What follow-up and long-term monitoring should this patient receive after completion of his cancer treatment?

■ SELF-STUDY ASSIGNMENTS

1. What are unfavorable prognostic factors for early and advanced HL, and how does this influence treatment?

2. What is the antiemetic regimen of choice to prevent acute nausea and vomiting for highly emetogenic chemotherapy?

3. What are the salvage therapy options for patients with relapsing HL?

4. What is the role for hematopoietic stem cell transplantation in HL?

CLINICAL PEARL

HL can be cured with chemotherapy, even in advanced stages. To achieve a cure, it is essential that a patient receives the appropriate treatment. This is based on several key factors, which include an accurate diagnosis of the type of HL with recommended immunostaining, determination of unfavorable prognostic factors, and use of combined chemotherapy and radiation treatment when appropriate.

REFERENCES

1. Eichenauer DA, Engert A. Advances in the treatment of Hodgkin lymphoma. Int J Hematol 2012;96:535–543.
2. Cheson BD, Fisher RI, Barrington SF, et al. Recommendations for initial evaluation, staging, and response assessment of Hodgkin and non-Hodgkin lymphoma: the Lugano classification. J Clin Oncol 2014;32:3059–3068.
3. Connors JM. Hodgkin lymphoma: special challenges and solutions. Hematol Oncol 2015;33:21–24.
4. NCCN Hodgkin Lymphoma Clinical Practice Guidelines in Oncology (Version V.2.2015). Available at: *http://www.nccn.org*. Accessed January 14, 2016.
5. Gordon LI, Hong F, Fisher RI, et al. Randomized phase III trial of ABVD versus Stanford V with or without radiation therapy in locally extensive and advanced-stage Hodgkin lymphoma: an intergroup study coordinated by the Eastern Cooperative Oncology Group (E2496). J Clin Oncol 2013;31:684–691.
6. von Tresckow B, Plutschow A, Fuchs M, et al. Dose-intensification in early unfavorable Hodgkin's lymphoma: final analysis of the German Hodgkin study group HD14 trial. J Clin Oncol 2012;30:907–913.
7. NCCN Antiemesis Clinical Practice Guidelines in Oncology (Version V.2.2015). Available at: *http://www.nccn.org*. Accessed January 14, 2016.
8. NCCN Myeloid Growth Factors Clinical Practice Guidelines in Oncology (Version V.1.2015). Available at: *http://www.nccn.org*. Accessed January 14, 2016.
9. Schaapveld M, Aleman BM, van Eggermond A, et al. Second cancer risk up to 40 years after treatment for Hodgkin's lymphoma. N Engl J Med 2015;373:2499–2511.
10. Hodgson DC. Long-term toxicity of chemotherapy and radiotherapy in lymphoma survivors: optimizing treatment for individual patients. Clin Adv Hematol Oncol 2015;13:103–112.

154

OVARIAN CANCER

Amber E. Proctor, PharmD

William C. Zamboni, PharmD, PhD

LEARNING OBJECTIVES

After completing this case study, the reader should be able to:

- Recognize the signs and symptoms of ovarian cancer.
- Describe the genetic factors associated with ovarian cancer.
- Recommend a pharmacotherapeutic plan for the chemotherapy of newly diagnosed and relapsed ovarian cancer.
- Describe the uses and potential pharmacologic advantages of pegylated liposomal doxorubicin.
- Recognize the dose-limiting and most common toxicities associated with the chemotherapeutic agents used in the treatment of ovarian cancer.

PATIENT PRESENTATION

Chief Complaint

"I'm very anxious about getting chemotherapy. My uncles have gone through chemotherapy for colorectal cancer and they became very sick. One of them was even admitted to the hospital due to the side effects. I don't want that to happen to me."

HPI

Edith Hillebrand is a 56-year-old woman who presents to the Gynecology Oncology clinic 1 week after surgery for stage IIIB (T2c N1 M0) serous epithelial ovarian adenocarcinoma. She originally presented to her PCP's office 1 month ago with complaints of a 3-day progressive worsening of LLE pain, swelling, and redness. The physician ordered a Doppler ultrasound of the LLE. Results indicated that she had a DVT in the popliteal vein extending to the iliac vein. Her last physical exam was performed more than 15 months prior. The physician performed a complete history and physical exam and identified a left adnexal mass, abdominal pain, bloating, and weight gain. CT scans of the abdomen and pelvis showed a large, soft tissue pelvic mass. Laboratory examination revealed a CA-125 level of 490 IU/mL.

Mrs Hillebrand underwent an exploratory laparotomy, TAH-BSO, omentectomy, and bilateral pelvic and periaortic lymph node dissection with comprehensive staging by a gynecologic oncologist. On entering the abdomen, there was a relatively small amount of ascitic fluid. A large left adnexal mass measuring 15 cm × 5 cm × 10 cm was discovered and removed. Multiple small tumor nodules (2 cm or less) outside the pelvis were also removed. Numerous adhesions were seen throughout the omentum and surrounding organs. At completion of the surgery, the surgeon noted that the patient was optimally debulked. Ascitic fluid, peritoneal washings, left adnexal mass, left and right ovaries, multiple pelvic and periaortic lymph nodes, and omentum were sent to pathology for further examination.

Gross examination of left and right ovaries revealed multiple adhesions extending from each ovary with interspersed broad regions of necrosis. Each ovary was serially sectioned for microscopic examination, which revealed numerous papillations of tumor cells destructively permeating the stroma (grade 2). Based on this information, Mrs Hillebrand was diagnosed with stage IIIB (T2c N1 M0) serous epithelial ovarian adenocarcinoma.

PMH

Hypothyroidism × 30 years
HTN × 22 years
Type 2 DM × 17 years
Dyslipidemia × 15 years
GERD × 10 years

FH

Married × 37 years with two children, a son age 35 and daughter age 32. Her father died of an MI at age 72, and her mother died at age 66 with ovarian cancer. Has two paternal uncles (age 80 and 76 years) alive with colorectal cancer.

SH

Consumes one glass of red wine with dinner every evening. Has a 20 pack-year history of cigarette smoking; quit 25 years ago. No recreational drug use.

Meds

Ibuprofen 200 mg, 1–2 tablets PO Q 6 H PRN headaches/muscle aches (OTC)
Levothyroxine 0.1 mg PO daily
Pantoprazole 40 mg PO daily
Atorvastatin 40 mg PO daily
Metformin 1,000 mg PO twice daily
Glyburide 10 mg PO twice daily
Lisinopril 40 mg PO daily

All

Penicillin (hives as a child)
Codeine ("sour stomach")

ROS

Somewhat fatigued lately, progressively worsening over the past 2 months. Reports to have struggled with weight loss for most of her adult life and reports a 10-kg weight gain over the past 4 months. She also reports requiring more sleep than usual, about 9–10 hours per night, but cannot recall when this change occurred. Her mood is depressed because of concern about her recent cancer diagnosis. She reports occasional headaches (~1 episode per month) relieved by OTC ibuprofen. Denies any changes in sight, smell, hearing, and taste. Also reports constipation and dry skin.

Physical Examination

Gen

The patient appears to be her stated age. Appears anxious in the office on exam.

VS

BP 135/85 mm Hg, P 110 bpm, RR 18, T 37.0°C; Ht 5′7″, Wt 70 kg

Skin

No erythema, rash, ecchymoses, or petechiae

LN

No cervical or axillary lymphadenopathy

HEENT

PERRLA, EOMI; TMs intact; fundus benign; OP dry

Breasts

Without masses, discharge, or adenopathy; no nipple or skin changes

Cor

RRR; no M/R/G

Pulm

CTA bilaterally

Abd

Soft, nontender; no HSM. Surgical wound healing well; no exudate or erythema; covered with 4 × 4 bandage with antibiotic ointment

Genit/Rect

Normal female genitalia; heme (–) dark brown stool; no rectal wall tenderness or masses

Ext

No C/C/E. Residual erythema and swelling in LLE from prior DVT; no signs of ulceration

Neuro

CN II–XII intact; sensation decreased to light touch and pinprick below the knees bilaterally; vibration sense diminished at the great toes bilaterally

Labs

Na 140 mEq/L	Hgb 12.8 g/dL	AST 25 IU/L
K 3.4 mEq/L	Hct 31%	ALT 40 IU/L
Cl 99 mEq/L	Plt 135 × 10³/mm³	T. bili 0.7 mg/dL
CO₂ 24 mEq/L	WBC 5.2 × 10³/mm³	Alb 4.0 units/L
BUN 20 mg/dL	Neutros 60%	CA-125 490 IU/mL
SCr 1.1 mg/dL	Bands 3%	
Glu 135 mg/dL	Lymphs 30%	
Ca 9.8 mg/dL	Monos 5%	
Mg 2.0 mg/dL	Eos 1%	
Phos 3.5 mg/dL	Basos 1%	

UA

WBC 1–5/hpf, RBC 0/hpf, 1+ ketones, 1+ protein, pH 5.0

Genetic Results

DNA analysis from a blood sample revealed that the patient is positive for BRCA1 gene mutation

Assessment/Plan

Mrs Hillebrand is a 56-year-old woman with advanced stage IIIB (T2c N1 M0) serous epithelial ovarian adenocarcinoma. She underwent optimal surgical debulking by a trained gynecologic oncologist and presents to the clinic for follow-up management. Based on the stage of diagnosis and risk for recurrence, first-line chemotherapy is recommended.

QUESTIONS

Problem Identification

1.a. What are the patient's drug therapy problems?

1.b. What information (signs, symptoms, and laboratory values) indicates the presence and severity of ovarian cancer?

1.c. What stage of ovarian cancer does this patient have, and how does the stage of disease affect the choice of therapy?

1.d. What is the significance of the size of residual tumor after primary cytoreductive surgery?

Desired Outcome

2   What are the goals of therapy for this patient?

Therapeutic Alternatives

3.a. How do her genetic results influence the choice of therapy and prognosis?

3.b. What are the first-line chemotherapy options for this patient?

3.c. What are the specific toxicities and logistical issues related to intraperitoneal (IP) therapy?

3.d. What is the role of bevacizumab in the first-line setting?

Optimal Plan

4.a. Which first-line chemotherapy regimen and ancillary treatment measures would you recommend for this patient?

4.b. Regardless of whether you recommended intravenous carboplatin, use the Calvert equation to calculate the carboplatin dose required to achieve a target AUC of 5 mg/mL · min.

■ CLINICAL COURSE (PART 1)

The patient and oncologist agreed to begin treatment with the combination of IV docetaxel and carboplatin on day 1 every 21 days for six cycles as first-line treatment of her ovarian cancer.

Outcome Evaluation

5 How would you monitor the therapy for efficacy and adverse effects?

■ CLINICAL COURSE (PART 2)

Mrs Hillebrand completed six cycles of docetaxel 75 mg/m^2 IV over 1 hour followed by carboplatin AUC 6 IV over 1 hour on day 1 every 21 days. She tolerated therapy very well with no dose reductions or delays. Her serum CA-125 level slowly declined over the course of treatment and was 12 IU/mL 3 weeks after her sixth cycle. Based on her CA-125 level and the negative CT scans following the fourth and sixth cycles, Mrs Hillebrand was defined as a clinical complete response. Her CA-125 levels were followed monthly.

Patient Education

6. What information would you provide to the patient about this therapy?

■ CLINICAL COURSE (PART 3)

Starting 1 month after treatment was discontinued, monthly CA-125 levels were 8, 10, 14, 20, 30, 43, and 88 IU/mL. A CT scan performed at 8 months after treatment discontinuation revealed a pelvic mass (6 cm × 5 cm × 4 cm) arising from the retroperitoneum and a 2-cm mass in the head of the pancreas. Laboratory data were normal except for a CA-125 level of 150 IU/mL. She was diagnosed with recurrent ovarian cancer.

Follow-Up Questions

1. Is it useful to treat early relapsed disease based only on a rising CA-125 level rather than delaying treatment until there are clinical signs of relapse?

2. What therapeutic options are available for this patient's relapsed disease?

3. Which of the chemotherapeutic regimens would you recommend for the patient's locally relapsed ovarian cancer? Provide the rationale for your answer.

■ CLINICAL COURSE (PART 4)

The decision was made to start IV carboplatin AUC 5 and pegylated liposomal doxorubicin 30 mg/m^2 on day 1 every 28 days. Mrs Hillebrand received two cycles of carboplatin and pegylated liposomal doxorubicin. Radiologic imaging just prior to the third cycle showed no evidence of disease progression. During her third cycle, she complained of having trouble putting on her shoes and pain in her feet on walking. On physical exam, the patient's feet were red, swollen, and cracked. Her CA-125 levels were 155, 158, and 160 IU/mL after each of her first three cycles of carboplatin plus pegylated liposomal doxorubicin.

Follow-Up Question

4. What are the potential adverse effects of pegylated liposomal doxorubicin therapy that require monitoring and patient education?

■ CLINICAL COURSE (PART 5)

The fourth cycle of therapy was delayed for 2 weeks and restarted when her skin lesions resolved. However, after her fourth cycle radiographic findings revealed evidence of disease progression, and a repeat CA-125 was 288 IU/mL.

Follow-Up Questions

5. Mrs Hillebrand has heard from her friends about medications that are more targeted to fight cancer. Are there any targeted agents available to treat her recurrent, platinum resistant ovarian cancer?

6. What other options are available for salvage therapy, and which would you choose for this patient? Provide the rationale for your answer.

■ SELF-STUDY ASSIGNMENTS

1. What are the pharmacologic advantages of IV therapy versus IP therapy?

2. Why is the size of the residual tumor important with regard to IP therapy?

3. What are the probable causes of paclitaxel and docetaxel hypersensitivity?

4. What are the issues related to maintenance therapy in patients with advanced ovarian cancer after achieving complete response to consolidative chemotherapy?

5. How might cytochrome P450 3A4/5 polymorphism potentially affect docetaxel therapy of ovarian cancer?

CLINICAL PEARL

Surgical cytoreduction followed by chemotherapy was chosen for Mrs Hillebrand, but what treatments are available for patients whose disease or health status prevents them from undergoing this approach? One option for patients with advanced age or poor performance status is neoadjuvant chemotherapy. Neoadjuvant chemotherapy is given prior to the primary treatment, which is surgery, with the goal of reducing tumor volume in hopes for a greater chance of a cure. It simplifies surgery by decreasing tumor volume, blood loss, and transfusions during surgery and can reduce surgical complications and length of stays.

REFERENCES

1. The NCCN Clinical Practice Guidelines in Oncology™ Ovarian Cancer (Version 2.2015). © 2015 National Comprehensive Cancer Network Inc. Available at: NCCN.org. Accessed November 23, 2015. To view the most recent and complete version of the NCCN guidelines, go online to NCCN.org.

2. Boyd J, Sonoda Y, Federici MG, et al. Clinicopathologic features of BRCA-linked and sporadic ovarian cancer. JAMA 2000;283:2260–2265.

3. Ozols RF, Bundy BN, Greer BE, et al. Gynecologic Oncology Group. Phase III trial of carboplatin and paclitaxel compared with cisplatin and paclitaxel in patients with optimally resected stage III ovarian cancer: a gynecologic oncology group study. J Clin Oncol 2003;21:3194–3200.

4. du Bois A, Luck HJ, Meier W, et al. Arbeitsgemeinschaft Gynakologische Onkologie Ovarian Cancer Study Group. A randomized clinical trial of cisplatin/paclitaxel versus carboplatin/paclitaxel as first-line treatment of ovarian cancer. J Natl Cancer Inst 2003;95:1320–1329.

5. Vasey PA, Jayson GC, Gordon A, et al. Scottish Gynaecological Cancer Trials Group. Phase III randomized trial of docetaxel–carboplatin versus paclitaxel–carboplatin as first-line chemotherapy for ovarian carcinoma. J Natl Cancer Inst 2004;96:1682–1691.

6. Armstrong DK, Bundy B, Wenzel L, et al. Gynecologic Oncology Group. Intraperitoneal cisplatin and paclitaxel in ovarian cancer. N Engl J Med 2006;354:34–43.

7. Perren TJ, Swart AM, Pfisterer J, et al. A phase 3 trial of bevacizumab in ovarian cancer. N Engl J Med 2011;365:2484–2496.

8. Burger RA, Brady MF, Bookman MA, et al. Incorporation of bevacizumab in the primary treatment of ovarian cancer. N Engl J Med 2011;365(26):2473–2483.

9. Rustin GJ, van der Burg ME, Griffin CL, et al. Early versus delayed treatment of relapsed ovarian cancer (MRC OV05/EORTC 55955): a randomised trial. Lancet 2010;376:1155–1163.

10. Wagner U, Marth C, Largillier R, et al. Final overall survival results of phase III GCIG CALYPSO trial of pegylated liposomal doxorubicin and carboplatin vs paclitaxel and carboplatin in platinum-sensitive ovarian cancer patients. Br J Cancer 2010;107:588–591.

11. Pujade-Lauraine E, Hilpert F, Weber B, et al. Bevacizumab combined with chemotherapy for platinum resistant recurrent ovarian cancer: The AURELIA open-label randomized phase III trial. J Clin Oncol 2014;32:1302–1308.

12. Kim G, Ison G, McKee AE, et al. FDA approval summary: olaparib monotherapy in patients deleterious germline BRCA-mutated advanced ovarian cancer treated with three or more lines of chemotherapy. Clin Cancer Res 2015;21(19):4257–4261.

155

ACUTE LYMPHOCYTIC LEUKEMIA

Ian's Unexpected Weight Loss .... Level II

Deborah A. Hass, PharmD, BCOP, BCPS

LEARNING OBJECTIVES

After completing this case study, the reader should be able to:

- Interpret the laboratory values that signify the response of acute lymphocytic leukemia (ALL) to chemotherapy.

- Describe the ancillary medications and supportive care measures that are necessary when administering chemotherapy to patients with ALL.

- Understand the appropriate medications needed to treat neutropenic fever.

- Identify the backbone of therapy for treatment of adult ALL.

- State why CNS prophylaxis is routinely done in adult patients with ALL.

PATIENT PRESENTATION

■ Chief Complaint

Episodic diaphoresis, dizziness, and progressively worsening weakness and dyspnea on exertion × 1 month.

■ HPI

Ian Hamilton is a 58-year-old man with a past medical history of diabetes, hyperlipidemia, and hypertension who presents with episodic diaphoresis, dizziness, and progressively worsening weakness and dyspnea on exertion for 1 month. He has lost 40 lb in the last 9 months; he recently has been trying to eat more but is still losing 2 lb per week. Flow cytometry done 3 days ago at an outside hospital showed blastic B cells consistent with pre-B-cell lymphoblastic leukemia. The patient was found to have normocytic anemia (Hgb 9.9 g/dL). He also had a CT of the chest/abdomen/pelvis completed at the outside hospital due to weight loss and occasional abdominal pain and sensation that his stomach is "churning," although no report was sent with his records. He denies diarrhea but admits to once having an episode of dry heaving. A CXR was unremarkable. The patient was previously taking Janumet for type 2 DM, but since this workup began he stopped it and per patient has had blood sugars in the 100–130s.

■ PMH

DM type 2
HTN
Dyslipidemia

■ FH

Father had MI at age 60 and leukemia at age 78, and expired shortly thereafter. Mother is alive with heart disease, skin cancer, an unknown GI malignancy, and a recent diagnosis of lymphoma. He has five brothers and two sisters. One brother died at age 48 from Hodgkin lymphoma, diagnosed at age 18. Another brother has multiple sclerosis. The other three brothers and both sisters are healthy.

■ SH

Denies tobacco, EtOH, and illicit drugs. Drives a waste management truck, has three children, and lives with his wife.

■ Meds

None

■ All

NKDA

■ ROS

Constitutional: Positive for sweats, fatigue, anorexia, and weight loss
HEENT: Negative
Respiratory: Positive for dyspnea

CV: Negative

GI: Positive for nausea and abdominal pain

GU: Negative

Heme/lymph: Negative

MS: Negative

Neuro: Positive for dizziness and weakness

■ Physical Examination

Gen

A & O × 3; NAD

VS

BP 124/58 mm Hg, P 106 bpm, RR 18, T 37.2°C; Wt 100.8 kg, Ht 5′11″, SpO$_2$: 98% (room air)

Skin

Normal, no rashes

HEENT

EOMI, no scleral icterus, no conjunctival pallor

Neck/Lymph Nodes

No cervical LAD

Lungs/Thorax

CTA bilaterally without crackles, wheezes, or rhonchi

CV

RRR; normal S$_1$, S$_2$; no murmurs, rubs, or gallops

Abd

Soft, obese, NT/ND, normoactive bowel sounds

Genit/Rect

Deferred

MS/Ext

No CCE

Neuro

UE/LE strength 5/5 bilaterally

■ Labs

Na 137 mEq/L	Hgb 9.9 g/dL	AST 16 IU/L
K 4.1 mEq/L	Hct 27.2%	ALT 10 IU/L
Cl 100 mEq/L	MCV 93.5 μmm^3	T. bili 0.5 mg/dL
CO$_2$ 28 mEq/L	RDW 17.1%	Alb 3 g/dL
BUN 19 mg/dL	Plt 95 × 10^3/mm^3	Fe 23 mcg/dL
SCr 1.2 mg/dL	WBC 7.1 × 10^3/mm^3	TIBC 252 mcg/dL
Glu 93 mg/dL	Segs 35%	T. sat 35%
	Bands 0.2%	Ferritin 159 ng/L
	Lymphs 5.2%	TSH 3.3 μIU/mL
	Monos 8.6%	PSA 0.52 ng/mL
	Myelos 1.6%	B$_{12}$ 311 ng/mL
	Blasts 49%	Folate 9.5 ng/mL

■ Peripheral Blood Flow Cytometry

Large population of abnormal blasts, ~49% of leukocyte population expressing CD45. Blasts have precursor B-cell phenotype, express CD19, CD22, CD34, CD38, HLA-DR, and terminal deoxynucleotidyl transferase (TdT). About 59% of blasts express CD20. Blasts are negative for surface IG, T-cell-related antigens, and myeloid antigens. The mature lymphocyte population consists of a mix of unremarkable T and B cells.

■ Assessment and Plan

1. Pre-B-cell lymphoblastic leukemia (Philadelphia chromosome negative):
   - Obtain LDH/uric acid
   - Bone marrow biopsy
   - MUGA scan
   - Central catheter placement
   - Will attempt to obtain CT report from outside hospital
   - Acute leukemia panel
2. Type 2 DM with controlled BS despite stopping meds recently:
   - Accuchecks QID
   - Diabetic diet
   - Obtain UA to check for proteinuria; patient recently on ACE inhibitor but taken off. SCr ranging from 0.9 to 1.2 mg/dL at outside hospital.
3. Nausea:
   - Ondansetron PRN
4. HTN:
   - Patient recently taken off meds due to weight loss; will monitor pressures and restart meds as needed
5. Thrombocytopenia:
   - Transfuse to keep platelets greater than 10.0 × 10^3/mm^3
6. Anemia:
   - Transfuse to keep hemoglobin greater than 8 g/dL
7. FEN:
   - Diabetic diet as above
   - Maintain K >4 mEq/L and Mg >2 mg/dL
8. VTE prophylaxis:
   - SCD boots

CLINICAL COURSE

Within 2 days of admission, the patient receives a BM biopsy, MUGA (EF = 60%), and PICC line placement. The results of the biopsy were as follows:

The vast majority of the cells in the aspirate and biopsy are large blasts with fine chromatin and many prominent cytoplasmic vacuoles. Nucleoli are not generally prominent, and flow cytometric studies clearly indicated that this is a neoplasm of immature B cells. In addition, strong TdT expression is seen by immunohistochemistry. CD20 is weakly to strongly expressed in about half of the neoplastic cells.

WHO classification: B lymphoblastic leukemia.

He is started on the following medications:

- Pantoprazole delayed-release tablet 40 mg PO daily.
- Ondansetron 8 mg PO Q 8 H PRN.
- 0.9% normal saline by continuous IV infusion.
- Allopurinol 300 mg PO daily.

Following recovery from the PICC line placement, the patient was started on the R-HyperCVAD regimen based on Ht 180 cm, Wt 100.8 kg, and BSA = 2.2 m².

CHEMOTHERAPY

■ Regimen 1:

Cyclophosphamide 300 mg/m² (660 mg) IV over 3 hours every 12 hours for six doses on Days 1–3.

Mesna 600 mg/m² (1320 mg) IV over 24 hours on Days 1–3, ending 12 hours after the last dose of cyclophosphamide.

Vincristine 2 mg IV on Days 4 and 11.

Doxorubicin 50 mg/m² (110 mg) IV on Day 4.

Dexamethasone 40 mg PO on Days 1–4 and 11–14.

Rituximab 375 mg/m² (825 mg) IV on Day 1. (Patient did not receive it on Day 1 to prevent tumor flare.)

■ Regimen 2

(He will alternate cycles every 21 days with the following regimen, for a total of six to eight cycles depending on patient tolerability and disease progression; patient-specific doses will be based on the patient's weight at that time):

Methotrexate 200 mg/m² IV over 2 hours, followed by 800 mg/m² IV over 22 hours on Day 1

Leucovorin 25 mg PO Q 6 H starting 24 hours after completion of the methotrexate infusion until methotrexate level is <0.05 µmol/mL

Cytarabine 3000 mg/m² IV over 2 hours every 12 hours for four doses on Days 2–3

Methylprednisolone 50 mg IV BID on Days 1–3

■ CNS prophylaxis:

Methotrexate 12 mg intrathecally on Day 2.

Cytarabine 100 mg intrathecally on Day 8.

Repeat with each cycle of chemotherapy, depending on the risk of CNS disease. The CNS prophylaxis is given with both regimens 1 and 2.

■ Additional medications with chemotherapy:

Ondansetron injection 8 mg IV push Q 12 H

Fluconazole 400 mg PO daily

Acyclovir 400 mg PO Q 12 H

Prochlorperazine 10 mg IV push Q 6 H PRN

Prochlorperazine 10 mg PO Q 6 H PRN

Lorazepam 0.5 mg PO Q 6 H PRN

CLINICAL COURSE

■ Day 2 of induction chemotherapy:

Blood glucose remained in the 90s with one reading at 77 early this morning. Patient denies any symptoms of hypoglycemia. Patient was started on a diabetic diet yesterday, which he has been tolerating. Given his recent weight loss, he may no longer have the same degree of insulin resistance as before. Continue to monitor BS levels. Hypoglycemic protocol is in place if patient's BS drops below 70.

■ Day 3 of induction chemotherapy:

Patient c/o mild nausea but still has good appetite and is eating well; encouraged use of PRN antiemetics. Patient tolerated intrathecal chemotherapy. No acute events overnight.

■ Day 4 of induction chemotherapy:

Patient spiked temp to 101°F. Denies any respiratory, urinary, or other symptoms. Started on cefepime 2 g IV Q 8 H.

■ Day 5 of induction chemotherapy:

Patient continues to complain of nausea but has not vomited. He is able to tolerate a little solid food but reports that his appetite is not what it was. Reports two episodes of watery, nonbloody diarrhea early this morning with no further episodes since then.

■ Day 6 of induction chemotherapy:

Patient reports that his appetite is improving. He still complains of nausea, which has improved only slightly, but he has had no episodes of vomiting. No further episodes of diarrhea. No acute events overnight. Patient will receive rituximab 375 mg/m² (825 mg) IV today.

■ Day 7 of induction chemotherapy:

Patient reported chills and shaking during rituximab infusion yesterday. Acetaminophen 650 mg PO and diphenhydramine 50 mg IV were given. Patient felt better after that. No further symptoms during the day. Patient's only complaint is lack of bowel movement for 2 days. He is also still nauseated but is able to tolerate a regular meal without any emesis. No acute events overnight.

■ Day 8 of induction chemotherapy:

Patient complains of severe hiccups throughout the day and night yesterday that prevented him from sleeping. He said that he also has epigastric discomfort associated with the hiccups. He has pain in the epigastric region that he rates as 7/10 in intensity with no radiation. It is neither sharp nor dull and feels like a "knot." He also feels very full and bloated. He says it feels better when he stands up and walks around and also subsides when the hiccups cease. No further episodes of diarrhea and no vomiting. Patient still nauseated but able to tolerate meals. He had one small BM yesterday. No acute events overnight.

■ Day 15 of induction chemotherapy:

The patient was discharged to home. He was instructed to call the hematology fellow on call at any sign of a fever or infection. He was also instructed to stay away from people who have active infections, such as an upper respiratory virus. He was told to avoid large crowds and not to do any gardening. This is all to decrease the risk of infection. He will return to the hospital in 6 days for cycle 2 of chemotherapy. He is sent home with the following prescriptions:

Fluconazole 400 mg PO daily

Acyclovir 400 mg PO Q 12 H

Prochlorperazine 10 mg PO Q 6 H PRN

QUESTIONS

Problem Identification

1.a. Create a list of the patient's drug therapy problems. What effect will this chemotherapy regimen have on his diabetes?

1.b. Why was the patient started on allopurinol prior to starting his chemotherapy?

Desired Outcome

2.a. What are the short-term goals of pharmacotherapy in this patient?

2.b. The patient will receive four cycles of R-HyperCVAD alternating with four cycles of high-dose methotrexate and cytarabine. What are the long-term goals of pharmacotherapy in this patient?

Therapeutic Alternatives

3.a. What nondrug therapies might be useful for this patient?

3.b. What other pharmacotherapeutic options are available for this patient's ALL?

Optimal Plan

4.a. Why was the patient started on fluconazole and acyclovir in the doses prescribed?

4.b. Why was the patient started on intrathecal chemotherapy with no current evidence of CNS disease?

4.c. Outline the optimal drug therapy regimen if the initial treatment fails and the alternative therapy you described in question 3.b. is used.

Outcome Evaluation

5. What laboratory parameters and other diagnostic tests indicate an adequate response to induction therapy?

Patient Education

6.a. What information should be provided to the patient about the potential beneficial and adverse effects from the chemotherapy agents used during induction therapy?

6.b. Assume that the patient does not understand why he has to have so many courses of chemotherapy. Explain why he cannot be treated with just one cycle of chemotherapy.

■ SELF-STUDY ASSIGNMENTS

1. Discuss the value of colony-stimulating factors in the prophylaxis or treatment of therapy-related complications in patients with ALL.

2. Discuss the response criteria used to determine if a patient with ALL has obtained a complete remission or partial remission.

3. Define the terms stable disease and progressive disease as they relate to ALL.

CLINICAL PEARL

First-line therapy for treatment of ALL must contain the backbone of an anthracycline derivative, vincristine, and a corticosteroid. Asparaginase is also a useful agent in this disease, due to the leukemic cell's unique lack of endogenous asparagine. *E. Coli* derived L-asparaginase is no longer available in the United States. It is available in pegylated formulations and Erwinia-derived formulations. Patients with Philadelphia chromosome-positive ALL are treated with BCR-ABL tyrosine kinase inhibitors such as imatinib or dasatinib *in addition* to the induction chemotherapy regimen, such as R-HyperCVAD which our patient received.

REFERENCES

1. Kantarjian H, Thomas D, O'Brien S, et al. Long-term follow-up results of hyperfractionated cyclophosphamide, vincristine, doxorubicin, and dexamethasone (Hyper-CVAD), a dose-intensive regimen, in adult acute lymphocytic leukemia. Cancer 2004;101:2788–2801.

2. Thomas DA, Cortes J, O'Brien S, et al. Hyper-CVAD program in Burkitt's-type adult acute lymphoblastic leukemia. J Clin Oncol 1999;17:2461–2470.

3. Freifeld AG, Bow EJ, Sepkowitz KA, et al. Clinical practice guideline for the use of antimicrobial agents in neutropenic patients with cancer: 2010 update by the Infectious Diseases Society of America. Clin Infect Dis 2011;52(4):e56–e93.

4. Wetzler M, Sanford BL, Kurtzberg J, et al. Effective asparagine depletion with pegylated asparaginase results in improved outcomes in adult acute lymphoblastic leukemia: Cancer and Leukemia Group B Study 9511. Blood 2007;109:4164–4167.

156

CHRONIC MYELOGENOUS LEUKEMIA

It's Not Always Sunny in Philadelphia . . . . Level II

Alexandra Shillingburg, PharmD, BCOP

Aaron Cumpston, PharmD, BCOP

LEARNING OBJECTIVES

After completing this case study, the reader should be able to:

- Identify the presenting signs and symptoms of chronic myelogenous leukemia (CML).

- Identify important prognostic indicators for CML.

- Discuss available treatment options for newly diagnosed CML and refractory or relapsed CML and recommend an appropriate therapy.

- Choose appropriate parameters to monitor efficacy and potential adverse effects of treatment for CML.

- Educate patients on dosing and administration, the importance of adherence, and the most common side effects of the selected therapy for CML.

- Discuss potential mechanisms of resistance to first-line therapy for CML and formulate a treatment strategy for these patients.

PATIENT PRESENTATION

■ Chief Complaint

"I'm here for my routine visit for my back pain, but I have been feeling pretty tired lately and have this dull pain in my abdomen."

■ HPI

Carl Boyd is a 55-year-old man with a history of chronic back pain secondary to injury 5 years ago; he presents for his annual appointment and physical. Today he complains of left-sided abdominal discomfort and fullness that has resulted in some decreased appetite and increasing fatigue and inactivity over the past 3 months. When questioned, he reports experiencing intermittent drenching night sweats for the past 2 months that seem to be more frequent now.

▨ PMH

Chronic back pain
Childhood asthma, last symptoms at age 21
Appendectomy 16 years ago

▨ FH

Father died at age 66 due to MI. Mother is living, 71 years old with osteoporosis, depression, and GERD. He has one sister, age 52, living in Maine with no known medical issues. Paternal grandfather had prostate cancer but passed away from unrelated causes. Patient has no natural children.

▨ SH

Married and has one stepson, age 19, who attends college overseas. He works as a nurse in a local long-term care facility, and his wife is a tax accountant. He has no smoking history but drinks alcohol on social occasions. He denies any illicit drug use.

▨ Meds

One-A-Day multivitamin PO once daily
Cyclobenzaprine 10 mg PO BID as needed
Ibuprofen 800 mg PO TID as needed
Oxycodone 10 mg every 6 H as needed

▨ All

NKA

▨ ROS

Positive for increased weakness and tiredness, frequent night sweats, mild shortness of breath on exertion, general musculoskeletal pain, and LUQ pain. Denies bleeding, headaches, vision changes, nausea, vomiting, chest pain, rashes, numbness or tingling in extremities, or urinary symptoms.

▨ Physical Examination

Gen

Caucasian man who appears his stated age and is in no obvious distress

VS

BP 122/60 mm Hg, P 63 bpm, RR 20, T 36.3°C; Wt 77.5 kg, Ht 180 cm, Pain Score 0

Skin

Skin warm and dry, no rashes and no lesions

HEENT

Head atraumatic and normocephalic; ENT without erythema or injection; mucous membranes moist; conjunctivae clear; PERRLA. No sinus discharge or tenderness. Lips, teeth, and gums without tenderness.

Neck

No JVD or thyromegaly appreciated

Lymph Nodes

No palpable cervical, supraclavicular, axillary, or inguinal adenopathy

Lungs

Diffuse expiratory wheezes bilaterally

CV

Regular rate and rhythm; S_1 and S_2 normal; 2/6 systolic murmur

Abd

Tender to palpation; tip of spleen palpable in LUQ. Normoactive bowel sounds. No hepatomegaly.

Rect

Deferred

MS/Ext

Normal gait, full range of motion in flexion and extension of the upper and lower extremities with 5/5 strength throughout. No cyanosis or edema; no synovitis or joint effusions.

Neuro

Grossly normal; CN II–XII intact; alert and oriented × 3

Psychiatric

Normal affect, behavior, memory, thought content, judgment, and speech

▨ Labs

Na 139 mEq/L	Hgb 10.3 g/dL	AST 24 IU/L	Ca 8.2 mg/dL
K 3.7 mEq/L	Hct 33.8%	ALT 38 IU/L	Mg 2.2 mEq/L
Cl 105 mEq/L	Plt 470 × 10³/mm³	Alk phos 72 IU/L	Phos 3.8 mg/dL
CO_2 27 mEq/L	WBC 123 × 10³/mm³	LDH 950 IU/L	Uric acid 6.5 mg/dL
BUN 28 mg/dL	PMNs 53%	T. bili 0.6 mg/dL	LAP absent
SCr 0.8 mg/dL	Bands 13%	T. prot 6.9 g/dL	
Glu 92 mg/dL	Lymphs 7%	Alb 3.5 g/dL	
Retic 2.3%	Myelos 9%		
	Metas 10%		
	Eos 4%		
	Basos 4%		

▨ Bone Marrow Biopsy

The bone marrow is markedly hypercellular (essentially 100% cellular) due to extensive proliferation of granulocytes. The granulocytic series are left-shifted; however, blasts are not increased and no Auer rods or significant dysplasia is noted. Erythroid precursors are slightly decreased and megakaryocytes are markedly increased with many small, hypolobate forms. Iron stores are decreased, and mild reticulin fibrosis is identified. Eosinophilia and basophilia are also present in the peripheral blood and bone marrow. FISH analysis is positive for BCR-ABL1 rearrangement.

Cytogenetic studies show translocation involving the long arms of chromosomes 9 and 22 [t(9q;22q)] (Philadelphia chromosome), with 95% of malignant cells analyzed found to be Ph-positive (see Fig. 156-1). This information is consistent with the characteristics of CML, and the morphologic features are consistent with chronic phase (CML-CP).

QUESTIONS

Problem Identification

1.a. What information in the patient's history is consistent with a diagnosis of CML-CP?

1.b. Describe the natural progression of CML.

1.c. List factors that signal a poor prognosis for CML patients in chronic phase.

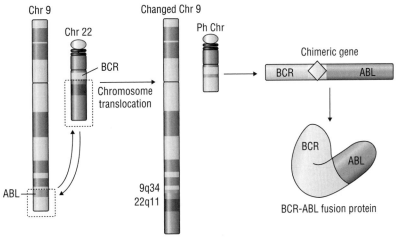

FIGURE 156-1. The chromosomal translocation responsible for chronic myeloid leukemia (CML). The Philadelphia chromosome (Ph) is result of the transloca-tion between chromosomes 9 and 22 which joins the ABL oncogene with the BCR gene. This fusion gene codes for a unique fusion protein that is constitutively active. *(Reprinted with permission from Morin PJ, Trent JM, Collins FS, Vogelstein B. Cancer genetics. In: Kasper DL, Fauci AS, Hauser SL, Longo DL, Jameson JL, Loscalzo J, eds. Harrison's Principles of Internal Medicine, 19th Ed. New York, McGraw-Hill, 2015.)*

Desired Outcome

2. What are long-term therapy goals for this patient?

Therapeutic Alternatives

3. What nonpharmacologic and pharmacologic alternatives should be considered for this newly diagnosed patient?

Optimal Plan

4. Considering all patient factors, describe the optimal initial treat-ment plan for this patient.

Outcome Evaluation

5. Describe parameters for monitoring disease response and toxic-ity for the treatment option you recommended.

Patient Education

6. What information should be given to the patient prior to treatment?

■ CLINICAL COURSE

The regimen you recommended was initiated. At the 2-week follow-up visit, the patient's WBC count was $34 \times 10^3/mm^3$. At the 4-week follow-up visit, his WBC count had decreased to $9 \times 10^3/mm^3$. After 3 months of treatment, his WBC count remained stable at $8.2 \times 10^3/mm^3$ and he had a minimal cytogenetic response as evi-denced by a bone marrow biopsy that revealed 70% Philadelphia chromosome-positive metaphases. After 6 months, he remained in complete hematologic response but minor cytogenetic response with 60% positive metaphases. Molecular analysis (PCR testing for the Philadelphia chromosome) also showed less than a major response. Because he experienced a suboptimal response, mutation testing was performed and revealed the presence of a Y253F muta-tion. Also, since beginning treatment with imatinib, the patient has noticed mild periorbital edema, moderate myalgias, and nausea. He presents to clinic today to discuss further treatment options with the healthcare team.

Follow-Up Questions

1. What are the possible mechanisms of resistance to imatinib?

2. What therapeutic options are available for this patient with a suboptimal response to imatinib 400 mg PO once daily?

3. Compare and contrast dasatinib, nilotinib, bosutinib, and pona-tinib in terms of efficacy and toxicity in patients with suboptimal responses to imatinib.

4. Is it possible to discontinue tyrosine kinase inhibitor (TKI) therapy and maintain remission, or will the patient need lifelong therapy?

5. How would your recommendations differ if the patient had a T315I mutation instead?

■ SELF-STUDY ASSIGNMENTS

1. Describe the hematologic and cytogenetic response criteria (complete, partial, minor, and no response) for therapy in patients with CML, including WBC count, splenomegaly, and percent of Ph+ marrow cells.

2. If this patient becomes pregnant, how should her therapy be revised?

3. Discuss the progress being made to develop treatments for patients with the T315I mutation.

CLINICAL PEARL

Mutation testing in patient with chronic phase CML is generally not performed unless the patient has a suboptimal or lack of response to imatinib because mutations can occasionally be found in patients without resistant disease.

REFERENCES

1. O'Brien SG, Guilhot F, Larson RA, et al. IRIS investigators. Ima-tinib compared with interferon and low-dose cytarabine for newly diagnosed chronic-phase chronic myeloid leukemia. N Engl J Med 2003;348:994–1004.

2. Deininger M, O'Brien SG, Guilhot F, et al. International random-ized study of interferon vs STI571 (IRIS) 8-year follow up: sustained survival and low risk for progression or events in patients with newly diagnosed chronic myeloid leukemia in chronic phase (CML-CP) treated with imatinib. ASH Annual Meeting Abstracts 2009;114:1126.

3. Jabbour E, Kantarjian HM, Saglio G, et al. Early response with dasat-inib or imatinib in chronic myeloid leukemia: 3-year follow-up from a randomized phase 3 trial (DASISION). Blood 2014;123:494–500.

4. Larson RA, Hochhaus A, Hughes TP, et al. Nilotinib vs imatinib in patients with newly diagnosed Philadelphia chromosome-positive chronic myeloid leukemia in chronic phase: ENESTnd 3-year follow-up. Leukemia 2012;26:2197–2203.

5. Rea D. Management of adverse events associated with tyrosine kinase inhibitors in chronic myeloid leukemia. Ann Hematol 2015;94(Suppl 2):S149–S158.

6. Hochhaus A, Kantarjian HM, Baccarani M, et al. Dasatinib induces notable hematologic and cytogenetic responses in chronic-phase chronic myeloid leukemia after failure of imatinib therapy. Blood 2007;109:2303–2309.

7. Baccarani M, Deininger MW, Rosti G, et al. European LeukemiaNet recommendations for the management of chronic myeloid leukemia: 2013. Blood 2013;122(6):872–884.

8. Cortes JE, Kantarjian HM, Brümmendorf TH, et al. Safety and efficacy of bosutinib (SKI-606) in chronic phase Philadelphia chromosome-positive chronic myeloid leukemia patients with resistance or intolerance to imatinib. Blood 2011;118:4567–4576.

9. Cortes JE, Kim DW, Pinilla-Ibarz J, et al. A phase 2 trial of ponatinib in Philadelphia chromosome-positive leukemias. N Engl J Med 2013;369:1783–1796.

10. Cortes J, Lipton JH, Rea D, et al. Phase 2 study of subcutaneous omacetaxine mepesuccinate after TKI failure in patients with chronic-phase CML with T315I mutation. Blood 2012;120:2573–2580.

157

KIDNEY CANCER

Molecular Therapies . . . . Level II

Daniel J. Crona, PharmD, PhD

Jessica J. Auten, PharmD, BCPS, BCOP

LEARNING OBJECTIVES

After completing this case study, the reader should be able to:

- Evaluate first-line pharmacotherapeutic options for patients with metastatic kidney cancer.

- Formulate a monitoring plan for a patient receiving treatment for metastatic kidney cancer based on patient-specific factors and the prescribed regimen.

- Recommend alternative pharmacotherapeutic treatment options for patients with relapsed or progressive metastatic kidney cancer.

- Provide appropriate and detailed educational information to patients about the targeted therapies for metastatic kidney cancer.

PATIENT PRESENTATION

Chief Complaint

"What treatment options do I have for my kidney cancer?"

HPI

Morgan Shepherd is a 65-year-old woman who presented 3.5 months ago to her primary care physician with complaints of back pain, cough, and weight loss. She did not respond to an initial course of antibiotics for assumed pyelonephritis and developed gross hematuria a few days later. She was subsequently referred to a urologist, who detected a mass on renal ultrasound. CT scan of chest, abdomen, and pelvis revealed a 7-cm left upper-pole kidney tumor, and several bilateral lung nodules. She was referred to a nearby cancer center for further evaluation. A core needle biopsy of the kidney mass revealed neoplastic cells, but the sample was too small and heterogeneous to definitively determine a specific histology. In order to relieve worsening symptoms and further elucidate a specific histopathology of the mass, she underwent radical nephrectomy of her left kidney. Pathologic examination revealed kidney cancer with a clear cell histologic etiology.

Now, 6 weeks later, the patient has recovered from surgery with resolution of back pain and hematuria. She presents to the outpatient oncology clinic for an appointment with the medical oncologist. A postsurgical CT scan reveals persistent lung metastases (unchanged in number or size). She is interested in pursuing systemic treatment of her metastatic renal carcinoma and would like to discuss available treatment options.

PMH

Hypertension
Dyslipidemia

FH

Her mother died at age 75 due to complications related to MI, and her father died at age 73 due to PE. She has one brother, age 58, who is alive and living with asthma, but who is otherwise healthy. She has no family history of cancer.

SH

Mrs Shepherd has been happily married for over 40 years. She has one grown son, age 33, who is alive and healthy. The patient reports an extensive smoking history (25 pack-years), but quit 5 years ago. She is overweight (BMI 29.3 kg/m²).

Meds

Hydrochlorothiazide 25 mg PO once daily
Enalapril 5 mg PO once daily
Atorvastatin 10 mg PO once daily

All

NKDA

ROS

No fever or chills; no headaches; no nausea or vomiting; feels very weak since the surgery

Physical Examination

Gen

WDWN Caucasian female in NAD

VS

BP 130/84 mm Hg, P 64 bpm, RR 18, T 37.0°C; Wt 82.4 kg, Ht 5′6″, BSA 1.96 m²

Skin

Olive complexion. Nephrectomy site is fully healed.

HEENT

PERRLA, EOMI; oropharynx without lesions

Neck/Lymph Nodes

Supple without adenopathy; thyroid without masses

Lung/Thorax

Slight wheezing in LUL

CV

RRR; normal S_1 and S_2; no MRG

Abd

Soft, NT/ND; (+) BS

Genit/Rect

Deferred

Ext

No clubbing, cyanosis, or edema

Neuro

A & O × 3; CN II–XII intact; DTRs 2+ throughout; motor and sensory levels intact; Babinski (–)

▨ Labs

Na 137 mEq/L	Hgb 12 g/dL	WBC 6.1×10^6/mm³	T. bili 0.8 mg/dL
K 4.0 mEq/L	Hct 36%	Neutros 66%	AST 25 IU/L
Cl 99 mEq/L	Plt 325×10^3/mm³	Bands 4%	ALT 27 IU/L
CO_2 25 mEq/L		Lymphs 26%	Alk phos 125 IU/L
BUN 20 mg/dL		Monos 4%	Alb 3.8 g/dL
SCr 2.0 mg/dL			LDH 220 IU/L
Glu 75 mg/dL			Ca 8.5 mg/dL
			Mg 2.0 mg/dL

▨ Assessment

A 65-year-old woman with metastatic clear cell kidney cancer, who is S/P resection of her primary tumor via radical nephrectomy, presents to the medical oncology clinic. Multiple subcentimeter metastatic lesions in lung persist; however, there continues to be no evidence of additional metastatic disease. Briefly, she is not a candidate for high-dose IL-2 based on inadequate results of pulmonary function testing (both FVC and FEV_1 were <65% of predicted values), a SCr value of 2.0 mg/dL, and diminished performance status. In addition, she had a conversation with her medical oncologist about the option of surveillance and forgoing systemic treatment for now. However, she is interested in hearing about her available pharmacotherapeutic options.

QUESTIONS

Problem Identification

1. What information in the patient's history (eg, signs, symptoms, and laboratory values) indicates the presence of kidney cancer? Also, list the factors in the patient's history that could determine the severity of her kidney cancer.

Desired Outcome

2. What are the goals of pharmacotherapy in this case?

Therapeutic Alternatives

3. What nonpharmacologic and pharmacologic alternatives should be considered as first-line treatment options for this patient?

Optimal Plan

4. Considering all patient factors, describe the optimal initial pharmacotherapeutic plan for this patient.

Outcome Evaluation

5. What clinical and laboratory parameters are necessary to evaluate the therapy for achievement of the desired therapeutic outcome and to detect or prevent adverse effects?

Patient Education

6. What information would you provide to the patient before initiation of treatment?

■ CLINICAL COURSE

Mrs Shepherd was started on the treatment you recommended and achieved partial regression of some of her metastatic pulmonary lesions. She experienced adverse effects, including hypertension (maximum BP was 160/95), hand–foot skin reaction, a slight yellowing of her skin, hair depigmentation, and peripheral edema. Hypertension was controlled by increasing her enalapril dosage to 10 mg per day.

Unfortunately after 9 months of treatment, today's follow-up CT scan indicates progression of the cancer. The patient expressed a desire to continue treatment and is here to inquire about available second-line treatment options.

Follow-Up Questions

1. Given this situation, what pharmacotherapeutic options are available at this time? Provide the rationale for your answer.

2. How would you monitor for the potential adverse effects of the treatment you recommended?

3. What education should the patient receive about the new regimen that you propose?

4. What alterations would you recommend to the patient's regimen if she were also receiving a strong inducer of hepatic CYP3A4 enzymes? What about a strong inhibitor of CYP3A4?

■ SELF-STUDY ASSIGNMENTS

1. Discuss the role of immunotherapies used in metastatic kidney cancer.

2. What role, if any, does adjuvant treatment play after surgery for localized kidney cancer?

3. What role does tumor histology play in treatment selection for metastatic kidney cancer?

CLINICAL PEARL

Until a decade ago, few effective treatment options were available to treat metastatic kidney cancer because most patients were unresponsive to traditional cytotoxic chemotherapy and radiation. Additionally, cytokine therapy (eg, interferon or high-dose IL-2) is toxic and rarely results in a durable remission. A deeper understanding of the molecular mechanisms involved in kidney cancer pathogenesis led to development and approval of eight targeted agents directed at signaling mechanisms in the VEGF or mTOR pathways. However, patients almost always progress after treatment with a first-line targeted agent, so treating patients with second-, third- and even fourth-line targeted agents is not uncommon.

REFERENCES

1. Hutson TE, Lesovoy V, Al-Shukri S, et al. Axitinib versus sorafenib as first-line therapy in patients with metastatic renal-cell carcinoma: a randomised open-label phase 3 trial. Lancet Oncol 2013;14:1287–1294.

2. Sternberg CN, Davis ID, Mardiak J, et al. Pazopanib in locally advanced or metastatic renal cell carcinoma: results of a randomized phase III trial. J Clin Oncol 2010;28:1061–1068.

3. Motzer R, Hutson TE, Cella D, et al. Pazopanib versus sunitinib in metastatic renal-cell carcinoma. N Engl J Med 2013;369:722–731.

4. Motzer RJ, Hutson TE, Tomczak P, et al. Overall survival and updated results for sunitinib compared with interferon alfa in patients with metastatic renal cell carcinoma. J Clin Oncol 2009;27:3584–3590.

5. Rini BI, Halabi S, Rosenberg JE, et al. Bevacizumab plus interferon alfa compared with interferon alfa monotherapy in patients with metastatic renal cell carcinoma: CALGB 90206. J Clin Oncol 2008;26:5422–5428.

6. Hudes G, Carducci M, Tomczak P, et al. Temsirolimus, interferon alfa, or both for advanced renal-cell carcinoma. N Engl J Med 2007;356:2271–2281.

7. Motzer RJ, Escudier B, Oudard S, et al. Efficacy of everolimus in advanced renal cell carcinoma: a double-blind, randomized, placebo-controlled phase III trial. Lancet 2008;372:449–456.

8. Rini BI, Escudier B, Tomczak P, et al. Comparative effectiveness of axitinib versus sorafenib in advanced renal cell carcinoma (AXIS): a randomised phase 3 trial. Lancet 2011;378:1931–1939.

9. Motzer RJ, Escudier B, McDermott DF, et al. Nivolumab versus everolimus in advanced renal-cell carcinoma. N Engl J Med 2015;373:1803–1813.

10. Choueiri TK, Escudier B, Powles T, et al. Cabozantinib versus everolimus in advanced renal-cell carcinoma. N Engl J Med 2015;373:1814–1823.

158

MELANOMA

You Have Been Exposed . . . . Level II

Jamie Poust, PharmD, BCOP

Sarah Norskog, PharmD

LEARNING OBJECTIVES

After completing this case study, the reader should be able to:

- Identify risk factors for developing melanoma.

- Determine treatment options for metastatic melanoma.

- Prepare educational information to provide to a patient receiving treatment for metastatic melanoma.

- Discuss ways to prevent melanoma.

PATIENT PRESENTATION

■ Chief Complaint

"I have been getting short of breath walking to work lately."

■ HPI

Douglas Kenney is a 52-year-old Caucasian man who presents with increasing shortness of breath and dyspnea on exertion. He denies chest pain and hemoptysis. He reports that he could not walk more than one block without having to stop to catch his breath today. He normally walks 10 blocks to and from work each day and has noted progressive shortness of breath each week for the past 2–4 weeks. He has a history of a left lower leg thrombosis diagnosed 2 months ago after returning home from a trip to Australia. He also has a history of Stage IIA melanoma (T3a, N0, M0) diagnosed 4 years ago.

■ PMH

GERD
Type 2 DM
DVT of the LLE, diagnosed 2 months ago
Melanoma (Stage IIA, superficial spreading, Breslow's thickness of 1.2 mm); diagnosed 4 years ago; left lower back—s/p wide surgical excision—sentinel lymph node biopsy was negative for melanoma

■ FH

Patient is oldest of three children; he has two sisters, both alive; one with type 2 diabetes mellitus. Mother is age 74 with a history of basal cell carcinoma and melanoma skin cancers and heart disease. Father deceased at age 71 secondary to pneumonia.

■ SH

The patient is employed as an architect and is married with one daughter (age 17). He has a history of smoking cigarettes, 0.5 pack per day for 4 years in college. He is a social drinker and reports no illicit drug use.

■ Meds

Lansoprazole 30 mg PO once daily
Glipizide 10 mg PO once daily
Metformin 1,000 mg PO twice daily
Enoxaparin 100 mg SC twice daily

■ All

NKDA

■ ROS

Denies fever, chills, rigors, and chest pain; (+) shortness of breath and DOE

■ Physical Examination

Gen

Slightly overweight Caucasian man in mild respiratory distress

VS

BP 129/72 mm Hg, P 92 bpm, RR 22, T 37.8°C; Wt 102.2 kg, Ht 5′10″

Skin

Fair skin, multiple scattered dysplastic nevi covering trunk and torso; left lower back melanoma excision site noted, which is well healed. Small bruises on abdomen and upper thighs related to enoxaparin injection sites.

HEENT

PERRLA, EOMI; normal sclera; clear oropharynx

Neck/Lymph Nodes

Supple; no lymphadenopathy or masses

Lung/Thorax

Decreased breath sounds in the left lower base

CV

RRR; no MRG

Abd

NTND; (+) BS

Genit/Rect

Deferred

MS/Ext

Normal ROM and sensation; LLE slightly larger than RLE

Neuro

A & O × 3; normal cranial nerves; normal reflexes and sensation

▨ Labs

Na 135 mEq/L	Hgb 15.8 g/dL	WBC 5.6 × 10⁶/mm³	T. bili 1.1 mg/dL
K 4.1 mEq/L	Hct 46%	Neutros 68%	AST 22 IU/L
Cl 100 mEq/L	RBC 5.2 × 10⁶/mm³	Bands 3%	ALT 28 IU/L
CO_2 25 mEq/L	Plt 322 × 10³/mm³	Eos 1%	Alk phos 165 IU/L
BUN 9 mg/dL		Lymphs 26%	Alb 4.2 g/dL
SCr 1.0 mg/dL		Monos 2%	LDH 187 IU/L
Glu 75 mg/dL			Ca 8.5 mg/dL
			Mg 2.1 mg/dL
			PO_4 3.6 mg/dL

▨ CT Chest

No pulmonary emboli. Two nodules consistent with metastasis found in the left lower lung; a small- to moderate-sized pleural effusion is also seen in the left lower lung.

▨ CT Abdomen

Solitary lesion consistent with metastasis seen in the right lobe of the liver

▨ CT-Guided Lung Biopsy

Tissue taken from left lower lobe is consistent with metastasis from melanoma. Tumor tissue testing reveals BRAF^{V600} wild type DNA.

▨ Assessment

A 52-year old man with recurrent melanoma metastatic to the liver and lungs with shortness of breath and dyspnea on exertion related to his metastatic disease and requires treatment of his disease.

QUESTIONS

Problem Identification

1.a. Create a list of the patient's drug therapy problems.

1.b. What information (signs, symptoms, and laboratory values) indicates the presence or severity of melanoma?

1.c. What risk factor(s) does this patient have for developing melanoma?

Desired Outcome

2. What are the goals for treatment of melanoma in this patient?

Therapeutic Alternatives

3.a. What therapeutic regimens are feasible options for this patient?

3.b. What nondrug therapies might be useful for this patient?

Optimal Plan

4. What therapeutic regimen (drug, dosage form, dose, schedule, and duration of therapy) do you suggest for treating this patient's metastatic melanoma?

Outcome Evaluation

5. What clinical and laboratory parameters are necessary to evaluate the therapy for achievement of the desired therapeutic outcome and to detect or prevent adverse effects?

Patient Education

6. What information would you provide to the patient about the agent(s) used to treat his metastatic melanoma?

▨ ADDITIONAL CASE QUESTION

1 Mr Kenney's daughter is concerned that she is at risk for developing melanoma. How can melanoma be prevented?

▨ SELF-STUDY ASSIGNMENTS

1. How would you manage immune-mediated adverse reactions caused by ipilimumab?

2. How long does he need to be anticoagulated for the DVT?

3. What is the ABCDE rule in helping to distinguish features of a normal mole from an abnormal mole?

CLINICAL PEARL

Measurement of serum LDH at the time of Stage IV diagnosis is important in determining prognosis. The 1-year overall survival rate for Stage IV patients with a normal LDH is 65% compared to only 32% in patients with an elevated LDH.

REFERENCES

1. Balch CM, Gershenwald JE, Soong S, et al. Final version of 2009 AJCC melanoma staging and classification. J Clin Oncol 2009;27:6199–6206.

2. NCCN Clinical Practice Guidelines in Oncology. Melanoma v.1.2016. Available at: *www.nccn.org.* Accessed November 1, 2015.

3. Robert C, Long GV, Brady B, et al. Nivolumab in previously untreated melanoma without BRAF mutation. N Engl J Med 2015;372:320–330.

4. Weber JS, D'Angelo SP, Minor D, et al. Nivolumab versus chemotherapy in patients with advanced melanoma who progressed after anti-CTLA-4 treatment (CheckMate 037): a randomized, controlled, open-label, phase 3 trial. Lancet Oncol 2015;16:375–384.

5. Robert C, Schachter J, Long GV, et al. Pembrolizumab versus ipilimumab in advanced melanoma. N Engl J Med 2015;372:2521–2532.

6. Robert C, Ribas A, Wolchok JD, et al. Anti-programmed-death-receptor-1 treatment with pembrolizumab in ipilimumab-refractory advanced melanoma: a randomized dose-comparison cohort of a phase 1 trail. Lancet 2014;384:1109–1117.

7. Postow M, Chesney J, Pavlick AC, et al. Nivolumab and ipilimumab versus ipilimumab in untreated melanoma. N Engl J Med 2015;372:2006–2017.

8. American Cancer Society. Melanoma Skin Cancer. Available at *http://www.cancer.org/acs/groups/cid/documents/webcontent/003120-pdf.pdf.* Accessed November 1, 2015.

159

HEMATOPOIETIC STEM CELL TRANSPLANTATION

Many Meds, Many Interactions ....Level III

Teresa C. Kam, PharmD, BCOP

LEARNING OBJECTIVES

After completing this case study, the reader should be able to:

- Understand the regimen-related toxicities of immunosuppression medications used for allogeneic stem cell transplantation (SCT).

- Differentiate the presenting features of immunosuppressive medication adverse events from other medications.

- Design appropriate pharmacotherapeutic plans for patients who develop toxicity from immunosuppression.

PATIENT PRESENTATION

Chief Complaint

The patient is being seen for follow-up in clinic and has developed bothersome tremors and headaches. He was seen recently by his PCP for dyslipidemia and hypertension and has had changes in his medication regimen.

HPI

Jacob Weber is a 45-year-old man who presents to the BMT clinic 75 days post HLA-matched unrelated donor allogeneic stem cell transplantation for high-risk AML. His preparative regimen consisted of thiotepa (5 mg/kg IV Q 12 H × 3 doses) and cyclophosphamide (60 mg/kg IV Q 24 H × 2 doses). His GVHD prophylaxis regimen consisted of tacrolimus and sirolimus, both starting on day 3. His hospital course was complicated by febrile neutropenia, acute kidney injury, mucositis, and diarrhea. These complications had resolved at the time of discharge approximately 6 weeks ago. Two weeks ago, he developed a skin rash and diarrhea and was diagnosed with grade 2 acute GVHD. He was started on prednisone 90 mg (1 mg/kg) orally BID, and fluconazole was switched to posaconazole 300 mg orally once daily. His PCP also added gemfibrozil 600 mg orally twice daily to his lipid regimen.

Today, his main complaints are headache and tremors with movement such as typing or holding a cup. He reports taking his hospital discharge dose of tacrolimus 2 mg orally twice daily and sirolimus 2 mg orally once daily.

PMH

High-risk AML treated with idarubicin and cytarabine induction, followed by high-dose cytarabine × 1 cycle. He was started on amlodipine at hospital discharge for newly-diagnosed hypertension. Dyslipidemia was managed previously with atorvastatin and recently with addition of gemfibrozil.

FH

Married with two children. Father is deceased from atherosclerotic heart disease.

Meds (at Day +75)

Posaconazole 300 mg PO daily
Esomeprazole 40 mg PO daily
Tacrolimus 2 mg PO twice daily
Prednisone 90 mg PO twice daily
Valacyclovir 500 mg PO twice daily
Amlodipine 10 mg PO daily
Prochlorperazine 10 mg PO Q 8 H PRN nausea/vomiting
Sirolimus 2 mg PO once daily
Dapsone 100 mg PO daily
Atorvastatin 10 mg PO daily
Gemfibrozil 600 mg PO BID
Triamcinolone 1% cream—apply twice daily to chest and shoulders

All

Sulfa → urticaria

ROS

Worsening "annoying" motor tremors that interfere with activities of daily living such as typing and drinking. Patient also reports dull headache that started about a week ago.

Physical Examination

Gen

Patient is a WDWN Caucasian male

VS

BP 158/76 mm Hg, P 92 bpm, T 37.4°C; O$_2$ sat 98% in room air; Wt 90 kg; Ht 5′10″

HEENT

Moist mucous membranes

Skin

Red rash on chest and shoulders

Neck/Lymph Nodes

Supple; no thyromegaly

Lungs

Clear without wheezes, rhonchi, or crackles

Heart

RRR; normal heart sounds; no M/R/G

Abd

Slight distention, RUQ tenderness, mild hepatomegaly

Ext

Grade I–II edema in LE bilaterally

Neuro

A & O × 3

■ Labs

Na 132 mEq/L	Hgb 8.8 g/dL	AST 55 IU/L
K 3.0 mEq/L	Hct 28%	ALT 61 IU/L
CL 112 mEq/L	Plt 110 × 10³/mm³	Alk phos 222 IU/L
CO₂ 19 mEq/L	WBC 4.1 × 10³/mm³	LDH 70 IU/L
BUN 22 mg/dL		T. bili 0.9 mg/dL
SCr 1.1 mg/dL		Alb 2.9 g/dL
Glu 124 mg/dL		Fasting LDL unknown
Mg 1.2 mg/dL		Fasting HDL 46 mg/dL
		Fasting Trig 800 mg/dL
		Tacrolimus 19.6 ng/mL (target 5–10 ng/mL)
		Sirolimus 20.5 ng/mL (target 5–10 ng/mL)

■ Assessment

New-onset tremors, headaches, hypokalemia, hypomagnesemia, and hypertriglyceridemia

QUESTIONS

Problem Identification

1.a. What are the likely causes for the patient's tremors and headache?

1.b. What are potential causes for development of hypertriglyceridemia?

1.c. What are the potential causes of hypokalemia and hypomagnesemia?

Desired Outcome

2. What are the therapeutic goals in this patient?

Therapeutic Alternatives

3. What treatment options exist for managing the patient's dyslipidemia?

Optimal Plan

4.a. Describe your pharmacotherapeutic plan for the patient's dyslipidemia.

4.b. Outline changes that should be made to the patient's immunosuppressive regimen.

4.c. What pharmacotherapeutic interventions should be implemented to treat this patient's electrolyte disturbances?

4.d. What changes, if any, should be made to the infection prophylaxis regimen?

Outcome Evaluation

5. What parameters should you monitor to assess the response to therapy and to detect adverse effects?

Patient Education

6. What information should be given to the patient and his family/caregivers?

■ FOLLOW-UP QUESTIONS

1. What options are available for prevention of graft-versus-host disease after allogeneic stem cell transplantation?

2. Which vaccinations and at what schedule should patients receive after allogeneic stem cell transplantation?

■ SELF-STUDY ASSIGNMENTS

1. What diseases are amenable to treatment with allogeneic SCT?

2. Aside from the complications reviewed in this case, derive a list of potential problems that could occur after allogeneic marrow transplantation.

CLINICAL PEARL

Allogeneic SCT is often associated with multiple medical conditions and drug interactions requiring careful evaluation to prevent further toxicity.

REFERENCES

1. Glotzbecker B, Duncan C, Alyea E, Campbell B, Soiffer R. Important drug interactions in hematopoietic stem cell transplantation: what every physician should know. Biol Blood Marrow Transplant 2012;18:989–1006.

2. Rosenbeck LL, Kiel PJ, Kalsekar I, et al. Prophylaxis with sirolimus and tacrolimus ± antithymocyte globulin reduces the risk of acute graft-versus-host disease without an overall survival benefit following allogeneic stem cell transplantation. Biol Blood Marrow Transplant 2011;17:916–922.

3. Cutler C, Logan BR, Nakamura R, et al. Tacrolimus/sirolimus vs tacrolimus/methotrexate for graft-versus-host disease prophylaxis after HLA-matched, related donor hematopoietic stem cell transplantation: results of Blood and Marrow Transplant Clinical Trials Network Trial 0402. Blood (ASH Annual Meeting Abstracts) 2012;120:abstract 739.

4. Griffith ML, Savani BN, Boord JB. Dyslipidemia after allogeneic stem cell transplantation: evaluation and management. Blood 2010;116:1197–1204.

5. Ullmann AJ, Lipton JH, Vesole DH, et al. Posaconazole or fluconazole for prophylaxis in severe graft-versus-host disease. N Engl J Med 2007;356:335–347.

6. Tomblyn M, Chiller T, Einsele H, et al. Guidelines for preventing infectious complications among hematopoietic cell transplantation recipients: a global perspective. Biol Blood Marrow Transplant 2009;15:1143–1238.

160

PARENTERAL NUTRITION

Getting Past the Obstruction . . . . Level III

Michael D. Kraft, PharmD, BCNSP

Melissa R. Pleva, PharmD, BCPS, BCNSP

LEARNING OBJECTIVES

After completing this case study, the reader should be able to:

- Describe how a bowel obstruction can lead to nutritional, fluid, and electrolyte abnormalities.

- Characterize the severity of malnutrition based on subjective and objective patient data.

- Identify potential complications related to parenteral nutrition (PN) in patients with malnutrition (eg, refeeding syndrome) and steps to avoid or manage such complications.

- Design a patient-specific PN prescription that is based on the nutritional diagnosis and other subjective and objective patient data.

- Construct and evaluate appropriate monitoring parameters for a hospitalized patient receiving PN.

PATIENT PRESENTATION

Chief Complaint

"My stomach hurts and I can't keep down any food or water."

HPI

Steven Brown is a 49-year-old man familiar to the GI Surgery Service with a history of a ventral hernia, hypertension, dyslipidemia, and type 2 DM. He presented to the ED earlier today with abdominal pain, nausea, vomiting, and inability to tolerate PO intake. Approximately 2 months ago, he underwent an exploratory laparotomy with small bowel resection and primary anastomosis for repair of a ventral hernia with incarcerated small bowel. His postoperative course was complicated by an anastomotic leak, peritonitis, and sepsis, and he was ultimately discharged to home after a 3-week hospital stay. For the past 4 days, he has had worsening abdominal pain and has been unable to tolerate any PO intake. His last bowel movement was 6 days ago. He has lost ~25 lb (~11 kg) from his weight prior to his surgery 2 months ago. This weight loss includes ~14 lb (~6.5 kg) since his prior discharge due to poor appetite and limited PO intake at home.

The surgical team decides to admit Mr Brown to the hospital. On admission, they obtain an abdominal CT scan, which demonstrates dilated loops of small bowel consistent with a small bowel obstruction (SBO) and negative for anastomotic leak or abscess. The team believes this SBO is likely due to adhesions from his prior surgery.

PMH

Ventral hernia
Hypertension
Dyslipidemia
Type 2 DM

PSH

Exploratory laparotomy, small bowel resection with primary anastomosis for repair of ventral hernia with incarcerated small bowel 2 months ago

FH

Remarkable for DM in his mother, HTN and CAD in his father

SH

Married, lives with his wife; construction worker. Drinks two to three alcoholic beverages per week; quit smoking 2 years ago, 25 pack-year history prior to quitting.

ROS

Reports feeling thirsty, no appetite. Complains of moderate abdominal pain, nausea, and vomiting. Also complains his abdomen feels "crampy" and is very bloated. Complains of not passing flatus or having a bowel movement in 6 days; urinating infrequently over the past 2 days, and urine is dark and concentrated. Feels lightheaded and dizzy if he stands up quickly. Denies chills, fevers, or other pain.

Meds Prior to Admission

Simvastatin 40 mg PO at bedtime
Hydrochlorothiazide 25 mg PO daily
Metoprolol 25 mg PO twice daily
Glyburide/metformin 10 mg/1000 mg PO twice daily with meals

All

NKDA

Physical Examination

Gen

African-American man, uncomfortable because of abdominal pain, appears malnourished

VS

BP 96/60 mm Hg, P 108 bpm, RR 18, T 37.7°C; Wt 71 kg (wt prior to surgery 2 months ago ~83 kg), Ht 71″ (180 cm)

Skin

Dry, flaking in some spots, poor turgor

HEENT

PERRLA, EOMI, anicteric sclerae, normal conjunctivae, mouth is dry, pharynx is clear, some evidence of wasting noted on temporal lobes, eyes appear sunken in, orbital ridge protruding somewhat, evidence of moderate–severe wasting of muscle and subcutaneous fat.

Lungs/Thorax

CTA and percussion bilaterally; bilateral protruding scapulae

CV

RRR, no murmurs

Abd

Distended; hypoactive (nearly absent) bowel sounds; diffuse tenderness throughout all four quadrants

Genit/Rect

No lesions, no internal masses

MS/Ext

(–) Cyanosis, (–) edema, 2+ dorsalis pedis and posterior tibial pulses bilaterally, evidence of moderate–severe wasting of muscle and subcutaneous fat, especially around large muscle groups (biceps, triceps, and quadriceps)

Neuro

A & O × 3; CN II–XII intact; motor 5/5 upper and lower extremity bilaterally; sensation intact and reflexes symmetric with downgoing toes

■ Labs on Admission

Na 132 mEq/L	Hgb 12.1 g/dL	AST 24 IU/L	Ca 8.2 mg/dL
K 3.3 mEq/L	Hct 35.9%	ALT 21 IU/L	Mg 1.4 mEq/dL
Cl 94 mEq/L	Plt 334 × 10³/mm³	Alk phos 41 IU/L	Phos 2.6 mg/dL
CO_2 34 mEq/L	WBC 7.5 × 10³/mm³	GGT 45 IU/L	PT 12.3 sec
BUN 17 mg/dL		T. bili 0.9 mg/dL	INR 0.8
SCr 0.5 mg/dL		T. prot 4.9 g/dL	
Glu 142 mg/dL		Alb 2.9 g/dL	

■ Radiology

A CT scan with contrast demonstrates dilated loops of small bowel consistent with SBO; negative for anastomotic leak; negative for abscess

■ Assessment

This is a 49-year-old man with a history of a ventral hernia, hypertension, dyslipidemia and type 2 DM, S/P exploratory laparotomy, small bowel resection with primary anastomosis, and repair of incarcerated ventral hernia 2 months ago, who is admitted with abdominal pain, nausea, vomiting, and inability to tolerate PO intake. His symptoms and CT scan are consistent with SBO. His history and physical exam also demonstrate evidence of malnutrition.

■ Clinical Course

Given that he has had recent abdominal surgery, as well as significant weight loss and evidence of malnutrition, the surgical team elects to manage his SBO conservatively (nonoperatively). Because of recent abdominal surgery, the team would like to avoid reentering the abdomen for surgical intervention at this time (the patient is likely to still have inflammation and adhesions from his prior operation, and additional surgical intervention can further increase inflammation and risk of complications [eg, adhesions, fistula]). The patient is made NPO, and home PO medications are held for now. An NG tube is placed for gastric decompression, and a PICC is inserted for administration of PN and IV fluids. The team gives the patient a 1000-mL IV fluid bolus with normal saline followed by normal saline at 100 mL/h. Once PN is initiated and the patient has been resuscitated, IV fluids will be decreased to maintain a total fluid intake of 100 mL/h. The surgical team obtains nutrition and pharmacy consults for PN recommendations.

QUESTIONS

Problem Identification

1.a. What clinical and laboratory data indicate the presence of malnutrition in this patient? Characterize the type and severity of malnutrition, and describe why he is at risk for nutritional deficiencies.

1.b. How can small bowel obstruction lead to malnutrition? What other nutritional disorders (eg, fluid, electrolytes, and micronutrients) can develop in patients with small bowel obstruction?

1.c. Create a list of this patient's drug therapy problems, as well as problems related to nutritional, fluid, and electrolyte status.

1.d. What are the limitations of serum albumin as a marker of nutritional status in acutely ill patients?

1.e. What additional nutrition assessment data should you obtain and why?

Desired Outcome

2. What are the goals of pharmacotherapy and nutrition support therapy in this patient?

Therapeutic Alternatives

3. What are the therapeutic options for nutrition support intervention in this patient? Is PN indicated? Provide the rationale for your answer.

Optimal Plan

4.a. What treatment would you recommend for this patient's current drug therapy problems and fluid, electrolyte, and acid–base problems?

4.b. What are the ranges of estimated daily goals for calories (kcal/kg per day), protein (g/kg per day), and hydration (mL per day or mL/kg per day) for this patient?

4.c. Design a goal PN formulation for this patient that includes the total volume (mL per day) and goal rate (mL/h), amino acids (g per day), dextrose (g per day), and IV fat emulsion (IVFE; g per day). Take into consideration the goals you developed in question 4.b., as well as the underlying nutrition problems identified previously (question 1.c.).

4.d. How would you initiate PN in this patient? How quickly would you advance to the goal infusion rate? Provide the rationale for your answers.

4.e. What other monitoring parameters would you suggest ordering at the initiation of the PN?

Outcome Evaluation

5.a. What parameters should be monitored to assess the efficacy and safety of PN in this patient? How frequently should each of these be monitored?

5.b. What specific parameter(s) should you monitor to assess this patient's nutritional status?

Patient Education

6. What information should be provided to the patient and family during his hospitalization regarding the PN?

■ CLINICAL COURSE

Mr Brown was managed conservatively with bowel rest, PN, NG tube decompression, and supportive care. His symptoms improved over 4–5 days, and he began having bowel sounds and passing flatus. On hospital day #7, he had a small bowel movement, and the team began to advance his diet and taper the PN.

Follow-Up Question

1. How should PN be tapered off in this patient? Develop a plan to taper PN based on PO intake in this patient.

■ SELF-STUDY ASSIGNMENTS

1. Mr Brown is at risk for a condition called refeeding syndrome. What is the refeeding syndrome? What are its signs, symptoms, and potential complications? How can it be prevented? How should it be treated if signs and symptoms develop?

2. What other specific postoperative complications can develop in surgical patients with moderate-to-severe malnutrition? How can preoperative nutrition support impact a malnourished surgical patient's risk for postoperative complications?

3. Calculate how many milliliters per day of dextrose 70%, amino acids 10%, and IVFE 20% stock solutions are needed to compound the daily PN prescription that you determined for this patient.

4. Using the calculated daily goals for amino acids, dextrose, and IVFE, determine the minimum PN volume that could be compounded for this patient. Assume it will be compounded using a 10% amino acid solution, 70% dextrose solution, and 20% IVFE, and use an estimate of 100 mL for all micronutrients and additives.

CLINICAL PEARLS

The refeeding syndrome can lead to serious complications, including death. It is one of the few true nutritional emergencies. A good rule of thumb in patients with moderate-to-severe malnutrition is to "start low and go slow" when initiating nutrition support (PN, enteral nutrition, or even an oral diet) to avoid complications, and aggressively correct serum electrolyte abnormalities (especially phosphorus, potassium [K], and magnesium [Mg]) *before* initiating nutrition support, as well as during therapy.

Achieving appropriate glycemic control while avoiding hyperglycemia and hypoglycemia can reduce morbidity and mortality. Previous data suggested that tight glycemic control (blood glucose 80–110 mg/dL) with insulin infusions in intensive care unit patients was associated with reduced mortality. However, achieving this goal while avoiding hypoglycemia can be a significant challenge, and severe hypoglycemia has been associated with increased patient morbidity and mortality. Results of subsequent studies and meta-analyses have challenged these initial findings. More recent guidelines suggest a goal serum glucose of 140–180 mg/dL for adult hospitalized patients receiving nutrition support, and hyperglycemia (>180 mg/dL), hypoglycemia (<70 mg/dL), and significant fluctuations in serum glucose should be avoided.[9]

REFERENCES

1. White JV, Guenter P, Jenson G, et al. Consensus statement: Academy of Nutrition and Dietetics and American Society for Parenteral and Enteral Nutrition: Characteristics recommended for the identification and documentation of adult malnutrition (undernutrition). JPEN J Parenter Enteral Nutr 2012;36:275–283.

2. Kudsk KA, Tolley EA, DeWitt RC, et al. Preoperative albumin and surgical site identify surgical risk for major postoperative complications. JPEN J Parenter Enteral Nutr 2003;27:1–9.

3. Kraft MD, Btaiche IF, Sacks GS. Review of the refeeding syndrome. Nutr Clin Pract 2005;20:625–633.

4. Foster NM, McGory ML, Zingmond DS, Ko CY. Small bowel obstruction: a population-based appraisal. J Am Coll Surg 2006;203:170–176.

5. Brown KA, Dickerson RN, Morgan LM, et al. A new graduated dosing regimen for phosphorus replacement in patients receiving nutrition support. JPEN J Parenter Enteral Nutr 2006;30:209–214.

6. The American Society for Parenteral and Enteral Nutrition. Task Force for the Revision of Safe Practices for Parenteral Nutrition. Safe practices of parenteral nutrition. JPEN J Parenter Enteral Nutr 2004;28:S39–S70.

7. Boullata JI, Gilbert K, Sacks G, et al. A.S.P.E.N. clinical guidelines: Parenteral nutrition ordering, order review, compounding, labeling, and dispensing. JPEN J Parenter Enteral Nutr 2014;38:334–377.

8. Ayers P, Adams S, Boullata J, et al. A.S.P.E.N. parenteral nutrition safety consensus recommendations. JPEN J Parenter Enteral Nutr 2014;38:296–333.

9. McMahon MM, Nystrom E, Braunschweig C, et al. A.S.P.E.N. Clinical Guidelines: nutrition support of adult patients with hyperglycemia. JPEN J Parenter Enteral Nutr 2013;37:23–36.

161

ADULT ENTERAL NUTRITION

Gut Check . . . . Level III

Carol J. Rollins, MS, RD, PharmD, BCNSP

Amanda E. Shearin, PharmD, BCPS

LEARNING OBJECTIVES

After completing this case study, the reader should be able to:

- List contraindications to enteral nutrition (EN) therapy.

- Calculate the protein, calorie, and fluid requirements for a patient who is to receive EN therapy.

- Recommend an appropriate enteral formula and feeding route.

- Implement an appropriate monitoring plan to achieve the desired nutritional endpoints and avoid complications.

- Design an appropriate regimen for administering medications via a feeding tube, including recommending alternate dosage forms for medications that cannot be crushed.

PATIENT PRESENTATION

Craig Baker is a 47-year-old man referred to the nutrition support team for evaluation and possible initiation of parenteral nutrition.

The history on the referral states: admission to the hospital 3 days ago with c/o nausea, vomiting, and abdominal pain, primarily in the epigastric and LUQ region. Continued c/o nausea and abdominal pain; no vomiting in the last 24 hours. He is currently NPO except for sips of water for comfort.

QUESTIONS

Problem Identification

1.a. What other information is necessary or would be helpful to evaluate the patient and provide recommendations for a nutrition support plan of care?

1.b. What is the appropriate timing for nutrition intervention?

1.c. Based on risk-versus-benefit considerations, is the consult for initiation of parenteral nutrition appropriate for this patient?

CLINICAL COURSE

After following appropriate procedures, you obtain the following additional information about the patient.

■ HPI

Mr Baker began having symptoms of nausea and epigastric/LUQ pain about a week (per patient) prior to hospital admission. He thought this would "go away on its own; like in the past," and then he began feeling weak and dizzy. He finally asked a friend to take him to the ED after he had several episodes of vomiting the day before admission. His history indicates five episodes with symptoms of nausea and abdominal pain in the last 8 months. With previous episodes, the pain was reported as less severe and lasted only a couple days; nausea occurred, but there was no vomiting; he was not weak or dizzy. He did not go to the hospital with the past episodes since the pain improved on its own.

In the ED, Mr Baker received 6 L of 0.9% NaCl for hydration; D5%/0.45% NaCl + 20 mEq KCl/L has been infusing at 150 mL/h since then. A CT scan in the ED indicated edema of the proximal pancreatic duct with possible stricture and a small pancreatic pseudocyst.

Height: 72 in. Weight: no admission weight available; weight on hospital day 2 was 84 kg. Patient states that he lost a few pounds when he was hospitalized 4 months ago but he "came right back up to 170–175 pounds" where his weight has been for many years.

■ PMH

HTN
GERD
PE 4 months ago for which he receives warfarin 4 mg PO daily

■ FH

Mother died from a stroke 8 years ago; she had DM and HTN. Father is healthy and works as an auto mechanic. Per patient, his father's only health complaints are "aching bones" and need for glasses to see his work. All four brothers are "healthy" as far as the patient knows.

■ SH

Divorced; no contact with his ex-wife or two grown children. He works full-time in an auto parts store. He smokes about two packs per week, down from about two packs per day for 15 years prior to the PE; alcohol consumption is typically a beer after work and occasional heavy "party" use (a few times per year). The patient

has private health insurance through his employer. Per the case manager, insurance coverage provides a drug benefit for oral medications but follows Medicare Parts A and B for hospitalization and home coverage.

■ ROS

From physician's note today:

Constitutional: Moderate pain and nausea.

ENT: No vision changes or eye pain. No tinnitus or ear pain. No throat pain. No problem with swallowing.

CV: No SOB, DOE, and chest pain.

Resp: No cough or sputum production.

GI: Continued persistent epigastric and LUQ abdominal pain; improved with fentanyl patch and more frequent breakthrough pain coverage. No emesis or diarrhea; complains of intermittent nausea and mild/moderate constipation.

GU: No nocturia or hematuria.

MS: (+) Abdominal pain; no other muscle aches or bone pain.

Skin: No rashes, nodules, or itching. Deep cut on the right heel is red, warm, and swollen; cultures sent today. Mr Baker says he probably stepped on a piece of glass from a cup he dropped the day before coming to the ED.

Neuro: No headaches, dizziness, unsteady gait, or seizures.

Endo: Blood glucose in 100–160 mg/dL range.

Heme/lymph nodes: No recent blood transfusions or swollen glands.

■ Meds

Metoprolol succinate tablet 200 mg PO daily
Morphine sulfate, immediate release 4 mg PO Q 2 H PRN pain
Fentanyl transdermal patch 50 mcg, change every 72 hours
Lansoprazole 15 mg PO every morning
Bisacodyl tablet 5 mg PO at bedtime
Moxifloxacin 400 mg PO daily × 7 days (start today)
Warfarin 5 mg PO daily

■ All

NKDA

■ Physical Examination

Gen

Well-developed Caucasian man; alert and conversant

VS

BP 144/88 mm Hg, P 88 bpm, RR 20, T 37.1°C; Wt 84 kg

Skin

No nodules, masses, or rash; no ecchymoses or petechiae. Venous access device in right hand.

HEENT

PERRLA; EOMs intact. Eyes anicteric. No mouth lesions; tongue normal size.

Neck

Neck supple; no thyromegaly or masses

Lymph Nodes

No cervical, supraclavicular, axillary, or inguinal adenopathy

Heart

RRR with no gallop, rubs, or murmur

Lungs

Clear

Abd

Tender to palpation; no masses palpable; no distension

Genit/Rect

Deferred

MS/Ext

No clubbing or cyanosis; 1+ bilateral ankle edema; 2+ sacral edema; no spine or CVA tenderness

Neuro

Cranial nerves intact; DTRs active and equal

■ Endoscopy Report

From yesterday: ERCP, unable to enter pancreatic duct due to swelling and edema surrounding the area; suspected stricture although this could not be visualized. Stent placement is not possible at this time. Recommendation for repeat CT in 2–3 weeks to determine if ERCP with stent placement or surgery is more appropriate. Continue patient on NPO except sips of clear liquids.

■ Labs

See Table 161-1.

■ Other

Peripheral blood smear: anisocytosis 3+, poikilocytosis 2+, macrocytosis 2+, microcytosis 1+, and hypersegmented neutrophils

■ Assessment

Acute pancreatitis with pseudocyst, probably secondary to pancreatic duct stricture, possibly related to alcohol. Intolerance to diet; tolerates limited volume (150–200 mL per day) of clear liquids daily. Per GI service note, Mr Baker is to remain NPO except for sips of clear liquids.

Problem Identification (Continued)

1.d. Create a drug therapy problem list for this patient.

1.e. What information indicates the presence or severity of malnutrition?

1.f. What type and degree of malnutrition does this patient exhibit? What evidence supports your assessment?

Desired Outcome

2.a. What are the goals of nutrition support in this patient?

2.b. What outcomes should be considered for the patient's other medical problems?

Therapeutic Alternatives

3.a. What are the potential alternatives for improving nutritional status in this patient other than initiating specialized nutrition support?

3.b. What are the potential routes for specialized nutrition support and the reason(s) why each is or is not appropriate for this patient?

3.c. By postponing invasive therapy (stent or surgery for the stricture) for several weeks, the potential of continuing nutrition support outside the hospital arises. Based on the information now available to you, does this patient meet criteria for home enteral therapy? Recall that his insurance follows Medicare guidelines for home coverage.

Optimal Plan

4.a. Estimate the protein, calorie, and fluid requirements for this patient.

4.b. What type of formula (eg, polymeric, monomeric) is most appropriate for this patient?

4.c. What administration regimen should be used for tube feedings?

4.d. Assuming that the patient is to continue his current medications during tube feedings, how should each of these be administered?

Outcome Evaluation

5. What clinical and laboratory parameters are necessary to evaluate the therapy for detection and/or prevention of adverse effects and to evaluate achievement of the desired response?

Patient Education

6. What information should be provided to the patient or his caregiver to enhance compliance, ensure successful therapy, and minimize adverse effects of EN therapy?

■ CLINICAL COURSE

After presenting literature related to nutrition support during acute pancreatitis to the medical team, EN therapy was discussed with the patient. The patient consented to feeding tube placement. A 1.2-cal/mL, 55.5-g protein/L, 300-mOsm/kg polymeric formula was started using an enteral infusion pump via nasojejunal tube at 35 mL/h for 8 hours, and then advanced to the goal rate of 70 mL/h. Basic metabolic panel results on day 2 of EN revealed electrolyte values WNL. The WBC decreased to $10.6 \times 10^3/mm^3$ with 75% segs, 9% bands, 14% lymphs, and 2% monos. The basic metabolic panel on day 3 of EN showed stable values and a prealbumin of 16 mg/dL. The plan for discharge to home was confirmed and arrangements for home EN were finalized. The plan is for his diet to continue as limited clear liquids (<240 mL per day) and repeat the CT scan in 2–3 weeks to assess the small pancreatic pseudocyst and potentially schedule him for surgery the following week for the pancreatic duct stricture.

TABLE 161-1	Lab Values				
Na 140 mEq/L	Hgb 8.5 g/dL	WBC $11.9 \times 10^3/mm^3$	AST 23 IU/L	T. chol 239 mg/dL
K 3.9 mEq/L	Hct 26.7%	Segs 67%	ALT 34 IU/L	Trig 105 mg/dL
Cl 109 mEq/L	RBC $2.65 \times 10^6/mm^3$	Bands 14%	Alk phos 287 IU/L	Ca 7.9 mg/dL
CO_2 26 mEq/L	Plt $265 \times 10^3/mm^3$	Lymphs 17%	LDH 154 IU/L	Mg 1.9 mg/dL
BUN 7 mg/dL	MCV 104 μm^3	Monos 2%	T. bili 0.9 mg/dL	Phos 3.5 mg/dL
SCr 0.9 mg/dL			T. prot 7.1 g/dL	Amylase 462 mg/dL
Glu 147 mg/dL			Alb 2.6 g/dL	Lipase 591 mg/dL

■ SELF-STUDY ASSIGNMENTS

1. Select a current patient you are following, and design an appropriate regimen for administering medications via a feeding tube, including alternate dosage forms for medications that cannot be crushed and proper dosage adjustments for different forms where necessary.

2. Educate an actual patient or do a mock education with a classmate about medication administration through a feeding tube.

3. Select a current patient you are following, and determine the potential cumulative sorbitol dose if all medications were changed to oral liquid dosage forms.

4. Identify the metabolic changes associated with refeeding syndrome and the characteristics that increase the risk of this complication.

CLINICAL PEARL

Medications administered through a feeding tube frequently clog the tube; avoid administration through the tube when possible. Administer medications orally if the patient can and will take them orally.

REFERENCES

1. White JV, Guenter P, Jensen G, Malone A, Schofield M. Academy of Nutrition and Dietetics Malnutrition Work Group; A.S.P.E.N. Malnutrition Task Force; A.S.P.E.N. Board of Directors. Consensus statement of the Academy of Nutrition and Dietetics/American, Society for Parenteral and Enteral Nutrition: characteristics recommended for the identification and documentation of adult malnutrition (undernutrition). J Acad Nutr Diet 2012;112:730–738.

2. Mirtallo JM, Patel M. Overview of parenteral nutrition. In: Mueller CM, ed. The A.S.P.E.N. Adult Nutrition Support Core Curriculum, 2nd ed. Silver Spring, MD, American Society for Parenteral and Enteral Nutrition; 2012:234–244.

3. McClave SA, Martindale RG, Vanek VW, et al. Guidelines for the provision and assessment of nutrition support therapy in the adult critically ill patient. Section K. Acute pancreatitis. J Parenter Enteral Nutr 2009;33:277–316.

4. Parrish CR, Krenitsky J, McClave SA. Pancreatitis. In: Mueller CM, ed. The A.S.P.E.N. Adult Nutrition Support Core Curriculum, 2nd ed. Silver Spring, MD, American Society for Parenteral and Enteral Nutrition; 2012:472–490.

5. Wojtylak FR, Hamilton K,. Reimbursement for home nutrition support. In: Ireton-Jones CS, DeLegge MH, eds. Handbook of Home Nutrition Support. Burlington, MA, Jones and Bartlett Learning, 2007:389–412.

6. Mascarenhas MR, Divito D, McClave S. Pancreatic disease. In: Merritt R, ed. The A.S.P.E.N. Nutrition Support Manual, 2nd ed. Silver Spring, MD, American Society for Enteral and Parenteral Nutrition; 2005:211–230.

7. Bankhead R, Boullata J, Brantley S, et al. Enteral nutrition practice recommendations. J Parenter Enteral Nutr 2009;33:122–167.

8. Makola D, Krenitsky J, Parrish C, et al. Efficacy of enteral nutrition for the treatment of pancreatitis using standard enteral formula. Am J Gastroenterol 2006;101:2347–2355.

9. Burkhardt O, Stass H, Thuss U, et al. Effects of enteral feeding on the oral bioavailability of moxifloxacin in healthy volunteers. Clin Pharmacokinet 2005;44:969–976.

10. Rollins CJ. Drug–nutrient interactions in patients receiving enteral nutrition. In: Boullata JI, Armenti VT, eds. Handbook of Drug–Nutrient Interactions. Totowa, NJ, Humana Press, 2009:515–552.

162

OBESITY

To Be Single and 23 Again (BMI That Is) . . . . Level II

Dannielle C. O'Donnell, BS, PharmD

LEARNING OBJECTIVES

After completing this case study, the reader should be able to:

- Identify common obesity-related comorbidities.

- Calculate body mass index (BMI), and use waist circumference to determine a patient's risk of obesity-related morbidity.

- Develop a pharmacotherapeutic plan and treatment strategy for obese patients.

- Provide patient counseling on the expected benefits, possible adverse effects, and drug interactions with weight loss medications.

PATIENT PRESENTATION

■ Chief Complaint

"I've been through a painful divorce. I think I'm ready to try and get out and meet someone and start over, but I must've eaten my way through all of the stress of the separation and legal proceedings. Who's gonna even look at me when I'm this size? I may have to take up smoking again. It was easier to stay skinny when I smoked."

■ HPI

Francine Mallory is a 35-year-old woman who has "yo-yo'd" with her weight over the years. She feels best at 55 kg, which was how much she weighed when she was 23 years old and got married. She states that she was a "chubby" kid who really worked in college to "get healthier" through exercise classes at the college gym. That was also when she started smoking. She and her ex-husband were smokers and stopped when she was 27 because they wanted a smoke-free home before starting a family. She remembers frustration that while she "did great going cold turkey with the cigs," she put on 12 kg in the first six smoke-free months. She "worked out like crazy" and dropped 7 kg before they conceived their first child at the age of 29. She delivered a healthy baby, although her pregnancy was complicated by a diagnosis of gestational diabetes and excessive weight gain (27 kg). Her hyperglycemia resolved postdelivery and she "was happy with how quickly most of the baby weight came off while nursing" but then she plateaued 8 kg above her prepregnancy weight and "just couldn't get the rest off. I don't have time to commit to exercising while juggling a job and family." She has now put on more weight during the stress and hectic lifestyle of the divorce. She now lives in an apartment with her 5-year-old. She says she has tried weight loss shakes but finds herself just starving and "pigging out" at the end of the day. She says she does not have time for a gym membership or money for a "fancy program" where they provide meals for you. She has bought some "herbal stuff" from a coworker that helped with end-of-day hunger, but thinks cigarettes would be even cheaper than that. To economize and work with her hectic single-mom schedule, they eat out quite a bit based on where the "kids eat free" meal nights are (ie, an all-you-can-eat buffet on Monday nights and a pancake house on Wednesday nights, drive-thru meals at least one other night each week).

■ **PMH**

GDM
Hemorrhoids
Insomnia
Tension headaches
Adjustment disorder post-divorce

■ **FH**

Mother had an MI at the age of 62 years; father died in an MVA at the age of 67. Maternal grandmother died at age 62 with diabetes. She states that her mother and grandmother were "big boned," and all women in her family have struggled with their weight. No other family members have a significant medical history, although she states that her 5 year old is "a big boy." She blames his dad, stating that when he has him all they do is eat junk food, and he uses the TV and video games as a babysitter.

■ **SH**

She is a single working mom and a previous smoker (1 ppd × 9 years). Stopped 6 years ago. She denies IVDA. She has previously had success with weight loss by focusing on exercising but is not exercising now.

■ **Diet**

Has never had formal diet instruction. Her diet appears to be low in fiber, high in saturated fat, sugars, and calories.

■ **Meds**

Tylenol PM PRN sleep (one to two times per week)
Anusol HC PRN
Ibuprofen 600 mg PO PRN HA and knee/hip pain one to two times a day most days of the week
Citalopram 20 mg PO once daily
Unknown "herbal" weight loss product—discontinued 3 months ago

■ **All**

Macrolides—rash

■ **ROS**

She complains of general fatigue and periods of weepiness that she attributes to the divorce and a preoccupation with food and her weight and feeling "undesirable" although the sadness is less since citalopram was increased from 10 to 20 mg 2 months ago. She denies symptoms of cold or heat intolerance; changes in skin, hair, or nails; nervousness; irritability; lethargy; muscle pain or weakness; palpitations; diarrhea or constipation; polyuria; polydipsia; chest pain; or shortness of breath. Despite being fatigued, she relates some difficulty sleeping and reports waking up feeling "unrested." She also complains of occasional right knee and hip pain and stiffness after walking, standing, or sitting for prolonged periods. She denies binge eating or purging.

■ **Physical Examination**

Gen

The patient is in NAD but looks tired and older than her stated age. She is clean in appearance and dressed appropriately for the weather.

VS

BP 148/88 mm Hg (consistent with previous clinic reading), P 80 bpm, RR 16, T 36.4°C; Wt 80 kg, waist 100 cm, Ht 5′3″

Skin

Warm, with normal distribution of body hair. No significant lesions or discolorations.

HEENT

NC/AT; PERRLA; EOMI; TMs intact

CV

RRR, S_1 and S_2 normal; no murmurs, rubs, or gallops

Pulm

CTA & P bilaterally

Abd

Obese with multiple striae; NT; ND; (+) BS; no palpable masses

Genit/Rect

Pelvic and rectal exams deferred

Ext

LE varicosities present. Pedal pulses 2+ bilaterally. Mild crepitus in R knee. No joint swelling or tenderness.

Neuro

A & O × 3; CN II–XII intact; Romberg test (–); sensory and motor levels intact; 2+ triceps tendons and DTR; Babinski (–)

■ **Labs (Fasting)**

Na 138 mEq/L	AST 24 IU/L
K 3.9 mEq/L	TSH 0.5 mIU/mL
Cl 96 mEq/L	*Fasting lipid profile*
CO_2 26 mEq/L	T. chol 208 mg/dL
BUN 13 mg/dL	LDL-C 109 mg/dL
SCr 1.0 mg/dL	HDL-C 38 mg/dL
Glu 115 mg/dL	Trig 305 mg/dL

■ **Assessment**

This is an obese, middle-aged woman with obesity-related complications including: hypertension (diagnosed today based on her 2 clinic readings), dyslipidemia, and impaired fasting glucose (metabolic syndrome). Knee and hip pain likely reflects early osteoarthritic changes caused or worsened by obesity. Poor quality sleep may be a sign of sleep apnea. With her history of GDM, she is at increased risk of developing type 2 DM in the next several years. Weight loss would decrease her risk of developing type 2 DM and can improve BP, lipids, and perhaps even osteoarthritic and sleep symptoms.

QUESTIONS

Problem Identification

1.a. Create a drug therapy problem list for this patient.

1.b. Calculate the patient's BMI. By using the BMI and any other markers of adiposity, categorize her obesity and stratify her risk.

1.c. What information (signs, symptoms, and laboratory values) indicates the presence or severity of obesity?

1.d. Could any of the patient's problems have been caused by her drug therapy?

1.e. What other medical conditions should be considered to exclude primary or secondary causes of her obesity?

Desired Outcome

2. What are the goals of therapy for the patient's obesity?

Therapeutic Alternatives

3.a. What nondrug therapies should be recommended for this patient?

3.b. What feasible pharmacotherapeutic alternatives (OTC or prescription) are available for treating this patient's obesity?

Optimal Plan

4.a. What drug(s), dosage form(s), dose(s), schedule(s), and duration would be most appropriate to treat this patient's obesity and why?

4.b. What alternatives would be appropriate if initial therapy fails?

Outcome Evaluation

5. What clinical and laboratory parameters are necessary to evaluate the therapy for achievement of the desired therapeutic outcome and to detect or prevent adverse effects?

Patient Education

6. What general and medication-specific information should be provided to the patient to enhance adherence, ensure successful therapy, and minimize adverse effects?

■ CLINICAL COURSE

Mrs Mallory returns for her second follow-up visit after 24 weeks. She is now working out at home regularly 30 minutes each evening (typically four nights a week) with a video after her son goes to bed. She also got a pedometer and does her best to get in 10,000 steps each day. Although they still eat out a lot, she is making significantly different choices, increasing her lean meats, decreasing carbohydrates and saturated fats, and abstaining from having seconds and having less frequent desserts. She has eliminated sugary beverages (sweet tea, sodas) and is having good success sticking to her plan of not eating anything after her son goes to bed. If she is really struggling, she makes herself some hot tea with sugar substitute and eats a rice cake. She is logging her daily food intake onto the pedometer App and has found it to be insightful to have to write down everything she eats and when she eats it.

While she had lost 4% of her weight at her first return visit, since that 3-month point, she has lost additional weight. She weighs 72.5 kg, and her waist circumference is 96 cm. Her FBG is now 102 mg/dL, and her fasting lipid profile includes total cholesterol 202 mg/dL, LDL-C 110 mg/dL, HDL-C 45 mg/dL, and triglycerides 235 mg/dL. Her blood pressure has improved to 142/82 mm Hg, having also initiated lisinopril 10 mg/day at her visit 6 months ago.

She states that she is as compliant with her lifestyle modifications as in previous weeks and is in much better spirits overall. She has noticed a definite improvement in her clothing fit, but she is starting to become frustrated again that she has not seen any additional improvement in the last 2 weeks and does not like how she looks.

She wants to know if there is something else she can take or if she could have the Lap-Band procedure. Although she is pleased with the improvement in her blood pressure and glucose, she is frustrated that her cholesterol did not improve more. She is wondering if it might further help her weight loss efforts if she picked up some of "that herbal dandelion tea from Paraguay" that her coworker sells for weight loss just to help move things along.

Follow-Up Questions

1. What changes, if any, should be made in her weight loss regimen today?

2. How would you educate her regarding her question about the herbal weight loss tea?

3. What pharmacotherapeutic changes, if any, should be made for her lipids, glucose, and/or blood pressure at this time? Is a medication indicated at this point to prevent or treat diabetes?

■ SELF-STUDY ASSIGNMENTS

1. List the limitations of height–weight charts or BMI determinations. What are the most accurate methods for quantifying body fat, and why are they not routinely employed?

2. Assume that you are a member of a pharmacy and therapeutics committee for a managed care corporation. Justify whether anti-obesity drugs should be a covered benefit, and, if so, which specific agent(s) should be added to the formulary.

3. Compile a compendium of common herbal and dietary supplements that claim weight loss benefits, and make a list of the evidence for their safety and efficacy.

4. Make a list of the various prescription weight loss medications that have been introduced and subsequently withdrawn from the US and EU markets and the reasons for the withdrawal.

CLINICAL PEARL

Taking psyllium with orlistat has been reported to decrease the frequency and severity of orlistat GI side effects such as oily stool and leakage.

REFERENCES

1. Jensen MD, Ryan DH, Apovian CM, et al. 2013 AHA/ACC/TOS guideline for the management of overweight and obesity in adults: a report of the American College of Cardiology/American Heart Association Task Force on Practice Guidelines and The Obesity Society. Circulation 2013;63(25 Pt B):2985–3023.

2. Apovian CM, Aronne LJ, Bessesen DH, et al. Pharmacological management of obesity: an Endocrine Society clinical practice guideline. J Clin Endocrinol Metab 2015;100(2):342–362.

3. Gonzalez-Campoy JM, St. Jeor ST, Castorino K, et al. Clinical practice guidelines for healthy eating for the prevention and treatment of metabolic and endocrine diseases in adults: Cosponsored by the American Association of Clinical Endocrinologists/the American College of Endocrinology and the Obesity Society. Endocr Pract 2013;19(Suppl 3):1–82.

4. Toplak H, Woodward E, Yumuk V, et al. 2014 EASO position statement on the use of anti-obesity drugs. Obes Facts 2015;8(3):166–174.

5. Dunican KC, Adams NM, Desilets AR. The role of pramlintide for weight loss. Ann Pharmacother 2010;44:538–545.

COMPLEMENTARY AND ALTERNATIVE THERAPIES (LEVEL III)

Cydney E. McQueen, PharmD

TO THE READER

Although use of many dietary supplements has leveled off or decreased in the last few years (with a few notable exceptions, such as vitamin D and fish oil), many patients are still interested in trying supplements, either in place of (alternative) or along with (complementary) prescription and OTC therapies. Patients have increased desire for knowledge on the potential benefits and risks of these therapies and are more often expecting pharmacists and other healthcare providers to provide information they can use to make decisions.

As part of providing appropriate care, clinicians have a duty to help individual patients avoid interactions with their drug therapies and prevent use of products unsafe for them because of other disease state contraindications. That is a fairly straightforward task when dealing with prescription and OTC therapies; there is so much information and research available that most problems and risks are well understood. If a patient is prescribed a contraindicated drug, we can ensure that he or she does not receive it. With dietary supplements, there is often not enough information available to make clear-cut judgments about risks. We also cannot prevent patients from taking supplements even if known to be unsafe or risky for them, because we do not control their access to those therapies. Instead, we are limited to providing as much guidance as possible to help maximize any possible benefit and minimize possible harm.

CASEBOOK QUESTIONS ABOUT DIETARY SUPPLEMENTS

The following questions regarding supplement therapy aid in the decision-making process and will be addressed in the section "Clinical Course" of the Casebook. It is assumed that necessary information about a patient's medical history and current drug regimen has already been obtained.

1. **What is the known or proposed mechanism of action?**

   - This might be a silly question for prescription medications, but many supplements are used with only a small amount of knowledge regarding their pharmacologic activities. Botanical supplements in particular are extremely complex and may have multiple activities, some synergistic to the desired effect and some in opposition or unrelated. When there is little or no definitive human evidence for either efficacy or safety, we must often extrapolate based on in vitro or animal data in order to provide patients with reasonable information or instructions. For example, if a plant extract has been shown to improve glucose uptake in tissue studies, then it is reasonable to expect that activity to some extent when taken by human beings. It would also be reasonable to offer cautions about use with sulfonylurea drugs or other hypoglycemic agents, even when no case studies or clinical trials have reported interactions. Depending on the risks if an interaction should happen, appropriate real-life statements to patients can range from: "If you use this supplement, you will have to do additional checks of your blood sugar for the first 2 weeks to make sure it's not interfering with your other medication" to "This particular supplement just isn't safe for you at all."

2. **How extensive or conclusive are the clinical trial data on effectiveness?**

   - When clinical trial data conclude that a supplement has beneficial effects, it may be less hazardous for a patient to try a supplement before a prescription drug with known adverse events. Whenever evidence of efficacy is lacking or contradictory, the severity of the patient's condition becomes more important in the risk/benefit equation. For example, a patient wishing to try a supplement for the common cold or athlete's foot is not at great risk of harm if the supplement is not effective—he or she will simply endure some unpleasant symptoms for a time, and then most likely use a standard medication. On the other hand, a patient with severe hypertension who tries an ineffective supplement may be at increased risk for a cardiovascular event.

3. **What is known about safety?**

   - This question relates back to what is known about the mechanism of action: whenever there is a lack of information from long-term clinical trials, decisions about safety must be based on extrapolation from basic science studies and isolated case reports. It must be kept in mind that safety issues can be both overemphasized and underemphasized and that information (and therefore reasonable recommendations) can change fairly rapidly. For example, ginger is often described as being associated with increased risk of bleeding. This is absolutely true at doses of 4 g per day or more but is unlikely at lower doses. However, even use at lower doses would become a major consideration in patients who have other medical conditions (eg, a clotting disorder) or if there are drug interactions involved (eg, warfarin or chronic NSAID use). One safety rule of thumb to keep in mind for counseling patients is that ALL supplements should be stopped 10–14 days prior to scheduled surgery to minimize risks of interactions or increased risk of bleeding.

4. **Does the product have any specific quality considerations?**

   - Two questions are associated with "quality." First, is the product the "right" product—that is, the same strength or standardization as that used in clinical trials that demonstrated any benefits? Second, is the product a "good quality product"—that is, contains what it is labeled to contain with no contaminants? The first question is answered by close attention to reliable information resources and clinical trials and to reading product labels to ensure the chosen product is the appropriate standardization or strength and doses are not subtherapeutic or toxic. Both of these extremes have occurred.

The second question is best addressed by advising patients to only purchase products from manufacturers that participate in quality seal programs or that have been tested by third-party laboratories. The first choice for a quality seal program is USP's Dietary Supplement Verification Program, but UL (Underwriters' Laboratories) and NSF International also have facility cGMP audit and certification programs. Third party laboratories with consumer-accessible information include ConsumerLab.com and Labdoor.com.

- Certain products are more likely to have specific problems with quality or carry additional risk. For example, melatonin is usually produced synthetically, but a few available products are from "natural sources," generally meaning extracted from the pituitary glands of cattle. Because the pituitary gland is in the brain, these products do carry a small but real risk of contamination with prion proteins associated with bovine spongiform encephalopathy, also known as mad cow disease.

5. **Would this be an appropriate treatment choice in this particular patient?**

- Each patient may have different motivations to try a treatment. If clinical or basic science supports potential benefit of a supplement for a given condition, the next thing to consider is the patient's own expectations of therapy and ability to self-monitor for both efficacy and safety. For example, a post-menopausal woman who suffers 10 severe hot flushes a week and wants to end them entirely will probably be disappointed with a supplement, whereas another woman who also has 10 severe hot flushes a week and would like to reduce their frequency and/or severity may be very happy with the same product. Expectations must be appropriate; only rarely will a supplement work as strongly or as quickly as a prescription drug.

6. **If the patient is going to use the product, what counseling information will allow him or her to maximize any possible benefit and minimize any harm?**

- Counseling information should cover the same categories of information as prescription drugs: dose, schedule, duration of therapy, side effects, and interactions. Unfortunately, because there is usually less information available about side effects and interactions, it is impossible to warn patients about every possibility. It is best to counsel patients to contact their healthcare providers if anything "unexpected or unusual" occurs. This provides protection for the patient and allows evaluation of any possible link to the supplement, which aids in expanding the supplement knowledge base.

- Specificity is important in counseling. For example, if a patient is going to use *Ginkgo biloba*, he or she needs to be told to watch for easy bruising, not just that the ginkgo may increase bleeding risk. Specificity is even more important when a patient chooses to take a supplement despite being counseled against it because of safety issues.

- In addition, there are extra categories of information to include in counseling that do not generally have to be addressed with prescription and OTC drugs: using the appropriate product and a high-quality product. For botanical supplements, it is generally necessary to specify information such as the standardization of an extract (eg, saw palmetto should be 160 mg of extract standardized to 85–95% fatty acids and sterols twice daily). For nonbotanical supplements, the salt form may need to be specified (eg, glucosamine sulfate for monotherapy has more evidence of efficacy than glucosamine hydrochloride for monotherapy and so is the preferred form).

OBTAINING CURRENT AND RELIABLE DIETARY SUPPLEMENT INFORMATION

Decisions made about using supplements are only as good as the information used in making the decisions. Unfortunately, incomplete or wrong information about dietary supplements is abundantly available in both electronic and print media, so using only reliable resources is vital. A brief list of recommended resources is provided at the end of this section, but practitioners need to know what to look for or to avoid as they come across new resources. The following questions and rules of thumb should be kept in mind:

- Avoid resources published or provided by manufacturers; their primary interest is selling the product.

- Investigate the authors or source of the information; is the resource actually created by trained professionals, or by a ghost-writing group?

- Are recommendations based on careful analysis of the quality of clinical trials? Recommendations based solely on the end results of trials are often wrong; it is not possible to get good decision-making data from a badly designed or poorly conducted trial.

- Are cautions (about interactions, contraindications, or adverse effects) based on all theoretical, animal, or human data available, or only on well-documented human trials or case reports? Although it may seem counterintuitive at first, there is such a lack of high-quality reports and information in humans that theoretical data (based on in vitro experiments or theorized mechanisms of action) or animal data becomes more important in generating cautions that help keep patients safe. Often these cautions should not be as strong, of course. If a supplement has been found to affect glucose utilization in tissue cultures, a diabetic patient starting to take the supplement may be warned appropriately to monitor blood glucose more frequently, whereas a case report of loss of glycemic control in two patients using the supplement would generate a strong warning not to use the supplement.

- Does the resource include up-to-date information? Supplement information changes rapidly, so publication dates can matter tremendously. For example, a well-researched, completely evidenced-based book on herbal toxicology contained an obsolete chapter on St. John's wort (SJW) when it rolled off the printing press in February 2000, due solely to new information about SJW's effects on cytochrome P-450 3A4 published in January 2000.

RECOMMENDED INFORMATION RESOURCES

Literature Search Strategies

One of the most essential resources is a comprehensive literature search, because this can retrieve the most current information. While it is recommended that more than one indexing system be used (such as both Medline and EMBASE), healthcare students and professionals often do not have access to anything other than Medline. Consequently, it is essential to use very thorough search strategies, as discussed here:

- Because pertinent articles can be incompletely or wrongly indexed, search using more than just MESH (or EMTREE) terms to ensure proper retrieval. For example, to search for saw palmetto, search the MESH term (*Serenoa*), and then perform keyword searches for the common name (saw palmetto), the botanical name (*Serenoa repens*), and any alternative botanical names (*Sabul serrulata*). Consider searching misspellings; the spelling "saw palmeto" may not be common, but "gingko" instead of "ginkgo," is very common. Combining the results of these searches with "OR" will optimize retrieval of articles that may be relevant.

- Search the relevant disease state and any closely related terms. Continuing the example, search "BPH," "benign prostatic hyperplasia," "prostatic hyperplasia," "prostate hypertrophy," and "prostatic hypertrophy" as both MESH (or EMTREE) terms and keywords. It may also be useful to search symptom or outcome measure terms, such as "urinary retention" or "micturition rate."

- After combining product and disease state searches, if the retrieval set is so large as to be impossible to review, limitations can be used. For clinical decision making, the most useful types of limitations are clinical trials, evidence-based reviews, meta-analyses, and systematic reviews. Because it is not uncommon for articles about dietary supplement trials to report results of both animal and human studies, it is not recommended that a limitation of "human only" be used, because that could eliminate appropriate articles based on indexing.

■ Electronic Database Resources

Electronic databases available for purchase include:

- Natural Medicines Comprehensive Database (www .naturaldatabase.com). It is the most comprehensive resource available and includes a wide range of individual and combination products. It contains evidence-based recommendations and summaries of clinical and basic science information that are regularly reviewed and updated. The site allows for easy checking of supplement–drug interactions. It is available for purchase by individuals as well as institutions. A consumer version is also available.

- ConsumerLab.com (www.consumerlab.com). This is a third-party laboratory that tests dietary supplements for compliance with labeled content and for appropriate dissolution and contaminants. No clinical recommendations are given; the site's utility is primarily limited to aiding in the choice of a high-quality product. However, there is an "Encyclopedia" providing some information on herbs and supplements, although it is less obviously evidenced-based and it is unknown how often the information is updated, so it should only be used as a "double-check" of information. It is inexpensive (about $40 per year) and is also appropriate for use by consumers.

Free electronic databases include:

- The Health Information site of the National Institutes of Health Office of Dietary Supplements (http://ods.od.nih.gov/ HealthInformation/). This is a government site with links to several useful informational resources including tips for using supplements and fact sheets on a number of dietary supplements.

- Memorial Sloan-Kettering Cancer Center Integrative Medicine Service Web site (http://www.mskcc.org/mskcc/ html/1979.cfm). It includes a database of individual supplements. Information is specifically focused on use of supplements in cancer patients, a population that has a high rate of use of complementary and alternative medicine therapies. The site includes more discussion of interactions with chemotherapeutic agents than other resources.

- Computer Access to Research on Dietary Supplements (CARDS; https://ods.od.nih.gov/Research/CARDS_Database .aspx). This is a database of federally funded clinical trials of supplements.

- The PubMed Dietary Supplement Subset (https://ods .od.nih.gov/Research/PubMed_Dietary_Supplement_Subset .aspx). This will automatically search Medline for dietary supplement-focused literature. The subset database is focused on medical use of plants, so it can be easier to search than other literature databases that contain citations for agricultural-focused studies.

- The Dietary Supplement Label Database (DSLD) became active in 2013 (http://dsld.nlm.nih.gov/dsld/). A project of both the National Library of Medicine and the Office of Dietary Supplements, it is a searchable database of labeling information for products both available and discontinued from the US market. It may be especially useful when gathering medication histories or when patients ask questions about brand name products that contain multiple ingredients.

■ Print Resources

Because of limitations on the timeliness of information in print resources, it is difficult to make strong recommendations. New print resources should be evaluated according to the criteria listed above to determine their usefulness.

CASE 26: DYSLIPIDEMIA

■ Garlic and Fish Oil for Dyslipidemia

Clinical Course

Mrs Thorngrass is already taking garlic capsules, but she is not sure about the type or dose. Because you are making changes to her current prescription regimen, you need to investigate the advisability of continuing the garlic. If Mrs Thorngrass does begin a statin drug as indicated, she would not be able to take red yeast rice, a common supplement used for dyslipidemia, because it contains mevacolin K, a lovastatin analog, and would be duplicative therapy. Would fish oil be a possible option for her?

■ FOLLOW-UP QUESTIONS

Garlic

1. What is the known or proposed mechanism of action?

2. How extensive or conclusive are the clinical trial data on effectiveness?

3. What is known about safety?

4. Does the product have any specific quality concerns?

5. Would this be an appropriate treatment choice in this particular patient?

6. If the patient is going to use the product, what counseling information will allow her to maximize any possible benefit and minimize any harm?

Fish Oil/Omega-3 Fatty Acids

1. What is the known or proposed mechanism of action?

2. How extensive or conclusive are the clinical trial data on effectiveness?

3. What is known about safety?

4. Does the product have any specific quality concerns?

5. Would this be an appropriate treatment choice in this particular patient?

6. If the patient is going to use the product, what counseling information will allow her to maximize any possible benefit and minimize any harm?

REFERENCES

1. Khoo YSK, Aziz A. Garlic supplementation and serum cholesterol: a meta-analysis. J Clin Pharm Ther 2009;34:133–145.

2. Mathew BC, Prasad NV, Prabodh R. Cholesterol-lowering effect of organosulphur compounds from garlic: a possible mechanism of action. Kathmandu Univ Med J 2004;2(2):100–102.

3. Zeng T, Zhang C-L, Zhao X-l, Xie K-Q. The role of garlic on the lipid parameters: a systematic review of the literature. Crit Rev Food Sci Nutr 2013;53:215–230.

4. Hosseini A, Hosseinzadeh H. A review on the effects of *Allium sativum* (Garlic) in metabolic syndrome. J Endocrinol Invest 2015;38:1147–1157.

5. Shouk R, Abdou A, Shetty K, et al. Mechanisms underlying the antihypertensive effects of garlic bioactives. Nutr Res 2015;34:106–115.

6. Dhawan V, Jain S. Garlic supplementation prevents oxidative DNA damage in essential hypertension. Mol Cell Biochem 2005;275:85–94.

7. Ried K, Toben C, Fakler P. Effect of garlic on serum lipids: an updated meta-analysis. Nutr Rev 2013;71(5):282–299.

8. Ried K. Garlic lowers blood pressure in hypertensive individuals, regulates serum cholesterol, and stimulates immunity: an updated meta-analysis and review. J Nutr 2016;146(2):389S–396S.

9. Rohner A, Ried K, Sobenin IA, et al. A systematic review and meta-analysis on the effects of garlic preparations on blood pressure in individuals with hypertension. Am J Hyperten 2015;28(3)414–423.

10. Xiong XJ, Wang PQ, Li SJ, et al. Garlic for hypertension; a systematic review and meta-analysis of randomized controlled trials. Phytomed 2015;22:352–361.

11. Ried K, Travica N, Sali A. The effect of aged garlic extract on blood pressure and other cardiovascular risk factors in uncontrolled hypertensives: the AGE at Heart trial. Integrated Blood Press Cont 2016;9:9–21.

12. Matsumoto S, Nakanishi R, Li D, et al. Aged garlic extract reduced low attenuation plaque in coronary arteries of patients with metabolic syndrome in a prospective randomized double-blind study. J Nutr 2016;146(2):427S–432S.

13. Borrelli F, Capasso R, Izzo AA. Garlic (*Allium sativum* L.): adverse effects and drug interactions in humans. Mol Nutr Food Res 2007;51:1386–1397.

14. Cho H-J, Yoon I-S. Pharmacokinetic interactions of herbs with cytochromeP450 and p-glycoprotein. Evid Based Complement Altern Med 2015:736431.

15. Fetterman Jr JW, Zdanowicz MM. Therapeutic potential of n-3 polyunsaturated fatty acids in disease. Am J Health Syst Pharm 2009;66:1169–1179.

16. Siriwardhana N, Kalupahana NS, Moustaid-Moussa N. Health benefits of n-3 polyunsaturated fatty acids: eicosapentaenoic acid and docosahexaenoic acid. Adv Food Nutr Res 2012;65:211–222.

17. Adkins Y, Kelley DS. Mechanisms underlying the cardioprotective effects of omega-3 polyunsaturated fatty acids. J Nutr Biochem 2010;21:781–792.

18. Schmidt S, Willers J, Stahl F, et al. Regulation of lipid metabolism-related gene expression in whole blood cells of normo- and dyslipidemic men after fish oil supplementation. Lipids Health Dis 2012;11:172.

19. Schmit S, Stahl F, Mutz K-O, Scheper T, Hahn A, Schuchardt JP. Different gene expression profiles in normo- and dyslipidemic men after fish oil supplementation: results from a randomized controlled trial. Lipids Health Dis 2012;11:105.

20. Puglisi MJ, Hasty AH, Saraswathi V. The role of adipose tissue in mediating the beneficial effects of dietary dish oil. J Nutr Biochem 2011;22:101–108.

21. Lewis A, Lookinland S, Beckstrand RL, et al. Treatment of hypertriglyceridemia with omega-3 fatty acids: a systematic review. J Am Acad Nurse Pract 2004;16(9):384–395.

22. Hartweg J, Farmer AJ, Perera R, et al. Meta-analysis of the effects of n-3 polyunsaturated fatty acids on lipoproteins and other emerging lipid cardiovascular risk markers in patients with type 2 diabetes. Diabetologia 2007;50(8):1593–1602.

23. Eslick GD, Howe PRC, Smith C, Priest R, Bensoussan A. Benefits of fish oil supplementation in hyperlipidemia: a systematic review and meta-analysis. Int J Cardiol 2009;136:4–16.

24. Pirillo A, Catapano AL. Omega-3 polyunsaturated fatty acids in the treatment of hypertriglyceridaemia. Intl J Cardiol 2013;7(2 Suppl 1): S16–S20. Available at: *http://dx.doi.org/10.1016/j.ijcard.2013.06.040*.

25. Leslie MA, Cohen CJA, Liddle DM, et al. A review of the effect of omega-3 polyunsaturated fatty acids on blood triacylglycerol levels in normolipidemic and borderline hyperlipidemic individuals. Lipids Health Dis 2015;14:53.

26. GISSI-Prevenzione Investigators. Dietary supplementation with n-3 polyunsaturated fatty acids and vitamin E after myocardial infarction: results of the GISSI-Prevenzione trial. Lancet 1999;354:447–455.

27. Khawaja OA, Gaziano JM, Djoussé L. N-3 fatty acids for prevention of cardiovascular disease. Curr Athersler Rep 2014;16450.

28. Minihane AM. Fish oil omega-3 fatty acids and cardio-metabolic health, alone or with statins. Eur J Clin Nutr 2013;67:536–540.

29. Lichtenstein AH, Appel LJ, Brands M, et al. Diet and lifestyle recommendations revision 2006: a scientific statement from the American Heart Association Nutrition Committee. Circulation 2006;114:82–96.

30. Lovaza [package insert]. Liberty Corner, NJ: Reliant Pharmaceuticals, Inc; August 2007. Available at: *www.lovaza.com*. Accessed May 2016.

31. Khandelwal S, Demonty I, Jeemon P, et al. Independent and interactive effects of plant sterols and fish oil n-3 long-chain polyunsaturated fatty acids on the plasma lipid profile of mildly hyperlipidaemic Indian adults. Br J Nutr 2009;02:722–732.

32. Foran SE, Flood JG, Lewandrowski KB. Measurement of mercury levels in concentrated over-the-counter fish oil preparations: is fish oil healthier than fish? Arch Pathol Lab Med 2003;127(12):1603–1605.

33. Smutna M, Kruzikova K, Marsalek P, Kopriva V, Svobodova Z. Fish oil and cod liver as safe and healthy food supplements. Neuroendocr Lett 2009;30(Suppl 1):156–162.

34. Hajeb P, Selamat J, Afsah-Hejri L, et al. Effect of supercritical fluid extraction on the reduction of toxic elements in fish oil compared with other extraction methods. J Food Protection 2015;78(1):172–179.

35. Melanson SF, Lewandrowski EL, Flood JG, et al. Measurement of organochlorines in commercial over-the-counter fish oil preparations: implications for dietary and therapeutic recommendations for omega-3 fatty acids and a review of the literature. Arch Pathol Lab Med 2005;129:74–77.

36. United States Pharmacopeia. Listing of dietary supplements enrolled in the Dietary Supplement Verification Program. Available at: *http://www.usp.org/usp-verification-services/usp-verified-dietary-supplements/verified-supplements*. Accessed May 2016.

CASE 40: NAUSEA AND VOMITING

■ Ginger for Nausea and Vomiting

Clinical Course

While discussing Mr Jones' antiemetic regimen, he says, "I remember that my sister used to take ginger to prevent sea sickness when she went on a cruise, and my cousin used ginger when he was having chemotherapy a few years ago. Would that be good for me to try?"

■ FOLLOW-UP QUESTIONS

Ginger

1. What is the known or proposed mechanism of action?

2. How extensive or conclusive are the clinical trial data on effectiveness?

3. What is known about safety?

4. Does the product have any specific quality concerns?

5. Would this be an appropriate treatment choice in this particular patient?

6. If the patient is going to use the product, what counseling information will allow him to maximize any possible benefit and minimize any harm?

REFERENCES

1. Lete I, Allué J. The effectiveness of ginger in the prevention of nausea and vomiting during pregnancy and chemotherapy. Integr Med Insights 2016;11:11–17.

2. Giacosa A, Morazzoni P, Bombardelli E, et al. Can nausea and vomiting be treated with ginger extract? Eur Rev Med Pharmacol Sci 2015;19:1291–1296.

3. Walstab J, Krüger D, Stark T, et al. Ginger and its pungent constituents non-competitively inhibit activation of human recombinant and native 5-HT$_3$ receptors of enteric neurons. Neurogastroenterol Motil 2013;25:439–448, e302.

4. Pillai AK, Sharma KK, Gupta YK, Bakshi S. Antiemetic effect of ginger powder versus placebo as an add-on therapy in children and young adults receiving high emetogenic chemotherapy. Pediatr Blood Cancer 2011;56:234–238.

5. Ryan JL, Heckler CE, Roscoe JA, et al. Ginger (Zingiber officinale) reduces acute chemotherapy-induced nausea: a URCC CCOP study of 576 patients. Support Care Cancer 2012;20:1479–1489.

6. Lee J, Oh H. Ginger as an antiemetic modality for chemotherapy-induced nausea and a systematic review and meta-analysis. Oncol Nurs Forum 2013;40(2):163–170.

7. Marx WM, Teleni L, McCarthy AL, et al. Ginger (Zingiber officinale) and chemotherapy-induced nausea and vomiting: a systematic literature review. Nutr Rev 2013;71(4):245–254.

8. Young HY, Liao JC, Chang YS, et al. Synergistic effect of ginger and nifedipine on human platelet aggregation: a study in hypertensive patients and normal volunteers. Am J Chin Med 2006;34:545–551.

CASE 69: PARKINSON DISEASE

■ Coenzyme Q10 for Parkinson Disease

Clinical Course

Ms Farmer has been taking coenzyme Q10 for about a month before coming in for re-evaluation. Unlike the kava and cowage, which could be actively worsening her symptoms or posing other safety problems, coenzyme Q10 might actually have some benefit for Parkinson disease. Should Ms Farmer continue taking the supplement?

■ FOLLOW-UP QUESTIONS

1. What is the known or proposed mechanism of action?

2. How extensive or conclusive is the clinical trial data on effectiveness?

3. What is known about safety?

4. Does the product have any specific quality concerns?

5. Would this be an appropriate treatment choice in this particular patient?

6. If the patient is going to use the product, what counseling information will allow her to maximize any possible benefit and minimize any harm?

REFERENCES

1. Morris G, Anderson G, Berk M, Maes M. Coenzyme Q10 depletion in medical and neuropsychiatric disorders: potential repercussions and therapeutic implications. Mol Neurobiol 2013;48:883–903.

2. Littarru GP, Tiano L. Clinical aspects of coenzyme Q10: an update. Nutrition 2010;26:250–254.

3. Isobe C, Abe T, Terayama Y. Levels of reduced and oxidized coenzyme Q-10 and 9-hydroxy-2'-deoxyguanosine in the cerebrospinal fluid of patients with living Parkinson's disease demonstrate that mitochondrial oxidative damage and/or oxidative DNA damage contributes to the neurodegenerative process. Neurosci Lett 2010;469:159–163.

4. Mischley LK, Allen J, Bradley R. Coenzyme Q10 deficiency in patients with Parkinson's disease. J Neurol Sci 2012;318:72–75.

5. Shults C, Oakes D, Kieburtz K, et al. Effects of coenzyme Q10 in early Parkinson's disease. Arch Neurol 2002;59(10):1541–1550.

6. Muller T, Buttner T, Gholipour A, Kuhn W. Coenzyme Q10 supplementation provides mild symptomatic benefit in patients with Parkinson's disease. Neurosci Lett 2003;341(3):201–204.

7. The NINDS NET-PD Investigators. A randomized clinical trial of coenzyme Q10 and GPI-1485 in early Parkinson disease. Neurology 2007;68:20–28.

8. Storch A, Jost WH, Vieregge P, et al. Randomized, double-blind, placebo-controlled trial on symptomatic effects of coenzyme Q10 in Parkinson disease. Arch Neurol 2007;64:E1–E7.

9. Seet RC-S, Lim ECH, Tan JJH, et al. Does high-dose coenzyme Q10 improve oxidative damage and clinical outcomes in Parkinson's disease? Antioxid Redox Signal 2014;21(2):211–217.

10. The Parkinson Study Group QE3 Investigators. A randomized clinical trial of high-dosage coenzyme Q10 in early Parkinson disease. JAMA Neurol 2014;71(5):543–552.

11. Smith RAJ, Murphy MP. Animal and human studies with the mitochondria-targeted antioxidant MitoQ. Ann NY Acad Sci 2010;1201:96–103.

12. Snow BJ, Rolfe FL, Lockhart MM, et al. A double-blind, placebo-controlled study to assess the mitochondria-targeted antioxidant MitoQ as a disease-modifying therapy in Parkinson's disease. Mov Dis 2010;25(11):1670–1674.

CASE 72: MIGRAINE HEADACHE

■ Butterbur and Feverfew for Prevention of Migraine

Clinical Course

While discussing possible alternatives to her valproic acid therapy, Ms Miller says that a friend who also has migraines had read about some herbal remedies used for migraine prevention. She asks whether any products like that could be used instead of or along with her prescription medications. Ms Miller is very interested in a more "natural" therapy, but only if it would reduce the number of migraines she experiences.

■ FOLLOW-UP QUESTIONS

Butterbur and Feverfew

1. What are the known or proposed mechanisms of action?

2. How extensive or conclusive are the clinical trial data on effectiveness of each?

3. What is known about safety of each?

4. Does either of the products have any specific quality concerns?

5. Would either product be an appropriate treatment choice in this particular patient?

6. If the patient is going to use either of the products, what counseling information will allow her to maximize any possible benefit and minimize any harm?

7. Between the two products, which might be a better choice for Ms Miller?

REFERENCES

1. Sutherland A, Sweet BV. Butterbur: an alternative therapy for migraine prevention. AJHP 2010;67:705–711.

2. Agosti R, Duke RK, Chrubasik JE, Chrubasik S. Effectiveness of *Petasites hybridus* preparations in the prophylaxis of migraine: a systematic review. Phytomedicine 2006;13:743–746.

3. Horak S, Koschak A, Stuppner H, Streissnig J. Use-dependent block of voltage-gated Cav2.1 Ca^{2+} channels by petasins and eudesmol isomers. J Pharmacol Exp Ther 2009;330:220–226.

4. Utterback G, Zacharias R, Timraz S, Mershman D. Butterbur extract: prophylactic treatment for childhood migraines. Compl Ther Clin Pract 2014;20:61–64.

5. Lipton RB, Göbel H, Einhäupl KM, et al. *Petasites hybridus* root (butterbur) is an effective preventative treatment for migraine. Neurology 2004;63:2240–2244.

6. Diener HC, Rahlfs VW, Danesch U. The first placebo-controlled trial of a special butterbur root extract for the prevention of migraine: reanalysis of efficacy criteria. Eur Neurol 2004;51:89–97.

7. Rajapakse T, Pringsheim T. Nutraceuticals in migraine: a summary of existing guidelines for use. Headache Curr 2016;56(4):808–816.

8. Loder E, Burch R, Rizzoli. The 2012 AHS/AAN guidelines for prevention of episodic migraine: a summary and comparison with other recent clinical practice guidelines. Headache 2012;52:930–945.

9. Giles M, Ulbricht C, Khalsa KP, Kirkwood CD, Park C, Basch E. Butterbur: an evidence-based systematic review by the Natural Standard Research Collaboration. J Herb Pharmacother 2005;5:119–143.

10. Anderson N, Meier T, Borlak J. Toxicogenomics applied to cultures of human hepatocytes enabled an identification of novel *Petasites hybridus* extracts for the treatment of migraine with improved hepatobiliary safety. Toxicol Sci 2009;112:507–520.

11. Wang YP, Yan J, Fu PP, Chou MW. Human liver microsomal reduction of pyrrolizidine alkaloid N-oxides to form the corresponding carcinogenic parent alkaloid. Toxicol Lett 2005;155:411–420.

12. Avula B, Wang YH, Wang M, et al. Simultaneous determination of sesquiterpenes and pyrrolizidine alkaloids from the rhizomes of *Petasites hybridus* (L.) G.M. et Sch. and dietary supplements using UPLC-UV and HPLC-TOF-MS methods. J Pharm Biomed Anal 2012;70:53–63.

13. Calhoun AH, Hutchinson S. Hormonal therapies for menstrual migraine. Curr Pain Headache Rep 2009;13:381–385.

14. Materazzi S, Benemei S, Fusi C, et al. Parthenolide inhibits nociception and neurogenic vasodilatation in the trigeminovascular systems by targeting the TRPA1 channel. Pain 2013;154:2750–2758.

15. Magni P, Ruscica M, Dozio E, et al. Parthenolide inhibits the LPS-induced secretion of IL-6 and NF-κB nuclear translocation in BV-2 microglia. Phytother Res 2012;26(9):1405–1409.

16. Jager AK, Krydsfeldt K, Rasmussen HB. Bioassay-guided isolation of apigenin with GABA-benzodiazepine activity from *Tanacetum parthenium*. Phytother Res 2009;23(11):1642–1644.

17. Pittler MH, Ernst E. Feverfew for preventing migraine. Cochrane Database Syst Rev 2000;(3):CD002286.

18. Pfaffenrath V, Diener HC, Fischer M, et al. The efficacy and safety of *Tanacetum parthenium* (feverfew) in migraine prophylaxis—a double-blind, multicentre, randomized placebo-controlled dose–response study. Cephalalgia 2002;22:523–532.

19. Diener HC, Pfeffenrath V, Schnitker J, Friede M, et al. Efficacy and safety of 6.25 mg t.i.d. feverfew CO_2-extract (MIG-99) in migraine

20. Ferro EC, Biagini AP, da Silva ÍEF, et al. The combined effect of acupuncture and *Tanacetum parthenium* on quality of life in women with headache: randomized study. Acupunct Med 2012;30:252–257.

21. Unger M, Frank A. Simultaneous determination of the inhibitory potency of herbal extracts on the activity of six major cytochrome P450 enzymes using liquid chromatography/mass spectrometry and automated online extraction. Rapid Commun Mass Spectrom 2004;18:2273–2281.

prevention—a randomized, double-blind, multicentre, placebo-controlled study. Cephalalgia 2005;25:1031–1041.

CASE 78: MAJOR DEPRESSION

St. John's Wort for Depression

Clinical Course

Mrs Flowers understands that she must stop the SJW she has been taking because of an interaction with her prescribed mirtazapine and Ortho-Novum, but she wonders if it would have been helpful if she had started it when she first began feeling depressed.

■ FOLLOW-UP QUESTIONS

1. What is the known or proposed mechanism of action?

2. How extensive or conclusive are the clinical trial data on effectiveness?

3. What is known about safety?

4. Does the product have any specific quality concerns?

5. Would this be an appropriate treatment choice in this particular patient?

6. If the patient is going to use the product, what counseling information will allow her to maximize any possible benefit and minimize any harm?

REFERENCES

1. Russo E, Scicchitano F, Whalley BJ, et al. *Hypericum perforatum*: pharmacokinetic, mechanism of action, tolerability, and clinical drug–drug interactions. Phytother Res 2014;28:643–655.

2. Crupi R, Abusamra YAK, Spina E, Calapai G. Preclinical data supporting/refuting the use of *Hypericum perforatum* in the treatment of depression. CNS Neurol Dis Drug Targ 2013;12(4):474–486.

3. Wang Y, Shi X, Qi Z. Hypericin prolongs action potential duration in hippocampal neurons by acting on K^+ channels. Br J Pharmacol 2010;159(7):1402–1407.

4. Butterweck V. Mechanism of action of St. John's wort in depression: What is known? CNS Drugs 2003;17:539–562.

5. Vance KM, Ribnicky DM, Hermann GE, et al. St. John's wort enhances the synaptic activity of the nucleus of the solitary tract. Nutrition 2014;30:S37–S42.

6. Schrader E. Equivalence of St. John's wort extract (Ze 117) and fluoxetine: a randomized, controlled study in mild–moderate depression. Int Clin Psychopharmacol 2000;15:61–68.

7. Szegedi A, Kohnen R, Dienel A, Kieser M. Acute treatment of moderate to severe depression with *Hypericum* extract WS 5570 (St. John's wort): randomized controlled double blind non-inferiority trial versus paroxetine. BMJ 2005;333:503–506.

8. Bjerkenstedt L, Edman GV, Alken RG, Mannel M. *Hypericum* extract LI 160 and fluoxetine in mild to moderate depression. Eur Arch Psych Clin Neurosci 2005;255:40–47.

9. Randlov C, Mehlsen J, Thomsen CF, et al. The efficacy of St. John's wort in patients with minor depressive symptoms or dysthymia—a double-blind placebo-controlled study. Phytomedicine 2006;13:215–221.

10. Hypericum Depression Trial Study Group. Effect of *Hypericum perforatum* (St. John's wort) in major depressive disorder. JAMA 2002;287:1807–1814.

11. Sarris J, Fava M, Schweitzer I, Mischoulon D. St. John's wort (*Hypericum perforatum*) versus sertraline and placebo in major depressive disorder: continuation data from a 26-week RCT. Pharmacopsychiatry 2012;45:275–278.

12. Rapaport MH, Nierenberg AA, Holand R, Dording C, Schettler PJ, Mischoulon D. The treatment of minor depression with St. John's wort or citalopram: failure to show benefit over placebo. J Psychiatr Res 2011;45:931–941.

13. Anghelescu IG, Kohnen R, Szegedi A, Klement S, Kieser M. Comparison of *Hypericum* extract WS 5570 and paroxetine in ongoing treatment after recovery from an episode of moderate to severe depression: results from a randomized multicenter study. Pharmacopsychiatry 2006;39:213–219.

14. Kaspar S, Volz HP, Möller HJ, Dienel A, Kieser M. Continuation and long-term maintenance treatment with *Hypericum* extract WS® 5570 after recovery from an acute episode of moderate depression—a double-blind, randomized, placebo-controlled long-term trial. Eur Neuropsychopharmacol 2008;18:803–813.

15. Gastpar M, Singer A, Zeller K. Comparative efficacy and safety of a once-daily dosage of *Hypericum* extract STW3-VI and citalopram in patients with moderate depression: a double-blind, randomized, multicenter, placebo-controlled study. Pharmacopsychiatry 2006;39:66–75.

16. Singer A, Schmit M, Hauke W, Stade K. Duration of response after treatment of mild to moderate depression with *Hypericum* extract STW 3-VI, citalopram, and placebo. Phytomedicine 2011;11:739–742.

17. Shelton RC. St. John's wort (*Hypericum perforatum*) in major depression. J Clin Psychol 2009;70(Suppl 5):23–27.

18. Sarris J. St. John's wort for the treatment of psychiatric disorders. Psychiatr Clin N Am 2013;36:65–72.

19. Mannel M, Kuhn U, Schmidt U, Ploch M, Murck H. St. John's wort extract LI160 for the treatment of depression with atypical features—a double-blind, randomized, and placebo-controlled trial. J Psychiatr Res 2010;44:760–767.

20. Rahimi R, Abdollahi M. An update on the ability of St. John's wort to affect the metabolism of other drugs. Expert Opin Drug Metab Toxicol 2012;8(6):691–708.

21. Beckman SE, Sommi RW, Switzer J. Consumer use of St. John's wort: a survey on effectiveness, safety, and tolerability. Pharmacotherapy 2000;20(5):568–574.

22. Kasper S, Gastpar M, Möller H-J, et al. Better tolerability of St. John's wort extract WS 5570 compared to treatment with SSRIs: a reanalysis of data from controlled clinical trials in acute major depression. Int J Clin Psychopharmacol 2010;25:204–213.

23. Kolding L, Pedersen LH, Henriksen TB, Olsen J, Grzeskowiak LE. *Hypericum perforatum* use during pregnancy and pregnancy outcome. Reprod Toxicol 2015;58:234–237.

CASE 80: GENERALIZED ANXIETY DISORDER

Kava for Anxiety

Clinical Course

Mr Johnson is still worried about both the side effects of prescription drugs to treat his anxiety and whether he will be able to afford them. He states that he has read a lot of information about kava that "it really works for anxiety." Mr Johnson says, "Maybe I was just using a bad product last time I tried it and that's why it didn't help much and hurt my stomach. Should I get a better product and try it again?"

FOLLOW-UP QUESTIONS

1. What is the known or proposed mechanism of action?

2. How extensive or conclusive are the clinical trial data on effectiveness?

3. What is known about safety?

4. Does the product have any specific quality concerns?

5. Would this be an appropriate treatment choice in this particular patient?

6. If the patient is going to use the product, what counseling information will allow him to maximize any possible benefit and minimize any harm?

REFERENCES

1. Singh YN, Singh NN. Therapeutic potential of kava in the treatment of anxiety disorders. CNS Drugs 2002;16:731–743.

2. Boonen G, Ferger B, Kuschinsky K, et al. Influence of genuine kavapyrone enantiomers on the GABA-A binding site. Planta Med 1998;64:504–506.

3. Sarris J, LaPorte E, Schweitzer I. Kava: a comprehensive review of efficacy, safety, and psychopharmacology. Aust NZ J Psychiatry 2011;45:27–35.

4. Sarris J, Kavanagh DJ. Kava and St. John's wort: current evidence for use in mood and anxiety disorders. J Altern Complement Med 2009;15:827–836.

5. Pittler M, Ernst E. Efficacy of kava extract for treating anxiety: systematic review and meta-analysis. J Clin Psychopharmacol 2000;20:84–89.

6. Pittler M, Ernst E. Kava extract versus placebo for treating anxiety. Cochrane Database Syst Rev 2003;1:CD003383.

7. Witte S, Loew D, Gaus W. Meta-analysis of the efficacy of the acetonic kava–kava WS®1490 in patients with non-psychotic anxiety disorders. Phytother Res 2005;19:183–188.

8. Woelk H, Kapoula S, Lehrl S, et al. Treatment of patients suffering from anxiety. Double-blind study: kava special extract versus benzodiazepines. Z Allegemeinmed 1993;69:271–277.

9. Boerner RJ, Sommer H, Berger W, et al. Kava–kava extract LI 150 is as effective as opipramol and buspirone in generalised anxiety disorder—an 8-week randomized, double-blind multi-centre clinical trial in 129 out-patients. Phytomedicine 2003;10:38–49.

10. Sarris J, Kavanagh DJ, Byrne G, et al. The kava anxiety depression spectrum study (KADSS): a randomized, placebo-controlled crossover trial using an aqueous extract of *Piper methysticum*. Psychopharmacology 2009;205:399–407.

11. Sarris J, Stough C, Bouseman CA, et al. Kava in the treatment of generalized anxiety disorder. A double-blind, randomized, placebo-controlled study. J Clin Psychopharmacol 2013;33(5):643–648.

12. Baker JD. Tradition and toxicity: evidential cultures in the kava safety debate. Social Stud Sci 2011;41(3):361–384.

13. Teschke R, Sarris J, Glass X, Schulze J. Kava, the anxiolytic herb: back to basics to prevent liver injury? Br J Clin Pharmacol 2011;71(3):445–448.

14. Kuchta K, Schmidt M, Nahrstedt A. German kava ban lifted by court: the alleged hepatotoxicity of kava (*Piper methysticum*) as a case of ill-defined herbal drug identity, lacking quality control, and misguided regulatory politics. Planta Med 2015;81(18):1647–1653.

15. Stevinson C, Huntley A, Ernst E. A systematic review of the safety of kava extract in the treatment of anxiety. Drug Saf 2002;25:251–261.

16. Sarris J, LaPorte E, Scholey A, et al. Does a medicinal dose of kava impair driving? A randomized, placebo-controlled, double-blind study. Traffic Injury Prevent 2013;14:13–17.

17. Mathews JM, Etheridge AS, Valentine JL, et al. Pharmacokinetics and disposition of the kavalactone kawain: interaction with kava extract and kavalactones in vivo and in vitro. Drug Metab Dispos 2005;33:1555–1563.

18. Gurley BJ, Swain A, Hubbard MA, et al. Supplementation with goldenseal (*Hydrastis canadensis*), but not kava kava (*Piper methysticum*), inhibits human CYP3A activity in vivo. Clin Pharmacol Ther 2008;83:61–69.

19. Maya D, Schneider Y, Wan DW, et al. Blame it on the kava? Am J Gastroenterol 2015;110(Suppl 1):S364.

CASE 84: TYPE 2 DIABETES MELLITUS: NEW ONSET

■ Fish Oil, Cinnamon, and α-Lipoic Acid for Type 2 Diabetes Mellitus

Clinical Course

While discussing Mr Giuliani's diagnosis with him, he states that his neighbor with diabetes told him that she just follows her diabetic diet and takes cinnamon and something called "alip acid" and does not have to take any prescriptions for her blood sugar. He also says that he has read about fish oil being used for diabetes. Mr Giuliani asks if he should start any of those to help get his blood sugar under control.

■ FOLLOW-UP QUESTIONS

1. What is the known or proposed mechanism of action for each?

2. How extensive or conclusive are the clinical trial data on effectiveness for each?

3. What is known about safety of each?

4. Do any of the products have any specific quality concerns?

5. Would anyone or these be an appropriate treatment choice in this particular patient?

6. If the patient is going to use any of these products, what counseling information will allow him to maximize any possible benefit and minimize any harm?

REFERENCES

1. Fetterman Jr JW, Zdanowicz MM. Therapeutic potential of n-3 polyunsaturated fatty acids in disease. Am J Health Syst Pharm 2009;66:1169–1179.

2. Balk EM, Lichtenstein AH, Chung M, et al. Effects of omega-3 fatty acids on serum markers of cardiovascular disease risk: a systematic review. Atherosclerosis 2006;189(1):19–30.

3. Schmidt S, Willers J, Stahl F, et al. Regulation of lipid metabolism-related gene expression in whole blood cells of normo- and dyslipidemic men after fish oil supplementation. Lipids Health Dis 2012;11:172.

4. Schmit S, Stahl F, Mutz K-O, Scheper T, Hahn A, Schuchardt JP. Different gene expression profiles in normo- and dyslipidemic men after fish oil supplementation: results from a randomized controlled trial. Lipids Health Dis 2012;11:105.

5. Puglisi MJ, Hasty AH, Saraswathi V. The role of adipose tissue in mediating the beneficial effects of dietary dish oil. J Nutr Biochem 2011;22:101–108.

6. Kabir M, Skurnik G, Naour N, et al. Treatment for 2 mo with n-3 polyunsaturated fatty acids reduces adiposity and some atherogenic factors but does not improve insulin sensitivity in women with type 2 diabetes: a randomized controlled study. Am J Clin Nutr 2007;86:1670–1679.

7. Zheng J-S, Huang T, Yang, J, Fu Y-Q. Marine n-3 polyunsaturated fatty acids are inversely associated with risk of type 2 diabetes in Asians: a systematic review and meta-analysis. PLos One 2012;7(9):e44525.

8. Rudkowska I. Fish oils for cardiovascular disease: impact on diabetes. Maturitas 2010;67:25–28.

9. Strand E, Pedersen ER, Svingen GFT, et al. Dietary intake of n-3 long-chain polyunsaturated fatty acids and risk of myocardial infarction in coronary artery disease patients with or without diabetes mellitus: a prospective cohort study. BMC Med 2013;11:216.

10. Hartweg J, Perera R, Montori VM, Dinneen SF, Neil AHAWM, Farmer AJ. Omega-3 polyunsaturated fatty acids (PUFA) for type 2 diabetes mellitus. Cochrane Database Syst Rev 2008;1:CD003205.

11. Lichtenstein AH, Appel LJ, Brands M, et al. Diet and lifestyle recommendations revision 2006: a scientific statement from the American Heart Association Nutrition Committee. Circulation 2006;114:82–96.

12. Mostad IL, Bjerve KS, Bjorgaas MR, Lydersen S, Grill V. Effect of n-3 fatty acids in subjects with type 2 diabetes: reduction of insulin sensitivity and time-dependent alterations from carbohydrate to fat oxidation. Am J Clin Nutr 2006;84:540–550.

13. Rafehi H, Ververis K, Karagiannis TC. Controversies surrounding the clinical potential of cinnamon for the management of diabetes. Diab Obes Metab 2012;14:493–499.

14. Medagama AB. The glycaemic outcomes of cinnamon, a review of the experimental evidence and clinical trials. Nutr J 2015;14:108.

15. Lu Z, Jia Q, Wang R, et al. Hypoglycemic activities of A- and B-type procyanidin oligomer-rich-extracts from different cinnamon barks. Phytomedicine 2011;18:298–302.

16. Leach MJ, Kumar S. Cinnamon for diabetes mellitus. Cochrane Database System Rev 2012;9:CD007170.

17. Akilen R, Tsiami A, Devendra D, Robinson N. Cinnamon in glycaemic control: systemic review and meta analysis. Clin Nutr 2012;31:609–615.

18. Davis PA, Yokoyama W. Cinnamon intake lowers fasting blood glucose: meta-analysis. J Med Food 2011;14(9):884–889.

19. Akilen R, Tsiami A, Devendra D, Robinson N. Glycated haemoglobin and blood pressure-lowering effect of cinnamon in multi-ethnic type 2 diabetic patients in the UK: a randomized, placebo-controlled, double-blind clinical trial. Diabetic Med 2010;27:1159–1167.

20. Lu T, Sheng H, Wu J, et al. Cinnamon extract improves fasting blood glucose and glycosylated hemoglobin level in Chinese patients with type 2 diabetes. Nutr Res 2012;32:408–412.

21. Allen RW, Schwartzman E, Baker WL, et al. Cinnamon use in type 2 diabetes: an updated systematic review and meta-analysis. Ann Fam Med 2013;11(5):452–459.

22. Wickenberg J, Lindstedt S, Berntorp K, et al. Ceylon cinnamon does not affect postprandial plasma glucose or insulin in subjects with impaired glucose tolerance. Br J Nutr 2012;107:1845–1849.

23. Beejmohum V, Peytavy-Izard M, Mignon C, et al. Acute effect of Ceylon cinnamon extract on postprandial glycemia: alpha-amylase inhibition, starch tolerance test in rats, and randomized crossover clinical trial in healthy volunteers. BMC Complement Altern Med 2014;14:351.

24. Chase CK, McQueen CE. The use of cinnamon in diabetes. Am J Health Syst Pharm 2007;64:1033–1035.

25. Kamenova P. Improvement of insulin sensitivity in patients with type 2 diabetes mellitus after oral administration of alpha-lipoic acid. Hormones 2006;5(4):251–258.

26. Rochette L, Ghibu S, Muresan A, Vergely C. Alpha-lipoic acid: molecular mechanisms and therapeutic potential in diabetes. Can J Physiol Pharmacol 2015;93:1021–1027.

27. Reljanovic M, Reichel G, Rett K, et al. Treatment of diabetic polyneuropathy with the antioxidant thioctic acid (α-lipoic acid): a two year multicenter randomized double-blind placebo-controlled trial (ALADIN II). Free Radic Res 1999;31:171–179.

28. Zeigler D, Ametov A, Barinov A, et al. Oral treatment with alpha-lipoic acid improves symptomatic diabetic polyneuropathy. Diab Care 2006;29:2365–2370.

29. Ziegler D, Low PA, Litchy WJ, et al. Efficacy and safety of antioxidant treatment with alpha-lipoic acid over 4 years in diabetic polyneuropathy. Diab Care 2011;34:2054–2060.

30. Ansar H, Mazloom Z, Kazemi F, Hajazi N. Effect of alpha-lipoic acid on blood glucose, insulin resistance, and glutathione peroxidase of type 2 diabetic patients. Saudi Med J 2011;32(6):584–588.

31. Porasuphatana S, Suddee S, Nartnampong A, et al. Glycemic and oxidative status of patients with type 2 diabetes mellitus following oral administration of alpha-lipoic acid: a randomized double-blinded placebo-controlled study. Asia Pac J Clin Nutr 2012;21(1):12–21.

32. de Oliveira AM, Rondó PHC, Luzia LA, D'Abronzo FH, Illison VK. The effects of lipoic acid and α-tocopherol supplementation on the lipid profile and insulin sensitivity of patients with type 2 diabetes mellitus: a randomized, double-blind, placebo-controlled trial. Diab Res Clin Pract 2011;92:253–260.

33. Segermann J, Hotze A, Ulrich H, Rao GS. Effect of alpha-lipoic acid on the peripheral conversion of thyroxine to triiodothyronine and

on serum lipid-, protein- and glucose levels. Arzneimittel Forschung 1991;41(12):1294–1298.

CASE 96: MANAGING MENOPAUSAL SYMPTOMS

▦ Black Cohosh and Soy for Menopausal Symptoms

Clinical Course

Because Mrs Peterson is considering stopping her HT due to her family history of breast cancer but still desires some relief from hot flushes, she asks for additional information on other alternatives. She has heard that black cohosh should not be used in women with breast cancer, but she has a friend who also has a family history of breast cancer who has been on black cohosh for about 9 months on the recommendation of her physician, although the friend must have a checkup with lab tests every 6 months. Mrs Peterson asks if black cohosh or soy would be an appropriate option to help keep her hot flushes under control.

■ FOLLOW-UP QUESTIONS

1. What are the known or proposed mechanisms of action?

2. How extensive or conclusive are the clinical trial data on effectiveness for each?

3. What is known about safety of each?

4. Do the products have any specific quality concerns?

5. Would either product be an appropriate treatment choice in this particular patient?

6. If the patient is going to use either of these products, what counseling information will allow her to maximize any possible benefit and minimize any harm?

REFERENCES

1. Butt DA, Deng LY, Lewis JE, et al. Minimal decrease in hot flashes desired by postmenopausal women in family practice. Menopause 2007;14:203–207.

2. Powell SL, Gödecke T, Nikolic D, et al. In vitro serotonergic activity of black cohosh and identification of N_ω-methylserotonin as a potential active constituent. J Agric Food Chem 2008;56:11718–11726.

3. Borrelli F, Izzo AA, Ernst E. Pharmacological effects of *Cimicifuga racemosa*. Life Sci 2003;73:1215–1229.

4. Johnson TL, Fahey JW. Black cohosh: coming full circle? J Ethnopharmacol 2012;141:775–779.

5. Wuttke W, Jarry H, Haunschild J, et al. The non-estrogenic alternative for the treatment of climacteric complaints; black cohosh (*Cimicifuga* or *Actaea racemosa*). J Ster Biochem Mol Biol 2014;139:302–310.

6. Ruhlen RL, Haubner J, Tracy JK, et al. Black cohosh does not exert an estrogenic effect on the breast. Nutr Cancer 2007;59:269–277.

7. Fritz H, Seely D, McGowan J, et al. Black cohosh and breast cancer: a systematic review. Integer Cancer Ther 2014;13(1):12–29.

8. Frei-Kleiner S, Schaffner W, Rahlfs VW, et al. *Cimicifuga racemosa* dried ethanolic extract in menopausal disorders: a double-blind placebo-controlled clinical trial. Maturitas 2005;51:397–404.

9. Borrelli F, Ernst E. Black cohosh (*Cimicifuga racemosa*) for menopausal symptoms: a systematic review of its efficacy. Pharmacol Res 2008;58:8–14.

10. Palacio C, Masi G, Mooradian AD. Black cohosh for the management of menopausal symptoms. A systematic review of clinical trials. Drugs Aging 2009;26:23–36.

11. Leach MJ, Moore V. Black cohosh (*Cimicifuga* spp.) for menopausal symptoms. Cochrane Database Syst Rev 2012;9:CD007244.

12. Shams T, Setia MS, Hemmings R, McCusker J, Sewitch Clampi A. Efficacy of black cohosh-containing preparations on menopausal symptoms: a meta-analysis. Altern Ther 2010;16:36–44.

13. Beer A-M, Osmers R, Schnitker J, et al. Efficacy of black cohosh (*Cimicifuga racemosa*) medicines for treatment of menopausal symptoms—comments on major statements of the Cochrane Collaboration report 2012 "black cohosh (*Cimicifuga* spp.) for menopausal symptoms (review)". Gynecol Endocrinol 2013;29(12):1022–1025.

14. Wuttke W, Seidlova-Wuttke D. News about black cohosh. Maturitas 2012;71;92–93.

15. Schellenberg R, Saller R, Hess L, et al. Dose-dependent effects of the *Cimicifuga racemosa* extract Ze 450 in the treatment of climacteric complaints: a randomized, placebo-controlled study. Evid Based Complement Altern Med 2012:260301.

16. Drewe J, Zimmermann C, Zahner. The effect of a *Cimicifuga racemosa* extracts Ze 450 in the treatment of climacteric complaints—an observational study. Phytomedicine 2013;20:659–666.

17. Mohannad-Alizadeh-Charandabi S, Shahnazi M, Nahaee J, Bayatipayan S. Efficacy of black cohosh (*Cimicifuga racemosa* L.) in treating early symptoms of menopause: a randomized clinical trial. Chin Med 2013;8(1):20.

18. Jiang K, Jin Y, Huang L, et al. Black cohosh improves objective sleep in postmenopausal women with sleep disturbance. Climacteric 2015;18:559–567.

19. Pockaj BA, Gallagher JG, Loprinzi CL, et al. Phase III double-blind, randomized, placebo-controlled crossover trial of black cohosh in the management of hot flashes: NCCTG trial N01CC. J Clin Oncol 2006;24(18):2836–2841.

20. Rostock M, Fischer J, Mumm A, Stammwitz U, Saller R, Bartsch HH. Black cohosh (*Cimicifuga racemosa*) in tamoxifen-treated breast cancer patients with climacteric complaints—a prospective observational study. Gynecol Endocrinol 2011;27(1):844–848.

21. Rebbeck TR, Troxel AB, Norman S, et al. A retrospective case–control study of the use of hormone-related supplements and association with breast cancer. Int J Cancer 2007;120:1523–1528.

22. Obi N, Chang-Claude J, Berger J, et al. The use of herbal preparations to alleviate climacteric disorders and risk of postmenopausal breast cancer in a German case–control study. Cancer Epidemiol Biomark Prev 2009;18(8):2207–2213.

23. Raus K, Brucker C, Gorkow C, Wuttke W. First-time proof of endometrial safety of the special black cohosh extract (*Actaea* or *Cimicifuga racemosa* extract) CR BNO 1055. Menopause 2006;13(4):678–691.

24. McKenzie SC, Rahman A. Bradycardia in a patient taking black cohosh. Med J Aust 2010;193:479–481.

25. Dinman S. Black cohash [sic]: a contraindication in general anesthesia. Plastic Surg Nursing 2006;26:42–43.

26. Borrelli F, Ernst E. Black cohosh (*Cimicifuga racemosa*): a systematic review of adverse events. Am J Obstet Gynecol 2008;199:455–456.

27. Teschke R, Schwarzenboeck A, Schmidt-Taenzer W, Wolff A, Hennermann K-H. Herb induced liver injury presumably caused by black cohosh; a survey of initially purported cases and herbal quality specifications. Ann Hepatol 2011;11(3):249–259.

28. Teschke F, Bahre R, Fuchs J, Wolff A. Black cohosh hepatotoxicity: quantitative causality evaluation in nine suspected cases. Menopause 2009;16(5):956–965.

29. Teschke F, Bahre R, Genthner A, et al. Suspected black cohosh hepatotoxicity—challenges and pitfalls of causality assessment. Maturitas 2009;63:302–314.

30. Naser B, Schnitker J, Minkin MJ, Garcia de Arriba S, Nolte K-U, Osmers R. Suspected black cohosh hepatotoxicity: no evidence by meta-analysis of randomized controlled clinical trials for isopropanolic black cohosh extract. Menopause 2022;18(4):366–375.

31. Enbom E, Le MD, Oesterich L, Rutgers J, French SW. Mechanism of hepatotoxicity due to black cohosh (*Cimicifuga racemosa*): histological, immunohistochemical and electron microscopy analysis of two liver biopsies with clinical correlation. Exp Mol Pathol 2014;96:279–283.

32. Setchell KDR, Brown N, Lydeking-Olsen E. The clinical importance of the metabolite equol—a clue to the effectiveness of soy and it's isoflavones. J Nutr 2002;132:3577–3584.

33. North American Menopause Society. The role of soy isoflavones in menopausal health: report of The North American Menopause Society/Wulf H. Utian Translational Science Symposium in Chicago, IL (October 2010). Menopause 2011;18(7):732–753.

34. Villaseca P. Non-estrogen conventional and phytochemical treatments for vasomotor symptoms: what needs to be known for practice. Climacteric 2012;15:115–124.

35. Duncan AM, Underhill KE, Xu X, et al. Modest hormonal effects of soy isoflavones in postmenopausal women. J Clin Endocrinol Metab 1999;84:3479–3484.

36. Ginsburg J, Prelevic GM. Lack of significant hormonal effects and controlled trials of phyto-oestrogens. Lancet 2000;355:163–164.

37. Schmidt M, Arjomand-Wölkart K, Birkhäuser MH, et al. Consensus: soy isoflavones as a first-line approach to the treatment of menopausal vasomotor complaints. Gynecol Endocrinol 2016;32(6):427–430.

38. Jacobs A, Wegewitz U, Sommerfeld C, Grossklaus R. Efficacy of isoflavones in relieving vasomotor menopausal symptoms—a systematic review. Mol Nutr Food Res 2009;53:1084–1097.

39. Howes LG, Howes JB, Knight DC. Isoflavone therapy for menopausal flushes: a systematic review and meta-analysis. Maturitas 2006;55:203–211.

40. Taku K, Melby MK, Kronenberg F, Kurzer MS, Messina M. Extracted or synthesized soybean isoflavones reduce menopausal hot flash frequency and severity: systemic review and meta-analysis of randomized controlled trials. Menopause; 2012;19(7):776–790.

41. Ghazanfarpour M, Sadeghi R, Roudsari RL. The application of soy isoflavones for subjective symptoms and objective signs of vaginal atrophy in menopause: a systematic review of randomized controlled trials. J Obstet Gynecol 2016;36:160–171.

42. Tranche S, Brotons C, de la Pisa BP, et al. Impact of a soy drink on climacteric symptoms: an open-label, crossover, randomized clinical trial. Gynecol Endocrinol 2016;32(6):477–482.

43. Ma D-F, Qin L-Q, Wang P-Y, Katoh R. Soy isoflavone intake increases bone mineral density in the spine of menopausal women: meta-analysis of randomized controlled trials. Clin Nutr 2008;27:57–64.

44. Zheng X, Lee S-K, Chun OK. Soy isoflavones and osteoporotic bone loss: a review with an emphasis on modulation of bone remodeling. J Med Food 2016;19(1):1–14.

45. Kwak HS, Park SY, Kim MG, et al. Marked individual variation in isoflavone metabolism after a soy challenge can modulate the skeletal effect of isoflavones in premenopausal women. J Korean Med Sci 2009;24:867–873.

46. Taku K, Melby MK, Kurzer MS, Mizuno S, Watanabe S, Ishimi Y. Effects of soy isoflavone supplements on bone turnover markers in menopausal women: systematic review and meta-analysis of randomized controlled trials. Bone 2010;47:413–423.

47. Ricci E, Cipriani S, Chiaffarino F, Malvezzi M, Parazzini F. Soy isoflavones and bone mineral density in perimenopausal and postmenopausal western women: a systematic review and meta-analysis of randomized controlled trials. J Women's Health 2010;19(9):1609–1617.

48. Wei P, Liu M, Chen Y, Chen D-C. Systematic review of soy isoflavone supplements on osteoporosis in women. Asian Pac J Trop Med 2012;5(3):243–248.

49. Divi RL, Chang HC, Doerge DR. Anti-thyroid isoflavones from soybean: isolation, characterization, and mechanisms of action. Biochem Pharmacol 1997;54:1087–1096.

50. van Duursen MB, Nijmeijer SM, de Morree ES, de Jong PC, van den Berg M. Genistein induces breast cancer-associated aromatase and stimulates estrogen-dependent tumor cell growth in in vitro breast cancer model. Toxicology 2011;89(2–3)67–73.

CASE 98: BENIGN PROSTATIC HYPERPLASIA

■ *Pygeum africanum* for BPH

Clinical Course

As the pharmacist in the team, you perform a literature search on the use of saw palmetto for BPH. You discover that there are reports of the dietary supplement both improving and worsening

symptoms of ED. In addition, your readings indicate that saw palmetto should really only be used by patients with mild-to-moderate BPH. Based on this information, you do not recommend use of saw palmetto for the patient's BPH symptoms. However, because the patient is requesting information on natural products you search for alternative dietary supplements that may provide some benefit for this patient's BPH without contributing to ED. Would *Pygeum africanum* be a reasonable option to consider?

■ FOLLOW-UP QUESTIONS

1. What is the known or proposed mechanism of action?

2. How extensive or conclusive is the clinical trial data on effectiveness?

3. What is known about safety?

4. Does the product have any specific quality concerns?

5. Would this be an appropriate treatment choice in this particular patient?

6. If the patient is going to use the product, what counseling information will allow him to maximize any possible benefit and minimize any harm?

REFERENCES

1. Suter A, Saller R, Riedi E, Heinrich M. Improving BPH symptoms and sexual dysfunctions with a saw palmetto preparation? Results from a pilot trial. Phytother Res 2013;27:218–226.

2. Boyle P, Robertson C, Lowe F, Roehrborn C. Updated meta-analysis of clinical trials of *Serenoa repens* extract in the treatment of symptomatic benign prostatic hyperplasia. Br Urol 2004;93:751–756.

3. Tacklind J, MacDonald R, Rutks I, et al. *Serenoa repens* for benign prostatic hyperplasia. Cochrane Database Syst Rev 2012;12:CD001423.

4. Scaglione F. How to choose the right *Serenoa repens* extract. Eur Urol Suppl 2015;14:e1464–e1469.

5. Quiles MT, Arbós MA, Fraga A, et al. Antiproliferative and apoptotic effects of the herbal agent *Pygeum africanum* on culture prostate stromal cells from patients with benign prostatic hyperplasia (BPH). Prostate 2010;70:1044–1053.

6. Papaioannou M, Schleich S, Roell D, et al. NBBS isolated from *Pygeum africanum* bark exhibits androgen antagonistic activity, inhibits AR nuclear translocation and prostate cancer cell growth. Invest New Drugs 2010;28:729–743.

7. Roell D, Baniahmad A. The natural compounds atraric acid and N-butylbenzene-sulfonamide as antagonists of the human androgen receptor and inhibitors of prostate cancer cell growth. Mol Cell Endocrinol 2011;332:1–8.

8. Edgar AD, Levin R, Constantinou CE, Denis L. A critical review of the pharmacology of the plant extract of *Pygeum africanum* in the treatment of LUTS. Neurourol Urodynam 2007;26:458–463.

9. Shenouda NS, Sakla MS, Newton LG, et al. Physterol *Pygeum africanum* regulates prostate cancer in vitro and in vivo. Endocrine 2007;31:72–81.

10. Breza J, Dzurny O, Borowka A, et al. Efficacy and acceptability of Tadenan® (*Pygeum africanum* extract) in the treatment of benign prostatic hyperplasia (BPH): a multicentre trial in central Europe. Cur Med Res Opin 1998;14:127–139.

11. Chatelain C, Autet W, Brackman F. Comparison of once and twice daily dosage forms of *Pygeum africanum* extract in patients with benign prostatic hyperplasia: a randomized, double-blind study, with long-term open label extension. Urology 1999;54:473–478.

12. Ishani A, MacDonald R, Nelson D, Rutks I, Wilt TJ. *Pygeum africanum* for the treatment of patients with benign prostatic hyperplasia: a systematic review and quantitative meta-analysis. Am J Med 2000;109:654–664.

13. Wilt T, Ishani A, Mac Donald R, Rutks I, Stark G. *Pygeum africanum* for benign prostatic hyperplasia. Cochrane Data Syst Rev 2002;(1):CD001044.

CASE 105: OSTEOARTHRITIS

▓ Glucosamine Sulfate, Glucosamine Hydrochloride, and Chondroitin for Osteoarthritis

Clinical Course

While discussing multiple treatment options with Mr Kansella, he says, "This may seem silly, but I have a neighbor a couple years older than me who was getting some pretty bad arthritis in both knees a few years ago. He says he hardly has any pain anymore because he's taking these glucosamine and chondroitin pills. He even started back to golfing! Is there any way those could help me with my pain?"

■ FOLLOW-UP QUESTIONS

1. What are the known or proposed mechanisms of action?

2. How extensive or conclusive is the clinical trial data on effectiveness of each of the products or their combinations?

3. What is known about safety?

4. Do the products have any specific quality concerns?

5. Would any of these be appropriate treatment choice in this particular patient?

6. If the patient is going to use the products, what counseling information will allow him to maximize any possible benefit and minimize any harm?

REFERENCES

1. Nagaoka I, Igarashi M, Sakamoto K. Biological activities of glucosamine and its related substances. Adv Food Nutr Res 2012;65:337–352.

2. Henrotin Y, Mobasheri A, Marty M. Is there any scientific evidence for the use of glucosamine in the management of human osteoarthritis? Arthritis Res Ther 2012;14:201. doi:10.1186/ar3657.

3. Volpi N. Anti-inflammatory activity of chondroitin sulphate: new functions from an old natural molecule. Inflammopharmacology 2011;19:299–306.

4. Martel-Pelletier J, Farran A, Montell E, et al. Discrepancies in composition and biological effects of different formulations of chondroitin sulfate. Molecules 2015;20:4277–4289.

5. Calamia V, Mateos J, Fernández-Puente P, et al. A pharmacoproteomic study confirms the synergistic effect of chondroitin sulfate and glucosamine. Sci Rep 2014;45069.

6. Lee YH, Woo J-H, Choi SJ, et al. Effect of glucosamine or chondroitin sulfate on the osteoarthritis progression: a meta-analysis. Rheumatol Int 2010;30:357–363.

7. Bruyére O, Altman RD, Reginster J-Y. Efficacy and safety of glucosamine sulfate in the management of osteoarthritis: evidence from real-life setting trials and surveys. Semin Arthritis Rheum 2016;45:S12–S17.

8. Wandel S, Jüni P, Tendal B, et al. Effects of glucosamine, chondroitin, or placebo in patients with osteoarthritis of hip or knee: network meta-analysis. BMJ 2010;34:c4675.

9. Sawitzke AD, Shi H, Finco MF, et al. Clinical efficacy and safety of glucosamine, chondroitin sulfate, their combination, celecoxib or placebo taken to treat osteoarthritis of the knee: 2-year results from GAIT. Ann Rheum Dis 2010;69:1459–1464.

10. Hochberg Mc. Structure-modifying effects of chondroitin sulfate in knee osteoarthritis: an updated meta-analysis of randomized placebo-controlled trials of 2-year duration. Osteoarthritis Cart 2010;18:S28–S31.

11. Gabay C, Medinger-Sadowski C, Gascon D, et al. Symptomatic effects of chondroitin 4 and chondroitin 6 sulfate on hand osteoarthritis. Arthritis Rheum 2011;63(11):3383–3391.

12. Hochberg MC, Martel-Pelletier J, Monfort J, et al. Combined chondroitin sulfate and glucosamine for painful knee osteoarthritis: a multi-centre, randomized, double-blind, non-inferiority trial versus celecoxib. Ann Rheum Dis 2016;75:37–44.

13. Provenza JR, Shinjo SM, Silva JM, et al. Combined glucosamine and chondroitin sulfate, once or three times daily, provides clinically relevant analgesia in knee osteoarthritis. Clin Rheumatol 2015;34:1455–1462.

14. Mazieres B, Combe B, Phan Van A, et al. Chondroitin sulfate in osteoarthritis of the knee: a prospective, double-blind, placebo-controlled multicenter clinical study. J Rheumatol 2001;28:173–181.

15. Villacis J, Rice TR, Bucci LR, et al. Do shrimp-allergic individuals tolerate shrimp-derived glucosamine? Clin Exp Allergy 2006;36:1457–1461.

CASE 108: ALLERGIC RHINITIS

▓ Butterbur Extract for Allergic Rhinitis

Clinical Course

James' mother is quite concerned about drowsiness associated with prescription treatments for his symptoms because he has a tendency to nap when he is supposed to be doing homework. Mrs Patrick uses butterbur extract for migraine prophylaxis and has heard that it is effective for allergy symptoms; she asks about using the same product for James.

■ FOLLOW-UP QUESTIONS

1. What is the known or proposed mechanism of action?

2. How extensive or conclusive are the clinical trial data on effectiveness?

3. What is known about safety?

4. Does the product have any specific quality concerns?

5. Would this be an appropriate treatment choice in this particular patient?

6. If the patient is going to use the product, what counseling information will allow him to maximize any possible benefit and minimize any harm?

REFERENCES

1. Thomet OA, Schapowal A, Heinisch IV, et al. Anti-inflammatory activity of an extract of *Petasites hybridus* in allergic rhinitis. Int Immunopharmacol 2002;2:997–1006.

2. Brattström A, Schapowal A, Maillet I, et al. Petasites extract Ze 339 (PET) inhibits allergen-induced Th2 responses, airway inflammation and airway hyperreactivity in mice. Phytother Res 2010;24:680–685.

3. Dumitru AF, Shamji M, Wagenmann M, et al. Petasol butanoate complex (Ze 339) relieves allergic rhinitis-induced nasal obstruction more effectively than desloratadine. J Allergy Clin Immunol 2011;127:1515–1521.

4. Lee DKC, Haggart K, Robb FM, Lipworth BJ. Butterbur, a herbal remedy, confers complementary anti-inflammatory activity in asthmatic patients receiving inhaled corticosteroids. Clin Exp Allergy 2004;34:110–114.

5. Giles M, Ulbricht C, Khalsa KP, Kirkwood CD, Park C, Basch E. Butterbur: an evidence-based systematic review by the Natural Standard Research Collaboration. J Herb Pharmacother 2005;5:119–143.

6. Guo R, Pittler MH, Ernst E. Herbal medicines for the treatment of allergic rhinitis: a systematic review. Ann Allergy Asthma Immunol 2007;99:483–495.

7. Schapowal A. Treating intermittent allergic rhinitis: a prospective, randomized, placebo and antihistamine-controlled study of butterbur extract Ze 339. Phytother Res 2005;19:530–537.

8. Schapowal A. Randomised controlled trial of butterbur and cetirizine for treating seasonal allergic rhinitis. BMJ 2002;324:144–146.

9. Lee DK, Gray RD, Robb FM, et al. A placebo-controlled evaluation of butterbur and fexofenadine on objective and subjective outcomes in perennial allergic rhinitis. Clin Exp Allergy 2004;34:646–649.

10. Nebel S, Kobi C, Zahner C. Effective treatment of early allergic and late inflammatory symptoms of allergic rhinitis with Ze 339 (Tesalin®): results of a non-interventional observational study. Planta Med 2014;80:16.

11. Danesch UC. *Petasites hybridus* (butterbur root) extract in the treatment of asthma—an open trial. Altern Med Rev 2004;9:54–62.

12. Anderson N, Meier T, Borlak J. Toxicogenomics applied to cultures of human hepatocytes enabled an identification of novel *Petasites hybridus* extracts for the treatment of migraine with improved hepatobiliary safety. Toxicol Sci 2009;112:507–520.

13. Wang YP, Yan J, Fu PP, Chou MW. Human liver microsomal reduction of pyrrolizidine alkaloid N-oxides to form the corresponding carcinogenic parent alkaloid. Toxicol Lett 2005;155:411–420.

CASE 125: INFLUENZA

■ **Elderberry for Influenza**

Clinical Course

As Mr Kharitonov is leaving, he thanks you and promises to follow your recommendations. He does say that he is worried about making anyone else sick, because of his son's upcoming wedding; "My cousins back in Russia keep telling me they use elderberry syrup to keep from getting sick during flu season. Could that help keep my wife from getting this flu?"

■ FOLLOW-UP QUESTIONS

1. What is the known or proposed mechanism of action?

2. How extensive or conclusive are the clinical trial data on effectiveness?

3. What is known about safety?

4. Does the product have any specific quality concerns?

5. Would this be an appropriate treatment choice in this particular patient or for the patient's wife?

6. If the patient is going to use the product, what counseling information will allow him to maximize any possible benefit and minimize any harm?

REFERENCES

1. Ulbricht C, Basch E, Cheung L, et al. An evidence-based systematic review of elderberry and elderflower (*Sambucus nigra*) by the Natural Standard Research Collaboration. J Dietary Suppl 2014;11(1):80–120.

2. Krawitz C, Abu Mraheil M, Stein M, et al. Inhibitory activity of a standardized elderberry liquid extract against clinically-relevant human respiratory bacterial pathogens and influenza A and B viruses. BMC Complement Altern Med 2011;11:16.

3. Kinoshita E, Hayashi K, Katayama H, et al. Anti-influenza virus effects of elderberry juice and its fractions. Biosci Biotechnol Biochem 2012;76(9):1633–1638.

4. Ivanova D, Tasinov O, Kiselova-Kaneva Y. Improved lipid profile and increased serum antioxidant capacity in healthy volunteers after *Sambucus nigra* L. fruit infusion consumption. Int J Food Sci Nutr 2014;65(6):740–744.

5. Murkovic M, Abuja PM, Bermann AR, et al. Effects of elderberry juice on fasting and postprandial serum lipids and low-density lipoprotein oxidation in healthy volunteers: a randomized, double-blind, placebo-controlled study. Eur J Clin Nutr 2004;58:244–249.

6. Zakay-Rones Z, Varsano N, Zlotnik M, et al. Inhibition of several strains of influenza virus in vitro and reduction of symptoms by an elderberry extract (*Sambucus nigra* L.) during an outbreak of influenza B Panama. J Altern Complement Med 1995;1:361–369.

7. Zakay-Rones Z, Thom E, Wollan T, et al. Randomized study of the efficacy and safety of oral elderberry extract in the treatment of influenza A and B virus infections. J Int Med Res 2004;32:132–140.

8. Rauš K, Pleschka S, Klein P, et al. Effect of an *Echinacea*-based hot drink versus oseltamivir in influenza treatment: a randomized, double-blind, double-dummy, multicenter, noninferiority clinical trial. Curr Therapeutic Res 2015;77:66–72.

9. Tiralongo E, Wee SS, Lea RA. Elderberry supplementation reduces cold duration and symptoms in air-travellers: a randomized, double-blind placebo-controlled clinical trial. Nutrients 2016;8(4):182.

10. Curtis PJ, Kroom PA, Hollands WJ, et al. Cardiovascular disease risk biomarkers and liver and kidney function are not altered in postmenopausal women after ingesting and elderberry extract rich in anthocyanins for 12 weeks. J Nutr 2009;139:2266–2271.

CONVERSION FACTORS AND ANTHROPOMETRICS*

CONVERSION FACTORS

■ SI Units

SI (*le Système International d'Unités*) units are used in many countries to express clinical laboratory and serum drug concentration data. Instead of employing units of mass (such as micrograms), the SI system uses moles (mol) to represent the amount of a substance. A molar solution contains 1 mol (the molecular weight of the substance in grams) of the solute in 1 L of solution. The following formula is used to convert units of mass to moles (mcg/mL to μmol/L or, by substitution of terms, mg/mL to mmol/L or ng/mL to nmol/L).

Micromoles per Liter (μmol/L)

$$\mu mol/L = \frac{\text{drug concentration (mcg/mL)} \times 1{,}000}{\text{molecular weight of drug (g/mol)}}$$

Milliequivalents

An equivalent weight of a substance is that weight which will combine with or replace 1 g of hydrogen; a milliequivalent is 1/1,000 of an equivalent weight.

Milliequivalents per Liter (mEq/L):

$$mEq/L = \frac{\text{weight of salt (g)} \times \text{valence of ion} \times 1{,}000}{\text{molecular weight of salt}}$$

$$\text{weight of salt (g)} = \frac{mEq/L \times \text{molecular weight of salt}}{\text{valence of ion} \times 1{,}000}$$

Approximate Milliequivalents

Weights of Selected Ions

Salt	mEq/g Salt	mg Salt/mEq
Calcium carbonate ($CaCO_3$)	20.0	50.0
Calcium chloride ($CaCl_2 \cdot 2H_2O$)	13.6	73.5
Calcium gluceptate ($Ca[C_7H_{13}O_8]_2$)	4.1	245.2
Calcium gluconate ($Ca[C_6H_{11}O_7]_2 \cdot H_2O$)	4.5	224.1
Calcium lactate ($Ca[C_3H_5O_3]_2 \cdot 5H_2O$)	6.5	154.1
Magnesium gluconate ($Mg[C_6H_{11}O_7]_2 \cdot H_2O$)	4.6	216.3
Magnesium oxide (MgO)	49.6	20.2
Magnesium sulfate ($MgSO_4$)	16.6	60.2
Magnesium sulfate ($MgSO_4 \cdot 7H_2O$)	8.1	123.2
Potassium acetate ($K[C_2H_3O_2]$)	10.2	98.1
Potassium chloride (KCl)	13.4	74.6
Potassium citrate ($K_3[C_6H_5O_7] \cdot H_2O$)	9.2	108.1
Potassium iodide (KI)	6.0	166.0
Sodium acetate ($Na[C_2H_3O_2]$)	12.2	82.0
Sodium acetate ($Na[C_2H_3O_2] \cdot 3H_2O$)	7.3	136.1
Sodium bicarbonate ($NaHCO_3$)	11.9	84.0
Sodium chloride (NaCl)	17.1	58.4
Sodium citrate ($Na_3[C_6H_5O_7] \cdot 2H_2O$)	10.2	98.0
Sodium iodide (NaI)	6.7	149.9
Sodium lactate ($Na[C_3H_5O_3]$)	8.9	112.1
Zinc sulfate ($ZnSO_4 \cdot 7H_2O$)	7.0	143.8

■ Valences and Atomic Weights of Selected Ions

Substance	Electrolyte	Valence	Molecular Weight
Calcium	Ca^{2+}	2	40.1
Chloride	Cl^-	1	35.5
Magnesium	Mg^{2+}	2	24.3
Phosphate	HPO_4^- (80%)	1.8	96.0[a]
(pH = 7.4)	$H2PO_4^-$ (20%)		
Potassium	K^+	1	39.1
Sodium	Na^+	1	23.0
Sulfate	SO_4^-	2	96.0[a]

[a]The molecular weight of phosphorus only is 31; that of sulfur only is 32.1.

*This appendix contains information from Appendices 1 and 2 of Anderson PO, Knoben JE, Troutman WG, et al (eds). *Handbook of Clinical Drug Data*, 10th ed. New York, McGraw-Hill, 2002:1053–1058, with permission.

Anion Gap

The anion gap is the concentration of plasma anions not routinely measured by laboratory screening. It is useful in the evaluation of acid–base disorders. The anion gap is greater with increased plasma concentrations of endogenous species (eg, phosphate, sulfate, lactate, and ketoacids) or exogenous species (eg, salicylate, penicillin, ethylene glycol, ethanol, and methanol). The formulas for calculating the anion gap are as follows:

$$\text{Anion gap} = (Na^+ + K^+) - (Cl^- + HCO_3^-)$$

or

$$\text{Anion gap} = Na^+ - (Cl^- + HCO_3^-)$$

where the expected normal value for the first equation is 11–20 mmol/L, and the expected normal value for the second equation is 7–16 mmol/L. Note that there is a variation in the upper and lower limits of the normal range.

Temperature

Fahrenheit to Centigrade: $(°F - 32) \times 5/9 = °C$
Centigrade to Fahrenheit: $(°C \times 9/5) + 32 = °F$
Centigrade to Kelvin: $°C + 273 = °K$

Calories

1 calorie = 1 kilocalorie = 1,000 calories = 4.184 kilojoules (kJ)
1 kilojoule = 0.239 calories = 0.239 kilocalories = 239 calories

Weights and Measures

Metric Weight Equivalents

1 kilogram (kg) = 1,000 grams
1 gram (g) = 1,000 milligrams
1 milligram (mg) = 0.001 gram
1 microgram (mcg) = 0.001 milligram
1 nanogram (ng) = 0.001 microgram
1 picogram (pg) = 0.001 nanogram
1 femtogram (fg) = 0.001 picogram

Metric Volume Equivalents

1 liter (L) = 1,000 milliliters
1 deciliter (dL) = 100 milliliters
1 milliliter (mL) = 0.001 liter
1 microliter (μL) = 0.001 milliliter
1 nanoliter (nL) = 0.001 microliter
1 picoliter (pL) = 0.001 nanoliter
1 femtoliter (fL) = 0.001 picoliter

Apothecary Weight Equivalents

1 scruple (℈) = 20 grains (gr)
60 grains (gr) = 1 dram (ʒ)
8 drams (ʒ) = 1 ounce (fl ʒ)
1 ounce (ʒ) = 480 grains
12 ounces (ʒ) = 1 pound (lb)

Apothecary Volume Equivalents

60 minims (m̦) = 1 fluidram (fl ʒ)
8 fluidrams (fl ʒ) = 1 fluid ounce (fl ʒ)
1 fluid ounce (ft ʒ) = 480 minims
16 fluid ounces (fl ʒ) = 1 pint (pt)

Avoirdupois Equivalents

1 ounce (oz) = 437.5 grains
16 ounces (oz) = 1 pound (lb)

Weight/Volume Equivalents

1 mg/dL = 10 mcg/mL
1 mg/dL = 1 mg%
1 ppm = 1 mg/L

Conversion Equivalents

1 gram (g) = 15.43 grains
1 grain (gr) = 64.8 milligrams
1 ounce (ʒ) = 31.1 grams
1 ounce (oz) = 28.35 grams
1 pound (lb) = 453.6 grams
1 kilogram (kg) = 2.2 pounds
1 milliliter (mL) = 16.23 minims
1 minim (m̦) = 0.06 milliliter
1 fluid ounce (fl oz) = 29.57 milliliter
1 pint (pt) = 473.2 milliliter
0.1 milligram = 1/600 grain
0.12 milligram = 1/500 grain
0.15 milligram = 1/400 grain
0.2 milligram = 1/300 grain
0.3 milligram = 1/200 grain
0.4 milligram = 1/150 grain
0.5 milligram = 1/120 grain
0.6 milligram = 1/100 grain
0.8 milligram = 1/80 grain
1 milligram = 1/65 grain

Metric Length Equivalents

2.54 cm = 1 inch
30.48 cm = 1 foot
1.6 km = 1 mile

ANTHROPOMETRICS

Creatinine Clearance Formulas

Formulas for Estimating Creatinine Clearance in Patients with Stable Renal Function

Cockcroft–Gault Formula

Adults (age 18 years and older)[1]:

$$\text{CLcr (males)} = \frac{(140 - \text{age}) \times \text{weight}}{Cr_s \times 72}$$

$$\text{CLcr (males)} = 0.85 \times \text{above value}^\dagger$$

where CLcr is creatinine clearance (in mL/minute), Cr_s is serum creatinine (in mg/dL), age is in years, and weight is in kilograms.

Children (age 1–18 years)[2]:

$$\text{CLcr} = \frac{0.48 \times \text{height} \times \text{BSA}}{Cr_s \times 1.73}$$

where BSA is body surface area (in m^2), CLcr is creatinine clearance (in mL/minute), Cr_s is serum creatinine (in mg/dL), and height is in centimeters.

---

†Some studies suggest that the predictive accuracy of this formula for women is better without the correction factor of 0.85.

Formula for Estimating Creatinine Clearance from a Measured Urine Collection

$$CLcr \text{ (mL/minute)} = \frac{U \times V^\ddagger}{P \times T}$$

where U is the concentration of creatinine in a urine specimen (in same units as P), V is the volume of urine (in mL), P is the concentration of creatinine in serum at the midpoint of the urine collection period (in same units as U), and T is the time of the urine collection period in minutes (eg, 6 hours = 360 minutes; 24 hours = 1,440 minutes).

MDRD Formula for Estimating Glomerular Filtration Rate (from the Modification of Diet in Renal Disease Study)[3]

Conventional calibration MDRD equation (used only with those creatinine methods that have not been recalibrated to be traceable to isotope dilution mass spectrometry, IDMS).

For creatinine in mg/dL:

$$X = 186 \text{ creatinine}^{-1.154} \times \text{age}^{-0.203} \times \text{constant}$$

For creatinine in µmol/L:

$$X = 32,788 \times \text{creatinine}^{-1.154} \times \text{age}^{-0.203} \times \text{constant}$$

where X is the glomerular filtration rate (GFR), constant for white males is 1 and for females is 0.742, and constant for African Americans is 1.21. Creatinine levels in µmol/L can be converted to mg/dL by dividing by 88.4.

IDMS-Traceable MDRD Equation (Used Only with Creatinine Methods That Have Been Recalibrated to Be Traceable to IDMS)

For creatinine in mg/dL:

$$X = 175 \times \text{creatinine}^{-1.154} \times \text{age}^{-0.203} \times \text{constant}$$

For creatinine in µmol/L:

$$X = 175 \times (\text{creatinine}/88.4)^{-1.154} \times \text{age}^{-0.203} \times \text{constant}$$

where X is the glomerular filtration rate (GFR), constant for white males is 1 and for females is 0.742, and constant for African Americans is 1.21.

■ Ideal Body Weight (IBW)

IBW is the weight expected for a nonobese person of a given height. The IBW formulas below and various life insurance tables can be used to estimate IBW. Dosing methods described in the literature may use IBW as a method in dosing obese patients.

Adults (age 18 years and older)[4]:

$$IBW \text{ (males)} = 50 + (2.3 \times \text{height in inches over 5 ft})$$

$$IBW \text{ (females)} = 45.5 + (2.3 \times \text{height in inches over 5 ft})$$

where IBW is in kilograms.

Children (age 1–18 years)[2]:

Under 5 feet tall:

$$IBW = \frac{\text{height}^2 \times 1.65}{1,000}$$

where IBW is in kilograms and height is in centimeters.

Five feet or taller:

$$IBW \text{ (males)} = 39 + (2.27 \times \text{height in inches over 5 ft})$$

$$IBW \text{ (females)} = 42.2 + (2.27 \times \text{height in inches over 5 ft})$$

where IBW is in kilograms.

REFERENCES

1. Cockcroft DW, Gault MH. Prediction of creatinine clearance from serum creatinine. Nephron 1976;16:31–41.
2. Traub SI, Johnson CE. Comparison of methods of estimating creatinine clearance in children. Am J Hosp Pharm 1980;37:195–201.
3. Levey AS, Bosch JP, Lewis JB, et al. A more accurate method to estimate glomerular filtration rate from serum creatinine: a new prediction equation. Modification of Diet in Renal Disease Study Group. Ann Intern Med 1999;130:461–470.
4. Devine BJ. Gentamicin therapy. Drug Intell Clin Pharm 1974;8:650–655.

$\ddagger$The product of $U \times V$ equals the production of creatinine during the collection period and, at steady state, should equal 20–25 mg/kg per day for ideal body weight (IBW) in males and 15–20 mg/kg per day for IBW in females. If it is less than this, inadequate urine collection may have occurred, and CLcr will be underestimated.

APPENDIX B
COMMON LABORATORY TESTS

The following table is an alphabetical listing of some common laboratory tests and their reference ranges for adults as measured in plasma or serum (unless otherwise indicated). Reference values differ among laboratories, so readers should refer to the published reference ranges used in each institution. For some tests, both SI units and conventional units are reported.

Laboratory	Conventional Units	Conversion Factor	SI Units
Acid phosphatase			
Male	2–12 units/L	16.7	33–200 nkat/L
Female	0.3–9.2 units/L	16.7	5–154 nkat/L
Activated partial thromboplastin time (aPTT)	25–40 s		
Adrenocorticotropic hormone (ACTH)	15–80 pg/mL or ng/L	0.2202	3.3–17.6 pmol/L
Alanine aminotransferase (ALT, SGPT)	7–53 IU/L	0.01667	0.12–0.88 µkat/L
Albumin	3.5–5.0 g/dL	10	35–50 g/L
Albumin:creatinine ratio (urine)			
Normal	Less than 30 mg/g creatinine		
Microalbuminuria	30–300 mg/g creatinine		
Proteinuria	Greater than 300 mg/g creatinine		
or	or		
Normal			
Male	Less than 2.0 mg/mmol creatinine		
Female	Less than 2.8 mg/mmol creatinine		
Microalbuminuria			
Male	2.0–20 mg/mmol creatinine		
Female	2.8–28 mg/mmol creatinine		
Proteinuria			
Male	Greater than 20 mg/mmol creatinine		
Female	Greater than 28 mg/mmol creatinine		
Aldosterone			
Supine	Less than 16 ng/dL	27.7	Less than 444 pmol/L
Upright	Less than 31 ng/dL	27.7	Less than 860 pmol/L
Alkaline phosphatase			
10–15 years	130–550 IU/L	0.01667	2.17–9.17 µkat/L
16–20 years	70–260 IU/L	0.01667	1.17–4.33 µkat/L
Greater than 20 years	38–126 IU/L	0.01667	0.13–2.10 µkat/L
Alpha-fetoprotein (AFP)	Less than 15 ng/mL	1	Less than 15 mcg/L
Alpha₁-antitrypsin	80–200 mg/dL	0.01	0.8–2.0 g/L
Amikacin, therapeutic	15–30 mg/L peak	1.71	25.6–51.3 µmol/L peak
	Less than or equal to 8 mg/L trough		Less than or equal to 13.7 µmol/L trough
Amitriptyline	80–200 ng/mL or mcg/L	3.4	272–680 nmol/L
Ammonia (plasma)	15.33–56.20 mcg NH₃/dL	0.5872	9–33 µmol NH₃/L
Amylase	25–115 IU/L	0.01667	0.42–1.92 kat/L
Androstenedione	50–250 ng/dL	0.0349	1.7–8.7 nmol/L
Angiotensin-converting enzyme	15–70 units/L	16.67	250–1,167 nkat/L
Anion gap	7–16 mEq/L	1	7–16 mmol/L
Anti–double-stranded DNA (anti-ds DNA)	Negative		
Anti-HAV	Negative		
Anti-HBc	Negative		
Anti-HBs	Negative		
Anti-HCV	Negative		
Anti–Sm antibody	Negative		
Antinuclear antibody (ANA)	Negative		
Apolipoprotein A-1			
Male	95–175 mg/dL	0.01	0.95–1.75 g/L
Female	100–200 mg/dL	0.01	1.0–2.0 g/L
Apolipoprotein B			
Male	50–110 mg/dL	0.01	0.5–1.10 g/L
Female	50–105 mg/dL	0.01	0.5–1.05 g/L

(continued)

Laboratory	Conventional Units	Conversion Factor	SI Units
Aspartate aminotransferase (AST, SGOT)	11–47 IU/L	0.01667	0.18–0.78 μkat/L
Beta$_2$-microglobulin	Less than 0.2 mg/dL	10	2 mg/L
Bicarbonate	22–26 mEq/L	1	22–26 mmol/L
Bilirubin			
Total	0.3–1.1 mg/dL	17.1	5.13–18.80 μmol/L
Direct	0–0.3 mg/dL	17.1	0–5.1 μmol/L
Indirect	0.1–1.0 mg/dL	17.1	1.71–17.1 μmol/L
Bleeding time	3–7 min		
Blood gases (arterial)			
pH	7.35–7.45	1	7.35–7.45
PaO$_2$	80–105 mm Hg	0.133	10.6–14.0 kPa
PaCO$_2$	35–45 mm Hg	0.133	4.7–6.0 kPa
HCO$_3$	22–26 mEq/L	1	22–26 mmol/L
O$_2$ saturation	Greater than or equal to 95%	0.01	0.95
Blood urea nitrogen	8–25 mg/dL	0.357	2.9–8.9 mmol/L
B-type natriuretic peptide (BNP)	0–99 pg/mL	1	0–99 ng/L
BUN-to-creatinine ratio	10:1 to 20:1		
C-peptide	0.51–2.70 ng/mL	330	170–900 pmol/L or
		0.33	0.172–0.900 nmol/L
C-reactive protein	Less than 0.8 mg/dL	10	Less than 8 mg/L
CA-125	Less than 35 units/mL	1	Less than 35 kilounits/L
CA 15-3	Less than 30 units/mL	1	Less than 30 kilounits/L
CA 19-9	Less than 37 units/mL	1	Less than 37 kilounits/L
CA 27-29	Less than 38 units/mL	1	Less than 38 kilounits/L
Calcium			
Total	8.6–10.3 mg/dL	0.25	2.15–2.58 mmol/L
	4.3–5.16 mEq/L	0.50	2.15–2.58 mmol/L
Ionized	4.5–5.1 mg/dL	0.25	1.13–1.28 mmol/L
	2.26–2.56 mEq/L	0.50	1.13–1.28 mmol/L
Carbamazepine, therapeutic	4–12 mg/L	4.23	17–51 μmol/L
Carboxyhemoglobin (nonsmoker)	Less than 2%	0.01	Less than 0.02
Carcinoembryonic antigen (CEA)			
Nonsmoker	Less than 2.5 ng/mL	1	Less than 2.5 mcg/L
Smoker	Less than 5 ng/mL		Less than 5 mcg/L
Cardiac troponin I (see troponin I)	Variable ng/mL	1	Variable mcg/L
CD4 lymphocyte count	31–61% of total lymphocytes		
CD8 lymphocyte count	18–39% of total lymphocytes		
Cerebrospinal fluid (CSF)			
Pressure	75–175 mm H$_2$O		
Glucose	40–70 mg/dL	0.0555	2.2–3.9 mmol/L
Protein	15–45 mg/dL	0.01	0.15–0.45 g/L
WBC	Less than 10/mm^3		
Ceruloplasmin	18–45 mg/dL	10	180–450 mg/L
		0.063	1.1–2.8 μmol/L
Chloride	97–110 mEq/L	1	97–110 mmol/L
Cholesterol			
Desirable	Less than 200 mg/dL	0.0259	Less than 5.18 mmol/L
Borderline high	200–239 mg/dL	0.0259	5.18–6.19 mmol/L
High	Greater than or equal to 240 mg/dL	0.0259	Greater than or equal to 6.2 mmol/L
Chorionic gonadotropin (β-hCG)	Less than 5 milliunits/mL	1	Less than 5 units/L
Clozapine	Minimum trough 300–350 ng/mL or mcg/L	3.06	918–1,071 nmol/L
CO$_2$ content	22–30 mEq/L	1	22–30 mmol/L
Complement component 3 (C3)	70–160 mg/dL	0.01	0.7–1.6 g/L
Complement component 4 (C4)	20–40 mg/dL	0.01	0.2–0.4 g/L
Copper	70–150 mcg/dL	0.157	11–24 μmol/L
Cortisol (fasting, morning)	5–25 mcg/dL	27.6	138–690 nmol/L
Cortisol (free, urinary)	10–100 mcg/day	2.76	28–276 nmol/day
Creatine kinase			
Male	30–200 IU/L	0.01667	0.50–3.33 μkat/L
Female	20–170 IU/L	0.01667	0.33–2.83 μkat/L
MB fraction	0–7 IU/L	0.01667	0.0–0.12 μkat/L
Creatinine clearance (CLcr) (urine)	85–135 mL/min/1.73 m^2	0.00963	0.82–1.3 mL/s/m^2
Creatinine			
Male 4–20 years	0.2–1.0 mg/dL	88.4	18–88 μmol/L
Female 4–20 years	0.2–1.0 mg/dL	88.4	18–88 μmol/L
Male (adults)	0.7–1.3 mg/dL	88.4	62–115 μmol/L
Female (adults)	0.6–1.1 mg/dL	88.4	53–97 μmol/L

(continued)

Laboratory	Conventional Units	Conversion Factor	SI Units
Cyclosporine			
Renal transplant	100–300 ng/mL or mcg/L	0.832	83–250 nmol/L
Cardiac, liver, or pancreatic transplant	200–350 ng/mL or mcg/L	0.832	166–291 nmol/L
Cryptococcal antigen	Negative		
D-dimers	Less than 250 ng/mL	1	Less than 250 mcg/L
Desipramine	75–300 ng/mL or mcg/L	3.75	281–1,125 mmol/L
Dexamethasone suppression test (DST) (overnight)	8:00 AM cortisol less than 5 mcg/dL	0.0276	Less than 0.14 μmol/L
DHEAS			
Male	170–670 mcg/dL	0.0271	4.6–18.2 μmol/L
Female			
Premenopausal	50–540 mcg/dL	0.0271	1.4–14.7 μmol/L
Postmenopausal	30–260 mcg/dL	0.0271	0.8–7.1 μmol/L
Digoxin, therapeutic	0.5–1.0 ng/mL or mcg/L	1.28	0.6–1.3 nmol/L
Erythrocyte count (blood) See under red blood cell count			
Erythrocyte sedimentation rate (ESR)			
Westergren			
Male	0–20 mm/h		
Female	0–30 mm/h		
Wintrobe			
Male	0–9 mm/h		
Female	0–15 mm/h		
Erythropoietin	2–25 mIU/mL	1	2–25 IU/L
Estradiol			
Male	10–36 pg/mL	3.67	37–132 pmol/L
Female	34–170 pg/mL	3.67	125–624 pmol/L
Ethanol, legal intoxication	Greater than or equal to 50–100 mg/dL	0.217	10.9–21.7 mmol/L
	Greater than or equal to 0.05–0.1%	217	
Ethosuccimide, therapeutic	40–100 mg/L or mcg/mL	7.08	283–708 μmol/L
Factor VIII or factor IX			
Severe hemophilia	Less than 1 IU/dL	0.01	Less than 0.01 units/mL
Moderate hemophilia	1–5 IU/dL	0.01	0.01–0.05 units/mL
Mild hemophilia	Greater than 5 IU/dL	0.01	Greater than 0.05 units/mL
Usual adult levels	60–140 IU/dL	0.01	0.60–1.40 units/mL
Ferritin			
Male	20–250 ng/mL	1	20–250 mcg/L
Female	10–150 ng/mL	1	10–150 mcg/L
Fibrin degradation products (FDP)	2–10 mg/L		
Fibrinogen	200–400 mg/dL	0.01	2.0–4.0 g/L
Folate (plasma)	3.1–12.4 ng/mL	2.266	7.0–28.1 nmol/L
Folic acid (RBC)	125–600 ng/mL	2.266	283–1,360 nmol/L
Follicle-stimulating hormone (FSH)			
Male	1–7 mIU/mL	1	1–7 IU/L
Female			
Follicular phase	1–9 mIU/mL	1	1–9 IU/L
Midcycle	6–26 mIU/mL	1	6–26 IU/L
Luteal phase	1–9 mIU/mL	1	1–9 IU/L
Postmenopausal	30–118 mIU/mL	1	30–118 IU/L
Free thyroxine index (FT$_4$I)	6.5–12.5		
Gamma glutamyl transferase (GGT)	0–30 IU/L	0.01667	0–0.5 μkat/L
Gastrin (fasting)	0–130 pg/mL	1	0–130 ng/L
Gentamicin, therapeutic	4–10 mg/L peak	2.09	8.4–21.0 μmol/L peak
	Less than or equal to 2 mg/L trough		Less than or equal to 4.2 μmol/L trough
Globulin	2.3–3.5 g/dL	10	23–35 g/L
Glucose (fasting, plasma)	65–109 mg/dL	0.0555	3.6–6.0 mmol/L
Glucose, 2-hour postprandial blood (PPBG)	Less than 140 mg/dL	0.0555	Less than 7.8 mmol/L
Granulocyte count	$1.8–6.6 \times 10^3/\mu L$	10^6	$1.8–6.6 \times 10^9/L$
Growth hormone (fasting)			
Male	Less than 5 ng/mL	1	Less than 5 mcg/L
Female	Less than 10 ng/mL	1	Less than 10 mcg/L
Haptoglobin	60–270 mg/dL	0.01	0.6–2.7 g/L
HBeAg	Negative		
HbsAg	Negative		
HBV DNA	Negative		
Hematocrit			
Male	40.7–50.3%	0.01	0.407–0.503
Female	36.1–44.3%	0.01	0.361–0.443

(continued)

Laboratory	Conventional Units	Conversion Factor	SI Units
Hemoglobin (blood)			
Male	13.8–17.2 g/dL	10	138–172 g/L
		Alternate SI: 0.62	8.56–10.67 mmol/L
Female	12.1–15.1 g/dL	10	121–151 g/L
		Alternate SI: 0.62	7.5–9.36 mmol/L
Hemoglobin A1C	4.0–6.0%	0.01	0.04–0.06
Heparin			
Via protamine titration method	0.2–0.4 mcg/mL		
Via anti-factor Xa assay	0.3–0.7 mcg/mL		
High-density lipoprotein (HDL) cholesterol	Greater than 35 mg/dL	0.0259	Greater than 0.91 mmol/L
Homocysteine	3.3–10.4 μmol/L		
Ibuprofen			
Therapeutic	10–50 mcg/mL	4.85	49–243 μmol/L
Toxic	100–700 mcg/mL or more	4.85	485–3,395 μmol/L or more
Imipramine, therapeutic	100–300 ng/mL or mcg/L	3.57	357–1071 nmol/L
Immunoglobulin A (IgA)	85–385 mg/dL	0.01	0.85–3.85 g/L
Immunoglobulin G (IgG)	565–1,765 mg/dL	0.01	5.65–17.65 g/L
Immunoglobulin M (IgM)	53–375 mg/dL	0.01	0.53–3.75 g/L
Insulin (fasting)	2–20 microunits/mL or milliunits/L	7.175	14.35–143.5 pmol/L
International normalized ratio (INR), therapeutic	2.0–3.0 (2.5–3.5 for some indications)		
Iron			
Male	45–160 mcg/dL	0.179	8.1–31.3 μmol/L
Female	30–160 mcg/dL	0.179	5.4–31.3 μmol/L
Iron binding capacity (total)	220–420 mcg/dL	0.179	39.4–75.2 μmol/L
Iron saturation	15–50%	0.01	0.15–0.50
Lactate (plasma)	0.7–2.1 mEq/L	1	0.7–2.1 mmol/L
	6.3–18.9 mg/dL	0.111	
Lactate dehydrogenase	100–250 IU/L	0.01667	1.67–4.17 μkat/L
Lead	Less than 25 mcg/dL	0.0483	Less than 1.21 μmol/L
Leukocyte count	3.8–9.8 × 10³/μL	10⁶	3.8–9.8 μ10⁹/L
Lidocaine, therapeutic	1.5–6.0 mcg/mL or mg/L	4.27	6.4–25.6 μmol/L
Lipase	Less than 100 IU/L	0.01667	1.7 μkat/L
Lithium, therapeutic	0.5–1.25 mEq/L	1	0.5–1.25 mmol/L
Low-density lipoprotein (LDL) cholesterol			
Desirable	Less than 130 mg/dL	0.0259	Less than 3.36 mmol/L
Borderline high risk	130–159 mg/dL	0.0259	3.36–4.11 mmol/L
High risk	Greater than or equal to 160 mg/dL	0.0259	Greater than or equal to 4.13 mmol/L
Luteinizing hormone (LH)			
Male	1–8 milliunits/mL	1	1–8 units/L
Female			
Follicular phase	1–12 milliunits/mL	1	1–12 units/L
Midcycle	16–104 milliunits/mL	1	16–104 units/L
Luteal phase	1–12 milliunits/mL	1	1–12 units/L
Postmenopausal	16–66 milliunits/mL	1	16–66 units/L
Lymphocyte count	1.2–3.3 × 10³/μL	10⁶	1.2–3.3 × 10⁹/L
Magnesium	1.3–2.2 mEq/L	0.5	0.65–1.10 mmol/L
	1.58–2.68 mg/dL	0.411	0.65–1.10 mmol/L
Mean corpuscular volume	80.0–97.6 μm³	1	80.0–97.6 fL
Mononuclear cell count	0.2–0.7 × 10³/μL	10⁶	0.2–0.7 × 10⁹/L
Nortriptyline, therapeutic	50–150 ng/mL or mcg/L	3.8	190–570 nmol/L
NT-ProBNP (see Pro-BNP)			
Osmolality (serum)	275–300 mOsm/kg	1	275–300 mmol/kg
Osmolality (urine)	250–900 mOsm/kg	1	250–900 mmol/kg
Parathyroid hormone (PTH), intact	10–60 pg/mL or ng/L	0.107	1.1–6.4 pmol/L
Parathyroid hormone (PTH), N-terminal	8–24 pg/mL or ng/L		
Parathyroid hormone (PTH), C-terminal	50–330 pg/mL or ng/L		
Phenobarbital, therapeutic	15–40 mcg/mL or mg/L	4.31	65–172 μmol/L
Phenytoin, therapeutic	10–20 mcg/mL or mg/L	3.96	40–79 μmol/L
Phosphate	2.5–4.5 mg/dL	0.323	0.81–1.45 mmol/L
Platelet count	140–440 × 10³/μL	10⁶	140–440 × 10⁹/L
Potassium (plasma)	3.3–4.9 mEq/L	1	3.3–4.9 μmol/L
Prealbumin (adult)	19.5–35.8 mg/dL	10	195–358 mg/L
Primidone, therapeutic	5–12 mcg/mL or mg/L	4.58	23–55 μmol/L
ProBNP	Less than 125 pg/mL or ng/L	0.118	Less than 14.75 pmol/L
Procainamide, therapeutic	4–10 mcg/mL or mg/L	4.23	17–42 μmol/L

(continued)

Laboratory	Conventional Units	Conversion Factor	SI Units
Progesterone			
Male	13–97 ng/dL	0.0318	0.4–3.1 nmol/L
Female			
Follicular phase	15–70 ng/dL		0.5–2.2 nmol/L
Luteal phase	200–2,500 ng/dL		6.4–79.5 nmol/L
Prolactin	Less than 20 ng/mL	1	Less than 20 mcg/L
Prostate-specific antigen (PSA)	Less than 4 ng/mL	1	Less than 4 mcg/L
Protein, total	6.0–8.0 g/dL	10	60–80 g/L
Prothrombin time (PT)	10–12 sec		
Quinidine, therapeutic	2–5 mcg/mL or mg/L	3.08	6.2–15.4 μmol/L
Radioactive iodine uptake (RAIU)	Less than 6% in 2 hours		
Red blood cell (RBC) count (blood)			
Male	4–6.2 × 10^6/μL	10^6	4–6.2 × 10^{12}/L
Female	4–6.2 × 10^6/μL	10^6	4–6.2 × 10^{12}/L
Pregnant			
Trimester 1	4–5 × 10^6/μL	10^6	4–5 × 10^{12}/L
Trimester 2	3.2–4.5 × 10^6/μL	10^6	3.2–4.5 × 10^{12}/L
Trimester 3	3.0–4.9 × 10^6/μL	10^6	3.0–4.9 × 10^{12}/L
Postpartum	3.2–5 × 10^6/μL	10^6	3.2–5.0 × 10^6/L
Red blood cell distribution width (RDW)	11.5–14.5%	0.01	0.115–0.145
Reticulocyte count			
Male	0.5–1.5% of total RBC count	0.01	0.005–0.015
Female	0.5–2.5% of total RBC count	0.01	0.005–0.025
Retinol-binding protein (RBP)	2.7–7.6 mg/dL	10	27–76 mg/L
Rheumatoid factor (RF) titer	Negative		
Salicylate, therapeutic	150–300 mcg/mL or mg/L	0.00724	1.09–2.17 mmol/L
	15–30 mg/dL	0.0724	
Sodium	135–145 mEq/L	1	135–145 mmol/L
Tacrolimus			
Renal transplant	6–12 ng/mL or mcg/L		
Liver transplant	4–10 ng/mL or mcg/L		
Pancreatic transplant	10–18 ng/mL or mcg/L		
Bone marrow transplant	10–20 ng/mL or mcg/L		
Testosterone (total)			
Men	300–950 ng/dL	0.0347	10.4–33.0 nmol/L
Women	20–80 ng/dL		0.7–2.8 nmol/L
Testosterone (free)			
Men	9–30 ng/dL	0.0347	0.31–1.04 nmol/L
Women	0.3–1.9 ng/dL		0.01–0.07 nmol/L
Theophylline			
Therapeutic	5–15 mcg/mL or mg/L	5.55	28–83 μmol/L
Toxic	20 or more mcg/mL or mg/L	5.55	111 or more μmol/L
Thrombin time	20–24 sec		
Thyroglobulin	Less than 42 ng/mL	1	Less than 42 mcg/L
Thyroglobulin antibodies	Negative		
Thyroxine-binding globulin (TBG)	1.2–2.5 mg/dL	10	12–25 mcg/L
Thyroid-stimulating hormone (TSH)	0.35–6.20 microunits/mL	1	0.35–6.20 milliunits/L
TSH receptor antibodies (TSH Rab)	0–1 unit/mL		
Thyroxine (T_4)			
Total	4.5–12.0 mcg/dL	12.87	58–155 nmol/L
Free	0.7–1.9 ng/dL	12.87	9.0–24.5 pmol/L
Thyroxine index, free (FT_4I)	6.5–12.5		
TIBC See Iron-binding capacity (total)			
Tobramycin, therapeutic	4–10 mcg/mL or mg/L peak	2.14	8.6–21.4 μmol/L
	Less than or equal to 2 mcg/mL mg/L trough	2.14	Less than or equal to 4.28 μmol/L
Transferrin	200–430 mg/dL	0.01	2.0–4.3 g/L
Transferrin saturation	30–50%	0.01	0.30–0.50
Triglycerides (fasting)	Less than 160 mg/dL	0.0113	Less than 1.8 mmol/L
Triiodothyronine (T_3)	45–132 ng/dL	0.0154	0.91–2.70 nmol/L
Triiodothyronine (T_3) resin uptake	25–35%		
Troponin I	Less than 0.6 ng/mL	1	Less than 0.6 g/L
Uric acid	3–8 mg/dL	59.48	179–476 μmol/L
Urinalysis (urine)			
pH	4.8–8.0		
Specific gravity	1.005–1.030		

(continued)

Laboratory	Conventional Units	Conversion Factor	SI Units
Protein	Negative		
Glucose	Negative		
Ketones	Negative		
RBC	1–2 per low-power field		
WBC	3–4 per low-power field		
Valproic acid, therapeutic	50–100 mcg/mL or mg/L	6.93	346–693 μmol/L
Vancomycin, therapeutic trough for CNS infections	20–40 mcg/mL or mg/L peak	0.690	14–28 μmol/L peak
	5–20 mcg/mL or mg/L trough	0.690	3–14 μmol/L trough
	15–20 mcg/mL or mg/L trough	0.690	10–14 μmol/L trough
Vitamin A (retinol)	30–95 mcg/dL	0.0349	1.05–3.32 μmol/L
Vitamin B$_{12}$	180–1,000 pg/mL	0.738	133–738 pmol/L
Vitamin D$_3$, 1, 25-dihydroxy	20–76 pg/m	2.4	48–182 pmol/L
Vitamin D$_3$, 25-hydroxy	10–50 ng/mL	2.496	25–125 nmol/L
Vitamin E (alpha tocopherol)	0.5–2.0 mg/dL	23.22	12–46 μmol/L
WBC count	$4–10 \times 10^3/\mu L$ or $4–10 \times 10^3/mm^3$	10^6	$4–10 \times 10^9/L$
WBC differential (peripheral blood)			
Polymorphonuclear neutrophils (PMNs)	50–65%		
Bands	0–5%		
Eosinophils	0–3%		
Basophils	1–3%		
Lymphocytes	25–35%		
Monocytes	2–6%		
WBC differential (bone marrow)			
Polymorphonuclear neutrophils (PMNs)	3–11%		
Bands	9–15%		
Metamyelocytes	9–25%		
Myelocytes	8–16%		
Promyelocytes	1–8%		
Myeloblasts	0–5%		
Eosinophils	1–5%		
Basophils	0–1%		
Lymphocytes	11–23%		
Monocytes	0–1%		
Zinc	60–150 mcg/dL	0.153	9.2–23.0 μmol/L

This table was reprinted with permission from: Chisholm-Burns MA, Wells BG, Schwinghammer TL, et al. (eds). Pharmacotherapy Principles and Practice. New York, McGraw-Hill, 2008.

APPENDIX C
PART I: Common Medical Abbreviations

Note: Many of the medical abbreviations contained in Part I of this appendix are used in the Casebook. A more extensive list of abbreviations is available on the Internet at *www.medilexicon.com* and other sites.

A & O	Alert and oriented
A & P	Auscultation and percussion; anterior and posterior; assessment and plan
A & W	Alive and well
A1C	Hemoglobin A1C
aa	Of each (*ana*)
AA	Aplastic anemia; Alcoholics Anonymous
AAA	Abdominal aortic aneurysm
AAL	Anterior axillary line
AAO	Awake, alert, and oriented
AAP	American Academy of Pediatrics
ABC	Absolute band count; absolute basophil count; aspiration, biopsy, and cytology; artificial beta cells
Abd	Abdomen
ABG	Arterial blood gases
ABI	Ankle brachial index
ABP	Arterial blood pressure
ABW	Actual body weight
ABx	Antibiotics
AC	Before meals (*ante cibos*)
ACC	American College of Cardiology
ACE	Angiotensin-converting enzyme
ACEI	Angiotensin-converting enzyme inhibitor
ACG	American College of Gastroenterology
ACL	Anterior cruciate ligament
ACLS	Advanced cardiac life support
ACR	Albumin:creatinine ratio, American College of Rheumatology
ACS	Acute coronary syndrome
ACT	Activated clotting time
ACTH	Adrenocorticotropic hormone
AD	Alzheimer's disease, right ear (*auris dextra*)
ADA	American Diabetes Association; adenosine deaminase
ADE	Adverse drug effect (or event)
ADH	Antidiuretic hormone
ADHD	Attention-deficit hyperactivity disorder
ADL	Activities of daily living
ADR	Adverse drug reaction
AED	Antiepileptic drug(s)
AF	Atrial fibrillation
AFB	Acid-fast bacillus; aortofemoral bypass; aspirated foreign body
Afeb	Afebrile
AFP	α-Fetoprotein
A/G	Albumin–globulin ratio
AGA	American Gastoenterological Association
AGE	Acute viral gastroenteritis
AHA	American Heart Association
AI	Aortic insufficiency
AIDS	Acquired immunodeficiency syndrome
AKA	Above-knee amputation; alcoholic ketoacidosis; all known allergies; also known as
AKI	Acute kidney injury
ALD	Alcoholic liver disease
ALFT	Abnormal liver function test
ALK	Anaplastic lymphoma kinase
ALL	Acute lymphocytic leukemia; acute lymphoblastic leukemia
ALP	Alkaline phosphatase
ALS	Amyotrophic lateral sclerosis
ALT	Alanine aminotransferase
AMA	Against medical advice; American Medical Association; antimitochondrial antibody
AMI	Acute myocardial infarction
AML	Acute myelogenous leukemia
Amp	Ampule
AMPA	α-amino-3-hydroxy-5-methyl-4-isoxazolepropionic acid
ANA	Antinuclear antibody
ANC	Absolute neutrophil count
ANLL	Acute nonlymphocytic leukemia
Anti-CCP	Anticyclic citrullinated peptide
AODM	Adult onset diabetes mellitus
A & O × 3	Awake and oriented to person, place, and time
A & O × 4	Awake and oriented to person, place, time, and situation
AOM	Acute otitis media
AP	Anteroposterior
APACHE	Acute Physiology and Chronic Health Evaluation
APAP	Acetaminophen (*N*-acetyl-*p*-aminophenol)
aPTT	Activated partial thromboplastin time
ARB	Angiotensin receptor blocker
ARC	AIDS-related complex
ARDS	Adult respiratory distress syndrome
ARF	Acute renal failure; acute respiratory failure; acute rheumatic fever
AROM	Active range of motion
AS	Left ear (*auris sinistra*)
ASA	Aspirin (acetylsalicylic acid)
ASCVD	Atherosclerotic cardiovascular disease
ASD	Atrial septal defect
ASH	Asymmetric septal hypertrophy
ASHD	Arteriosclerotic heart disease
AST	Aspartate aminotransferase
ATG	Antithymocyte globulin
ATN	Acute tubular necrosis
AU	Each ear (*auris uterque*)
AV	Arteriovenous; atrioventricular
AVM	Arteriovenous malformation
AVR	Aortic valve replacement

AWMI	Anterior wall myocardial infarction
BAC	Blood alcohol concentration
BAL	Bronchioalveolar lavage
BBB	Bundle branch block; blood–brain barrier
BC	Blood culture
BCACP	Board Certified Ambulatory Care Pharmacist
BCG	Bacillus Calmette Guerin
BCNP	Board Certified Nuclear Pharmacist
BCNSP	Board Certified Nutrition Support Pharmacist
BCNU	Carmustine
BCOP	Board Certified Oncology Pharmacist
BCP	Birth control pill
BCPP	Board Certified Psychiatric Pharmacist
BCPS	Board Certified Pharmacotherapy Specialist
BCR-ABL	Breakpoint cluster region-Abelson
BE	Barium enema
BID	Twice daily (*bis in die*)
BKA	Below-knee amputation
BM	Bone marrow; bowel movement
BMC	Bone marrow cells
BMD	Bone mineral density
BMR	Basal metabolic rate
BMT	Bone marrow transplantation
BNP	Brain natriuretic peptide
BP	Blood pressure
BPD	Bronchopulmonary dysplasia
BPH	Benign prostatic hyperplasia
bpm	Beats per minute
BPRS	Brief Psychiatric Rating Scale
BR	Bedrest
BRBPR	Bright red blood per rectum
BRM	Biological response modifier
BRP	Bathroom privileges
BS	Bowel sounds; breath sounds; blood sugar
BSA	Body surface area
BSO	Bilateral salpingo-oophorectomy
BTFS	Breast tumor frozen section
BUN	Blood urea nitrogen
BV	Bacterial vaginosis
Bx	Biopsy
C & S	Culture and sensitivity
CA	Cancer; calcium
CABG	Coronary artery bypass graft
CAD	Coronary artery disease
CAH	Chronic active hepatitis
CAM	Complementary and alternative medicine
CAPD	Continuous ambulatory peritoneal dialysis
CAT	COPD Assessment Test
CBC	Complete blood count
CBD	Common bile duct
CBG	Capillary blood gas; corticosteroid binding globulin
CBT	Cognitive-behavioral therapy
CC	Chief complaint
CCA	Calcium channel antagonist
CCB	Calcium channel blocker
CCE	Clubbing, cyanosis, edema
CCK	Cholecystokinin
CCMS	Clean catch midstream
CCNU	Lomustine
CCPD	Continuous cycling peritoneal dialysis
CCT	Central corneal thickness
CCU	Coronary care unit
CD	Crohn's disease

CDAD	*Clostridium difficile*-associated diarrhea
CDC	Centers for Disease Control and Prevention
CEA	Carcinoembryonic antigen
CF	Cystic fibrosis
CFS	Chronic fatigue syndrome
CFU	Colony-forming unit
CHD	Coronary heart disease
CHF	Congestive heart failure
CHO	Carbohydrate
CHOP	Cyclophosphamide, hydroxydaunorubicin (doxorubicin), Oncovin (vincristine), prednisone
CI	Cardiac index
CK	Creatine kinase
CKD	Chronic kidney disease
CKD-EPI	Chronic Kidney Disease—Epidemiology Collaboration
CKD-MBD	Chronic kidney disease—mineral and bone disorder
CLcr	Creatinine clearance
CLL	Chronic lymphocytic leukemia
CM	Costal margin
CMG	Cystometrogram
CML	Chronic myelogenous leukemia
CMV	Cytomegalovirus
CN	Cranial nerve
CNS	Central nervous system
c/o	Complains of
CO	Cardiac output; carbon monoxide
COC	Combined oral contraceptive
COLD	Chronic obstructive lung disease
COMT	Catechol-*O*-methyl transferase
COPD	Chronic obstructive pulmonary disease
CP	Chest pain; cerebral palsy
CPA	Costophrenic angle
CPAP	Continuous positive airway pressure
CPK	Creatine phosphokinase
CPP	Cerebral perfusion pressure
CPR	Cardiopulmonary resuscitation
CR	Complete remission
CRF	Chronic renal failure; corticotropin-releasing factor
CRH	Corticotropin-releasing hormone
CRI	Chronic renal insufficiency; catheter-related infection
CRNA	Certified Registered Nurse Anesthetist
CRNP	Certified Registered Nurse Practitioner
CRP	C-reactive protein
CRTT	Certified Respiratory Therapy Technician
CS	Central Supply
CSA	Cyclosporine
CSC	Corrected serum calcium
CSF	Cerebrospinal fluid; colony-stimulating factor
CSW	Cerebral salt wasting
CT	Computed tomography; chest tube
CTA	Clear to auscultation
CTB	Cease to breathe
cTnI	Cardiac troponin I
CTZ	Chemoreceptor trigger zone
CV	Cardiovascular
CVA	Cerebrovascular accident; costovertebral angle
CVAT	Costovertebral angle tenderness
CVC	Central venous catheter
CVP	Central venous pressure
CVVH-DF	Continuous venovenous hemodiafiltration
Cx	Culture; cervix
CXR	Chest x-ray

CYP	Cytochrome P-450 enzymes
D & C	Dilatation and curettage
d4T	Stavudine
D$_5$NS	5% Dextrose in normal saline
D$_5$W5	% Dextrose in water
DAA	Direct acting antivirals
DAS	Disease activity score
DBP	Diastolic blood pressure
D/C	Discontinue; discharge
DCC	Direct current cardioversion
ddC	Zalcitabine
ddI	Didanosine
DES	Diethylstilbestrol
DEXA	Dual-energy X-ray absorptiometry
DI	Diabetes insipidus
DIC	Disseminated intravascular coagulation
Diff	Differential
DIOS	Distal intestinal obstruction syndrome
DIP	Distal interphalangeal
DJD	Degenerative joint disease
DKA	Diabetic ketoacidosis
DKD	Diabetic kidney disease
dL	Deciliter
DM	Diabetes mellitus
DMARD	Disease-modifying antirheumatic drug
DNA	Deoxyribonucleic acid
DNR	Do not resuscitate
DO	Doctor of Osteopathy
DOA	Dead on arrival; date of admission; duration of action
DOAC	Direct oral anticoagulant (also see NOAC)
DOB	Date of birth
DOE	Dyspnea on exertion
DOT	Directly observed therapy
DP	Dorsalis pedis
DPGN	Diffuse proliferative glomerulonephritis
DPI	Dry powder inhaler
DRE	Digital rectal examination
DRG	Diagnosis-related group
DRSP	Daily record of severity of problem
DS	Double strength
DSM	Diagnostic and Statistical Manual of Mental Disorders
DSHEA	Dietary Supplement Health and Education Act (1994)
DST	Dexamethasone suppression test
DTIC	Dacarbazine
DTP	Diphtheria-tetanus-pertussis
DTR	Deep-tendon reflex
DVT	Deep-vein thrombosis
Dx	Diagnosis
DXA	Dual-energy X-ray absorptiometry (DEXA)
eAG	Estimated average glucose
EBL	Endoscopic band ligation
EBV	Epstein-Barr virus
EC	Enteric-coated
ECF	Extended care facility
ECG	Electrocardiogram
ECMO	Extracorporeal membrane oxygenator
ECOG	Eastern Cooperative Oncology Group
ECT	Electroconvulsive therapy
ED	Emergency Department
EEG	Electroencephalogram
EENT	Eyes, ears, nose, throat
EF	Ejection fraction

EGD	Esophagogastroduodenoscopy
EGFR	Epidermal growth factor receptor
EIA	Enzyme immunoassay
EKG	Electrocardiogram
EMG	Electromyogram
EML4-ALK	Echinoderm microtubule–associated protein-like 4–anaplastic lymphoma kinase
EMS	Emergency medical services
EMT	Emergency medical technician
Endo	Endotracheal; endoscopy
EOMI	Extraocular movements (or muscles) intact
EPO	Erythropoietin
EPS	Extrapyramidal symptoms
EPT	Early pregnancy test; expedited partner therapy
ER	Estrogen receptor; emergency room
ERCP	Endoscopic retrograde cholangiopancreatography
ERT	Estrogen replacement therapy
ESKD	End-stage kidney disease
ESLD	End-stage liver disease
ESA	Erythropoiesis-stimulating agent
ESR	Erythrocyte sedimentation rate
ESRD	End-stage renal disease
ESWL	Extracorporeal shockwave lithotripsy
ET	Endotracheal
ETOH	Ethanol
EVL	Endoscopic variceal ligation
FB	Finger-breadth; foreign body
FBDSI	Functional Bowel Disorder Severity Index
FBS	Fasting blood sugar
FDA	Food and Drug Administration
FDC	Fixed dose combinations
FDP	Fibrin degradation products
FEF	Forced expiratory flow (rate)
FEM-POP	Femoral-popliteal
FE$_{NA}$	Fractional excretion of sodium
FEV$_1$	Forced expiratory volume in 1 second
FFP	Fresh frozen plasma
FH	Family history
FiO$_2$	Fraction of inspired oxygen
FISH	Fluorescence in situ hybridization
fL	Femtoliter
FM	Face mask
FOBT	Fecal occult blood test
FOC	Fronto-occipital circumference
FODMAPs	Fermentable oligo-, di- and monosaccharides and polyols
FOI	Flight of ideas
FPG	Fasting plasma glucose
FPIA	Fluorescence polarization immunoassay
FRAX	Fracture Risk Assessment Tool
FSH	Follicle-stimulating hormone
FTA	Fluorescent treponemal antibody
f/u	Follow-up
FUDR	Floxuridine
FUO	Fever of unknown origin
Fx	Fracture
G6PD	Glucose-6-phosphate dehydrogenase
GABA	γ-aminobutyric acid
GABHS	Group A beta-hemolytic streptococcus
GAD	Generalized anxiety disorder
GB	Gallbladder
GBS	Group B *Streptococcus*; Guillain–Barré syndrome
GC	Gonococcus

G-CSF	Granulocyte colony-stimulating factor
GDM	Gestational diabetes mellitus
GE	Gastroesophageal; gastroenterology
GERD	Gastroesophageal reflux disease
GFR	Glomerular filtration rate
GGT	γ-Glutamyltransferase
GGTP	γ-Glutamyl transpeptidase
GI	Gastrointestinal
GM-CSF	Granulocyte-macrophage colony-stimulating factor
GN	Glomerulonephritis; graduate nurse
gr	Grain
GT	Gastrostomy tube
gtt	Drops (*guttae*)
GTT	Glucose tolerance test
GU	Gastric ulcer, genitourinary
GVHD	Graft-versus-host disease
GVL	Graft-versus-leukemia
Gyn	Gynecology
H & H	Hemoglobin and hematocrit
H & P	History and physical examination
HA or H/A	Headache
HAART	Highly active antiretroviral therapy
HAM-D	Hamilton Rating Scale for Depression
HAV	Hepatitis A virus
Hb, hgb	Hemoglobin
HbA$_{1C}$	Hemoglobin A1C
HBeAg	Hepatitis B early antigen
HBIG	Hepatitis B immune globulin
HBP	High blood pressure
HBsAg	Hepatitis B surface antigen
HBV	Hepatitis B virus
HC	Hydrocortisone; home care
HCC	Hepatocellular carcinoma
HCG	Human chorionic gonadotropin
HCM	Hypercalcemia of malignancy
HCO$_3$	Bicarbonate
Hct	Hematocrit
HCTZ	Hydrochlorothiazide
HCV	Hepatitis C virus
Hcy	Homocysteine
HD	Hodgkin's disease; hemodialysis
HDL	High-density lipoprotein
HE	Hepatic encephalopathy
HEC	High-emetic-risk chemotherapy
HEENT	Head, eyes, ears, nose, and throat
HEPA	High-efficiency particulate air
HF	Heart failure
HFA	Hydrofluoroalkane
H. flu	*Haemophilus influenzae*
HGH	Human growth hormone
HH	Hiatal hernia
HHS	Hyperosmolar hyperglycemic state
Hib	*Haemophilus influenzae* type b
HIV	Human immunodeficiency virus
HJR	Hepatojugular reflux
HL	Hodgkin lymphoma
HLA	Human leukocyte antigen; human lymphocyte antigen
HMG-CoA	Hydroxy-methylglutaryl coenzyme A
H/O	History of
HOB	Head of bed
HPA	Hypothalamic–pituitary axis
HPF	High-power field

HPI	History of present illness
HPV	Human papilloma virus
HR	Heart rate
HRQOL	Health-related quality of life
HRT	Hormone replacement therapy
HS	At bedtime (*hora somni*)
HSCT	Hematopoietic stem cell transplantation
HSM	Hepatosplenomegaly
HSV	Herpes simplex virus
HTN	Hypertension
HVPG	Hepatic venous pressure gradient
Hx	History
I & D	Incision and drainage
I & O	Intake and output
IABP	Intra-arterial balloon pump
IBD	Inflammatory bowel disease
IBS	Irritable bowel syndrome
IBS-C	Irritable bowel syndrome with constipation
IBS-D	Irritable bowel syndrome with diarrhea
IBS-SSS	Irritable Bowel Syndrome Symptom Severity Score
IBW	Ideal body weight
ICD	Implantable cardioverter defibrillator
ICP	Intracranial pressure
ICS	Intercostal space
ICU	Intensive care unit
ID	Identification; infectious disease
IDDM	Insulin-dependent diabetes mellitus
IFN	Interferon
Ig	Immunoglobulin
IgA	Immunoglobulin A
IgD	Immunoglobulin D
IHC	Immunohistochemistry
IHD	Ischemic heart disease
IJ	Internal jugular
IM	Intramuscular; infectious mononucleosis
IMV	Intermittent mandatory ventilation
INH	Isoniazid
INR	International normalized ratio
IOP	Intraocular pressure
IOR	Ideas of reference
IP	Intraperitoneal
IPG	Impedance plethysmography
IPI	International prognostic index
IPN	Interstitial pneumonia
IPPB	Intermittent positive pressure breathing
IPS	Idiopathic pneumonia syndrome
IRB	Institutional Review Board
ISA	Intrinsic sympathomimetic activity
ISDN	Isosorbide dinitrate
ISH	Isolated systolic hypertension
ISMN	Isosorbide mononitrate
IT	Intrathecal
ITP	Idiopathic thrombocytopenic purpura
IU	International unit
IUD	Intrauterine device
IV	Intravenous; Roman numeral IV; symbol for Class 4 controlled substances
IVC	Inferior vena cava; intravenous cholangiogram
IVDA	Intravenous drug abuse
IVF	Intravenous fluids
IVIG	Intravenous immunoglobulin
IVP	Intravenous pyelogram; intravenous push
IVPB	Intravenous piggyback

IVSS	Intravenous Soluset
IWMI	Inferior wall myocardial infarction
JODM	Juvenile-onset diabetes mellitus
JRA	Juvenile rheumatoid arthritis
JVD	Jugular venous distention
JVP	Jugular venous pressure
K	Potassium
kcal	Kilocalorie
KCL	Potassium chloride
KDIGO	Kidney Disease: Improving Global Outcomes
KOH	Potassium hydroxide
KRAS	Kirsten rat sarcoma viral oncogene homolog
KUB	Kidney, ureters, bladder
KVO	Keep vein open
L	Liter
LAD	Left anterior descending; left axis deviation
LAO	Left anterior oblique
LAP	Leukocyte alkaline phosphatase
LBBB	Left bundle branch block
LBP	Low back pain
LCM	Left costal margin
LDH	Lactate dehydrogenase
LDL	Low-density lipoprotein
LE	Lower extremity
LES	Lower esophageal sphincter
LFT	Liver function test
LHRH	Luteinizing hormone-releasing hormone
LIMA	Left internal mammary artery
LLE	Left lower extremity
LLL	Left lower lobe
LLQ	Left lower quadrant (abdomen)
LLSB	Left lower sternal border
LMD	Local medical doctor
LMP	Last menstrual period
LMWH	Low molecular weight heparin
LOA	Looseness of association
LOC	Loss of consciousness; laxative of choice
LOS	Length of stay
LP	Lumbar puncture
LPF	Low-power field
LPN	Licensed practical nurse
LPO	Left posterior oblique
LPT	Licensed physical therapist
LR	Lactated Ringer's
LS	Lumbosacral
LTCF	Long-term care facility
LUE	Left upper extremity
LUL	Left upper lobe
LUQ	Left upper quadrant
LVEF	Left ventricular ejection fraction
LVH	Left ventricular hypertrophy
MAOI	Monoamine oxidase inhibitor
MAP	Mean arterial pressure
MAR	Medication administration record
mcg	Microgram
MCH	Mean corpuscular hemoglobin
MCHC	Mean corpuscular hemoglobin concentration
MCL	Midclavicular line
MCP	Metacarpophalangeal
MCV	Mean corpuscular volume
MD	Medical doctor
MDI	Metered-dose inhaler
MDRD	Modified Diet in Renal Disease

MEFR	Maximum expiratory flow rate
mEq	Milliequivalent
mg	Milligram
MHC	Major histocompatibility complex
MI	Myocardial infarction; mitral insufficiency
MIC	Minimum inhibitory concentration
MICU	Medical intensive care unit
MIDAS	Migraine Disability Assessment
mL	Milliliter
MM	Multiple myeloma
MMA	Methylmalonic acid
MMEFR	Maximal midexpiratory flow rate
MMR	Measles-mumps-rubella
MMSE	Mini mental state examination
MOM	Milk of magnesia
MoCA	Montreal Cognitive Assessment
MPV	Mean platelet volume
MRG	Murmur/rub/gallop
MRI	Magnetic resonance imaging
MRSA	Methicillin-resistant *Staphylococcus aureus*
MRSE	Methicillin-resistant *Staphylococcus epidermidis*
MS	Mental status; mitral stenosis; musculoskeletal; multiple sclerosis; morphine sulfate
MSE	Mental status exam
MSM	Men who have sex with men
MSW	Master of social work
MTD	Maximum tolerated dose
MTP	Metatarsophalangeal
MTX	Methotrexate
MUD	Matched unrelated donor
MUGA	Multiple gated acquisition
MVA	Motor vehicle accident
MVI	Multivitamin
MVR	Mitral valve replacement; mitral valve regurgitation
MVS	Mitral valve stenosis; motor, vascular, and sensory
NAAT	Nucleic acid amplification test
NAD	No acute (or apparent) distress
NAFLD	Nonalcoholic fatty liver disease
NASH	Nonalcoholic steatohepatitis
N/C	Noncontributory; nasal cannula
NC/AT	Normocephalic/atraumatic
NDDI-E	Neurological Disorders Depression Inventory for Epilepsy
NG	Nasogastric
NGT	Nasogastric tube
NGTD	No growth to date (on culture)
NHL	Non-Hodgkin's lymphoma
NIDDM	Non–insulin-dependent diabetes mellitus
NIH	National Institutes of Health
NKA	No known allergies
NKDA	No known drug allergies
NL	Normal
NMDA	*N*-methyl-D-aspartate
NNRTI	Nonnucleoside reverse transcriptase inhibitor
NOAC	Nonwarfarin (also New, Novel, or Non-vitamin K) oral anticoagulant
NOS	Not otherwise specified
NPH	Neutral protamine Hagedorn; normal pressure hydrocephalus
NPN	Nonprotein nitrogen
NPO	Nothing by mouth (*nil per os*)
NRAS	Neuroblastoma RAS viral (v-ras) oncogene homolog
NRTI	Nucleoside reverse transcriptase inhibitor

NS	Neurosurgery; normal saline
NSAID	Nonsteroidal antiinflammatory drug
NSCLC	Nonsmall cell lung cancer
NSR	Normal sinus rhythm
NSS	Normal saline solution
NSVD	Normal spontaneous vaginal delivery
NTG	Nitroglycerin
NT/ND	Nontender/nondistended
N/V	Nausea and vomiting
NVD	Nausea/vomiting/diarrhea; neck vein distention; nonvalvular disease; neovascularization of the disk
NYHA	New York Heart Association
O & P	Ova and parasites
OA	Osteoarthritis
OB	Obstetrics
OBS	Organic brain syndrome
OCD	Obsessive–compulsive disorder
OCG	Oral cholecystogram
OCT	Ocular coherence tomography
OD	Right eye (*oculus dexter*); overdose; Doctor of Optometry
OGT	Oral glucose tolerance test
OHTx	Orthotopic heart transplantation
OIH	Opioid-induced hyperalgesia
OLTx	Orthotopic liver transplantation
OME	Otitis media with effusion
ONJ	Osteonecrosis of the jaw
OOB	Out of bed
OPD	Outpatient department
OPG	Ocular plethysmography
OPV	Oral poliovirus vaccine
OR	Operating room
ORT	Oral rehydration therapy
OS	Left eye (*oculus sinister*)
OSA	Obstructive sleep apnea
OT	Occupational therapy
OTC	Over-the-counter
OU	Each eye (*oculus uterque*)
P	Pulse, plan, percussion, pressure
P & A	Percussion and auscultation
P & T	Peak and trough
PA	Physician assistant; posterior–anterior; pulmonary artery
PAC	Premature atrial contraction
PaCO$_2$	Arterial carbon dioxide tension
PAH	Pulmonary arterial hypertension
PaO$_2$	Arterial oxygen tension
PAOP	Pulmonary artery occlusion pressure
PARP	Poly ADP ribose polymerase
PAT	Paroxysmal atrial tachycardia
PBI	Protein-bound iodine
PBSCT	Peripheral blood stem cell transplantation
PC	After meals (*post cibum*)
PCA	Patient-controlled analgesia
PCI	Percutaneous coronary intervention
PCKD	Polycystic kidney disease
PCN	Penicillin
PCOS	Polycystic ovarian syndrome
PCP	Primary care physician; phencyclidine; *Pneumocystis (carinii) jiroveci* pneumonia
PCWP	Pulmonary capillary wedge pressure
PDA	Patent ductus arteriosus
PDE	Phosphodiesterase

PE	Physical examination; pulmonary embolism
PEEP	Positive end-expiratory pressure
PEFR	Peak expiratory flow rate
PEG	Percutaneous endoscopic gastrostomy; polyethylene glycol
PERLA	Pupils equal, react to light and accommodation
PERRLA	Pupils equal, round, and reactive to light and accommodation
PET	Positron emission tomography
PFT	Pulmonary function test
pH	Hydrogen ion concentration
PharmD	Doctor of Pharmacy
PHQ	Patient health questionnaire
PI	Principal investigator; protease inhibitor
PICC	Peripherally inserted central catheter
PID	Pelvic inflammatory disease
PIP	Proximal interphalangeal
PKU	Phenylketonuria
PMD	Private medical doctor
PMH	Past medical history
PMI	Point of maximal impulse
PMN	Polymorphonuclear leukocyte
PMS	Premenstrual syndrome
PNC-E	Postnecrotic cirrhosis-ethanol
PND	Paroxysmal nocturnal dyspnea
PNH	Paroxysmal nocturnal hemoglobinuria
po	By mouth (*per os*)
POAG	Primary open-angle glaucoma
POD	Postoperative day
POS	Polycystic ovarian syndrome
PP	Patient profile
PPBG	Postprandial blood glucose
ppd	Packs per day
PPD	Purified protein derivative
PPE	Personal protective equipment
PPH	Past psychiatric history
PPI	Proton pump inhibitor
PPN	Peripheral parenteral nutrition
pr	Per rectum
PR	Progesterone receptor; partial remission
PRA	Panel-reactive antibody; plasma renin activity
PRBC	Packed red blood cells
PRN	When necessary; as needed (*pro re nata*)
PSA	Prostate-specific antigen
PSCT	Peripheral stem cell transplant
PSE	Portal systemic encephalopathy
PSH	Past surgical history
PSVT	Paroxysmal supraventricular tachycardia
PT	Prothrombin time; physical therapy; patient; posterior tibial
PTA	Prior to admission
PTCA	Percutaneous transluminal coronary angioplasty
PTE	Pulmonary thromboembolism
PTH	Parathyroid hormone
PTHrP	Parathyroid hormone-related peptide
PTSD	Posttraumatic stress disorder
PTT	Partial thromboplastin time
PTU	Propylthiouracil
PUD	Peptic ulcer disease
PVC	Premature ventricular contraction
PVD	Peripheral vascular disease
Q	Every (*quaque*)
QA	Quality assurance

QD	Every day (*quaque die*)	SBGM	Self blood glucose monitoring
QI	Quality improvement	SBO	Small bowel obstruction
QID	Four times daily (*quater in die*)	SBP	Systolic blood pressure; spontaneous bacterial peritonitis
QNS	Quantity not sufficient		
QOD	Every other day	SC	Subcutaneous; subclavian
QOL	Quality of life	SCID	Severe combined immunodeficiency
QOLIE	Quality of Life in Epilepsy	SCLC	Small cell lung cancer
QS	Quantity sufficient	SCr	Serum creatinine
R & M	Routine and microscopic	SDP	Single donor platelets
RA	Rheumatoid arthritis; right atrium	SEM	Systolic ejection murmur
RADT	Rapid antigen detection test	SG	Specific gravity
RAIU	Radioactive iodine uptake	SGOT	Serum glutamic oxaloacetic transaminase
RANKL	Receptor activator of nuclear factor-κβ ligand	SCT	Stem cell transplantation
RAO	Right anterior oblique	SGPT	Serum glutamic pyruvic transaminase
RBBB	Right bundle branch block	SH	Social history
RBC	Red blood cell	SIADH	Syndrome of inappropriate antidiuretic hormone secretion
RCA	Right coronary artery		
RCM	Right costal margin	SIDS	Sudden infant death syndrome
RDA	Recommended daily allowance	SIMV	Synchronized intermittent mandatory ventilation
RDP	Random donor platelets	SIRS	Systemic inflammatory response syndrome
RDS	Respiratory distress syndrome	SJS	Stevens–Johnson syndrome
RDW	Red cell distribution width	SL	Sublingual
REM	Rapid eye movement	SLE	Systemic lupus erythematosus
RES	Reticuloendothelial system	SMBG	Self-monitoring of blood glucose
RF	Rheumatoid factor; renal failure; rheumatic fever	SNF	Skilled nursing facility
Rh	Rhesus factor in blood	SNRI	Serotonin–norepinephrine reuptake inhibitor
RHD	Rheumatic heart disease	SNS	Sympathetic nervous system
RLE	Right lower extremity	SOS	Sinusoidal obstruction syndrome
RLL	Right lower lobe	SOB	Shortness of breath; side of bed
RLQ	Right lower quadrant (abdomen)	S/P	Status post
RLS	Restless legs syndrome	SPEP	Serum protein electrophoresis
RML	Right middle lobe	SPF	Sun protection factor
RN	Registered nurse	SPS	Sodium polystyrene sulfonate
RNA	Ribonucleic acid	SRI	Serotonin reuptake inhibitor
R/O	Rule out	SRMD	Stress-related mucosal damage
ROM	Range of motion	SSKI	Saturated solution of potassium iodide
ROS	Review of systems	SSRI	Selective serotonin reuptake inhibitor
RPGN	Rapidly progressive glomerulonephritis	STAT	Immediately; at once
RPh	Registered pharmacist	STD	Sexually transmitted disease
RPR	Rapid plasma reagin	STI	Sexually transmitted infection
RR	Respiratory rate; recovery room	SUP	Stress ulcer prophylaxis
RRR	Regular rate and rhythm	SV	Stroke volume
RRT	Registered respiratory therapist	SVC	Superior vena cava
RSV	Respiratory syncytial virus	SVR	Supraventricular rhythm; systemic vascular resistance
RT	Radiation therapy	SVRI	Systemic vascular resistance index
RTA	Renal tubular acidosis	SVT	Supraventricular tachycardia
RTC	Return to clinic	SW	Social worker
RT-PCR	Reverse transcriptase-polymerase chain reaction	SWI	Surgical wound infection
RUE	Right upper extremity	Sx	Symptoms
RUL	Right upper lobe	T	Temperature
RUQ	Right upper quadrant (abdomen)	T & A	Tonsillectomy and adenoidectomy
RVH	Right ventricular hypertrophy	T & C	Type and crossmatch
S_1	First heart sound	TAH	Total abdominal hysterectomy
S_2	Second heart sound	TB	Tuberculosis
S_3	Third heart sound (ventricular gallop)	TBG	Thyroid-binding globulin
S_4	Fourth heart sound (atrial gallop)	TBI	Total body irradiation; traumatic brain injury
SA	Sinoatrial	T. bili	Total bilirubin
SAAG	Serum ascites–albumin gradient	T/C	To consider
SAD	Seasonal affective disorder	TCA	Tricyclic antidepressant
SAH	Subarachnoid hemorrhage	TCN	Tetracycline
SaO_2	Arterial oxygen percent saturation	TED	Thromboembolic disease
SBE	Subacute bacterial endocarditis	TEE	Transesophageal echocardiogram
SBFT	Small bowel follow-through	TEN	Toxic epidermal necrolysis

TENS	Transcutaneous electrical nerve stimulation
TFT	Thyroid function test
TG	Triglyceride
THA	Total hip arthroplasty
THC	Tetrahydrocannabinol
TIA	Transient ischemic attack
TIBC	Total iron-binding capacity
TID	Three times daily (*ter in die*)
TIH	Tumor-induced hypercalcemia
TIPS	Transjugular intrahepatic portosystemic shunt
TKA	Total knee arthroplasty
TKI	Tyrosine kinase inhibitor
TLC	Therapeutic lifestyle changes
TLI	Total lymphoid irradiation
TLS	Tumor lysis syndrome
TM	Tympanic membrane
TMJ	Temporomandibular joint
TMP/SMX	Trimethoprim-sulfamethoxazole
TMs	Tympanic membranes
TNF	Tumor necrosis factor
TnI	Troponin I (cardiac)
TnT	Troponin T
TNTC	Too numerous to count
TOD	Target organ damage
TPN	Total parenteral nutrition
TPR	Temperature, pulse, respiration
T. prot	Total protein
TSH	Thyroid-stimulating hormone
TSS	Toxic shock syndrome
TTP	Thrombotic thrombocytopenic purpura
TUIP	Transurethral incision of the prostate
TURP	Transurethral resection of the prostate
Tx	Treat; treatment
UA	Urinalysis; uric acid
UC	Ulcerative colitis
UCD	Usual childhood diseases
UDS	Urine drug screen
UE	Upper extremity

UFC	Urinary free cortisol
UFH	Unfractionated heparin
UGI	Upper gastrointestinal
UOQ	Upper outer quadrant
UPDRS	Unified Parkinson's Disease Rating Scale
UPT	Urine pregnancy test
URI	Upper respiratory infection
USP	United States Pharmacopeia
UTI	Urinary tract infection
UV	Ultraviolet
VA	Veterans' Affairs
VAMC	Veterans' Affairs Medical Center
VBL	Variceal band ligation
VDRL	Venereal Disease Research Laboratory
VF	Ventricular fibrillation
VL	Viral load
VLDL	Very low-density lipoprotein
VNA	Visiting Nurses' Association
VO	Verbal order
VOD	Veno-occlusive disease
VP-16	Etoposide
V_A/Q	Ventilation/perfusion
VRE	Vancomycin-resistant *Enterococcus*
VS	Vital signs
VSS	Vital signs stable
VT	Ventricular tachycardia
VTE	Venous thromboembolism
WA	While awake
WBC	White blood cell
W/C	Wheelchair
WDWN	Well-developed, well-nourished
WHO	World Health Organization
WNL	Within normal limits
W/U	Work-up
Y-BOCS	Yale-Brown Obsessive–Compulsive Scale
yo	Year-old
yr	Year
ZDV	Zidovudine

PART II: Prevent Medication Errors by Avoiding These Dangerous Abbreviations, Symbols, and Dose Designations

Institute for Safe Medication Practices

ISMP'S LIST OF *ERROR-PRONE ABBREVIATIONS, SYMBOLS,* AND *DOSE DESIGNATIONS*

The abbreviations, symbols, and dose designations found in this table have been reported to ISMP through the ISMP National Medication Errors Reporting Program (ISMP MERP) as being frequently misinterpreted and involved in harmful medication errors. They should **NEVER** be used when communicating medical information. This includes internal communications, telephone/verbal prescriptions, computer-generated labels, labels for drug storage bins, medication administration records, as well as pharmacy and prescriber computer order entry screens.

Abbreviations	Intended Meaning	Misinterpretation	Correction
μg	Microgram	Mistaken as "mg"	Use "mcg"
AD, AS, AU	Right ear, left ear, each ear	Mistaken as OD, OS, OU (right eye, left eye, each eye)	Use "right ear," "left ear," or "each ear"
OD, OS, OU	Right eye, left eye, each eye	Mistaken as AD, AS, AU (right ear, left ear, each ear)	Use "right eye," "left eye," or "each eye"
BT	Bedtime	Mistaken as "BID" (twice daily)	Use "bedtime"
cc	Cubic centimeters	Mistaken as "u" (units)	Use "mL"
D/C	Discharge or discontinue	Premature discontinuation of medications if D/C (intended to mean "discharge") has been misinterpreted as "discontinued" when followed by a list of discharge medications	Use "discharge" and "discontinue"
IJ	Injection	Mistaken as "IV" or "intrajugular"	Use "injection"
IN	Intranasal	Mistaken as "IM" or "IV"	Use "intranasal" or "NAS"
HS	Half-strength	Mistaken as bedtime	Use "half-strength" or "bedtime"
hs	At bedtime, hours of sleep	Mistaken as half-strength	
IU**	International unit	Mistaken as IV (intravenous) or 10 (ten)	Use "units"
o.d. or OD	Once daily	Mistaken as "right eye" (OD-oculus dexter), leading to oral liquid medications administered in the eye	Use "daily"
OJ	Orange juice	Mistaken as OD or OS (right or left eye); drugs meant to be diluted in orange juice may be given in the eye	Use "orange juice"
Per os	By mouth, orally	The "os" can be mistaken as "left eye" (OS-oculus sinister)	Use "PO," "by mouth," or "orally"
q.d. or QD**	Every day	Mistaken as q.i.d., especially if the period after the "q" or the tail of the "q" is misunderstood as an "i"	Use "daily"
qhs	Nightly at bedtime	Mistaken as "qhr" or every hour	Use "nightly"
qn	Nightly or at bedtime	Mistaken as "qh" (every hour)	Use "nightly" or "at bedtime"
q.o.d. or QOD**	Every other day	Mistaken as "q.d." (daily) or "q.i.d." (four times daily) if the "o" is poorly written	Use "every other day"
q1d	Daily	Mistaken as q.i.d. (four times daily)	Use "daily"
q6PM, etc.	Every evening at 6 PM	Mistaken as every 6 hours	Use "daily at 6 PM" or "6 PM daily"
SC, SQ, sub q	Subcutaneous	SC mistaken as SL (sublingual); SQ mistaken as "5 every;" the "q" in "sub q" has been mistaken as "every" (eg, a heparin dose ordered "sub q 2 hours before surgery" misunderstood as every 2 hours before surgery)	Use "subcut" or "subcutaneously"
ss	Sliding scale (insulin) or ½ (apothecary)	Mistaken as "55"	Spell out "sliding scale;" use "one-half" or "½"
SSRI	Sliding scale regular insulin	Mistaken as selective-serotonin reuptake inhibitor	Spell out "sliding scale (insulin)"
SSI	Sliding scale insulin	Mistaken as Strong Solution of Iodine (Lugol's)	
i/d	One daily	Mistaken as "tid"	Use "1 daily"
TIW or tiw	3 times a week	Mistaken as "3 times a day" or "twice in a week"	Use "3 times weekly"
U or u**	Unit	Mistaken as the number 0 or 4, causing a 10-fold overdose or greater (eg, 4U seen as "40" or 4u seen as "44"); mistaken as "cc" so dose given in volume instead of units (eg, 4u seen as 4 cc)	Use "unit"
UD	As directed ("ut dictum")	Mistaken as unit dose (eg, diltiazem 125 mg IV infusion "UD" misinterpreted as meaning to give the entire infusion as a unit [bolus] dose)	Use "as directed"

(continued)

Dose Designations and Other Information	Intended Meaning	Misinterpretation	Correction
Trailing zero after decimal point (eg, 1.0 mg)**	1 mg	Mistaken as 10 mg if the decimal point is not seen	Do not use trailing zeros for doses expressed in whole numbers
"Naked" decimal point (eg, .5 mg)**	0.5 mg	Mistaken as 5 mg if the decimal point is not seen	Use zero before a decimal point when the dose is less than a whole unit
Abbreviations such as mg. or mL. with a period following the abbreviation	mg mL	The period is unnecessary and could be mistaken as the number 1 if written poorly	Use mg, mL, etc. without a terminal period
Drug name and dose run together (especially problematic for drug names that end in "l" such as Inderal 40 mg; Tegretol 300 mg)	Inderal 40 mg Tegretol 300 mg	Mistaken as Inderal 140 mg Mistaken as Tegretol 1300 mg	Place adequate space between the drug name, dose, and unit of measure
Numerical dose and unit of measure run together (eg, 10 mg, 100 mL)	10 mg 100 mL	The "m" is sometimes mistaken as a zero or two zeros, risking a 10- to 100-fold overdose	Place adequate space between the dose and unit of measure
Large doses without properly placed commas (eg, 100000 units; 1000000 units)	100,000 units 1,000,000 units	100000 has been mistaken as 10,000 or 1,000,000; 1000000 has been mistaken as 100,000	Use commas for dosing units at or above 1000, or use words such as 100 "thousand" or 1 "million" to improve readability

Drug Name Abbreviations	Intended Meaning	Misinterpretation	Correction
To avoid confusion, do not abbreviate drug names when communicating medical information. Examples of drug name abbreviations involved in medication errors include:			
APAP	acetaminophen	Not recognized as acetaminophen	Use complete drug name
ARA A	vidarabine	Mistaken as cytarabine (ARA C)	Use complete drug name
AZT	zidovudine (Retrovir)	Mistaken as azathioprine or aztreonam	Use complete drug name
CPZ	Compazine (prochlorperazine)	Mistaken as chlorpromazine	Use complete drug name
DPT	Demerol-Phenergan-Thorazine	Mistaken as diphtheria-pertussis-tetanus (vaccine)	Use complete drug name
DTO	Diluted tincture of opium, or deodorized tincture of opium (Paregoric)	Mistaken as tincture of opium	Use complete drug name
HCl	hydrochloric acid or hydrochloride	Mistaken as potassium chloride (The "H" is misinterpreted as "K")	Use complete drug name unless expressed as a salt of a drug
HCT	hydrocortisone	Mistaken as hydrochlorothiazide	Use complete drug name
HCTZ	hydrochlorothiazide	Mistaken as hydrocortisone (seen as HCT250 mg)	Use complete drug name
MgSO$_4$**	magnesium sulfate	Mistaken as morphine sulfate	Use complete drug name
MS, MSO$_4$**	morphine sulfate	Mistaken as magnesium sulfate	Use complete drug name
MTX	methotrexate	Mistaken as mitoxantrone	Use complete drug name
PCA	procainamide	Mistaken as patient controlled analgesia	Use complete drug name
PTU	propylthiouracil	Mistaken as mercaptopurine	Use complete drug name
T3	Tylenol with codeine No. 3	Mistaken as liothyronine	Use complete drug name
TAC	triamcinolone	Mistaken as tetracaine, Adrenalin, cocaine	Use complete drug name
TNK	TNKase	Mistaken as "TPA"	Use complete drug name
ZnSO$_4$	zinc sulfate	Mistaken as morphine sulfate	Use complete drug name

Stemmed Drug Names	Intended Meaning	Misinterpretation	Correction
"Nitro" drip	nitroglycerin infusion	Mistaken as sodium nitroprusside infusion	Use complete drug name
"Norflox"	norfloxacin	Mistaken as Norflex	Use complete drug name
"IV Vanc"	intravenous vancomycin	Mistaken as Invanz	Use complete drug name

Symbols	Intended Meaning	Misinterpretation	Correction
ℨ	Dram	Symbol for dram mistaken as "3"	Use the metric system
♏	Minim	Symbol for minim mistaken as "mL"	
x3d	For three days	Mistaken as "3 doses"	Use "for three days"
> and <	Greater than and less than	Mistaken as opposite of intended; mistakenly use incorrect symbol; "< 10" mistaken as "40"	Use "greater than" or "less than"
/ (slash mark)	Separates two doses or indicates "per"	Mistaken as the number 1 (eg, "25 units/10 units" misread as "25 units and 110" units)	Use "per" rather than a slash mark to separate doses
@	At	Mistaken as "2"	Use "at"
&	And	Mistaken as "2"	Use "and"

(continued)

Symbols	Intended Meaning	Misinterpretation	Correction
+	Plus or and	Mistaken as "4"	Use "and"
°	Hour	Mistaken as a zero (eg, q2° seen as q 20)	Use "hr," "h," or "hour"
Φ or Ø	zero, null sign	Mistaken as numerals 4, 6, 8, and 9	Use 0 or zero, or describe intent using whole words

**These abbreviations are included on The Joint Commission's "minimum list" of dangerous abbreviations, acronyms, and symbols that must be included on an organization's "Do Not Use" list, effective January 1, 2004. Visit *www.jointcommission.org* for more information about this Joint Commission requirement.

Reprinted with permission from the Institute for Safe Medication Practices (*www.ismp.org*), 200 Lakeside Drive; Suite 200, Horsham, PA 19044-2321. Report medication errors or near misses to the ISMP Medication Errors Reporting Program (MERP) at 1-800-FAIL-SAF(E) or online at *www.ismp.org*.

43

PEDIATRIC GASTROENTERITIS

One Thing You *Should* Try at Home . . . . Level II

William McGhee, PharmD

Laura M. Panko, MD, FAAP

CASE SUMMARY

A 3-day history of vomiting, diarrhea, and other symptoms causes a young mother to seek medical attention at the emergency department for her 9-month-old daughter. The patient has signs of moderate dehydration on physical and laboratory examination. The presumed diagnosis is viral gastroenteritis. Students should understand that replacement of fluid and electrolyte losses is critical to the effective treatment of acute diarrhea. Oral rehydration therapy (ORT) with carbohydrate-based solutions is the primary treatment for diarrhea in children with mild-to-moderate dehydration. When caregivers are properly instructed, therapy can begin at home which may potentially prevent an ED visit or hospital stay. IV fluids are often needed for cases of severe dehydration. Fluid losses should be replenished, and early refeeding with age-appropriate diets is essential to reduce stool volume after completion of rehydration therapy. Although antidiarrheal and antiemetic products are available, they have limited effectiveness, can cause adverse effects, and, most important, may divert attention from appropriate fluid and electrolyte replacement. Ondansetron can be used in patients with intractable vomiting who present to the ED after failed attempts at ORT. Families should have a commercially available oral rehydration solution (ORS) at home to start treatment as soon as vomiting and diarrhea begins. The availability of two oral rotavirus vaccines has dramatically reduced morbidity and mortality of rotavirus-induced diarrhea in countries where universal immunization has been adopted. Its use and effectiveness will continue to grow as support increases from public health agencies.

QUESTIONS

Problem Identification

1.a. Create a list of the patient's drug therapy problems.

- This patient has typical viral gastroenteritis and diarrhea, a common pediatric problem. The peak incidence occurs between 6 and 24 months of age and is characterized by the acute onset of emesis, progressing to watery diarrhea as the vomiting resolves. A number of viruses cause viral gastroenteritis, but rotavirus and norovirus are the most common. Prior to the introduction of rotavirus vaccines in 2006 and 2008,

rotavirus was the most common cause of pediatric gastroenteritis in the United States causing approximately 55,000–70,000 hospitalizations per year, 200,000 emergency room (ER) visits, and 400,000 outpatient physician visits among children younger than 5 years of age.[1] Mortality due to rotavirus gastroenteritis in the United States is uncommon with an estimated 20–60 deaths per year. Worldwide, the incidence of rotavirus diarrhea has increased over the past 30 years and is responsible for approximately 450,000 deaths in 2008 in children younger than 5 years of age, accounting for 37% of all diarrhea-related mortality and 5% of all deaths in children ≤5 years of age.[2]

- Currently, norovirus is the leading cause of gastroenteritis in the United States. Norovirus results in 19–21 million cases of gastroenteritis per year, 10–15% of severe gastroenteritis cases in children under 5 years of age, 56,000–71,000 hospitalizations per year, and 570–800 deaths (the latter accounting for children and the elderly). Additionally, norovirus was responsible for about 50% of all reported GI outbreaks in the United States and Europe.[3]

- Rotavirus is transmitted by the fecal–oral route, and spread of the virus is common in hospitals and daycare settings. Infection occurs when ingested virus infects enterocytes in the small intestine, leading to cell damage or death and loss of brush border digestive enzymes. Approximately 48 hours after exposure, infected children develop fever, vomiting, and watery diarrhea. Fever and vomiting usually subside in 1–2 days, but diarrhea can continue for several days, leading to significant dehydration. Dehydration, and the corresponding electrolyte losses, is the primary cause of morbidity in gastroenteritis. Children with poor nutrition also are at risk for complications. Approximately 65% of hospitalizations and 85% of diarrhea-related deaths occur in the first year of life.

- Norovirus is transmitted via the fecal–oral route, the vomitus–oral route, by contact with contaminated surfaces, and via consumption of contaminated food and water. The virus is very contagious and only a small number of ingested viral particles are required to cause disease. Disease is characterized by the abrupt onset of vomiting and watery diarrhea, abdominal cramping, and nausea. Fever and body aches can occur. Symptoms last from 1–3 days, though more prolonged illness can occur in the young, elderly, and hospitalized populations. Outbreaks have occurred in long-term facilities, schools, and cruise ships and as a result of contaminated food and water sources. Norovirus infection doses not result in long lasting immunity.[3]

- The patient has moderate dehydration (acute weight loss of 9%, from 9.0 kg [19.8 lb] to 8.2 kg [18.0 lb]) as well as clinical and laboratory evidence of dehydration with metabolic acidosis.

1.b. What information (signs, symptoms, laboratory values) indicates the presence or severity of gastroenteritis?

- Table 43-1 is a dehydration assessment tool to help categorize the degree of dehydration. Dehydration is categorized clinically into mild, moderate, and severe, but rarely does a child fall entirely into one category or another. When a child does not fit

TABLE 43-1 Clinical Assessment Guidelines for Dehydration in Children of All Ages

Parameter	Mild	Moderate	Severe
Weight loss (%)	3–5	6–9	≥10
Body fluid loss (mL/kg)	30–50	50–100	>100
Stage of shock	Impending	Compensated	Uncompensated
Heart rate	Normal	Increased	Increased
Blood pressure	Normal	Normal	Normal to reduced
Respiratory rate	Normal	Normal	Increased
Skin turgor	Normal	Decreased	"Tenting"
Anterior fontanelle	Normal	Sunken	Sunken
Capillary refill (s)	<2	2–3	>3
Mucous membranes	Slightly dry	Dry	Dry
Tearing	Normal/absent	Absent	Absent
Eye appearance	Normal	Sunken orbits	Deeply sunken orbits
Mental status	Normal	Normal to listless	Normal to lethargic to comatose
Urine volume	Slightly decreased	<1 mL/kg/hour	<1 mL/kg/hour
Urine specific gravity	1.020	1.025	>1.035
BUN	Upper normal	Elevated	High
Blood pH	7.40–7.22	7.30–6.92	7.10–6.8
Thirst	Slightly increased	Moderately increased	Very thirsty or too lethargic to indicate

into one category, the category with the most signs should be used. In assessing the degree of dehydration, changes in mental status, skin turgor, mucous membranes, and eyes are important assessment tools because they correlate with the degree of dehydration better than other signs and symptoms.

- The most accurate indicator of the degree of dehydration is actual weight loss. Fortunately, the patient had a physician's office visit 5 days earlier during which she was weighed; therefore, the actual weight loss (0.8 kg, 1.8 lb, or 9%) was documented, indicating moderate dehydration.

- By history, the patient had a 3-day history of fever, vomiting, and diarrhea of acute onset; resulting in increased fluid losses, further supported by a history of decreased wet diapers.

- She has a social history of daycare attendance, where several of her daycare mates had similar illnesses recently. Attendance at daycare and other sick contacts with similar symptoms is part of a typical history in pediatric gastroenteritis. Children can be infected, but asymptomatic and transmit the infection unknowingly. In addition, on the day she presented to the ER, her mother developed abdominal discomfort and loose stools.

- On physical examination, she was sleepy but arousable and her mental status was normal, which makes severe dehydration less likely. Her skin turgor had mild "tenting," and the capillary refill was increased, at 2–3 seconds. Her tongue and lips were dry, and there were scant tears. Her eyes were moderately sunken and the anterior fontanelle was sunken. She was tachypneic and tachycardic.

- Her labs indicated metabolic acidosis (total carbon dioxide [CO_2] 14 mEq/L and Cl 113 mEq/L), and her urinalysis showed a specific gravity of 1.029 (indicating moderate dehydration). Ketones were 2+ in the urine, indicating fat breakdown in a hypocaloric diet. Her serum sodium was 137 mEq/L, indicating isotonic dehydration (defined as serum sodium between 130 and 150 mEq/L), and her BUN was slightly high, at 23 mg/dL.

Desired Outcome

2. What are the goals of pharmacotherapy in this case?

- The goals of appropriate pharmacotherapy of dehydration include reversing dehydration, restoring normal urine output, and maintaining adequate nutrition.

- Replacement of fluid and electrolyte losses is the critical element of effective treatment. This is necessary to prevent clinically significant water, electrolyte, and acid–base disturbances.

- Reinstitution of an age-appropriate diet is essential to ensure adequate nutrition and to reduce stool volume. Further morbidity and unnecessary hospitalization may be prevented.

- Other secondary goals may include providing symptomatic relief and treating any curable causes of diarrhea.

Therapeutic Alternatives

3.a. What nondrug therapies might be useful for this patient?

- ORT with carbohydrate-based solutions is the mainstay of treatment of fluid and electrolyte losses caused by diarrhea in children with mild-to-moderate dehydration. It can be used regardless of the patient's age, causative pathogen, or initial serum sodium concentration. The basis for the effectiveness of ORT is the phenomenon of glucose–sodium cotransport, where sodium ions given orally are absorbed along with glucose (and other organic molecules) from the lumen of the intestine into the bloodstream. Once these molecules are absorbed, free water naturally follows. Any of the commercially available ORSs can be used successfully to rehydrate otherwise healthy children with mild-to-moderate dehydration. These products are formulated on physiologic principles and should be close to isotonic to avoid unnecessary shifts in fluid. They are to be distinguished from other nonphysiologic clear liquids that are commonly but inappropriately used to treat dehydration. Clear liquids to avoid include colas, ginger ale, apple juice, chicken broth, and sports beverages. This patient was treated inappropriately because in addition to an ORS (Pedialyte®), she received a variety of clear liquids including water, cola, and diluted apple juice. These liquids have unacceptably low electrolyte concentrations, and the soda and juice are inappropriate due to high osmolalities contributed to by high glucose concentrations. (See Table 43-2 for direct comparison of commercially available ORS and other commonly used beverages for ORT.) Despite being the first choice for rehydration in children with mild-to-moderate acute viral gastroenteritis (AGE), ORS can be difficult to administer to infants and young children due to salty taste and poor palatability. Recent product taste tests indicate that palatability can be significantly improved with the addition of sucralose over rice-based (Enfalyte®) solutions. Pedialyte® and Pediatric Electrolyte® contain sucralose and were significantly more palatable than the comparable rice based solution.

- *Early feeding of age-appropriate foods.* Carbohydrate-based ORT is highly effective in replacing fluid and electrolyte losses, but has no effect on stool volume or duration of diarrhea, which can be discouraging to parents. Early feeding of patients should be instituted as soon as oral rehydration is completed (within 4–6 hours after the onset of rehydration). Early feeding can reduce the duration of diarrhea by approximately 0.5 day. Therefore, children with diarrhea requiring rehydration should be fed with age-appropriate diets immediately after completing ORT. Optimal ORT incorporates early feeding of age-appropriate foods. Unrestricted diets generally do not worsen the symptoms of mild or moderate diarrhea and decrease the stool output compared with ORT alone. For breastfed infants, continued breastfeeding reduces the number and volume of diarrhea stools and reduces the duration of rotavirus-induced diarrhea. Supplementation with ORT between regular feedings should be considered to ensure adequate fluid intake. In addition, most children being fed milk-based formulas tolerate them well. Children who do not tolerate them, however, can be changed to a soy-based formula for the duration of diarrhea. Older children can resume a normal diet for their age once ORT is complete.

- The principles of ORT include two phases of treatment: (1) a rehydration phase in which water and electrolytes are administered with an appropriate ORS; and (2) reintroduction of age-appropriate diets as soon as rehydration is complete (replacement of ongoing fluid losses from continued diarrhea and vomiting is necessary with ORS). Despite published guidelines from the American Academy of Pediatrics (AAP) and the Centers for Disease Control and Prevention (CDC) and other studies stating that ORT is appropriate, preferred, and at least equivalent therapy to IV hydration for mild-to-moderate dehydration in infants and children, many healthcare providers in the United States overuse IV hydration, prolong rehydration, delay reintroduction of age-appropriate diets, and withhold ORT inappropriately, especially in children who are vomiting. Continuing education of healthcare workers and reemphasizing the value of oral rehydration versus IV rehydration is essential for the success of ORT.

3.b. What feasible pharmacotherapeutic alternatives are available for treating this patient's diarrhea?

- Antidiarrheal compounds have been used to treat pediatric gastroenteritis. Their proposed purpose is to shorten the course of diarrhea and to relieve discomfort by reducing stool output and electrolyte losses. However, despite a large number of antidiarrheal compounds available, none has proven efficacy in the routine treatment of acute diarrhea associated with pediatric gastroenteritis. Their usefulness remains to be proven, and evidence-based guidelines do not recommend their use. These agents have a variety of proposed mechanisms; their possible benefits and limitations are outlined below:

  ✓ *Antimotility agents (opioids and opioid/anticholinergic combination products)* delay GI transit and increase gut capacity and fluid retention. *Loperamide* with ORT significantly reduces the volume of stool losses, but this reduction is not clinically significant. Loperamide also may have an unacceptable rate of side effects (lethargy, respiratory depression, altered mental status, ileus, abdominal distention). *Anticholinergic agents* (eg, atropine or mepenzolate bromide) may cause dry mouth that can alter the clinical evaluation of

dehydration. Infants and children are especially susceptible to toxic effects of anticholinergics. Antimotility agents can worsen the course of diarrhea in shigellosis, antibiotic-associated pseudomembranous colitis, and *Escherichia coli* O157:H7-induced diarrhea. Most important, reliance on antidiarrheal compounds can shift the focus of treatment away from appropriate ORT and the early feeding of the child. They are not recommended by the AAP to treat acute diarrhea in children because of the modest clinical benefit, limited scientific evidence of efficacy, and concern for toxic effects.

  ✓ *Antisecretory agents (bismuth subsalicylate)* may have an adjunctive role for acute diarrhea. Bismuth subsalicylate decreases intestinal secretions secondary to cholera and *E. coli* toxins, decreases frequency of unformed stools, decreases total stool output, and reduces the need for ORT. However, the benefit is modest, and it requires dosing every 4 hours. Also, pediatric patients may absorb salicylate (but the effect on Reye's syndrome is unknown). This treatment is not recommended by the AAP because of modest benefit and concern for toxicity.

  ✓ *Adsorbent drugs (polycarbophil)* bind bacterial toxins and water, but their effectiveness remains unproven. There is no conclusive evidence of decreased duration of diarrhea, number of stools, or total stool output. Major toxicity is not a concern with these products, but they may adsorb nutrients, enzymes, and drugs. These products are not recommended by the AAP because of lack of efficacy.

- *Probiotics* are oral supplements or food products that contain sufficient viable microorganisms (usually *Lactobacillus*, *Bifidobacterium*, and *Streptococcus* genera) to alter the microflora of the patient and to produce beneficial health effects. Their use is widespread and growing significantly as they are marketed in supermarkets, retail outlets, and on the Internet. In 2014, retail sales for probiotics were $30 billion and are projected to grow. Of growing concern is the use of probiotics in patients with AGE without professional medical advice. Probiotics are fermentive, obligatory, or facultative anaerobes that typically produce lactic acid. When administered in appropriate amounts, they treat diarrheal disease presumably by inhibiting enteric pathogens by producing antimicrobial substances, decreasing adhesion of pathogens to enterocytes, decreasing toxin production, and/or stimulating specific immunoglobulin A-related immune responses to pathogens.

  The results of multiple meta-analyses have moved probiotics from alternative medicine status to an evidence-based role in treating acute gastroenteritis especially when caused by rotavirus. A recent meta-analysis reviewed 63 studies (56 in infants and young children) that included more than 8000 patients.[4] Conclusions from this analysis were: (1) probiotics significantly reduced the duration of diarrhea by approximately 24 hours; (2) probiotics significantly reduced the risk of diarrhea exceeding 3 days in duration; (3) they significantly reduced stool frequency on day 2 by approximately one diarrhea episode; and (4) no adverse drug reactions were attributable to probiotics. The authors concluded that "used alongside of rehydration therapy, probiotics seem to be safe and have clear beneficial effects in shortening the duration of diarrhea and reducing stool frequency in acute infectious diarrhea." The most widely studied probiotics with consistently helpful results were *Lactobacillus* GG (LGG) and *Saccharomyces boulardii*, which appear to be beneficial in treating rotavirus-related diarrhea.

Based on the results of these meta-analyses and other recent trials, probiotics have a limited role in the treatment of AGE and guidelines for treating AGE now include them. The guidelines of European Society for Pediatric Gastroenterology, Hepatology, and Nutrition/European Society for Pediatric Infectious Diseases concluded that "probiotics may be an effective adjunct to the management of diarrhea." Probiotics with proven clinical efficacy administered in appropriate dosages might be used adjunctively along with rehydration therapy for the treatment of AGE in children.[5] The AAP recognizes that randomized controlled trials in healthy children in developed countries provide good data on the benefit of probiotics in children with acute gastroenteritis and concludes that there is evidence to support the use of probiotics (specifically LGG) early in the course of acute gastroenteritis to reduce the duration by 1 day.

However, not all experts support the widespread use of probiotics in AGE and some question whether there is sufficient evidence to support their incorporation into AGE treatment guidelines especially in outpatient settings where the vast majority of patients with AGE are treated. Few studies include large numbers of children in outpatient settings. In addition, the widespread use of rotavirus vaccine in the United States and many countries has changed the epidemiology of AGE. The greatest success from probiotic use among inpatients is demonstrated in rotavirus AGE; its benefits against other pathogens such as norovirus are unknown. Other concerns exist against the widespread use of probiotics. The benefit from probiotics is strain and dose dependent; LGG has been the most effective probiotic to date. Although probiotics are generally recognized as safe, there are reports of bacteremia and fungemia occurring in immunosuppressed patients treated with probiotics. In addition, and perhaps of greater significance, because they are categorized as nutraceuticals, the FDA has no authority to regulate or standardize the production or purity of probiotics. There is great variability in product content, and when tested, some formulations have contained no bacteria. Therefore, because of these concerns, the use of probiotics for the treatment of pediatric gastroenteritis must be undertaken carefully. Only probiotics with proven clinical efficacy administered in appropriate dosages should be used which the general public and most physicians do not know. Patients must be cautioned that they are to be given adjunctively, *in addition to rehydration*. Practitioners must not allow the focus of treatment to shift away from appropriate ORT and the early feeding of the child. In summary, at the present time, probiotics reduce the duration of diarrhea by approximately 24 hours and significantly reduce the risk of diarrhea exceeding 3 days in duration. However, their use must be undertaken with caution. Further studies are needed to clarify their role especially after a decade of use of rotavirus vaccines and in outpatient settings. The establishment of approved standardized probiotics and well defined dosage and treatment regimens (along with the full understanding that their usefulness is only to shorten the duration of diarrhea) is necessary and once established, will expand their role in acute gastroenteritis. Note: the reversal of dehydration and the use of ORS remains the standard of care in AGE.

- *Antiemetic drugs* are widely used in dehydrated patients with vomiting, despite their use generally being discouraged. They are used with the intent of reducing vomiting and the severity of dehydration, improving the efficiency of ORT in patients who are vomiting. Ondansetron, almost exclusively (≥97% of surveyed emergency room physicians) is the most commonly used drug to stop vomiting in the child with gastroenteritis. There is no evidence for the usefulness of most other antiemetics. The additional cost of using ondansetron was recently justified in a US cost analysis, where the appropriate use of ondansetron in eligible children was estimated to prevent nearly 30,000 IV insertions, 7220 hospitalizations, and save society $65.6 million annually.[6] In the most recent Cochrane analysis (10 trials, 1,479 participants, 5 different treatment regimens including dexamethasone, dimenhydrinate, granisetron, metoclopramide, and ondansetron), there was clear evidence that IV or oral ondansetron compared with placebo significantly increased the proportion of patients with cessation of vomiting and reduced the immediate hospital admission rate and the need for IV rehydration therapy.[7] Use of ondansetron was associated with a risk of prolonged diarrhea, but there was no significant increase in return visits to the ED related to diarrhea. Of note, there was no evidence for using other antiemetics except granisetron and its value was only limited. Although this Cochrane analysis and previous reports concluded that healthcare policymakers should consider using ondansetron in selected patients with mild-to-moderate dehydration with uncontrolled vomiting, only the Canadian Pediatric Society recommends that ondansetron be considered for children between 6 months and 12 years of age with uncontrolled vomiting related to mild or moderate acute gastroenteritis or who have failed ORT. However, recognizing the usefulness of ondansetron, a recent survey of pediatric-trained emergency room physicians reported that 86% would use ondansetron in patients who failed oral rehydration.[8] Thus, when the decision is made to treat a child with mild-to-moderate acute gastroenteritis with an antiemetic drug because of uncontrolled vomiting, there is clear evidence to use ondansetron to decrease vomiting episodes, reduce the need for IV rehydration, and reduce the need for immediate hospitalization.[7] Since ondansetron can prolong the QT interval under certain circumstances, the safety of a one-time dose of oral ondansetron was recently reported. A recent review of the FDA and all global ADR databases revealed no reported cardiac arrhythmias after a one-time dose of oral ondansetron. The use of a single one-time dose of ondansetron is now generally recognized to be safe.[9]

- *Zinc supplementation* is recommended for treating acute diarrhea in malnourished children in developing countries. In those areas, zinc deficiency occurs in children not only because of increased stool losses with diarrhea but also because of prior reduced intake of animal foods, excess dietary phytates that decrease zinc absorption, and poor food intake. Oral zinc has ion absorption and antisecretory effects that result in reduced duration and severity of diarrhea as determined by stool output and frequency. Multiple meta-analyses have been published supporting the usefulness of zinc supplementation in children with AGE. The latest review identified 19 RCTs comparing oral zinc with placebo in children 1 month to 5 years of age. Most were from developing countries where zinc deficiency is common. In children >6 months, zinc supplementation reduced the duration of diarrhea and reduced the risk of diarrhea persisting until day 7. However, for children <6 months, zinc supplementation had no effect on the mean duration of diarrhea and actually may increase the risk of diarrhea persisting until day 7. Thus, children older than 6 months in developing countries should benefit from the use of zinc in the treatment of AGE. Both UNICEF and the World Health Organization (WHO) recommend that all children with diarrhea in developing countries be treated with zinc in addition to ORT, which is estimated to save 400,000 lives per year. There is insufficient evidence to justify the use of zinc for well-nourished children with gastroenteritis.

Optimal Plan

4.a. What drug(s), dosage forms, schedule, and duration of therapy are best for this patient?

- Treatment of a child with dehydration is directed primarily by the degree of dehydration present. Four potential treatment situations based on the severity of the dehydration are presented below. This patient had diarrhea with moderate dehydration (6–9% loss of body weight).

  ✓ *Diarrhea without dehydration.* ORT may be given in doses of 10 mL/kg to replace ongoing stool losses. Some children might not take the ORT because of its salty taste. For these few patients, freezer pops are available in a variety of flavors. ORT may not be necessary if fluid consumption and age-appropriate feeding adequately meets maintenance fluid requirements and losses over the duration of illness. Infants should continue to breastfeed or take regular-strength formula. Older children can usually drink full-strength milk and consume an unrestricted, age-appropriate diet:

  ✓ *Diarrhea with mild dehydration (3–5% weight loss).* Correct dehydration with ORT, 50 mL/kg over a 4-hour period. Reassess the status of dehydration and volume of ORT at 2-hour intervals. Concomitantly replace continuing losses from stool or emesis at 10 mL/kg for each stool; estimate emesis loss and replace with fluid. Children with emesis can usually tolerate ORT, but it is necessary to administer ORT in small 5- to 10-mL aliquots (one to two teaspoonfuls) every 1–2 minutes. Feeding should start immediately after rehydration is complete, using the feeding guidelines described previously.

  ✓ *Diarrhea with moderate dehydration (6–9% weight loss).* Although the patient presented to the emergency department, ORT is still the initial treatment of choice to reverse moderate dehydration, and it can usually be administered at home. Compared with IV rehydration, oral rehydration can be initiated more quickly and is equally effective. To correct the dehydration, administer ORT, 100 mL/kg, plus replacement of ongoing losses (10 mL/kg for each stool, plus estimated losses from emesis as above) during the first 4 hours. Assess rehydration status hourly and adjust the amount of ORT accordingly. Close supervision is required, but this can be done at home. Rapid restoration of blood volume helps to correct acidosis and to increase tissue perfusion. Resume feeding of age-appropriate diet as soon as rehydration is completed.

  ✓ *Diarrhea with severe dehydration (≥10% weight loss).* Severe dehydration and uncompensated shock should be treated aggressively with IV isotonic fluids to restore intravascular volume. Inadequately treated gastroenteritis and dehydration in pediatric patients, especially in infants, can cause life-threatening severe dehydration and should be considered a medical emergency. The patient may be in shock and should be referred to an emergency department. Administer 20-mL/kg aliquots of normal saline or lactated Ringer's solution over 15–30 minutes (even faster in uncompensated shock). Reassess the patient's status after each completed fluid bolus. Repeat boluses of up to 80 mL/kg total fluid may be used. Isotonic fluid replacement may be discontinued when blood pressure is restored, heart rate is normalized, peripheral pulses are strong, and skin perfusion is restored. Urine output is the best indicator of restored intravascular

volume and should be at least 1 mL/kg/hour. If the patient does not respond to rapid IV volume replacement, other underlying disorders should be considered, including septic shock, toxic shock syndrome, myocarditis, cardiomyopathy, pericarditis, and other underlying diseases. ORT may be instituted to complete rehydration when the patient's status is stable. Estimate the degree of remaining dehydration and treat according to the above guidelines. IV access should be maintained until it is certain that IV therapy will not be reinstituted. After ORT is complete, resume age-appropriate feeding following the guidelines outlined previously.

4.b. What is the efficacy and safety record of the available rotavirus vaccines, and what impact have they had on preventing rotavirus-induced diarrhea?

- Because rotavirus-induced disease kills approximately 450,000 children each year in developing countries and accounts for one-third of hospitalizations for diarrhea worldwide, preventing it through rotavirus immunization is the most effective way to lower its impact throughout the world. Rotavirus vaccination is safe, is associated with few adverse effects, and has been effective in reducing the burden of rotaviral disease in countries that have adopted universal rotavirus vaccination as recommended by the WHO and other authorities. In 1999, initial efforts to reduce the worldwide health burden of gastroenteritis through rotavirus vaccination suffered a setback when the first available rotavirus vaccine (Rotashield®) was removed from the market because of a 30-fold increased risk of intussusception (in week 1 after dose 1). Since then, two oral rotavirus vaccines were approved for use in the United States without evidence of a significantly increased rate of intussusception.

  ✓ RotaTeq® (RV5), a live oral human–bovine rotavirus vaccine, became available in 2006. It contains five live reassortant rotavirus strains active against rotavirus gastroenteritis caused by G1, G2, G3, and G4 serotypes and has proven efficacy in preventing rotavirus-induced diarrhea caused by these common serotypes. It is given as a three-dose series at 2, 4, and 6 months of age (the first dose can be given as early as 6 weeks, but the series needs to be initiated by 14 weeks, 6 days; the maximum age for the last dose is 8 months, 0 days). It is a liquid formulation requiring no reconstitution and is supplied as a single 2-mL dose in a squeezable plastic tube.

  ✓ Rotarix® (RV1) became available in the United States in 2008. It contains a single human rotavirus strain (RIX4414) active against G1, G2, G3, and G9 serotypes. It is given to infants as a two-dose series at 2 and 4 months (it can be initiated as early as 6 weeks with the second dose given as late as 8 months, 0 days). It is available as a vial of lyophilized vaccine with a prefilled oral applicator of diluent. It has latex in the tip and should be avoided in persons with a latex allergy.

- The safety and efficacy of RV5 and RV1 were determined from 11 randomized, controlled, prelicensure trials in 146,000 infants including three trials for RV5 and seven trials for RV1. An increased risk of intussusception was not initially found with either vaccine. Further post-marketing data have identified a small increased risk of intussusception in infants administered the currently licensed rotavirus vaccines, reported as 1 excess case per 30,000–100,000 vaccinated infants. The risk is greatest in the week following the first or second dose of the vaccine. It should be noted that this risk is lower than that reported with the Rotashield® vaccine. Efficacy against any rotavirus gastroenteritis ranged from 74 to 87%, and efficacy against severe disease ranged from 85 to 98%. Both vaccines reduced hospitalizations, emergency department visits, and physician visits. RV1 rotavirus vaccine was implemented into the immunization programs of several Latin American and European countries and results of its effectiveness have been reported for Brazil and Mexico,[9] where it is estimated that RV1 prevented approximately 80,000 hospitalizations and 1300 deaths per year from diarrhea in these two countries. The most recent global experience data report that RV1 and RV5 vaccination programs are 48–77% effective in reducing severe disease in young infants. Vaccine effectiveness for the RV5 rotavirus vaccine was recently reported from its use in a large urban population in the United States.[10] This case-control study of vaccine effectiveness was conducted using active surveillance at a large pediatric hospital. In this study, three doses of RV5 were 85–89% effective in preventing rotavirus gastroenteritis resulting in ED care or inpatient admission and conferred 100% protection against severe disease requiring hospitalization. Continued monitoring of the effectiveness of rotavirus vaccines in vaccinated children is necessary to determine if immunity wanes as the child grows older. Also, long-term surveillance is necessary to determine any effect that rotavirus vaccination might have on rotavirus epidemiology to assess any impact on the development of rotavirus strains against which vaccines might become less protective. More recent surveillance in the United States and other countries have found RV5 vaccine reassortant strains in stool samples of children with diarrhea and in some cases, have been postulated to have caused the diarrhea illness.

- The AAP recommends routine immunization of infants in the United States with rotavirus vaccine and does not express a preference for either RV5 or RV1. The vaccine series can be completed by using a combination of the two vaccines if one is unavailable but requires a three-dose series if one dose was RV5. Either vaccine can be substituted to complete the vaccine series.

Outcome Evaluation

5.a. What clinical and laboratory parameters should be monitored to evaluate therapy for achievement of the desired therapeutic outcome?

- Vital signs should normalize with appropriate therapy. Concurrent fever, agitation, pain, or respiratory illnesses can contribute to ongoing abnormalities in vital signs. Tachycardia is usually the first sign of mild dehydration (see Table 43-1). With increasing acidosis and fluid loss, the respiratory rate increases and breathing becomes deeper (hyperpnea). Hypotension is usually a sign of severe dehydration.

- Central nervous system (CNS) alterations should be reversed. No CNS changes occur in mild dehydration; some patients may appear listless with moderate dehydration, and severely dehydrated patients appear quite ill with lethargy or irritability.

- Skin and mucous membrane changes as well as delays in capillary refill should normalize. Mucous membranes should appear moist rather than dry (the latter can be seen in all degrees of dehydration). Normal capillary refill is <2 seconds and usually is not altered in mild dehydration. Capillary refill in moderately dehydrated patients is 2–3 seconds and >3 seconds in severely dehydrated patients. Skin turgor (elasticity) should be normal. There is no change in mild dehydration, but it decreases in moderate dehydration, with "tenting" occurring in patients with severe dehydration. The anterior fontanelle should no longer be sunken, which is seen in moderate-to-severe dehydration.

- The eyes should appear normal. No change occurs in mild dehydration, but in moderate-to-severe dehydration, tearing will be absent and the eyes will appear sunken.

- Laboratory tests should be ordered when clinically appropriate. Most dehydration occurring with pediatric gastroenteritis is isotonic, and serum electrolyte determinations are unnecessary. However, some patients with moderate dehydration (those whose histories and physical examinations are inconsistent with routine gastroenteritis), those with prolonged inappropriate intake of hypotonic or hypertonic solutions (see Table 43-2), and all severely dehydrated patients should have serum electrolytes determined and corrected.

- Urine output and specific gravity should normalize. In general, normal urine output for children is >1 mL/kg/hour. Progressive decreases in urine volume and increases in specific gravity are expected with increasing severity of dehydration. Urine output will be decreased to <1 mL/kg/hour in both moderate and severe dehydration (see Table 43-1). Specific gravity is 1.020 in mild dehydration, 1.025 in moderate dehydration, and maximal in patients with severe dehydration. Adequate rehydration should normalize both urine output and specific gravity. During rehydration, lung sounds should be assessed periodically. Lung sounds should remain clear. The development of crackles indicates fluid overload and requires careful

TABLE 43-2	Composition of Commercial Oral Rehydration Solutions (ORS) and Commonly Consumed Beverages					
Solution	CHO (gm/L)	Sodium (mmol/L)	Potassium (mmol/L)	Chloride (mmol/L)	Base (mmol/L)	Osmolarity (mOsm/L)
ORS						
WHO 2002	13.5	75	20	65	30	245
WHO 975	20	90	20	80	30	311
ESPGHN	16	60	20	60	30	240
Enfalyte®	30	50	25	45	34	200
Pedialyte®	25	45	20	35	30	250
Rehydralyte®	25	75	20	65	30	305
CeraLyte®	40	50–90	20	N/A	30	220
Commonly used beverages (not appropriate for diarrhea treatment)						
Apple juice	120	0.4	44	45	N/A	730
Coca-Cola®	112	1.6	N/A	N/A	13.4	650

CHO, carbohydrate; ESPGHN, European Society of Pediatric Gastroenterology, Hepatology and Nutrition; gm, gram; mmol, millimoles; mOsm, milliosmoles; WHO, World Health Organization.

reevaluation of the patient's clinical status prior to administering additional fluids.

Patient Education

6. What information should be provided to the child's parents to enhance compliance, ensure successful therapy, and minimize adverse effects?

- Treatment of diarrhea due to gastroenteritis in your child should begin at home. It is a good plan for you to keep ORS at home at all times (especially in rural areas and underserved urban neighborhoods where access to health care may be delayed) and to use it as instructed by your doctor. Sometimes doctors instruct new parents about this treatment at the first newborn visit. Be careful of information obtained from sources on the Internet. Much of the information available is not consistent with the accepted medical guidelines for the use of ORT in pediatric gastroenteritis.

- Infants with diarrhea should receive a medical evaluation for diarrhea. Additionally, any infant or young child with diarrhea and fever should be evaluated to rule out serious illness.

- Early home management with ORT results in fewer complications such as severe dehydration and poor nutrition, as well as fewer office or ER visits.

- Any of the commercial ORSs can be used to effectively rehydrate your child. However, rehydration alone does not reduce the duration of diarrhea or the volume of stool output. Early feeding after rehydration is necessary and can reduce the duration of diarrhea by as much as half a day.

- An effective oral rehydration strategy always combines early feeding with an age-appropriate diet after rehydration. This corrects dehydration, improves nutritional status, and reduces the volume of stool output.

- Vomiting usually does not preclude the use of oral rehydration. Consistent administration of small amounts (one to two teaspoonfuls) of an ORS every 1–2 minutes can provide as much as 10 oz/hour of rehydration fluid. You have to resist your child's desires for larger amounts of liquid. Otherwise, further vomiting may occur.

- If your child does not stop vomiting after the appropriate administration of oral rehydration (as above) and appears to be severely dehydrated, contact your doctor, who might refer you to the ER for IV rehydration therapy.

- Oral rehydration is insufficient therapy for bloody diarrhea (dysentery). Contact your doctor if this occurs.

- Additional treatments, including antidiarrheal compounds, antiemetics, and antimicrobial therapy, are usually not necessary in the treatment of pediatric gastroenteritis. Most children can be successfully rehydrated with ORS without the use of medicines for nausea and vomiting. If vomiting is uncontrolled, contact your doctor as a nausea medicine, ondansetron, could be used. Probiotics can decrease the number of days of diarrhea if given to your child soon after diarrhea starts. However, giving probiotics to your child should not take the place of ORS. A diet normal for your child should be started soon after vomiting stops.

- Proper hand-washing technique, diaper-changing practices, and personal hygiene can help to prevent spread of the disease to other family members.

- The child should be kept out of daycare until the diarrhea stops.

REFERENCES

1. Fischer TK, Viboud C, Parashur U, et al. Hospitalizations and deaths from diarrhea and rotavirus among children <5 years of age in the United States, 1993–2003. J Infect Dis 2007;195:1117–1125.
2. Tate JR, Burton AH, Boschi-Pinto C, et al. 2008 estimate of worldwide rotavirus-associated mortality in children younger than 5 years before the introduction of universal rotavirus vaccination programs: a systematic review and meta-analysis. Lancet Infect Dis 2012;12:136–141.
3. Centers for Disease Control and Prevention. Updated norovirus outbreak management and disease prevention guidelines. MMWR Morb Mortal Wkly Rep 2011;60(3):1–15.
4. Allen SJ, Martinez EG, Gregorio GV, Dans LF. Probiotics for treating acute infectious diarrhea. Cochrane Database Syst Rev 2010;(11):CD003048. doi:10.1002/14651858.CD003048.pub3.
5. Guarino A, Albano F, Ashkenazi S, et al. European Society for Paediatric Gastroenterology, Hepatology, and Nutrition/European Society for Paediatric Infectious Diseases evidence-based guidelines for the management of acute gastroenteritis in children in Europe. J Pediatr Gastroenterol Nutr 2008;46(Suppl 2):S81–S122.
6. Freedman SB, Steiner MJ, Chan KJ. Oral ondansetron administration in emergency departments to children with gastroenteritis: an economic analysis. PLoS Med 2010;7(10):e10000350. doi:10.1371/journal/pmed.1000350.
7. Carter B, Fedorowicz Z. Antiemetic treatment for acute gastroenteritis in children: an updated Cochrane systematic review with meta-analysis and mixed treatment comparison in a Bayesian framework. BMJ Open 2012;2:e000622. doi:10.1136/bmjopen-2011-000622.
8. Nunez J, Liu DR, Nager AL. Dehydration treatment practices among pediatrics-trained and non-pediatrics trained emergency physicians. Pedatric Emergency Care 2012;28:322–328.
9. Freedman SB, Uleryk E, Rumantir M, Finkelstein Y. Ondansetron and the risk of cardiac arrhythmias: a systematic review and postmarketing analysis. Annals of Emergency Medicine 2014;64:19–25.
10. Boom JA, Tate JE, Sahni LC, et al. Effectiveness of pentavalent rotavirus vaccine in a large urban population in the United States. Pediatrics 2010;125:e199–e207. doi: 10.1542/peds.2012-3804.

127

DIABETIC FOOT INFECTION

Let's Nail That Infection . . . . Level II

Renee-Claude Mercier, PharmD, BCPS-AQ ID, PhC, FCCP

Paulina Deming, PharmD, PhC

CASE SUMMARY

In this 67-year-old Hispanic man with poorly controlled type 2 diabetes mellitus and several comorbid conditions, an ingrown toe nail has become infected, causing significant erythema and swelling of the right foot with purulent discharge from the wound. Physical and laboratory findings, including an elevated white blood cell (WBC), ESR, and fever, suggest a potential systemic infection secondary to cellulitis. The patient undergoes incision and drainage of the lesion, and tissue is submitted to the laboratory for culture. Empiric antimicrobial treatment must be initiated before results of wound culture and sensitivity testing are known. Because of this patient's comorbidities and the size and severity of the wound, parenteral antibiotic therapy should be initiated. Since this is an acutely infected wound, aerobic gram-positive bacteria (especially *Staphylococcus aureus*) are the most likely causative organisms. However, broad-spectrum coverage for gram-negative and anaerobic bacteria should also be instituted due to the location of the wound (bottom of foot), its size and severity, foul-smelling drainage, and the patient's diabetes. This patient does have risk factors for hospital-acquired methicillin-resistant *S. aureus* (HA-MRSA) infection (ie, recent hospitalization and existing chronic illnesses), and empiric coverage of this organism should be considered. When tissue cultures are reported as positive for *S. aureus* (MRSA) and *Bacteroides fragilis*, the reader is asked to narrow to more specific therapy, which includes parenteral vancomycin or either oral or parenteral linezolid or tedizolid with anaerobic coverage (metronidazole or clindamycin). Second-line agents include daptomycin, telavancin, ceftaroline, oritavancin, or dalbavancin all in combination with a drug with anaerobic coverage (metronidazole or clindamycin). This infection will require 2–3 weeks of therapy, so the patient will most likely be discharged on outpatient antibiotic therapy. Although parenteral therapy using any of a variety of agents, or oral linezolid or tedizolid, may be completed as an outpatient, attention must be given to the patient's social and economic situation. Better glycemic control and education regarding techniques for proper foot care are important components of a comprehensive treatment plan for this patient.

QUESTIONS

Problem Identification

1.a. Create a list of the patient's drug therapy problems.

- Cellulitis and infection of the right foot in a patient with diabetes, requiring treatment.

- Poorly controlled type 2 diabetes mellitus, as evidenced by an A1C of 11.8% (goal <7%) and recent episode of hyperglycemic hyperosmolar state. Metformin is contraindicated in this patient due to his SCr of 2.4 mg/dL. However, his renal function may improve with hydration, and this should be monitored.

- Nonadherence with medication administration and home glucose monitoring.

- Renal insufficiency secondary to diabetic nephropathy, appropriately treated with lisinopril, may necessitate dosing adjustment of antimicrobial agents.

- Hyperlipidemia, appropriately treated with atorvastatin.

- History of alcohol abuse; patient may have liver dysfunction, and the use of metronidazole should elicit discussion on the potential for a disulfiram drug reaction.

- Fungal infection of toenails, requiring treatment.

- Language barrier requiring additional resources (ie, translator) to optimize patient education.

- Recent travel abroad in Mexico where antibiotics are not controlled and antibiotic resistance is much higher. Patient could have been self-treating his infection or could have acquired more resistant pathogens.

1.b. What signs, symptoms, or laboratory values indicate the presence of an infection?

- Swollen, sore, and red foot

- Purulent foul-smelling drainage with cellulitis

- 2+ edema of the foot increasing in amplitude

- Elevated WBC count ($17.3 \times 10^3/mm^3$)

- X-ray showing tissue swelling from first metatarsal to midfoot consistent with cellulitis

1.c. What risk factors for infection does the patient have?

- Patient with ingrown toenail; attempted self-treatment.

- He is a patient with poorly controlled diabetes.

- Vascular calcifications in the foot per x-ray indicate a decreased blood supply.

- He has decreased sensation of bilateral lower extremities.

- Poor foot care (presence of fungus and overgrown toenails).

- Recent hospitalization and travel to Mexico (poor water purity).

1.d. What organisms are most likely involved in this infection?

- Aerobic isolates: *S. aureus*, *Streptococcus* spp., *Enterococcus* spp., *Proteus mirabilis*, *Escherichia coli*, *Klebsiella* spp., and *Pseudomonas aeruginosa*

- Anaerobic isolates: *Peptostreptococcus* and *B. fragilis*[1]

Desired Outcome

2. What are the therapeutic goals for this patient?

- Eradicate the bacteria.

- Prevent the development of osteomyelitis and the need for amputation.

- Preserve as much normal limb function as possible.

- Improve control of diabetes mellitus.

- Prevent infectious complications.

Therapeutic Alternatives

3.a. What nondrug therapies might be useful for this patient?

- Deep culture of the wound for both anaerobes and aerobes

- Appropriate wound care by experienced podiatrists (incision and drainage, debridement of the wound, and toenail clipping), nurses (wound care, dressing changes of wound, and foot care teaching), and physical therapists (whirlpool treatments, wound debridement, and teaching about minimal weight-bearing with a walker or crutches)

- Bed rest, minimal weight-bearing, leg elevation, and control of edema

- Proper education about wound care and the importance of good diabetes control, glucometer use, adherence to the medication regimens, and foot care in the patient with diabetes

3.b. What feasible pharmacotherapeutic alternatives are available for the empiric treatment of diabetic foot infection?

- Based on the most recent 2012 clinical practice guideline for the diagnosis and treatment of diabetic foot infections, treatment differs based on infection severity (mild vs moderate vs severe)[1]:

  Mild: Local infection involving only the skin and subcutaneous tissues without systemic signs. Erythema >0.5 cm and ≤2 cm.

  ✓ Oral antimicrobial therapy may be used in mild, uncomplicated diabetic foot infections *only*.[1,2] The following agents could be considered as preferred oral options because they target *S. aureus* and *Streptococcus* spp.:

  - *Amoxicillin/clavulanate monotherapy*

  - *Dicloxacillin*

  - *Clindamycin*

- Cephalexin
- Levofloxacin

If MRSA coverage is needed, then use either *doxycycline* or *trimethoprim/sulfamethoxazole* (activity against streptococci is uncertain).

Although these regimens cover the most likely causative organisms, it is important to note that except for levofloxacin none of the antibiotics given above cover *P. aeruginosa*.

Moderate: Local infection with erythema >2 cm, or involving structures deeper than skin and subcutaneous tissues, and *no* systemic inflammatory response signs (SIRS).

Severe: Local infection with SIRS, which would include at least two of the following:

✓ Temperature >38°C or <36°C

✓ Heart rate >90 bpm

✓ Respiratory rate >20 breaths/minute or $PaCO_2$ <32 mm Hg

✓ WBC count >12,000 or <4,000 cells/μL or ≥10% immature forms

- Treatment of **moderate** infection may be with oral agents or initial parenteral therapy while **severe** infections should be treated with parenteral agents.[1] Consider coverage for MSSA, streptococci, Enterobacteriaceae, and obligate anaerobes. Options for IV monotherapy could be:

✓ *Piperacillin/tazobactam.*

✓ *Imipenem/cilastatin.*

✓ *Meropenem.*

✓ *Doripenem.*

✓ *Cefepime* or *levofloxacin* could be used; however, additional coverage against obligate anaerobes should be considered with either *metronidazole* or *clindamycin. Levofloxacin* is also not optimal for *S. aureus* coverage.

- These agents cover all of the most likely causative organisms, including anaerobes and *P. aeruginosa*. However, imipenem/cilastatin is a potent β-lactamase inducer, so therapy with the other agents may be preferable initially.

The following agents could also be used as IV therapy, but they do not cover *P. aeruginosa*:

✓ *Ampicillin/sulbactam*

✓ *Ertapenem*

✓ *Cefoxitin* or *cefotetan*

✓ Third-generation cephalosporin (*ceftriaxone/cefotaxime*) plus IV *clindamycin combination*

- A combination of *clindamycin IV* plus either *aztreonam* or *an oral* or *IV fluoroquinolone (ciprofloxacin* or *levofloxacin)* could be used in patients with moderate-to-severe infections who are allergic to penicillin. *Moxifloxacin* is also now recommended for treatment of moderate infections and offers the advantage of once-daily dosing, no need of renal adjustments, and being relatively broad spectrum including most obligate anaerobic organisms.

- MRSA may be a suspected causative organism in some cases. There are two genetically distinct types of MRSA that can be of concern in diabetic foot infections: community-associated MRSA (CA-MRSA) and HA-MRSA. While acquisition of HA-MRSA is associated with well-defined risk factors (history of prolonged hospital or nursing home stay, past antimicrobial use, indwelling catheters, pressure sores, surgery, or dialysis), risk factors for acquisition of CA-MRSA are not as well established. CA-MRSA is susceptible to more antibiotics than HA-MRSA.[3]

- *Vancomycin IV, daptomycin IV, linezolid or tedizolid oral or IV, ceftaroline IV,*[4] *dalbavancin IV,* or *oritavancin IV* may be used if HA-MRSA is a suspected causative organism. Persons who are at high risk for HA-MRSA wound infection include those who: (a) have a previous history of HA-MRSA infection/colonization; (b) have positive nasal cultures for HA-MRSA; (c) have a recent history (within the last year) of prolonged hospitalization or intensive care unit stay; or (d) receive frequent and/or prolonged courses of broad-spectrum antibiotics.[5,6] Should the above stated agents be used empirically, gram-negative and anaerobic coverage will need to be added to provide adequate empiric coverage.

- Should CA-MRSA be more of a concern (eg, in a patient with no HA-MRSA risk factors who is admitted from an area where the CA-MRSA rate is relatively high), the antibiotic regimen should include any of those agents active against HA-MRSA: *clindamycin, sulfamethoxazole/trimethoprim,* or *doxycycline* or *minocycline.*[3]

- Aminoglycosides should generally be avoided in diabetic patients as they are at increased risk for the development of diabetic nephropathy and renal failure.

- *Becaplermin 0.01% gel (Regranex)* is approved by the FDA for the treatment of diabetic ulcers on the lower limbs and feet. Becaplermin is a genetically engineered form of platelet-derived growth factor, a naturally occurring protein in the body that stimulates diabetic ulcer healing. It is to be used as adjunctive therapy, *in addition to* infection control and wound care. In one clinical trial, becaplermin applied once daily in combination with good wound care significantly increased the incidence of complete healing when compared with placebo gel (50% vs 35%, respectively). Becaplermin gel also significantly decreased the time to complete healing of diabetic ulcers by 32% (about 6 weeks faster). The incidence of adverse events, including infection and cellulitis, was similar in patients treated with becaplermin gel, placebo gel, or good diabetic wound care alone.[7] Further studies are needed to assess which patients might best benefit from becaplermin use, particularly considering its cost (average wholesale price $1104.68 per 15-gram tube at the time of this writing).

3.c. What economic and social considerations are applicable to this patient?

- A simplified drug regimen (monotherapy and less frequent dosing, whenever possible) should be selected because of his history of poor medication adherence.

- The patient receives his health care primarily at First Choice Clinic. This may become an important consideration in selecting his future therapeutic plan.

- For this patient to receive appropriate wound care and home IV therapy if judged necessary, the healthcare team must establish that his family or a home healthcare nurse will be able to provide assistance.

Optimal Plan

4. Outline a drug regimen that would provide optimal initial empiric therapy for the infection.

- This diabetic foot infection has significant involvement of the skin and skin structures with deep tissue involvement. Moreover, the area of cellulitis and induration exceeds 2 cm (4 cm × 5 cm). Because this is an acutely infected wound, aerobic gram-positive bacteria (especially *S. aureus*) are the most likely causative organisms.[1] However, broad-spectrum coverage for gram-negative and anaerobic bacteria should also be instituted due to the location of the wound (bottom of foot), foul-smelling discharge, its size and severity, and the patient's diabetes. This patient does have risk factors for HA-MRSA infection (ie, recent hospitalizations and existing chronic illnesses), and empiric coverage of this organism should be considered as well. Initial empiric IV therapy is recommended in severe diabetic foot infections such as this one.

- A number of treatment options are appropriate for empiric therapy of diabetic foot infection in this patient. The antimicrobial therapy selection may be based on institutional cost and drug availability through the formulary system. It should also be adjusted for the patient's renal function. This patient's calculated creatinine clearance, based on total body weight (patient's weight is below ideal body weight), is 25 mL/minute. Antimicrobial resistance within the area and based on patient's prior culture and susceptibility should also be taken into consideration when selecting an empiric regimen.[8]

- All antibiotic regimens appropriate for this patient include two or more antibiotics (one to cover HA-MRSA and other gram-positive bacteria, and one or two to cover gram-negative and anaerobic bacteria). It would be best to limit it to no more than two antibiotics to optimize nursing ease and patient adherence and to minimize drug costs and toxicity.

- To cover HA-MRSA, one of the following agents would be preferred:
  ✓ Vancomycin 1 g IV Q 48 H (or other dosing regimen to achieve vancomycin trough of 10–15 mg/L);
  ✓ Linezolid 600 mg PO Q 12 H; or
  ✓ Tedizolid 200 mg PO Q 24 H; or
  ✓ Daptomycin 240 mg IV Q 48 H is a second-line option.
  ✓ Telavancin (10 mg/kg [600 mg] Q 48 H) is also a second-line option.
  ✓ Ceftaroline 300 mg IV every 12 hours is also a second-line option (covers some common gram-negative organisms).
  ✓ Dalbavancin 1125 mg IV infused over 30 minutes as a single dose is a second-line option.
  ✓ Oritavancin 1200 mg IV infused over 3 hours as a single dose is a second-line option. (Although dosing adjustment in severe renal impairment CrCl <30 mL/minute has not been studied).

- To cover gram-negative bacteria and anaerobes, one of the following agents would be preferred (dosed for renal dysfunction when indicated):
  ✓ Piperacillin/tazobactam 2.25 g IV Q 6 H;
  ✓ Ampicillin/sulbactam 3 g IV Q 8 H;
  ✓ Ertapenem 500 mg IV Q 24 H;
  ✓ Imipenem/cilastatin 250 mg IV Q 6 H;
  ✓ Meropenem 1 g IV Q 12 H; or
  ✓ Doripenem 250 mg IV Q 12 H.

- Other acceptable IV alternatives for gram-negative and anaerobic coverage, with dose adjustments appropriate for Mr Chavez's renal function, include the combination of either clindamycin or metronidazole plus either a third or fourth-generation cephalosporin (ceftazidime or cefepime), aztreonam, or a fluoroquinolone. However, this would cause the patient to be on a three-drug empiric regimen (including the antibiotic active against HA-MRSA), which may be more costly, inconvenient, and associated with more adverse drug reactions than monotherapy or dual therapy options (eg, clindamycin and cephalosporins are more highly associated with *Clostridium difficile* colitis than other antibiotics).

Outcome Evaluation

5.a. What clinical and laboratory parameters are necessary to evaluate your therapy for achievement of the desired therapeutic outcomes and monitoring for adverse effects?

- Regardless of the drug chosen, improvement in the signs and symptoms of infection and healing of the wound with prevention of limb amputation are the primary end points.

- Observe for decreased swelling, induration, and erythema. Improvement should be observed after 72–96 hours of appropriate antimicrobial therapy and surgical debridement.

- A decrease in cloudy drainage and formation of new scar tissue are signs of positive response to therapy that may take as long as 7–14 days to be seen.

- Obtain a WBC count and differential every 48–72 hours for the first week or until normalization if <1 week, and weekly thereafter until the end of therapy. Continue monitoring until therapy is completed because neutropenia is associated with many antibiotics (eg, ampicillin/sulbactam, vancomycin).

- Vancomycin used at high dose (trough goal of 15–20 mg/L) has been associated with higher incidence of renal dysfunction, and Mr Chavez already has an impaired renal function that increases the risk. Routine weekly SCr levels may be recommended to prevent vancomycin-associated nephrotoxicity and ototoxicity that can develop with accumulation of the drug should the patient's renal function worsen. It would be reasonable to order a weekly vancomycin trough level also to ensure that an adequate trough level (~10–15 mg/L) is being achieved.

- ESR and CRP would be excellent makers of inflammation to follow while on therapy. Baseline levels then weekly should be drawn and normalization of the levels are anticipated by the end of therapy and predictors of positive outcomes.

- Question the patient to detect any unusual side effects related to the drug or infusion (eg, rash, nausea, vomiting, and diarrhea) daily for the first 3–5 days and then weekly thereafter.

5.b. What therapeutic alternatives are available for treating this patient after results of cultures are known to contain MRSA and *B. fragilis*?

- Once the culture results are available and the involved organism(s) is (are) considered pathogenic and responsible for the infectious process, therapy should be targeted at the specific organism(s).
  ✓ Vancomycin given IV is often considered the drug of choice for skin and soft tissue infections caused by MRSA, as it has established efficacy, is generally well tolerated, and is inexpensive.
  ✓ Linezolid is at least as effective as vancomycin in MRSA skin and soft tissue infections and has the advantage of oral administration, but it is expensive.[9] A weekly CBC must be obtained from patients receiving linezolid as it carries a significant risk of thrombocytopenia that may require treatment discontinuation (0.3–10.0%).
  ✓ Daptomycin is a lipopeptide antibiotic approved for the treatment of complicated skin and soft tissue infections due to susceptible organisms including MRSA. It is expensive and

its use is generally restricted to prevent the development of resistance.

✓ Telavancin has been approved for the treatment of complicated skin and soft tissue infections due to susceptible organisms including MRSA. It is fairly expensive, has been associated with renal dysfunction, and should be reserved for resistant bacteria or failure of first-line therapy.

✓ Ceftaroline has been approved for the treatment of complicated skin and soft tissue infections due to susceptible organisms including MRSA. Covers Enterobacteriaceae, but lacks coverage against anaerobes, extended-spectrum beta-lactamase (ESBL), AMP C or *Klebsiella pneumoniae* carbapenemase (KPC) producing strains and *P. aeruginosa*. Administered at least twice daily, but lacks data in diabetic foot infection and should be reserved for patients failing first-line agents.

✓ Dalbavancin and oritavancin are approved as single dose agent IV for the treatment of acute bacterial skin and soft tissue infection caused by gram-positive bacteria. Neither agent has activity against gram-negative organisms. Oritavancin has to be infused over 3 hours compared to 30 minutes for dalbavancin. Both agents are well tolerated although oritavancin has more drug and laboratory interactions than dalbavancin and it has not yet been studied in patient like Mr Chavez who have a CrCl of 25 mL/minute. Both agents are also very expensive.

- None of the above agents have anaerobic coverage, and, therefore, metronidazole or clindamycin will need to be added. Either agent could be used orally or parenterally. Metronidazole may be associated with a disulfiram reaction if the patient consumes alcohol again. Clindamycin has an increased risk of *C. difficile* colitis.

✓ Tigecycline has activity against MRSA, and it would provide activity against *B. fragilis*. However, tigecycline should only be considered when other therapies cannot be used as it failed to meet noninferiority in a diabetic foot infection trial.

5.c. Design an optimal drug treatment plan for treating the mixed infection while he remains hospitalized.

- The patient's therapy should be narrowed to vancomycin 1 g IV Q 48 H. After the third dose, a vancomycin trough level should be recommended and therapy adjusted to maintain a trough ≥10 mg/L. Metronidazole 500 mg PO Q 8 H should be initiated to cover the *B. fragilis*.

- The patient's infection should be assessed daily for changes in swelling, induration, and erythema. Temperature should be assessed at least twice daily and a WBC obtained daily if it was initially increased. Improvements in these physical signs and laboratory parameters should be observed after 72–96 hours of appropriate antimicrobial therapy and surgical debridement. If the area of swelling and erythema increases, or if response to therapy appears inadequate, it may be necessary to broaden therapy so that gram-negative bacteria are covered as well. Response to therapy is often patient dependent, and in some cases improvement may not be seen until after 7–10 days of treatment.

- The duration of therapy is controversial. The latest guidelines recommend continuing antibiotic therapy until, but not beyond, resolution of all signs and symptoms of infection, but not through complete healing of the wound. Wound healing in diabetic patients is often very slow. Therapy should be continued for at least 2–3 weeks total in severe infection.

- The patient should remain hospitalized until he is afebrile for 24–48 hours, has signs of improvement and positive response to therapy (decreased swelling, redness, purulent drainage; normalization of the WBC, ESR, or CRP), and outpatient wound care has been established, either by proper teaching to the patient (and his family) or through home healthcare services.

5.d. Design an optimal pharmacotherapeutic plan for completion of his treatment after he is discharged from the hospital.

- The decision about completion of therapy with IV versus oral therapy is often based on clinical experience because few clinical trials have been performed on long-term treatment of diabetic foot infections.[10]

- In this patient, continued use of IV vancomycin would probably be the best choice. Either the drug could be infused at home, most likely with the wife's or daughter's assistance and frequent nursing care visits, or the patient may be required to visit a home infusion clinic to receive therapy, depending on what is economically feasible. Discharge planning should be involved in this case to ensure a smooth transition to outpatient therapy.

- The patient should be seen in clinic at least once weekly while on therapy to assess therapeutic efficacy and safety. At each visit, a CBC should be obtained to evaluate for vancomycin-associated neutropenia or thrombocytopenia. A SCr should be obtained as well, and, if any significant changes in renal function are observed, the vancomycin dose should be adjusted or the drug stopped and changed to a non-nephrotoxic agent. ESR or CRP should be monitored weekly as a marker of inflammation and response to therapy.

Patient Education

6. What information should be provided to the patient to enhance adherence, ensure successful therapy, and minimize adverse effects with IV vancomycin and oral metronidazole?

- We will need to see you in the clinic each week to make sure the antibiotic is working. At these visits, we will draw some blood so that we can check for side effects of the medication.

- Vancomycin should be infused slowly, over 1–2 hours, to prevent flushing and blood pressure decreases that are associated with rapid infusion.

- Contact your physician or me if any unusual side effects, such as rash, shortness of breath, diminished hearing or ringing in the ears, or decreased urine production, occur while taking this medicine.

- Contact your home healthcare provider if pain, redness, or swelling is observed at the IV site.

- Avoid alcohol intake as you may experience a significant drug interaction with metronidazole that could be characterized by intense flushing, breathlessness, headache, increased or irregular heart rate, low blood pressure, nausea, and vomiting.

- *Note:* The patient needs to be made aware that osteomyelitis and limb amputation are possible consequences of these infections in diabetic patients. He also needs to be provided with personnel resources (telephone numbers and addresses) to contact if unusual reactions occur while on therapy, if infection worsens, or if he has questions or concerns. Adherence to outpatient clinic follow-up visits is of prime importance for success in this case.

REFERENCES

1. Lipsky BA, Berendt AR, Cornia PB, et al. 2012 Infectious Diseases Society of America clinical practice guideline for the diagnosis and treatment of diabetic foot infections. Clin Infect Dis 2012;54:132–173.

2. Levin ME. Management of the diabetic foot: preventing amputation. South Med J 2002;95:10–20.

3. Echániz-Aviles G, Velazquez-Meza ME, Vazquez-Larios Mdel R, Soto-Noguerón A, Hernández-Dueñas AM. Diabetic foot infection caused by community-associated methicillin-resistant *Staphylococcus aureus* (USA300). J Diabetes 2015;7(6):891–892.

4. Lipsky BA, Cannon CM, Ramani A, et al. Ceftaroline fosamil for treatment of diabetic foot infections: the CAPTURE study experience. Diabetes Metab Res Rev 2015;31(4):395–401.

5. Lipsky BA, Tabak YP, Johannes RS, Vo L, Hyde L, Weigelt JA. Skin and soft tissue infections in hospitalised patients with diabetes: culture isolates and risk factors associated with mortality, length of stay and cost. Diabetologia 2010;53:914–923.

6. Liu C, Bayer A, Cosgrove SE, et al. Clinical Practice Guidelines by the Infectious Diseases Society of America for the Treatment of Methicillin-Resistant *Staphylococcus aureus* infections in Adults and Children. Clin Infect Dis 2011;52:1–38.

7. Martí-Carvajal AJ, Gluud C, Nicola S, et al. Growth factors for treating diabetic foot ulcers. Cochrane Database Syst Rev 2015;(10):CD008548. doi:10.1002/14651858.CD008548.pub2.

8. Guillamet CV, Kollef MH. How to stratify patients at risk for resistant bugs in skin and soft tissue infections? Curr Opin Infect Dis 2016;29(2):116–123.

9. Weigelt J, Itani K, Stevens D, Lau W, Dryden M, Knirsch C. Linezolid versus vancomycin in the treatment of complicated skin and soft tissue infections. Antimicrob Agents Chemother 2005;46:2260–2266.

10. Nicolau DP, Stein GE. Therapeutic options for diabetic foot infections: a review with an emphasis on tissue penetration characteristics. J Am Podiatr Med Assoc 2010;100:52–63.